FETAL AND NEONATAL
SECRETS

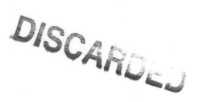

FETAL AND NEONATAL

SECRETS

Third Edition

Richard A. Polin, MD
Professor of Pediatrics
Columbia University
College of Physicians and Surgeons
Director, Division of Neonatology
Morgan Stanley Children's Hospital of New York–Presbyterian
New York, New York

Alan R. Spitzer, MD
Senior Vice President for Research, Education, and Quality
Pediatrix Medical Group
Sunrise, Florida

ELSEVIER
SAUNDERS

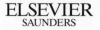
SAUNDERS

1600 John F. Kennedy Blvd.
Ste 1800
Philadelphia, PA 19103-2899

FETAL AND NEONATAL SECRETS, THIRD EDITION   ISBN: 978-0-323-09139-8
Copyright © 2014, 2007, 2001 by Saunders, an imprint of Elsevier Inc.

Notices

Knowledge and best practice in this field are constantly changing. As new research and experience broaden our understanding, changes in research methods, professional practices, or medical treatment may become necessary.

Practitioners and researchers must always rely on their own experience and knowledge in evaluating and using any information, methods, compounds, or experiments described herein. In using such information or methods they should be mindful of their own safety and the safety of others, including parties for whom they have a professional responsibility.

With respect to any drug or pharmaceutical products identified, readers are advised to check the most current information provided (i) on procedures featured or (ii) by the manufacturer of each product to be administered, to verify the recommended dose or formula, the method and duration of administration, and contraindications. It is the responsibility of practitioners, relying on their own experience and knowledge of their patients, to make diagnoses, to determine dosages and the best treatment for each individual patient, and to take all appropriate safety precautions.

To the fullest extent of the law, neither the Publisher nor the authors, contributors, or editors, assume any liability for any injury and/or damage to persons or property as a matter of products liability, negligence or otherwise, or from any use or operation of any methods, products, instructions, or ideas contained in the material herein.

Library of Congress Cataloging-in-Publication Data
Fetal and neonatal secrets / [edited by] Richard A. Polin, Alan R. Spitzer. -- 3rd ed.
    p. ; cm. -- (Secrets series)
  Includes bibliographical references and index.
  ISBN 978-0-323-09139-8 (pbk.)
  I. Polin, Richard A. (Richard Alan) II. Spitzer, Alan R. III. Series: Secrets series.
  [DNLM: 1. Fetal Diseases--Examination Questions. 2. Fetal Diseases--Outlines. 3. Infant, Newborn, Diseases--Examination Questions. 4. Infant, Newborn, Diseases--Outlines. WQ 18.2]
  RJ254
  618.92'01--dc23   2013004157

Content Strategy Director: Madelene Hyde
Senior Content Strategist: James Merritt
Content Development Specialist: Kimberly Hodges
Publishing Services Manager: Patricia Tannian
Project Manager: Amanda Mincher
Design Direction: Steven Stave

Printed in China

Last digit is the print number: 9 8 7 6 5 4 3 2 1

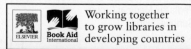

Working together
to grow libraries in
developing countries

www.elsevier.com • www.bookaid.org

To my wife, Helene; my children, Allison and her husband Ted, Mitchell, Jessica and her husband Zac, and Gregory; and my beautiful grandchildren, Lindsey, Eli, Willa, Jasper, and Casey. Without their love and support I could never have accomplished as much as I have as a physician and a teacher.

Richard A. Polin, MD

This book is dedicated to better outcomes for neonates everywhere and to my amazing grandchildren, Jacob, Matthew, Brianna, Molly, and Morgan, and their equally marvelous parents, Steve, Jen, Kevin, Sara, Jeff, and Lauren. I am also eternally indebted to my incredible wife of 42 years, Elaine, who knows more about children and how to make them smile than anyone else I know.

Alan R. Spitzer, MD

CONTRIBUTORS

Saima Aftab, MD
Assistant Professor, Department of Pediatrics
and Neonatology, Perelman School of
Medicine, University of Pennsylvania; Attending
Neonatologist, Department of Neonatology, The
Children's Hospital of Philadelphia, Philadelphia,
Pennsylvania

K.J.S. Anand, MBBS, DPhil
Professor, Department of Pediatrics, Anesthesiology,
Anatomy, and Neurobiology, Division Chief,
Pediatric Critical Care Medicine, Department of
Pediatrics, The University of Tennessee Health
Science Center; Medical Director, Pediatric
Intensive Care Unit, Le Bonheur Children's
Hospital, Memphis, Tennessee

Victoria R. Barrio, MD, FAAD, FAAP
Associate Clinical Professor, Department of
Pediatrics and Medicine—Dermatology, University
of California, San Diego; Rady Children's Hospital,
San Diego, California

Marisa Censani, MD
Pediatric Endocrinology Fellow, Department of
Pediatric Endocrinology, Columbia University
Medical Center, New York, New York

Michael F. Chiang, MD
Knowles Professor, Department of Ophthalmology
and Medical Informatics and Clinical
Epidemiology, Oregon Health and Science
University, Portland, Oregon

Robert D. Christensen, MD
Research Director, Department of Women and
Newborns, Intermountain Healthcare, Salt Lake
City, Utah

Wendy K. Chung, MD, PhD
Assistant Professor, Department of Pediatrics and
Medicine, Columbia University; Director of Clinical
Genetics, New York Presbyterian Hospital, New
York, New York

Robert Ryan Clancy, MD
Professor of Neurology and Pediatrics, University
of Pennsylvania School of Medicine; Senior
Attending Physician, Children's Hospital of
Philadelphia, Philadelphia, Pennsylvania

Reese H. Clark, MD
Vice President and Co-Director, the Center for
Research, Education, and Quality, Pediatrix
Medical Group, Sunrise, Florida

Mitchell I. Cohen, MD, FACC, FHRS
Clinical Associate Professor, Department of
Pediatrics, University of Arizona School of
Medicine—Phoenix Campus; Section Chief,
Pediatric Cardiology, Phoenix Children's Hospital,
Phoenix, Arizona

C. Andrew Combs, MD, PhD
Associate Director of Research, Center for Research,
Education, and Quality, Obstetrix Medical Group,
Mednax, Inc., San Jose, California

Lawrence F. Eichenfield, MD, FAAD, FAAP
Professor of Pediatrics and Medicine—Dermatology,
University of California, San Diego School of
Medicine; Chief, Pediatric and Adolescent
Dermatology, Rady Children's Hospital, San Diego,
California

Jacquelyn R. Evans, MD
Professor of Clinical Pediatrics, Department of
Pediatrics and Neonatology, Perelman School of
Medicine, University of Pennsylvania; Associate
Division Chief, Department of Pediatrics
and Neonatology, The Children's Hospital of
Philadelphia, Philadelphia, Pennsylvania

Karin M. Fuchs, MD
Assistant Clinical Professor, Department of Obstetrics
and Gynecology, Columbia University; Attending
Physician, Division of Maternal Fetal Medicine,
Columbia University Medical Center, New York,
New York

Mary Pat Gallagher, MD
Assistant Professor of Clinical Pediatrics, Department of Pediatrics, Columbia University; Assistant Attending, Pediatrics, Morgan Stanley Children's Hospital of New York–Presbyterian, New York, New York

Alejandro Garcia, MD
Resident, General Surgery, Columbia University Medical Center, New York, New York

Thomas J. Garite, MD
Vice President and Co-Director of Obstetrics and Gynecology, University of California, Irvine, Orange, California; Editor in Chief, American Journal of Obstetrics and Gynecology; Director of Research and Education, Obstetrics, Pediatrix Medical Group, Sunrise, Florida

Daniel A. Greninger, MD
Instructor, Pediatric Ophthalmology and Strabismus, Department of Ophthalmology, Oregon Health and Science University, Portland, Oregon

R. Whit Hall, MD
Professor, Department of Pediatrics and Neonatology, University of Arkansas for Medical Sciences; Professor, Neonatology, Department of Pediatrics and Neonatology, Arkansas Children's Hospital, Little Rock, Arkansas

Qusai Hammouri, MBBS, MD
Director, Pediatric Orthopedics, North Shore Long Island Jewish, Staten Island University Hospital, Staten Island, New York

Karen D. Hendricks-Muñoz, MD, MPH
Professor and Chair of Neonatal Medicine, Pediatrics, Medical College of Virginia, Virginia Commonwealth University; Chief of Neonatal Medicine, Pediatrics, Children's Hospital of Richmond at Virginia Commonwealth Health Systems, Richmond, Virginia

Joshua E. Hyman, MD
Associate Professor, Orthopedic Surgery, Columbia University College of Physicians and Surgeons; Attending, Orthopedic Surgery, Morgan Stanley Children's Hospital of New York–Presbyterian, New York, New York

Beatriz Larru, MD, PhD
Fellow, Division of Infectious Diseases, Children's Hospital of Philadelphia, Philadelphia, Pennsylvania

Joel E. Lavine, MD, PhD
Professor, Department of Pediatrics, Columbia University; Chief, Pediatric Gastroenterology, Hepatology, and Nutrition, Morgan Stanley Children's Hospital of New York–Presbyterian, New York, New York

Christopher L. Lindblade, MD
Co-Director of Fetal Cardiology, Department of Cardiology, Phoenix Children's Hospital, Phoenix, Arizona

John M. Lorenz, MD
Professor of Clinical Pediatrics, Department of Pediatrics, College of Physicians and Surgeons, Columbia University; Attending Neonatologist, Department of Pediatrics, Morgan Stanley Children's Hospital of New York–Presbyterian, New York, New York

William Middlesworth, MD
Assistant Professor, Department of Surgery and Pediatrics, Columbia University; Assistant Attending Surgeon, Morgan Stanley Children's Hospital of New York–Presbyterian, New York, New York

Kimberly D. Morel, MD, FAAD, FAAP
Associate Professor of Clinical Dermatology and Clinical Pediatrics, Departments of Dermatology and Pediatrics, Columbia University and Morgan Stanley Children's Hospital of New York–Presbyterian, New York, New York

Sharon E. Oberfield, MD
Professor and Director of Pediatrics, Department of Pediatrics, Division of Pediatric Endocrinology, Diabetes, and Metabolism, Columbia University, New York, New York

Carol C. Prendergast, EdD
Institutional Advancement, Syracuse University, Syracuse, New York

Fabio Savorgnan, MD
Fellow, Department of Pediatrics, University of Tennessee, Memphis, Tennessee

Sarah A. Taylor, MD
Fellow, Department of Pediatrics, Columbia University; Fellow, Pediatric Gastroenterology, Hepatology, and Nutrition, Morgan Stanley Children's Hospital of New York–Presbyterian, New York, New York

Patricia L. Weng, MD

Assistant Professor of Clinical Pediatrics, Department of Pediatrics, Columbia University; Department of Pediatrics, Morgan Stanley Children's Hospital of New York–Presbyterian, New York, New York

Courtney J. Wusthoff, MD

Assistant Professor, Department of Neurology and Neurological Sciences, Stanford University; Co-Director, Neonatal Neuro-Intensive Care Unit, Pediatric Neurology, Lucile Packard Children's Hospital, Palo Alto, California

Theoklis E. Zaoutis, MD, MSCE

Professor, Department of Pediatrics and Epidemiology, Perelman School of Medicine, University of Pennsylvania; Associate Chief, Division of Infectious Diseases, The Children's Hospital of Philadelphia, Philadelphia, Pennsylvania

PREFACE TO THE THIRD EDITION

Although "secrets" is used in the title of our book, this word belies the book's purpose and content. Throughout much of history, the traditional way of learning medicine was to obtain an apprenticeship with a skilled medical practitioner for an ill-defined period of time. In that way, one learned the "secrets"—useful or not; correct or incorrect—that a single practitioner had acquired over many years of practice. In the United States, that system remained in place until the early-1900s when modern medical schools were developed. Our current system of education has evolved considerably since that time, but it has never abandoned the idea of students learning from wise clinicians. Although modern students and trainees now have nearly unlimited access to a broad range of information, that does not diminish the value of "great clinicians," whose wisdom is now passed on through seminars, books, and journals, many of which are available electronically. *Fetal and Neonatal Secrets* is an up-to-date collection of questions and answers that deals with a wide variety of common and uncommon neonatal diseases. In essence, it brings the great clinician—in this case, many outstanding clinicians and educators—directly to the reader so that he or she can learn the "secrets" from these talented individuals, as if the reader were an apprentice on their rounds. As in the previous editions, we have included facts that would qualify as trivia because of the enjoyment value they bring to learning. If used appropriately—and gently—by students and trainees, they are perfect for challenging teachers with information in areas that may be outside of their expertise. In summary, the book is meant to be both useful and fun. It is not meant to be encyclopedic, but we hope it will spur all students to challenge existing dogma and to search for better ways to care for critically ill neonates.

Richard A. Polin, MD

Alan R. Spitzer, MD

PREFACE TO THE FIRST EDITION

From the time we become physicians until the time we retire from medicine, we are guided by the phrase widely attributed to Hippocrates: *primum non nocere*, "first do no harm." Although the origins of that exact phrase are unclear, Hippocrates certainly conveyed that meaning in his oath: "I will prescribe regimen for the good of my patients according to my ability and my judgment and never do harm to anyone." Fundamental to the concept of "doing good" is the acquisition of medical knowledge that allows each of us to practice according to the highest possible standards. In the first two years of medical school, knowledge is transferred predominantly by large group lectures and required readings. Once we enter the clinical years, the process of acquiring new information begins to change. We continue to read textbooks, but journal articles become increasingly important sources of the newest information, and much information is transmitted to us through "personal communications" by individuals who are further along in their training. For the medical student, that often means an intern or resident, and for the senior resident, a fellow or an attending. This apprenticeship aspect of medicine has been an intrinsic part of the field since its inception. Even in this era of rapidly intensifying technologic advances, "see one, do one, teach one" remains a cornerstone of bedside medical education.

With this concept in mind, *Fetal and Neonatal Secrets* is designed to serve as a primer for the bedside teaching that remains such an important part of medical education. While it can be read from cover to cover (e.g., to prepare for a certifying examination), we believe that the information in the book should be shared wherever health care providers congregate to provide care (inpatient service, clinics, operating room) to the fetus and newborn infant. Although the word "secrets" connotes a sense of privacy, we hope that this book reveals rather than obscures secrets, and that the cumulative wisdom shared by the many experienced contributors serves to enlighten the reader. Furthermore, we would love to see these secrets used by the youngest members of the health care team to challenge those more experienced, as well as by professors to make their residents and students think. We fear that we may need to tote around a copy of this book on rounds ourselves, as our house staff, fellows, and nurse practitioners may throw down the gauntlet to test us on a daily basis! Although we have tried to make this book as comprehensive and practical as possible, the reader will encounter many facts that might be considered trivial (e.g., what is the ductus of Botallo?), but we hope that the reader is forgiving in this respect. The retention of important information has always seemed to be enhanced by its association with interesting, but less essential information (the Mary Poppins approach—"a spoonful of sugar helps the medicine go down"). Where would medicine be without mnemonics? In any event, we hope you find this book useful in your daily practice, but more important, we want you to have some fun along the way.

Richard A. Polin, MD

Alan R. Spitzer, MD

ACKNOWLEDGMENTS

In my development as a physician, I have been exposed to many wonderful teachers, scientists, and physicians. However, because of the enormous influence they have had on my career, I would like to acknowledge four individuals by name: Bill Speck (my lifelong friend—no one has ever cared more about resident and student education), John Driscoll (the master clinician who first excited me about neonatology and who remains my role model for the warm, compassionate physician), Bill Fox (my coeditor for *Fetal and Neonatal Physiology,* who demonstrated to me the importance and fun in doing clinical research and who periodically reminds me how to stay focused on the important things in life), and Mark Ditmar (my coeditor of *Pediatric Secrets,* whose combination of humor, knowledge, and compassion has allowed me to achieve a balance in medicine and who has shown me how "academic" and wonderful the practice of general pediatrics can be). I am indebted to all of them.

Finally, I would like to thank my developmental editor at Elsevier, Kimberly Hodges, for helping with the organization and development of this book, and my friend and senior editor at Elsevier, Linda Belfus, for hooking me on the Secrets series and allowing me to put my love of education into print.

Richard A. Polin, MD

A career in medicine is never static, but rather constantly evolving. As a result, the people and experiences that influence one's life in medicine often change in unexpected ways. In recent years, I have served as the course director for NEO—the Conference for Neonatology held annually in Orlando. As part of this meeting, we initiated the "Legends of Neonatology" awards, which I have the honor of presenting each year. In preparing for that evening, I have had the chance to venture back into the history of neonatology, relearning the origins of much of what we do today and examining the careers of some of the greatest figures in modern neonatal medicine, whose contributions have saved and enhanced the lives of countless infants. The impact of these individuals on my perspective on medicine has been immeasurable, and learning about their lives and the challenges that many of them had to overcome to achieve at the highest levels of our specialty has often left me in awe in ways that I would never have anticipated. To date, we have honored the following: Maria Delivoria-Papadopoulos, Mary Ellen Avery, Mildred Stahlman, Lu-Ann Papile, Avroy Fanaroff, Marshall Klaus, Jerrold Lucey, Robert Bartlett, William Norwood, George Gregory, John Clements, Forrest Bird, Stanley Dudrick, Abraham Rudolph, and William Oh. Upcoming are Lilly Dubowitz, Jeffrey Maisels, and Jen-Tien Wung. Each and every one of these figures faced incredible obstacles along their paths but believed in themselves and believed that their work would profoundly improve outcomes for children. Their courage and the quality of their work have been a model that I will always deeply admire and forever aspire to match.

I would be remiss, however, if I did not also thank several other people for their inspiration as role models. Roger Medel, the CEO of MEDNAX, Inc. (Pediatrix Medical Group), serves as a wise and understanding leader for those of us in my current position and has provided me with the opportunity to achieve certain goals in my career that would never have been possible otherwise. My current partner, Reese Clark, is the ultimate clinical scientist—thoughtful, insightful, knowledgeable, and scrupulously honest. Anyone who reads a paper with his name on it can rest assured that no one has ever provided data and its interpretation in a more ethically precise and clear manner. A former mentor, Bill Fox at the Children's Hospital of Philadelphia, has always been a great friend and huge supporter of my work; without him my career would have been very different and far less successful. Lastly, my coeditor of this book, Richard Polin, is without question the consummate clinician, educator, and investigator. I was most fortunate to spend a dozen years at the earliest stage of my career in the office next to Rich at CHOP, and if there was ever a perfect learning experience, that was it. To all of these people, I will forever be indebted.

Alan R. Spitzer, MD

CONTENTS

TOP 100 SECRETS

These secrets are 100 of the top board alerts. They summarize the concepts, principles, and most salient details of fetal and neonatal medicine.

1. About 10% of neonates will need some degree of resuscitative support at the time of birth.
2. Cold stress can adversely affect the resuscitation of a newborn infant in the delivery room.
3. With the elimination of silver nitrate eye prophylaxis at the time of delivery (causing a chemical conjunctivitis), the presence of any red eye, or a discharge from the eye of a neonate, must be evaluated and treated immediately.
4. Without pulse oximeter screening, congenital heart disease may be missed during the immediate newborn period in about 50% of neonates with the condition.
5. The average caloric content of breast milk is 20 calories per ounce but can range from 8 to 30 calories per ounce, primarily depending on the fat content.
6. For the first 6 months of life, breast milk alone provides adequate nutrition for virtually any term neonate.
7. Vaginal bleeding in newborn female infants is not uncommon and usually occurs because of withdrawal of maternal hormones that are present during pregnancy.
8. In the first 3 to 4 months of life, a newborn infant should gain about one ounce per day on average.
9. By 4 to 5 months of age, a healthy term infant should weigh double his or her birth weight.
10. Sonographic assessments of fetal weight are associated with a significant (approximately 10% to 20%) margin of error.
11. Absence of end-diastolic flow in the umbilical artery is indicative of increased placental resistance, whereas reversal of flow is suggestive of worsening fetal status and impending demise.
12. The biophysical profile is an antenatal test that uses five parameters—fetal movement, fetal breathing, fetal tone, amniotic fluid volume, and fetal heart rate monitoring—to assess fetal well-being; depending on the gestational age, a score of ≤6 out of 10 warrants additional surveillance or consideration of delivery.
13. In twin-twin transfusion syndrome (TTTS), selective laser photocoagulation of connecting arteriovenous anastomoses decreases the inter-twin transfusion and enhances survival.
14. *In utero* fetal therapy has been successfully performed for diseases such as primary pleural effusion, lower urinary tract obstruction, neural tube defect, hypoplastic left heart syndrome, congenital cystic adenomatoid malformation (CCAM), and sacrococcygeal teratoma; fetal intervention for congenital diaphragmatic hernia (CDH) is currently investigational.
15. Screening all pregnant women for aneuploidy using analysis of free fetal DNA in maternal blood is a new option that should decrease the need for amniocentesis and chorionic villous sampling.
16. Multiple courses of antenatal corticosteroids (ACS) to accelerate fetal lung maturity are no longer recommended. However, using a second course of ACS has been shown to be an effective and safe alternative for women who have gone beyond a week or two from their previous course of ACS and are threatening to deliver prematurely.
17. Weekly intramuscular progesterone has been shown to reduce the risk of prematurity in mothers with a history of previous spontaneous (not medically indicated) premature birth.
18. Screening with endovaginal ultrasound for a short cervix and treating those with a cervical length of <2 cm with daily vaginal progesterone is an option for all pregnant women to reduce the rate of premature birth.
19. Doppler flow studies of the fetal umbilical artery have been shown to be of value to determine risk of impending fetal death in growth-restricted fetuses.

20. Developmental care, such as paying attention to light, sound, handling, and touch in the neonatal intensive care unit (NICU), has become a standard of care that can improve the medical outcome of critically ill infants.
21. Including parents as part of the care team and in the provision of skin-to-skin care (Kangaroo Mother Care) reduces infant pain and stress and improves the medical outcome.
22. The senses continue to develop in the NICU, beginning with touch and ending with vision. Negative or positive environmental influences can have an impact on normal development of the senses.
23. Hearing loss is the most common congenital condition in the United States. All infants should receive hearing screening during the newborn period.
24. The four modes of heat loss in the neonate are conduction, convection, evaporation, and radiation.
25. A subgaleal hemorrhage presents as a balottable mass on the head of a newborn, and unlike a cephalohematoma or a caput succadeneum, it can be life threatening.
26. For infants whose mothers are HBsAg-positive, hepatitis B immune globulin (HBIG) and hepatitis B vaccine should be given as soon as possible after birth.
27. Failure of a term infant to pass meconium within the first 48 hours after birth should prompt an evaluation for intestinal obstruction.
28. The umbilical cord generally dries up and sloughs by 2 weeks after birth. Persistence of the cord beyond 30 days should prompt consideration of a migration abnormality of neutrophils, factor XIII deficiency, or presence of a persistent omphalomesenteric duct or patent urachus.
29. The absence of a murmur in the neonatal period does not rule out congenital heart disease.
30. Maintaining patency of the ductus arteriosus is important in severe right and left heart obstructive lesions.
31. The most common cyanotic congenital heart lesion in the newborn period is d-transposition of the great vessels.
32. Tetralogy of Fallot is the most common cyanotic lesion presenting outside of the newborn period.
33. Erythema toxicum is a benign condition. Erythema toxicum is no alien to the nursery; it is present in 50% of term newborns. It is much less prevalent in premature infants and occurs in only approximately 5%.
34. The standard recommendation for milia, sebaceous gland hyperplasia, transient neonatal pustular melanosis, erythema toxicum, and sucking blisters is to reassure the family that the condition will resolve over time. No other interventions are needed.
35. If a dermatitis involves the axillae or groin, it is more likely to be seborrheic dermatitis. If extensor surfaces such as forearms and shins are involved, atopic dermatitis is more likely. Both atopic dermatitis and seborrheic dermatitis involve scalp and posterior auricular areas, although seborrheic dermatitis has large, yellowish scale; when severe, it characteristically extends down to the forehead and eyebrow areas.
36. "Blueberry muffin baby" is a term used to describe neonates whose skin resembles a blueberry muffin (i.e., the skin shows diffuse, dark blue to violaceous purpuric macules and papules). The spots represent dermal hematopoiesis and are a sign of serious systemic disease—often a congenital infection.
37. Infantile hemangiomas are common vascular tumors that arise during the neonatal period. They are often not visible at birth but are noticed within the first weeks of life. Hemangiomas occur more frequently in female children, with a female-to-male incidence of 2 to 5:1. In addition, they arise more commonly in premature infants, low-birth-weight (LBW) infants, and infants born to mothers with advanced maternal age, placenta previa, and preeclampsia.
38. The chronological age at which hemangiomas are noted to begin proliferation in preterm infants is the same as for fullterm infants.
39. The most common cause of hypercalcemia during the neonatal period is excessive administration of calcium. The most common cause of hypermagnesemia during the newborn period is excessive maternal administration of magnesium.
40. Treatment for congenital hypothyroidism should begin as soon as possible after birth to prevent neurologic impairment. The *in utero* effects of hypothyroidism are variable and may have adverse consequences, even with early postnatal treatment. Early neonatal screening is therefore essential.

41. The most common cause of congenital adrenal hyperplasia and sexual ambiguity at birth in female infants is 21-hydroxylase deficiency.

42. A neonate requires approximately 4 to 8 mg/kg/min of glucose for maintenance of blood glucose levels. Under certain stress conditions, even higher rates may be necessary.

43. The most common cause of severe recurrent hypoglycemia in neonates is hyperinsulinemia.

44. Most premature infants lose weight after birth as the result of catabolism secondary to low caloric intake and a physiologic decrease in the extracellular water volume that is independent of caloric intake.

45. Insensible water loss decreases with increasing gestational and postnatal age, exposure to antenatal steroids, and increasing ambient humidity.

46. There is minimal evidence documenting the value of sodium bicarbonate infusions to correct acidemia due to lactic acidosis. In fact, data in animals, children, and adults suggest that correction of lactic acidosis with sodium bicarbonate infusions may be detrimental.

47. Cystic kidney disease in the neonate may present with a wide spectrum of clinical abnormalities, including hypertension, respiratory distress, oliguria, myocardial dysfunction, and prematurity.

48. Hypertension in the neonatal period is most likely secondary to renovascular etiology.

49. Significant bilious emesis in a newborn infant should be evaluated with an upper gastrointestinal tract series to assess for malrotation and midgut volvulus.

50. In an infant with constipation who does not pass meconium in the first 48 hours of life, Hirschsprung disease should be considered.

51. For term infants, human milk is superior to formula because it provides an ideal source of nutrition as well as other very important non-nutritive functions; it augments the infant's immune response (via immunoglobulins, α-lactalbumin, and lactoferrin), enhances the absorption of minerals, promotes motility and a faster gastric emptying time, stimulates the development of favorable gut flora, and relates to a lower incidence of necrotizing enterocolitis (NEC).

52. One should maintain a high index of suspicion for zinc deficiency in LBW infants presenting with severe diaper rash and oral lesions. LBW infants have greater requirements for zinc but lack sufficient stores and are susceptible to deficiency without supplementation.

53. Gastroesophageal reflux (GER) occurs in up to 50% of infants with emesis and is characterized as the "happy spitter." GER needs to be differentiated from gastroesophageal reflux disease (GERD), in which the infant's growth is affected and treatment with medication and a more elemental formula should be considered.

54. The evaluation of cholestatic jaundice (conjugated bilirubin >2.0 mg/dL or greater than 15% the total bilirubin) should first include a consideration for sepsis or a urinary tract infection. If negative, one should proceed to imaging studies such as the DISIDA scan to assess for biliary atresia, a diagnosis that, if made in a timely manner and treated surgically within 8 weeks of life, results in improved outcomes.

55. Patchy alternations in skin pigmentation in females suggest the possibility of genetic mosaicism or X-linked disorders that result from differential lyonization.

56. Thumb and radial ray abnormalities with or without café-au-lait spots may be the first indication of Fanconi anemia, a condition that may ultimately require bone marrow transplantation. The condition is autosomal recessive and most common in Jewish families.

57. All genetic problems in the child are not necessarily inherited from the parents. Many genetic problems occur *de novo,* or new, to the child and suggest a low risk of recurrence for future pregnancies. However, such genetic problems can be passed on to the children of the affected child with the *de novo* mutation.

58. Although the risk of Down syndrome is highest with mothers older than age 35 years, the majority of cases occur with women younger than age 35 because they have the majority of pregnancies.

59. A chromosome microarray study has replaced a karyotype as the first line genetic test for newborns with major congenital anomalies, dysmorphic features, or both and can also be used prenatally.

60. Genomic tests including chromosome microarray and whole exome sequencing are useful to identify genetic etiologies for rare familial conditions as well as conditions with no family history that are due to *de novo* mutations.

61. Once sepsis is suspected in a neonate, antimicrobial treatment should begin promptly after cultures have been obtained, even when there are no obvious risk factors for sepsis. Because group B *Streptococcus* (GBS) and *Escherichia coli* remain the most common pathogens of early-onset sepsis in the United States, a synergistic combination of ampicillin and an aminoglycoside (usually gentamicin) is suitable for the initial treatment of early-onset sepsis.

62. When meningitis is caused by enteric organisms, cefotaxime is preferred and is often paired with an aminoglycoside. Gram-negative meningitis is usually treated for at least 3 weeks. Because there is synergism between ampicillin and aminoglycosides for most GBS, *Listeria monocytogenes,* and enterococci, combination therapy is recommended for the treatment of meningitis due to Gram-positive organisms until the cerebrospinal fluid is sterilized. The total duration of treatment is usually 14 days.

63. Risk factors for systemic candidiasis in neonates include extreme prematurity, indwelling central lines, histamine blockers, and long-term use of broad spectrum antibiotics.

64. Data in infants with symptomatic congenital cytomegalovirus involving the central nervous system (CNS) suggest that the prognosis at 1 to 2 years of age may be improved if infected infants are treated with parental ganciclovir for 6 weeks. Valganciclovir given orally provides the same systemic levels of intravenous ganciclovir.

65. Approximately 50% of infants surviving neonatal herpes simplex virus (HSV) experience cutaneous recurrences. Use of oral acyclovir suppressive therapy for the 6 months following treatment of acute neonatal HSV diseases has been shown to improve neurodevelopmental outcomes in infants with HSV CNS involvement and to prevent skin recurrences in all infants infected with HSV regardless of their neonatal manifestations.

66. In infants born prematurely, gestational age at delivery is an important determinant of neurodevelopmental outcome. Infants born at <25 weeks are at a 50% to 75% risk for death or neurodisability. However, this risk is influenced significantly by gender, exposure to steroids, multiple gestation, birth weight, and NICU course.

67. Therapeutic hypothermia has been shown to reduce the risk of neurodevelopmental disability following hypoxic-ischemic encephalopathy. To be effective, this treatment should be started within 6 hours of birth.

68. More than 80% of electroencephalogram (EEG)-confirmed seizures are "subclinical" or subtle, having no visible outward signs detectable by caregivers. Accurate detection and diagnosis of neonatal seizures requires EEG monitoring.

69. Most neonatal seizures are symptomatic of acute illness and very rarely due to primary infantile epilepsy. Frequent causes of neonatal seizures include stroke and hypoxic-ischemic encephalopathy followed by infection and metabolic disruptions.

70. Central hypotonia is hypotonia resulting from a CNS lesion. This should not be confused with "axial" or "truncal" hypotonia, which describes hypotonia primarily affecting the core trunk muscles.

71. Premature infants ≤30 weeks gestational age with birth weight (BW) <1500 g or infants with BW between 1500 and 2000 g at request of the neonatologist should be screened for retinopathy of prematurity (ROP).

72. Intermittent strabismus (eye misalignment) commonly occurs in the newborn period. However, any eye misalignment that persists beyond the third month of life should be referred to an ophthalmologist.

73. Any midline dimple (especially a deep or assymetric pit), subcutaneous mass, hemangioma, nevus, tuft of hair, or areas of hypopigmentation or hyperpigmentation might indicate occult spinal dysraphism and a tethered cord. Coccygeal pits are generally benign. The presence of two or more midline skin lesions is the strongest predictor of spinal dysraphism. An ultrasound of the spine is indicated whenever occult spinal sysraphism is suspected. Magnetic resonance imaging is an alternative imaging study.

74. The most important orthopedic radiograph for a newborn child suspected of having a genetic skeletal dysplasia is the lateral cervical spine. More than 150 distinct osteochondrodysplasias have been identified. Each has distinctive features, but many also have similar radiographic findings. One of the most common is agenesis or hypoplasia of the upper cervical spine elements. This can lead to

instability and places the child at great risk of spinal cord injury during ordinary handling. Detection of cervical instability is mandatory to allow proper stabilization and protection.

75. Ultrasound of the hip is the study of choice for suspected developmental dislocation of the hip in neonates and infants younger than 4 months of age. In children of this age, the ossific nucleus of the femoral head is completely cartilaginous and therefore will not be seen on x-ray. After 4 months of age, radiographs should be obtained.

76. The initial treatment for clubfoot is weekly manipulation and casting using the Ponseti method. Approximately 6 to 10 casts are required. A brace is worn for 3 to 4 years to maintain the correct position. With this technique, approximately 80% to 90% of idiopathic clubfeet will be successfully treated. Those feet that cannot be corrected with this method will require surgical correction.

77. The clavicle is the bone that is most frequently fractured in newborns. This injury, which stems from excessive traction during delivery, generally results in a greenstick fracture. This fracture usually heals quite nicely without any therapy, although the callus formation may be notable.

78. Pain thresholds increase progressively during late gestation and in the postnatal period. Preterm neonates have much greater sensitivity to pain than term neonates, and they manifest prolonged periods of hyperalgesia after tissue injury.

79. In addition to supportive therapy and the slow weaning of opioids, some pharmacologic agents (e.g., methadone) with a relatively long half-life can be used to manage opioid withdrawal. We do not recommend the use of drugs such as paregoric, camphorated tincture of opium, phenobarbital, or chlorpromazine for opioid withdrawal, because of major side effects and lack of standardization. Therapeutic goals are to decrease the severity of withdrawal signs to a tolerable degree, to enable regular cycles of sleeping and feeding, and to decrease the agitation caused by medical interventions or nursing care.

80. Procedural pain should be avoided whenever possible. Procedural pain can be minimized with an appropriate awareness program involving nursing, respiratory therapy, physicians, and most importantly, parents. The most common sources of minor procedural pain are heel sticks and tracheal suctioning. Pain resulting from heel sticks can be lessened with 25% sucrose, and discomfort from tracheal suctioning can be treated with facilitated tucking. More pronounced pain should be treated with opiates. Remifentanil, for example, is a good choice for short-term procedures such as intubation, whereas more prolonged pain should be treated with a longer acting opiate, such as morphine or fentanyl. Anxietolytics such as midazolam can be used as adjuncts, but they do not treat pain. Circumcision should be performed with sucrose and local anesthetic nerve block before the procedure and acetaminophen after the procedure.

81. Managing the airway is always the most critical aspect of resuscitation. Most neonates who require support in the delivery room will respond to stimulation, opening of the airway, and gentle ventilation with a bag and mask.

82. Electronic fetal monitoring has not been shown to be any better than intermittent auscultation of the fetal heart rate. There are no well-controlled trials that show any decline in deaths or cerebral palsy (CP) rates that can be attributed to electronic fetal heart rate monitoring. Although the use of fetal heart rate monitoring has become a standard practice, its prognostic value remains unclear at the present time.

83. Immediate bag-and-mask ventilation is contraindicated when there is thick meconium in the hypopharynx and trachea or if a CDH is known or suspected. In all instances, however, the resuscitator must weigh the advantages of bag-and-mask therapy with the risks. At times, immediate intubation for suctioning or to avoid abdominal distention may be required.

84. Surfactant should be given within the first 1 to 2 hours of life to infants with severe respiratory distress syndrome who require intubation. There is no benefit to prophylactic administration of surfactant.

85. Infants with diaphragmatic hernia do not appear to share the benefits of inhaled nitric oxide that infants with other causes of hypoxemic respiratory failure experience. Indeed, there are suggestions that outcomes may be worse in infants with CDH who received inhaled nitric oxide compared with control subjects.

86. The definitive randomized trial establishing the effectiveness of neonatal extracorporeal membrane oxygenation (ECMO) was conducted by the National Health Service in the United Kingdom. Thirty of 93

infants (32%) referred to ECMO centers died compared with 54 of 92 (59%) who received conventional care. The relative risk for reduced mortality with ECMO was 0.55 (95% CI, 0.39-0.77; P<0.0005).

87. Caffeine is the preferred treatment for apnea of prematurity because of its once-a-day dosing and fewer side effects than other treatments. Caffeine therapy for apnea of prematurity reduces the rates of cerebral palsy and cognitive delay at 18 months of age. The improved outcomes seen at 18 months were not seen at 5 years after birth, but the trends toward improvement in outcome still favored use of caffeine over placebo for the treatment of apnea.

88. CDH was once thought to be a surgical emergency; now repair is deferred intentionally to allow for normal physiological changes to occur to the postnatal circulation. Current recommendations are for a period of stabilization until the neonate's clinical condition improves. If the baby requires ECMO preoperatively, surgical repair is usually done before decannulation but delayed until the ECMO settings have been lowered and the patient is considered ready to come off ECMO.

89. Plain abdominal radiographs (supine and decubitus) should be performed if congenital intestinal obstruction is suspected. A normal gas pattern with no dilation of intestinal loops and air in the rectum lowers the likelihood of obstruction. A "double bubble" sign is pathognomonic for complete duodenal obstruction. Several dilated loops of intestine with air fluid levels and a lack of distal gas are indicative of a high intestinal obstruction. Many dilated loops of intestine suggest a distal small bowel or colonic obstruction.

90. In development, Hirschsprung disease results from the failure of the parasympathetic nervous system to fully invest the digestive tract. Normally, ganglion cells migrate cranial to caudal during fetal development. Arrest of this process anywhere along its length results in aganglionic intestine, which occur distal to this point.

91. Meconium ileus is obstruction of the distal ileum due to thick and viscid meconium occurring in 10% to 20% of neonates with cystic fibrosis. Meconium plug is caused by meconium blocking the left colon in otherwise healthy babies. The small left colon syndrome is most common in infants of diabetic mothers and produces an obstruction from a temporarily dysfunctional, small-caliber left colon. A contrast enema with barium is usually diagnostic as well as therapeutic for both meconium plug and the small left colon syndrome (through its mechanical effect), although subsequent testing for Hirschsprung disease or cystic fibrosis may be indicated.

92. If an inguinal hernia is asymptomatic, some surgeons will wait several months to repair, but most recommend repairing an inguinal hernia before the baby's discharge from the nursery to prevent complications. If the infant is premature and has diminished respiratory reserve (e.g., bronchopulmonary dysplasia), the operative procedure can be done under spinal or epidural anesthesia, in most cases without having to intubate the baby.

93. Non-pharmacological methods for relieving pain in the neonate include swaddling, non-nutritive sucking, sucrose administration, and limiting environmental stressors, such as light and noise.

94. There are four primary shunts present in the fetal circulation: the ductus arteriosus, the ductus venosus, the fossa ovalis, and the placenta.

95. The two most common innocent murmurs in the neonate are the closing patent ductus arteriosus and peripheral pulmonic stenosis.

96. Symmetric intrauterine growth retardation, in which all growth parameters are reduced, is more worrisome for long-term development than asymmetric growth retardation, in which head sparing occurs.

97. The main causes of intrauterine hydrocephalus are aqueductal stenosis and Arnold–Chiari type II malformation, as seen in myelomeningocele and Dandy-Walker malformation.

98. The three primary forms of cerebral hemorrhage in the neonate are subdural or subarachnoid hemorrhage (usually a problem of term infants), intraventricular hemorrhage (usually seen in premature infants), and intraparenchymal hemorrhage (which may occur in any infant).

99. Central line infections in neonates can be reduced to a negligible rate (<1/1000 line days) with careful attention to sterile line placement, maintenance of the catheter site and hub, and infrequent interruptions of line continuity.

100. Normal 1 and 5-minute Apgar scores (both >7) do not eliminate the possibility of cerebral palsy developing in an infant

CHAPTER 1

CARE OF THE TERM INFANT

Alan R. Spitzer, MD

1. How is a term infant defined?

The World Health Organization (WHO) defines a term infant as one who is greater than 37 weeks' gestation. Recent evidence, however, has demonstrated that infants born at 37 weeks' gestation behave differently from infants delivered at 39 and 40 weeks' gestation. The more mature term infant (39 or 40 weeks) has fewer respiratory problems, less difficulty with feeding and hyperbilirubinemia, reduced birth injury, a greater ability to respond to infection, and an overall reduction in rates of neonatal complications.

Given that infants born before 37 weeks have even greater liability for problems, the recognition that true term status begins at about 39 weeks' gestation has led the American College of Obstetrics and Gynecology (ACOG) and the American Academy of Pediatrics (AAP) to recommend that no infants be delivered electively before 39 weeks.

American Academy of Pediatrics and the American College of Obstetricians and Gynecologists. Guidelines for perinatal care, 6th ed. Elk Grove Village, IL and Washington, DC: AAP and ACOG; 2007.
Clark S, Miller D, Belfort M, et al. Neonatal and maternal outcomes associated with elective delivery. Am J Obstet Gynecol 2009;200:156.e1-156.e4.

2. What is the average birth weight of a term infant?

The mean birth weight of a term infant is approximately 3400 grams, or approximately 7 pounds, 7 ½ ounces. Mean length, which is sometimes difficult to measure accurately, is approximately 52 to 53 centimeters, or 20 inches, and head circumference averages 34 centimeters, or approximately 13.5 inches. Of note is the fact that birth weight in recent years has declined slightly, even though premature births have been declining.

Donahue SM, Kleinman KP, Gillman MW, et al.Trends in birth weight and gestational length among singleton term births in the United States. 1990–2005. Obstet Gynecol 2010 Feb;115(2 Pt 1):357–64.

3. How often is neonatal resuscitation necessary for a term infant?

Approximately 10% of all infants need some assistance at birth (e.g., stimulation, oxygen), and approximately 1% need extensive assistance (e.g., positive pressure ventilation, fluids, drugs) at the time of birth.

American Academy of Pediatrics, The American College of Obstetrics and Gynecology. Care of the neonate in guidelines for perinatal care, 6th ed. 2007;205.

4. What are the critical skills needed by any individual called upon to resuscitate a neonate?

- The ability to rapidly and accurately evaluate the newborn's condition
- Knowledge of the risk factors that may predispose the neonate to resuscitation
- Indications for neonatal resuscitation
- Skill in airway management
- Skill in umbilical catheter placement
- Skill in insertion of chest tubes
- Understanding of the capabilities of the resuscitation team
- Knowledge of the hospitals' facilities for neonatal care

TABLE 1-1. THE APGAR SCORE			
	0	1	2
Skin color	Blue or pale all over	Blue extremities, body pink (acrocyanosis)	No cyanosis, body and extremities pink
Pulse rate	Absent	<100	≥100
Reflex irritability	No response to stimulation	Grimace/feeble cry when stimulated	Cry or pull away when stimulated
Muscle tone	None	Some flexion	Flexed arms and legs that resist extension
Breathing	Absent	Weak, irregular, gasping	Strong, lusty cry

5. What is an Apgar Score?

The Apgar score is a clinical assessment developed by Dr. Virginia Apgar at Columbia University during the early 1950s. Dr. Apgar was a great pioneer for women in medicine, and her development of the Apgar score is just one of her many landmark contributions to medicine. Although she was an anesthesiologist, she was very concerned about the status of newborn infants immediately after delivery. Her score, which was designed to evaluate both the immediate and long-term well-being of a neonate, has been reassessed periodically and still appears to be as valid today as when it was first introduced.

The Apgar score is determined at 1 and 5 minutes of life and consists of the measures listed in Table 1-1. These measures are scored 0, 1, or 2, then totaled.

It is rare for an infant to have an Apgar score of 10 (the highest possible score) in the absence of oxygen administration because the exposure of most newborn infants to the environmental temperature of the delivery room will cause some acrocyanosis of the hands and feet, reducing the potential score to 9. An Apgar score above 7 is considered good, one between 4 and 7 demands close observation, and one that is 3 or lower usually requires some intervention. Even with the changes that have occurred in modern medicine, the Apgar score has retained its value.

Finster M, Wood M. The Apgar score has survived the test of time. Anesthesiology. 2005 Apr;102(4):855–7.

5a. How should the Apgar change in the immediate postnatal period?

One of the other important aspects of the Apgar score is the change between 1 and 5 minutes of life. For vigorous term infants the Apgar score does not change significantly between 1 and 5 minutes of life. Changes in the Apgar score, however, are useful for assessing the response to resuscitation. For example, a newborn infant who has a 1-minute Apgar score of 3 and a 5-minute score of 8 has probably had some terminal difficulty at the time of delivery that has been quickly surmounted. On the other hand, the neonate with Apgar scores of 3 and 4 at 1 and 5 minutes is not responding well and may need further intervention. When an infant's 5-minute score is 5 or lower, it has become customary to continue to provide Apgar scores every 5 minutes up to 20 minutes of life or until the score is above 7. Slow improvement in an Apgar score may be associated with some element of hypoxia or ischemia during the delivery, but there are many other reasons for low Apgar scores. A low Apgar score at 1 or 5 minutes has a poor positive predictive accuracy for later disabilities.

6. What should be done to prepare for the delivery of a term infant?

When called to the delivery of a term infant, the clinician should first make sure that all possible tools that might be needed for resuscitation and maintenance of a thermal neutral environment are ready. Although the great majority of term infants in an uncomplicated pregnancy do not require any intervention, it is important to be prepared for any possibility. In addition, a number of other routine items are necessary. On arrival in the delivery room the following items should be checked:

- The radiant warmer should be turned on, and a temperature probe that can be attached to the skin should be available.
- Several dry towels and blankets should be heated under the radiant warmer for the infant.
- A resuscitation bag or a T-piece device should be available with masks of several sizes. If the gestational age of the infant is known, the most appropriate mask size can be chosen (typically a size 1 for term infants).
- An oxygen source should be available. In most instances resuscitation with 21% oxygen can be used initially if respiratory intervention is required.
- A laryngoscope and endotracheal (ET) tubes should be available. For the term infant, a 0 or 1 laryngoscope blade is appropriate, and a 3.5 FR ET tube should be used. Note: Although it may be easier to insert a smaller ET tube, this approach ignores the fact that work of breathing will be dramatically increased with a tube that is too small for the size of the infant.
- Umbilical catheters, size 3.5 and 5 FR, should be available along with D10W fluid and lactated Ringer's solution. Feeding tubes should also be available for insertion into the stomach to drain the contents or air.
- A pulse oximeter should be available. In term infants needing resuscitation, the pulse oximeter provides valuable information (heart rate and oxygen saturation levels) regarding whether the interventions are succeeding.
- A medication box should be present with all medications that might be necessary for resuscitation of a neonate. Although the use of medications such as bicarbonate and calcium have fallen out of favor, there are unique situations in which these solutions may be needed as well as pressor drugs, such as epinephrine, Prostaglandin E1 for ductal dilation, and narcotic antagonists such as naloxone. Rarely are any other medications required in the delivery room.
- Suction for the removal of meconium and the emptying of stomach contents must be present.
- An umbilical cord clamp and scissors should be on hand.
- Erythromycin eye ointment should be present for prevention of gonococcal ophthalmia.
- Vitamin K_1 for the prevention of vitamin K–dependent hemorrhagic disease of the newborn should be on hand.

7. **Why is temperature control of the delivery room so important for a term infant?**
   Immediately before delivery the fetus is bathed in amniotic fluid and maintained at a temperature identical to that of the mother. Within seconds after birth, however, the neonate is exposed to a temperature drop of approximately 10° C. The fluid bathing the skin starts to evaporate, further depressing body temperature. Exposure to cold stress initiates a metabolic response in which brown fat lining the vertebrae, the kidneys, and the adrenal gland is consumed. Metabolism of brown fat raises body temperature (the neonate does not have a developed shivering mechanism to accomplish an increase in body heat) but also leads to increased acid in the blood. Cooling may also increase pulmonary vascular resistance, resulting in hypoxemia and respiratory distress.

   Similarly, excessive heat administration may produce the same kind of changes. Delivery room heat usually comes from keeping a baby under the radiant warmer for a period of time without a temperature probe. In such cases the warmer will continue to emanate heat because it is not being servo controlled to the skin. The increased metabolic rate from the heat exposure can also cause the infant to become tachypneic. In infants with perinatal depression and possible hypoxic ischemic encephalopathy, hyperthermia should be prevented because it may increase the risk of neurodevelopmental disability.

   The thermal neutral environment is usually in the range of 36° to 37.5° C skin temperature. Both term and preterm infants suffer similarly when under environmental stress, but the large surface to body mass ratio of the premature infant exaggerates the adverse consequences (Fig. 1-1).

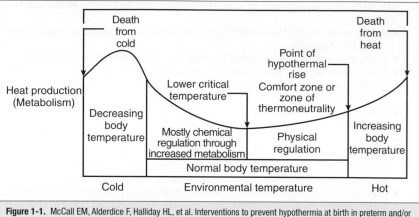

Figure 1-1. McCall EM, Alderdice F, Halliday HL, et al. Interventions to prevent hypothermia at birth in preterm and/or low birthweight infants. Cochrane Database Syst Rev 2010 Mar 17;3:CD004210.

8. **What should the first step be after the delivery of a term infant, once the baby is handed to the clinician?**
    Assuming that the obstetrician has clamped the baby's umbilical cord and the baby appears to be vigorous (i.e., the baby is crying, breathing, centrally pink), the infant should be brought immediately to the radiant warmer and dried thoroughly. A quick weight should be obtained once the baby is dry. All wet blankets and towels should be discarded and the infant clothed in a warmed diaper and dry top. A knit cap should be added to prevent loss of heat from the scalp.

9. **Why is eye prophylaxis important?**
    Historically, one of the most important issues with regard to newborn infants was the possibility of developing gonococcal ophthalmia as a result of passing through the birth canal of a mother infected with *Neisseria gonorrheae.* Gonococcal ophthalmia can produce a severe purulent conjunctivitis that may result in permanent loss of vision and generalized neonatal sepsis. The eye discharge resulting from this infection typically begins during the first 5 days of life.
    Eye prophylaxis previously consisted of treatment with silver nitrate drops to the eyes. However, silver nitrate itself causes a significant, though temporary, chemical conjunctivitis. In the past decade it has been replaced by the administration of antibiotic ointment, such as 1% tetracycline or 0.5% erythromycin in single-use ampules.

10. **What are other causes of neonatal conjunctivitis?**
    Neonatal conjunctivitis may be produced by a variety of infectious agents in addition to *N. gonorrheae.* *Chlamydia trachomatis* is now the most common form of neonatal conjunctivitis, occurring in approximately 0.5% to 2.5% of all term births in the United States. This infection typically appears between 3 days and 6 weeks of life with an eye discharge, which is occasionally accompanied by pneumonia (10% to 20% of patients). The agents used to prevent *N. gonorrheae* infection do not prevent chlamydial conjunctivitis.
    Other infectious agents capable of causing an eye infection in the newborn infant include *Staphylococcus,* Group A and B *Streptococcus, Pneumococcus, Pseudomonas aeruginosa,* and herpes simplex virus.

Zuppa AA, D'Andrea V, Catenazzi P, et al. Ophthalmia neonatorum: what kind of prophylaxis? J Matern Fetal Neonatal Med 2011 Jun;24(6):769–73.

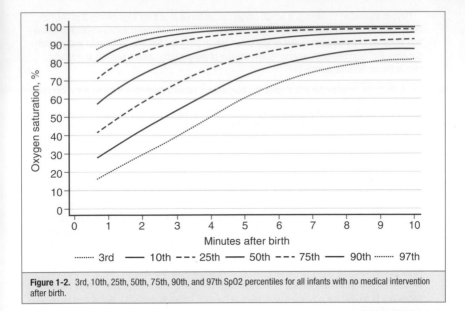

Figure 1-2. 3rd, 10th, 25th, 50th, 75th, 90th, and 97th SpO2 percentiles for all infants with no medical intervention after birth.

11. **Is footprinting for identification purposes necessary in the delivery room?**
    The use of footprints has been a tradition in hospitals for decades and is mandated in most states. Although the value of footprinting is debatable and the manner in which footprints are obtained is often haphazard, footprints occasionally prove valuable if the identity of the infant in the hospital is in question. Footprinting ideally should be done as soon as possible after delivery, but it can be deferred if the infant develops signs of disease that require intervention or if immediate maternal contact is desired. Footprints should be obtained before the child leaves the delivery room area. The long-term value of footprints is essentially negligible beyond the immediate neonatal period. More sophisticated methods to identify infants using DNA are coming into use.

12. **How long does it take for a baby to reach 95% oxygen saturation?**
    Studies from a number of investigators in recent years have contradicted the traditional concept that babies become well saturated within a few breaths after birth. In fact, the transition usually requires between 10 and 12 minutes, or longer occasionally, before a term infant's saturation reaches approximately 93% to 95% (Fig. 1-2).

13. **Why is oxygen saturation screening performed before hospital discharge?**
    For many years babies with congenital heart disease arrived in the delivery room with no prenatal diagnosis. Such infants commonly presented with severe cyanosis and respiratory distress, often beginning within minutes of birth. With the introduction of antenatal ultrasound screening during the early 1980s, the number of babies who were born undiagnosed dropped dramatically. It was evident, however, that some critical cardiac diagnoses could be overlooked on ultrasound examination and not manifest until some time later (even after hospital discharge of the infant), placing the baby at some jeopardy. Ductal-dependent lesions, in which the systemic circulation is oxygenated through blood flowing through a patent ductus arteriosus, may result in sudden cardiovascular collapse in affected infants as the ductus closes, with a risk of death. Lesions that can provoke this sudden deterioration include coarctation of the aorta, hypoplastic left heart syndrome, aortic stenosis, and transposition of the great vessels.

Oxygen saturation screening, in which oxygen saturation is less than 95% on day 2 of life, has been demonstrated to identify many of the infants who are not diagnosed during physical examination. Because of the apparent value of this screening, in 2011 the Secretary of Health and Human Services, Kathleen Sebelius, recommended the use of oxygen saturation screening in newborn infants before hospital discharge.

Bradshaw EA, Martin GR. Screening for critical congenital heart disease: advancing detection in the newborn. Curr Opin Pediatr 2012 Oct;24(5):603–8.

Mahle WT, Martin GR, Beekman RH 3rd, et al. Section on Cardiology and Cardiac Surgery Executive Committee. Endorsement of Health and Human Services recommendation for pulse oximetry screening for critical congenital heart disease. Pediatrics 2012 Jan;129(1):190–2.

14. Is there any downside to oxygen saturation screening?

A number of infants will not consistently demonstrate saturation levels at 95% or above in the 2 days before discharge from the nursery for a variety of reasons, most of which are not reflective of congenital heart disease. Preliminary data collected by Pediatrix Medical Group suggest that approximately 0.5% of all infants will fail initial screening. According to some observations, infants born at higher altitudes (>4000 feet) appear to have a false-positive rate of nearly 50% during initial screening. All infants who screen positive should be followed up with the currently recommended cardiac echocardiogram. This requirement presents substantial difficulties for many nurseries. In addition, many of the community hospitals around the country that offer maternity services do not have ready access to a cardiologist who can perform this study. It may become necessary to modify the screening procedure in the near future to prevent a prohibitive increase in the cost of care.

Bradshaw EA, Cuzzi S, Kiernan SC, et al. Feasibility of implementing pulse oximetry screening for congenital heart disease in a community hospital. J Perinatol 2012;32:710–5.

15. When should a healthy neonate first be fed?

The introduction of feedings has undergone significant changes during the past several decades. During the mid-1900s, it was thought that early feeding was not a good idea, and many neonates were not placed at the breast or approached with a bottle for 8 to 12 hours after birth. The sudden removal of a continuous source of nutrients from the placenta (especially glucose) during this time placed some neonates at risk for hypoglycemia. In fact, the definition of hypoglycemia has itself changed in recent years as the long-term outcome of hypoglycemic infants has become more of a concern. Few physicians would now consider a blood glucose level below 40 mg/dL acceptable for a term neonate, whereas it was not uncommon to see infants' blood glucose levels at 30 to 40 mg/dL several decades ago in the early hours after delivery. To promote successful breastfeeding, the AAP and the WHO have recommended that breastfeeding be initiated within the first hour after birth.

With the increased enthusiasm for breastfeeding of newborn infants, babies are often placed at the mother's breast within minutes of delivery. Although mother's milk is scanty at this time and it takes approximately 2 to 3 days for full milk flow to appear, the provision of the high fatty content of colostrum (the earliest milk that is secreted from the breast), together with the immunoprotective characteristics (e.g., white blood cells, antibodies) of colostrum, appears to be very advantageous for newborns and greatly reduces the incidence of hypoglycemia.

Eidelman AI, Schanler RJ. American Academy of Pediatrics Section on Breastfeeding. Breastfeeding and the use of human milk. Pediatrics 2012;129:e834.

16. What are the contraindications to breastfeeding?

Although breastfeeding is clearly best, it is not always possible. Infants with galactosemia should not nurse; instead, they must be fed a lactose-free formula. In the United States mothers with human immunodeficiency virus (HIV) should also not nurse or provide expressed milk because they may pass on the virus to the infant. Mothers with active untreated tuberculosis or active herpes simplex lesions on the breast should also not breastfeed, but they may use expressed milk because these organisms are not transmitted through the milk. Mothers who require antimetabolites or chemotherapy should not breastfeed as long as they are receiving those medications. Radioactive materials acquired during the performance of a medical study are temporary contraindications to nursing. Whereas most drugs are secreted into breast milk, they rarely form an absolute contraindication to nursing. Drug effects, however, should be carefully checked using a reliable resource to ensure that the infant is not unnecessarily exposed to a potentially hazardous medication.

Eidelman AI, Schanler RJ. American Academy of Pediatrics Section on Breastfeeding. Breastfeeding and the use of human milk. Pediatrics 2012;129:e832.

Schaefer C, Peters PWJ, Miller RK. Drugs during pregnancy and lactation: treatment options and risk assessment, 2nd ed. London: Academic Press; 2007.

Weiner CP, Buhimschi C. Drugs for pregnant and lactating women. Philadelphia: Saunders; 2009.

17. **What are the immunologic differences between breast milk and formula?**
Manufacturers of formula have long established that infants grow quite satisfactorily on any of the commercially available infant formulas. Nevertheless, it is evident that breast milk and formula are different in terms of their appearance and their composition. The most striking difference is the immunoprotective aspect of breast milk, which contains white cells and antibodies that appear to be quite valuable in preventing neonatal infections of a variety of types, especially in the respiratory system and the gastrointestinal tract.

Hurley WL, Theil PK. Perspectives on immunoglobulins in colostrum and milk. Nutrients 2011;3:442–74.

18. **What nutritional differences exist between breast milk and formula?**
It is difficult to state these differences precisely because breast milk is not a fixed entity. A mother's milk is said to "mature" over the course of the first weeks of an infant's life, with the composition changing to some degree during that period. Furthermore, breast milk changes even during the course of a single feeding between what is referred to as the *foremilk* (the early part of a feeding) and the *hindmilk* (the later part of a feeding). The gradual and progressive transition to hindmilk during a feed results in a higher fatty content, which aids in allowing the infant to feel satiated and initiates the termination of feeding. Over the first weeks of an infant's life, breast milk caloric density usually drops from approximately 20 to 25 calories per ounce on average to approximately 15 to 17 calories per ounce. In addition, levels of sodium and calcium decline.

Variations in the composition of breast milk among individual mothers can be quite dramatic. Some women will have relatively modest fat content in their milk, resulting in a caloric content as low as 9 to 10 calories per ounce. In contrast, other mothers produce rich, creamy breast milk, with a high fat content and a caloric density that may reach 30 calories per ounce.

Jacobi SK, Odle J. Nutritional factors influencing intestinal health of the neonate. Adv Nutr 2012;3:687–96.

19. **What is meant by bioavailability of nutrients?**
The concept of bioavailability, or the capacity to extract nutrients from food sources, is an important one. Because the composition of breast milk and that of formula differ, it is essential that the food substances, minerals, and vitamins in formula are accessible so that they can be utilized by the neonate. It has been shown that some important minerals (e.g., iron [Fe]) are not as bioavailable in formula as they are in breast milk. Term infants fed only breast milk beyond 6 months will rarely show evidence of iron deficiency anemia, even though the iron content of breast milk is lower than that of iron-fortified formula (0.3 mg/L versus approximately 12 mg/L).

Similarly, protein in breast milk is more bioavailable than protein in formula, and the concentration of protein in formula is correspondingly higher than the amount of protein in breast milk (formula contains approximately 2 to 2.1 g protein/100 kcal versus 1.5 g protein/100 kcal of breast milk). Similar differences between formula and breast milk exist for other vitamins and minerals, as well, to overcome the reduced bioavailability in formula.

20. **What type of protein is in breast milk?**
Breast milk is composed of approximately 60% whey (lactalbumin) protein and 40% casein. Formula is generally 80% casein and 20% lactalbumin.

21. **How do you know if a mother is producing an adequate volume of breast milk?**
When a mother first gets her milk supply, her breasts will feel significantly engorged, usually beginning on the second day after delivery. Placing the infant to the breast will allow the expression of the let-down reflex at this time. This response results in the formation of milk droplets on the nipple opposite from the the breast at which the baby is nursing. When this response occurs, the milk supply is usually considered adequate.

22. **How much time should an infant spend at the breast?**
Although most term neonates take to nursing right away, some are a bit slower to master the technique. In addition, the nipple needs to be toughened gradually so that the mother does not experience any discomfort while nursing. Therefore the duration of nursing should be limited to 5 minutes at one breast before the infant nurses from the other breast. Many babies will initially need some encouragement to keep nursing because they fall asleep early in the feeding. A little bit of stimulation, such as gently rubbing the shoulders or face, or repositioning the infant will usually be adequate to prompt the baby to resume nursing. Because newborns are "demand" feeders, feeding intervals are often irregular. Ideally, in the first few days a newborn should have between 8 and 12 feedings per day. Once the milk supply is well established, the infant usually will gain interest in feeding. As that occurs, the time spent on each breast can be progressively increased, although a maximum of approximately 10 minutes is generally a good idea during the first 2 weeks of nursing. After that time, mother and infant usually develop a comfortable pattern that no longer calls for watching the clock.

23. **A 3-week-old baby who is nursing falls asleep after approximately 10 minutes at the breast. Has this baby nursed long enough?**
Once a mother has established a solid breast milk supply, an infant will meet the bulk of its nutritional and fluid needs (>90%) within 10 minutes of nursing. It is important, however, that a mother empty her breasts regularly on both sides to reduce the risk of cracking of the nipples and mastitis. If the infant nurses on one side and then falls asleep, the mother should try to awaken the baby and place the baby on the other breast for some time, although the added nutrition will be modest.

24. **What should a mother do if she cannot get the baby to nurse as long as she wishes?**
In general, neonates regulate their intake needs quite well, and if the baby cannot be aroused with gentle stimulation, he or she is probably satiated. For comfort, however, the mother might elect to use a breast pump to express some milk from the side that has not been nursed. That milk can be saved and refrigerated in a clean bottle, allowing the father to get up in the middle of the night and share in the feeding responsibilities.

25. **Is breast milk really enough for a 3-month-old infant?**
There is little question that breast milk suffices for the overwhelming majority of infants. Nearly all infants will grow and gain weight well at 3 months of age even when fed milk from a mother who produces very low-fat, watery breast milk. Solid foods and cereals need not be introduced into the infant's diet until a minimum of 4 to 6 months of age.

26. **"I enjoy nursing my baby, but she wakes up for feeding every 1½ to 2 hours. I am getting exhausted. What do I do?"**
Many neonates, both from a nutritional and a comfort perspective, derive great pleasure from nursing. As a result, they often become avid feeders and want to nurse around the clock. This behavior may be especially true for infants whose mothers have breast milk with lower fat content because

these babies need to nurse more often to feel satiated. For those mothers, however, the joy of nursing soon gives way to chronic fatigue caused by awakening throughout the night to nurse.

During the daytime the interval between feedings should be lengthened progressively by simply distracting the infant. Talking to the baby, allowing the baby to watch the mother working around the house, reading simple stories to the baby, and so forth will often buy an additional hour or so between feedings. This timing change will usually form a new behavioral pattern that is less taxing for the mother. Expressing breast milk so that the father can participate in feeding is an ideal and obvious means of reducing the constant demands placed on the mother. The pediatrician should monitor the baby's weight to ensure that the increased intervals between feedings do not adversely affect the infant. They rarely do.

27. "What can I do about that ugly dried umbilical cord?"
The umbilical cord usually takes approximately 10 to 14 days to separate and fall off. Infants whose cords remain on longer may, in rare cases, have an immune deficiency that interferes with and delays this process. Until it falls off, the umbilical cord should simply be kept clean. In the past parents were told to clean the cord with alcohol frequently, but some evidence suggests that this may actually delay cord separation and offers no real advantage. Therefore the cord should be gently cleaned with warm water once or twice a day. Diapers should be folded down below the cord level so that the rough cord edges do not irritate or scrape the periumbilical area. If the cord becomes contaminated with urine or stool, it should be washed carefully with warm water and then dried well. Parents should avoid the tendency to pull the cord off, even when it appears to be hanging by a thin thread because doing so may result in omphalitis.

Takada H, Yoshikawa H, Imaizumi M, et al. Delayed separation of the umbilical cord in two siblings with Interleukin-1 receptor–associated kinase 4 deficiency: rapid screening by flow cytometer. J Pediatr 2006;148:546–8.

28. What causes an umbilicus to continue to ooze, even after the cord has fallen off?
In the majority of cases, continued oozing from an umbilical cord is caused by an umbilical granuloma (Fig. 1-3).

The granuloma represents a cord remnant but does not appear to be associated with any known disease states. It is pinkish-white and secretes a thin, watery mucous discharge. It is easily treated

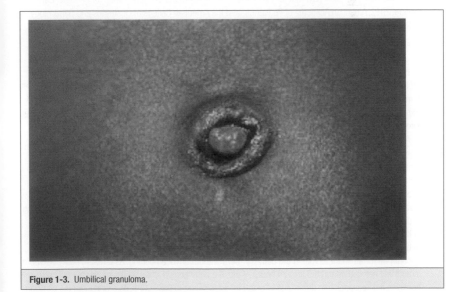

Figure 1-3. Umbilical granuloma.

by application of silver nitrate to the granuloma. It is important to avoid the surrounding umbilical area when applying the silver nitrate.

Caution should be exercised when examining the umbilicus to ensure that no other conditions exist that may affect the infant's well-being. A patent urachus—a connection between the umbilicus and the bladder—may secrete urine in the area. An omphalomesenteric sinus—a connection between the umbilicus and the bowel—may secrete stool though the umbilicus. Some infants may also have a small omphalocele in the area, and this should not be cauterized. All these lesions require surgical intervention.

29. What is omphalitis?

Omphalitis is cellulitis of the umbilicus or periumbilical area. It is marked by a red, indurated area around the umbilicus; fever; irritability; and a generally ill-appearing neonate. It typically appears during the latter part of the first or second week of life, just before cord separation. In addition to generalized sepsis, the greatest risk to the infant is spread to the abdominal fascial plane or penetration into the connecting vascular system (causing portal vein thrombosis). Omphalitis can be life-threatening and is usually caused by gram-positive organisms, especially *Staphylococcus aureus*.

Saleem S. Application of 4% chlorhexidine solution for cord cleansing after birth reduces neonatal mortality and omphalitis. Evid Based Med 2012. [Epub ahead of print]

30. What is the difference between omphalitis and funisitis?

As previously noted, omphalitis is a cellulitis of the periumbilical area that begins after birth. Funisitis is an infection of the umbilical cord tissue itself that typically begins *in utero* and is often associated with chorioamnionitis. Both the umbilical vessels and Wharton jelly of the cord may be involved in funisitis.

31. Should babies be circumcised?

Circumcision refers to the removal of the foreskin of the penis. The most recent recommendations of the AAP state that "the preventive health benefits of elective circumcision of newborn males outweigh the risks of this procedure. Benefits include significant reductions in the risk of urinary tract infection in the first year of life and, subsequently, in the heterosexual risk of HIV and other sexually transmitted infections. Although health benefits are not great enough to recommend routine circumcision for all newborn males, the benefits of circumcision are sufficient to justify access to this procedure for families choosing it and to warrant third-party payment for circumcision of newborn males." (Guidelines for Perinatal Care, 7th Edition, 2012, American Academy of Pediatrics, and the American College of Obstetrics and Gynecology, p. 286). Ritual circumcision is part of a number of religions, and cultural differences should be respected.

AAP Task Force on Circumcision. Pediatrics 2012;130;e756–e785.

32. Why does a 3-day-old infant have vaginal bleeding?

All infants are exposed to the mother's circulating hormones *in utero,* especially progesterone. In female infants the withdrawal of those hormones from the infant's circulation leads to a shedding of the immature uterine lining and a form of temporary menses, which, although often frightening to the parents, is completely benign.

A related phenomenon, referred to as "witch's milk," may also occur. This is a milky discharge from the infant's nipples during the first days of life, again related to high levels of circulating hormones transferred from the mother's circulation.

33. How often should a term infant void?

If you practice pediatric medicine for any length of time, you have received a call from a nurse informing you that a baby has not voided for ____ hours (the number of hours varies). The problem with voiding in the neonatal period is that it is a complex phenomenon that depends on fluid volume at the time of birth and a variety of other factors, many of which are not easily measurable. Furthermore, it is not uncommon for an infant to void in the delivery room without anyone noticing. As a result, many newborn infants will not void during the first 24 hours of life. If a baby goes beyond 24 hours without voiding, however, it is reasonable to determine why the infant is failing to pass urine. As a first step, the clinician should attempt to palpate the bladder. If the bladder is obstructed (the posterior urethral valves in a male infant is the most common site), the bladder will be easily felt and sometimes observed as a bulge above the symphysis pubis. If there is a concern about a urinary tract anomaly or renal failure, laboratory studies (blood urea nitrogen, creatinine, and electrolyte concentrations) and an ultrasound of the urinary tract should be obtained. The management of neonates with suspected renal failure is complex and should always include consultation with a pediatric nephrologist and, when appropriate, a urologist.

34. What is a normal stool pattern for a term infant?
There is essentially no such thing as a "normal" stool pattern in healthy term neonates. As with voiding, many infants will not pass an initial stool for a day or more.

34a. What are the characteristics of the neonatal stool?
The first several bowel movements consist of a tenacious black, tarry substance called meconium. Meconium comprises swallowed amniotic fluid, desquamated intestinal cells, and digestive enzymes. After the first few passages of meconium, the stool begins to change, as does the nature of the bowel movements, depending on the diet of the infant. The breastfed infant often has stools that become golden yellow, then yellow-green. They are fairly soft and occasionally become watery. These stools generally have little odor. In contrast, the formula-fed infant will have more solidly formed stools that are significantly harder and more odorous.

34b. How often do well term infants pass stool?
Breastfed infants may pass stool up to eight times daily with each feeding and be perfectly well. The formula-fed infant generally passes stool only once or twice a day, although they may do so more frequently on occasion.

35. Is there any alternative to disposable diapers for an environmentally conscious family?
Few products represent as much of a dilemma as disposable diapers. How mankind managed to survive without them for millions of years is difficult to imagine. Many parents today would never think of going out of the house without them. However, the plastics used in their manufacture are not biodegradable and are considered harmful to the environment. Cloth diapers are an acceptable alternative to disposable diapers and are available through diaper services in most communities. The cost is often less or comparable to that of disposable diapers. For the environmentally conscious family, the cloth diaper is preferable to the constant use of disposables.

36. Why do babies need to be tested immediately after birth for certain metabolic and genetic diseases?
Neonatal metabolic screening represents one of the most important changes in the care of the newborn infant during the past several decades. Starting with the initial metabolic defect of phenylketonuria (PKU), an increasing number of abnormalities can now be detected shortly after birth. During the 1950s it was recognized that infants with PKU could be treated effectively with dietary restriction that resulted in a normal outcome if the disease could be picked up early in life. Guthrie then developed a bacterial inhibition test (the Guthrie assay) for the detection of PKU. Beginning in 1961 states began to adopt newborn screening for PKU, which was soon followed by tests to detect congenital hypothyroidism. Additional tests were added by many states in their screening programs until the implementation of tandem mass screening technology during the past decade replaced most of these individual tests with a single test performed on a dried blood spot on filter paper. All 50 states now mandate screening for certain genetic and metabolic diseases.

37. "Why can't my baby go home from the hospital?"
There are three primary goals that otherwise healthy infants must meet to be discharged from the hospital after birth: (1) the ability to feed adequately; (2) the ability to maintain body temperature in a room air temperature environment; and (3) absence of any cardiorespiratory abnormality that may

place an infant at risk. The infant must also have passed stool and voided. Although the preceding goals are relatively easy for the term infant to meet, a variety of common issues may delay discharge. These include hyperbilirubinemia, hypoglycemia, suspected septicemia, infant apnea, anemia, and signs of substance withdrawal. Because many of these topics are discussed in depth elsewhere in this book, they will not be presented in detail here. Although parents whose infants cannot be discharged at 48 hours are often greatly distressed, a clear and sympathetic explanation of the reasons this is necessary usually alleviates their concerns. Providing a comfortable place for the mother to visit during the delayed discharge should also be a high priority of care.

38. **"My baby's feet turn in; what should I do? Will my baby be pigeon-toed?"**
The typical *in utero* position of a fetus is with the head placed towards the cervix and the legs positioned towards the fundus. Most commonly, the legs are flexed and crossed most of the time, with the tibia overlying one another. The feet may also tuck into the creases created by the leg flexion, and this position, depending on the site of placental implantation, may place some pressure on the tibia as the fetus matures. It is often interesting to try to flex the newborn's legs into the "position of comfort," or the position in which the neonate spent most of its time before birth. As a result, the tibia often turns in slightly, which is referred to as *tibial torsion*. This toeing-in from the tibial torsion usually disappears soon after the child starts to walk, and very few children are left pigeon-toed. As the feet can be brought to a neutral midline position, no intervention is usually necessary.

39. **How much weight should an infant gain in the weeks after hospital discharge?**
After an initial period of weight loss, primarily caused by the loss of the excess extracellular fluid that is present at birth, the infant will begin to gain weight toward the middle to end of the first week of life and should attain birth weight no later than 2 weeks after delivery. Weight gain usually approximates intrauterine weight gain and averages about 1 ounce (30 grams) per day. Weight gain begins to slow down at approximately 5 to 6 weeks of age. A commonly cited rule of thumb is that an infant's birth weight should double at 4 to 5 months of life and triple at approximately 1 year of age. However, the variability among completely normal children can be significant.

40. **Why do breastfed babies require vitamin D supplementation?**
Although breast milk is the best nutritive substance for infants, studies have demonstrated a high incidence of deficient vitamin D levels in breastfed infants. Breast milk can be low in vitamin D as a result of a lack of maternal sun exposure (particularly in the winter and in northern latitudes), increased use of sunscreen, and dress habits that prevent skin exposure. The AAP recommends that any breastfeeding infant be given 400 IU of vitamin D daily beginning within a few days of life. In breastfed infants who are receiving supplemental formula, vitamin D supplementation should still be provided unless the infant is consuming 1 liter of formula per day (the amount needed to provide 400 IU).

Wagner CL, Greer CR. American Academy of Pediatrics Committee on Breastfeeding; American Academy of Pediatrics Committee on Nutrition. Prevention of rickets and vitamin D deficiency in infants, children and adolescents. Pediatrics 2008;122:1142–1152.

41. **Should pacifier use be discouraged for breastfeeding infants?**
Pacifier use has previously been discouraged in breastfed infants because studies have demonstrated an association with less successful breastfeeding. However, pacifier use has also been shown to be associated with a reduction in the incidence of sudden infant death syndrome (SIDS). Thus it is now recommended that all formula-fed infants be given a pacifier at nap or at bedtime. For breastfeeding infants the use of a pacifier is also recommended at bedtime, but its use should not begin until breastfeeding has been well-established, which is typically 3 to 4 weeks after birth.

O'Connor NR, Tanabe KO, Siadaty MS, et al. Pacifiers and breastfeeding: a systematic review. Arch Pediatr Adolesc Med 2009;163:378–382.
Hauck FR, Omojokun OO, Siadaty MS. Do pacifiers reduce the risk of sudden infant death syndrome? A meta-analysis. Pediatrics 2005;116:e716-e723.

CHAPTER 2

FETAL GROWTH AND DEVELOPMENT

Karin M. Fuchs, MD

1. **What screening is available for fetal growth assessment?**

   Fetal growth assessments can be made clinically by assessing the fundal height; clinical assessment of fetal weight can be made by performing Leopold maneuvers (Fig. 2-1).

   Fundal height is measured from the upper edge of the symphysis pubis to the top of the uterine fundus. Between 20 and 34 weeks of gestation, fundal height measurements (in centimeters) approximate the gestational age (in weeks). A discrepancy between measured and expected fundal height measurements of 3 centimeters or more is suggestive of fetal growth restriction.

   Leopold maneuvers involve the palpation of the fetus through the maternal abdomen. Advantages of Leopold maneuvers include the fact that the procedure is relatively easy to perform and does not incur the expense of ultrasound; disadvantages include a low sensitivity for macrosomia. In general, clinical estimates of fetal weight are more likely to *under*estimate the weight of macrosomic infants than to overestimate the weight.

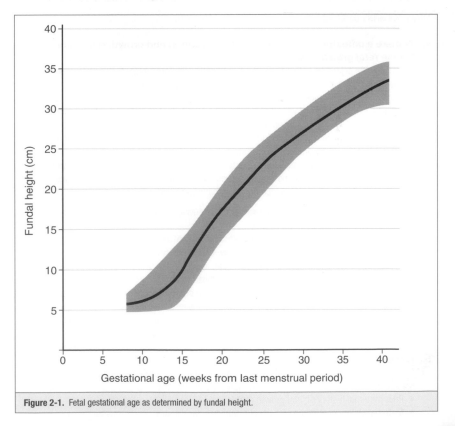

Figure 2-1. Fetal gestational age as determined by fundal height.

2. **How is ultrasound used to assess fetal growth?**

Ultrasound is generally used to evaluate possible fetal growth abnormalities. Biometric measurements used to assess fetal growth are as follows:
- Biparietal diameter (BPD)
- Head circumference (HC)
- Abdominal circumference (AC)
- Femur length (FL)

When a single sonographic measurement is used, the BPD or FL is generally the most reliable indicator of fetal age, whereas the AC is the most sensitive indicator of fetal growth.

When fetal growth is estimated, several individual biometric parameters are commonly entered into a standard formula to calculate a composite weight. Because two-dimensional estimates of fetal weight do not account for variation in fetal body composition and because of the margin of error inherent in sonographic measurement of fetal biometries, sonographic assessments of fetal weight are associated with a significant (~10% to 20%) margin of error.

ACOG practice bulletin No. 101: Ultrasonography in Pregnancy. Obstet Gynecol 2009;113:451–61.
ACOG practice bulletin No. 22: Fetal Macrosomia. Obstet Gynecol 2000;96(3).

3. **What is the difference between *macrosomia* and *large for gestational age*?**

Macrosomia is a term used to describe excessive fetal growth. No threshold weight has been universally accepted, but common definitions include a birth weight above 4000 or 4500 grams. In contrast to macrosomia, which is determined solely by birth weight, the term *large for gestational age* is used to describe any fetus with an estimated weight above the 90th percentile for a given gestational age.

ACOG practice bulletin No. 22: Fetal Macrosomia. Obstet Gynecol 2000;96(3).

4. **Is there a difference between growth retardation and growth restriction? Define *fetal growth restriction*.**

Because of the pejorative nature of the term *retardation,* the term *restriction* has been substituted. Intrauterine growth restriction (IUGR) is a deviation in the rate of growth of a fetus that is less than its genetically predetermined growth potential. Prenatally, *intrauterine growth restriction* is often defined as an estimated fetal weight that is less than the 10th percentile for a given gestational age.
- Symmetric IUGR is characterized by equal reduction in head, abdominal, and skeletal dimensions. It is indicative of an insult during the period of most active cell division, as seen in chromosomal or congenital abnormalities.
- Asymmetric IUGR is distinguished by a reduction in abdominal circumference but sparing of head and skeletal growth. It most likely represents an insult during cell growth caused by extrinsic factors such as uteroplacental insufficiency or maternal vascular disease.

ACOG practice bulletin No. 12: Intrauterine Growth Restriction. Obstet Gynecol 2000;95(1).

5. **How do you differentiate a growth-restricted infant from a small-for-gestational-age (SGA) infant and a low-birth-weight (LBW) infant?**

Both *IUGR* and *SGA* refer to fetal growth potential. In contrast to IUGR, which is diagnosed using *estimated* fetal weights, *SGA* refers to an infant whose *birthweight* is below a preset weight cutoff, typically the 10th percentile for gestational age, when compared with reference population norms.

The LBW classification refers to any infant who weighs less than 2500 grams at birth, independent of gestational age. This category includes term (≥37 weeks' gestation) SGA infants as well as premature infants who may be SGA or of appropriate size relative to their gestational age.

6. **Name the major risk factors for fetal growth restriction.**

Factors that affect fetal growth are typically categorized as fetal, placental, or maternal in origin and are summarized in Table 2-1. Common examples include the following:
- Prior maternal history of fetal growth restriction
- Maternal history of immunologic or collagen vascular disease

- Maternal TORCH infection: *T*oxoplasmosis, *O*ther (syphilis and other viruses), *R*ubella, *C*ytomegalovirus, and *H*erpes simplex virus
- Maternal hypertension or preeclampsia
- Genetic abnormalities in the fetus, including some aneuploidies and genetic syndromes
- Teratogens: cigarette smoke, Retin-A, warfarin, alcohol

TABLE 2-1. RISK FACTORS FOR INTRAUTERINE GROWTH RESTRICTION

MATERNAL	PLACENTAL	FETAL
Poor or inadequate nutritional intake	Mosaicism	Chromosomal abnormalities
Medical disease	Abnormal implantation	Trisomy 13, 18, and 21
Preeclampsia	Previa	Turner syndrome
Chronic hypertension	Accreta	**Genetic syndromes**
Collagen vascular disease	**Abnormal morphology**	Russell–Silver
Diabetes mellitus with vascular disease	Small size	Cornelia de Lange
Thrombophilia (congenital or acquired)	Bilobed, battledore, or circumvallate	**Congenital malformations**
Asthma	Velamentous cord insertion	Anencephaly
Cyanotic heart disease	**Lesions**	Congenital heart defect
Genetic disorder	Chorioangiomata	Congenital diaphragmatic hernia
Environment	Abruptio placentae	Gastroschisis
High altitude	**Infarction**	Omphalocele
Emotional or physical stress	Secondary to maternal chronic disease	Renal abnormalities
Medications and drugs	Chronic abruption	Multiple malformations
Warfarin	**Infection**	**Multiple gestation**
Anticonvulsants	Chorionitis	Twin-twin transfusion syndrome
Retin-A	Chorioamnionitis	**Infection**
Cigarette smoking	Funisitis	TORCH infections: Toxoplasmosis, other (syphilis and other viruses), rubella, cytomegalovirus, and herpes simplex virus
Alcohol		
Cocaine		
Heroin		
Prior obstetric complications		
Spontaneous abortion		
Stillbirth		
Intrauterine growth restriction, low birth weight, or premature offspring		

- Maternal pregestational diabetes
- Placental insufficiency
- Placental infarction
- Idiopathic factors

ACOG practice bulletin No. 12: Intrauterine Growth Restriction. Obstet Gynecol 2000;95(1).

7. **What is the initial work-up when fetal growth restriction is suspected?**
   - Fetal Doppler studies to screen for placental insufficiency as an etiology
   - Assessment of fetal aneuploidy risk and consideration of fetal karyotyping
   - Maternal serology (i.e., TORCH studies) for evidence of recent seroconversion, consideration of amniotic fluid viral DNA testing
   - Evaluation for preeclampsia

ACOG practice bulletin No. 12: Intrauterine Growth Restriction. Obstet Gynecol 2000;95(1).

8. **What role does Doppler ultrasonography have in the management of a growth-restricted fetus?**
   In pregnancies at risk for IUGR, Doppler analysis is used to evaluate placental resistance and fetal status and may improve fetal and neonatal outcomes. Normal umbilical arterial Doppler flow is reassuring and rarely associated with significant morbidity. Absence of end-diastolic flow in the umbilical artery is indicative of significant placental resistance; reversal of flow is suggestive of worsening fetal status and impending demise. Abnormalities in venous circulation (e.g., ductus venosus a-wave reversal) represent worsening circulatory compromise and may reflect a greater risk of fetal death than abnormalities in the arterial circulation.

ACOG practice bulletin No. 101: Ultrasonography in Pregnancy. Obstet Gynecol 2009;113:451–61.
ACOG practice bulletin No. 12: Intrauterine Growth Restriction. Obstet Gynecol 2000;95(1).
ACOG practice bulletin No. 9: Antepartum Fetal Surveillance. Obstet Gynecol 1999;94(4).
Turan S, Miller J, Baschat AA. Integrated testing and management in fetal growth restriction. Semin Perinatol 2008 Jun;32(3):194–200.

9. **Describe the "brain-sparing effect."**
   The brain-sparing effect observed in asymmetric IUGR refers to the fetal adaptive response to chronic hypoxia, in which the fetus preferentially redistributes its blood flow to the brain, myocardium, and adrenal glands. A decreased middle cerebral artery pulsatility index may provide direct evidence of brain sparing.

10. **How should one follow up a fetus at risk for growth restriction?**
    Once IUGR is suspected, fetal well-being should be closely monitored with serial antenatal testing (biophysical profile ± non-stress test; Doppler studies); the frequency of testing will be influenced by the gestational age as well as the maternal and the fetal condition. The timing of delivery is based on fetal maturity, signs of fetal distress, or worsening maternal disease.

ACOG practice bulletin No. 101: Ultrasonography in Pregnancy. Obstet Gynecol 2009;113:451–61.
ACOG practice bulletin No. 12: Intrauterine Growth Restriction. Obstet Gynecol 2000;95(1).
ACOG practice bulletin No. 9: Antepartum Fetal Surveillance. Obstet Gynecol 1999;94(4).
Turan S, Miller J, Baschat AA. Integrated testing and management in fetal growth restriction. Semin Perinatol 2008 Jun;32(3):194–200.

11. **What are the delivery implications for a growth-restricted fetus?**
    The timing of delivery is determined by the gestational age and clinical status of the fetus. For an IUGR fetus at term or near term, delivery is indicated if fetal lung maturity has been documented, there has been minimal fetal growth observed over serial ultrasounds, significant fetal compromise is evident on testing or Doppler study, or maternal status is worsening (e.g., hypertension). The IUGR

fetus is at increased risk of metabolic acidosis and hypoxia, which may be apparent in the fetal heart tracing; continuous monitoring is indicated in labor.

ACOG practice bulletin No. 12: Intrauterine Growth Restriction. Obstet Gynecol 2000;95(1).
    Turan S, Miller J, Baschat AA. Integrated testing and management in fetal growth restriction. Semin Perinatol 2008 Jun;32(3):194–200.
    Galan HL. Timing delivery of the growth-restricted fetus. Semin Perinatol 2011 Oct;35(5):262–9.

12. **What is the ponderal index (PI)?**

    The PI is a widely used measurement of the infant's relative thinness or fatness independent of race, gender, and gestational age. It is calculated from the following formula: (weight × 100)/ length³ with weight in grams and length in centimeters. Normal PI values range between 2.32 and 2.85. The PI is normal in symmetric IUGR, low in asymmetric IUGR, and high in the macrosomic fetus.

13. **List the primary short-term and long-term morbidities observed in growth-restricted infants.**

    An IUGR infant is initially at risk for perinatal asphyxia, intraventricular hemorrhage, meconium aspiration, respiratory distress syndrome, impaired thermoregulation, fasting and alimented hypoglycemia, hypocalcemia, hyperviscosity–polycythemia syndrome, immunodeficiency, and necrotizing enterocolitis. The potential long-term complications are cerebral palsy, behavioral and learning problems, and altered postnatal growth.

ACOG practice bulletin No. 12: Intrauterine Growth Restriction. Obstet Gynecol 2000;95(1).

14. **Describe the "fetal origins hypothesis" of adult disease (Barker hypothesis).**

    David Barker and colleagues postulated that impaired fetal growth may be a key determinant of later development of adult diseases such as obesity, insulin resistance, type 2 diabetes mellitus, and cardiovascular disease. Poor fetal nutrition results in developmental adaptations that permanently alter subsequent postnatal physiology and thereby "program" an infant's future predisposition to disease.

15. **How does *postmaturity* differ from *dysmaturity*?**

    Postmaturity refers to an infant born of a post-term pregnancy, defined as a pregnancy beyond 42 weeks of gestation. *Dysmaturity* may occur in term or preterm infants and describes an infant who exhibits characteristics of placental insufficiency, such as loss of subcutaneous fat and muscle mass or meconium staining of the amniotic fluid, skin, and nails.

16. **When in gestation do the five senses develop in the fetus?**

    - Touch: Between 8 and 15 weeks of gestation, the fetal somatosensory system develops in a cephalocaudal pattern. By 32 weeks of gestation, the fetus consistently responds to temperature, pressure, and pain.
    - Taste: Taste buds are morphologically mature by 13 weeks of gestation. By 24 weeks of gestation, gustatory responses may be present.
    - Hearing: Auditory function begins at 20 weeks of gestation, when the cochlea becomes functional. By 25 weeks of gestation, response to intense vibroacoustic stimuli can be elicited. Sensitivity and frequency resolution approach adult level by 30 weeks of gestation and are indistinguishable from the adult by term.
    - Sight: Pupillary response to light appears as early as 29 weeks of gestation and is present consistently by 32 weeks of gestation.
    - Smell: By 28 to 32 weeks of gestation, premature infants appear to respond to concentrated odor.

Lasky RE, Williams AL. The development of the auditory system from conception to term. NeoReviews 2005;6:141–152.
    Lecanuet JP, Schaal B. Fetal sensory competencies. Eur J Obstet Gynecol 1996;68:1–23.

17. **What features constitute the biophysical profile (BPP)?**
    The BPP is an antenatal test that is used to assess fetal well-being before birth. Five parameters are assessed:
    - Fetal breathing movements (one or more episodes of rhythmic fetal breathing movement of 30 seconds or more within 30 minutes)
    - Gross body movements (three or more discrete body or limb movements within 30 minutes)
    - Fetal tone (one or more episodes of extension of a fetal extremity with return to flexion, or opening or closing of a hand)
    - Qualitative amniotic fluid volume (a single pocket of amniotic fluid exceeding 2 cm)
    - Reactive fetal heart rate by nonstress test
    The presence of a normal assessment is scored as 2 points, and the absence of the finding is scored as 0. The maximum score is 10, and the minimum score is 0. If all of the ultrasound measurements are normal (i.e., BPP = 8), fetal heart monitoring may be omitted because it will not improve the test's predictive accuracy. If oligohydramnios is detected, further fetal evaluation is necessary, regardless of the BPP.

    ACOG practice bulletin No. 9: Antepartum Fetal Surveillance. Obstet Gynecol 1999;94(4).

18. **How is fetal breathing detected before birth?**
    A regular pattern of fetal breathing movements is observed by 20 to 21 weeks of gestation. Fetal breathing movement is controlled by centers on the ventral surface of the fourth ventricle. As a result, the presence of fetal breathing indicates an intact central nervous system. Fetal breathing movements appear to assist the movement of fetal lung fluid into the amniotic cavity and also tone the respiratory muscles for the initiation of breathing at the time of birth.

    ACOG practice bulletin No. 9: Antepartum Fetal Surveillance. Obstet Gynecol 1999;94(4).

19. **How does one differentiate pathologic absence of fetal breathing movements from periodic breathing that occurs during fetal sleep?**
    Fetal sleep cycles are generally approximately 20 minutes in length. Accordingly, to account for the possibility of fetal sleep during an observation period, a BPP must be performed over a minimum of 30 minutes before absence of fetal breathing can be diagnosed.

    ACOG practice bulletin No. 9: Antepartum Fetal Surveillance. Obstet Gynecol 1999;94(4).

20. **When should the BPP be used?**
    The BPP is applicable in cases of acute or chronic intrauterine hypoxia. In response to hypoxia, the individual components of the BPP theoretically disappear in the inverse of their appearance. Nonreactive fetal heart rate activity should be the first sign of fetal compromise, followed by absence of fetal breathing movements, gross body movement, and, lastly, tone.
    Whereas the other BPP parameters reflect more acute changes, amniotic fluid volume assessment is a measure of chronic fetal status. Oligohydramnios may be seen in response to impaired uteroplacental perfusion.

    ACOG practice bulletin No. 9: Antepartum Fetal Surveillance. Obstet Gynecol 1999;94(4).

21. **How does the BPP relate to the umbilical venous pH?**
    Figure 2-2 reveals the relationship between the fetal BPP and mean umbilical venous pH.

    Manning FA, Snijders R, Harman CR, et al. Fetal biophysical profile score. VI: Correlation with antepartum umbilical venous fetal pH. Am J Obstet Gynecol 1993;169:755–763.

22. **What is the relationship between the fetal BPP and neonatal outcome?**
    Figure 2-3 depicts the relationship between the fetal BPP and risk of any perinatal morbidity, meconium aspiration, and major congenital anomaly. A normal BPP is never associated with fetal acidemia.

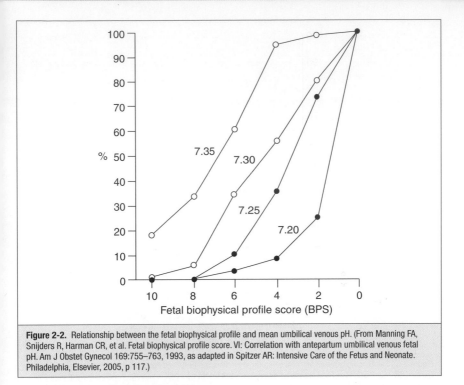

Figure 2-2. Relationship between the fetal biophysical profile and mean umbilical venous pH. (From Manning FA, Snijders R, Harman CR, et al. Fetal biophysical profile score. VI: Correlation with antepartum umbilical venous fetal pH. Am J Obstet Gynecol 169:755–763, 1993, as adapted in Spitzer AR: Intensive Care of the Fetus and Neonate. Philadelphia, Elsevier, 2005, p 117.)

The perinatal mortality rate is 0.8 per 1000 live births after a normal BPP. However, a BPP of 0 is almost always associated with fetal compromise.

23. **How are major and minor anomalies defined?**
    Fetal anomalies can be classified as either major or minor. Minor anomalies are those that may have cosmetic significance but rarely require medical or significant surgical treatment. In contrast, major anomalies are those that have a serious impact on the health, development, or functional ability of the affected individual. Although some women—such as those with diabetes, those born with a congenital anomaly, or those who have had a prior affected child—are at higher risk of having a baby with a birth defect, the majority of infants with congenital anomalies are born to women with no risk factors.

24. **What are the advantages of prenatal screening for anomalies?**
    The goal of prenatal screening is the early detection of major birth defects before delivery. Prenatal detection of anomalies allows time for referral to a tertiary care facility for consultation with appropriate pediatric subspecialists, delivery planning, and coordination of neonatal care.

25. **What are the primary methods of prenatal screening for anomalies?**
    2D ultrasound is the primary tool used to screen for fetal structural abnormalities. Although the majority of anomalies are detected in the second or third trimester, some major birth defects can be diagnosed already in the first trimester. Measurement of the nuchal translucency between 11 and 14 weeks of gestation can be used as an early screening tool for aneuploidy, fetal congenital heart disease, and other structural anomalies.

ACOG practice bulletin No. 101: Ultrasonography in Pregnancy. Obstet Gynecol 2009;113:451–61.

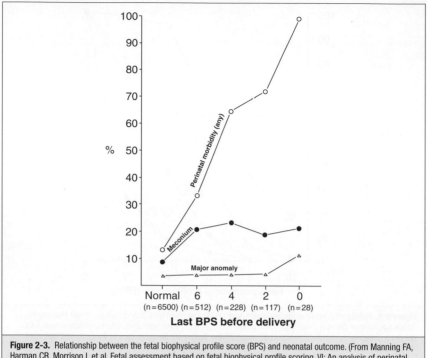

Figure 2-3. Relationship between the fetal biophysical profile score (BPS) and neonatal outcome. (From Manning FA, Harman CR, Morrison I, et al. Fetal assessment based on fetal biophysical profile scoring. VI: An analysis of perinatal morbidity and mortality. Am J Obstet Gynecol 1990;162:703–709, as adapted in Spitzer AR: Intensive Care of the Fetus and Neonate. Philadelphia: Elsevier; 2005. p 118.)

26. What factors affect the prenatal detection of fetal anomalies?

Although many birth defects can be diagnosed prenatally, some major and many minor anomalies are not detected until birth (or later). Several factors can affect the ability to detect a fetal malformation prenatally. In general, major anomalies are generally more likely to be detected before birth than minor abnormalities, but some major anomalies—such as congenital heart disease and orofacial clefts—have relatively low detection rates despite routine prenatal screening. In addition to the nature of the ultrasound facility and the experience of the sonographer or sonologist, ultrasound detection rates can also be affected by maternal factors, such as obesity and abdominal wall scarring, which can make it difficult to see fetal structures prenatally. Furthermore, some anomalies cannot be detected early in gestation either because the structure is not developed at the time the ultrasound is performed or because the abnormality may develop after the scan was done.

ACOG practice bulletin No. 101: Ultrasonography in Pregnancy. Obstet Gynecol 2009;113:451–61.

27. Aside from two-dimensional ultrasound, what other imaging tools can be used to diagnose anomalies prenatally?

In some cases, three-dimensional ultrasound or fetal magnetic resonance imaging (MRI) may be used to further characterize a structural abnormality or to screen for other malformations. In particular, fetal MRI may be used to evaluate abnormalities of the fetal brain because it can sometimes detect abnormalities that cannot be seen with ultrasound alone.

Fetal echocardiogram is recommended in all cases of suspected fetal congenital heart disease as well as in women at increased risk of fetal cardiac anomalies (e.g., personal or family history of congenital heart disease, pregestational diabetes, conception by way of in vitro fertilization, presence of other fetal structural anomalies).

Merz E, Abramowicz JS. 3D/4D ultrasound in prenatal diagnosis: is it time for routine use? Clin Obstet Gynecol 2012 Mar;55(1):336–51.

We JS, Young L, Park IY, et al. Usefulness of additional fetal magnetic resonance imaging in the prenatal diagnosis of congenital abnormalities. Arch Gynecol Obstet 2012;286(6):1443–52.

28. Define twin-twin transfusion syndrome (TTTS).

TTTS is defined as the presence of oligohydramnios in one amniotic sac and polyhydramnios in the other sac in a monochorionic diamniotic twin gestation. TTTS results from an unbalanced interfetal transfusion from a net unidirectional flow through arteriovenous anastomoses deep within the shared placenta. The severity of clinical presentation is modulated by the degree of bidirectional flow from superficial anastomoses.

Mosquera C, Miller RS, Simpson LL. Twin-twin transfusion syndrome. Semin Perinatol 2012 Jun;36(3):182–9.

29. What are the complications of TTTS?

Complications specific to the recipient twin are polycythemia, systemic hypertension, biventricular cardiac hypertrophy, and congestive heart failure. The donor twin is at risk for growth failure, anemia, high-output cardiac failure, and hydrops. Both twins are at increased risk of congenital anomalies, in utero demise, and cerebral palsy.

Mosquera C, Miller RS, Simpson LL. Twin-twin transfusion syndrome. Semin Perinatol 2012 Jun;36(3):182–9.

30. What is the Quintero staging system? How does it aid in the management of TTTS?

The Quintero staging system grades the severity of TTTS and may aid in determining the prognosis and selection of treatment modalities.

- **Stage I:** Oligo-polyhydramnios sequence and visible donor-twin bladder
- **Stage II:** "Stuck twin" phenomenon and empty (nonvisible) donor-twin bladder
- **Stage III:** Critically abnormal Doppler studies in either twin
- **Stage IV:** Fetal hydrops in one or both twins
- **Stage V:** In utero fetal demise of one or both twins

Mosquera C, Miller RS, Simpson LL. Twin-twin transfusion syndrome. Semin Perinatol 2012 Jun;36(3):182–9.

31. What are the available treatment modalities for TTTS?

- Serial amnioreduction of the recipient twin amniotic sac increases perfusion to the "stuck twin" by decreasing pressure on the donor amniotic sac.
- Selective laser photocoagulation of connecting arteriovenous anastomoses decreases the intertwin transfusion (Fig. 2-4). This is the only intervention that may be potentially curative.
- Amniotic intertwin septostomy restores normal amniotic fluid pressure gradient by allowing hydrostatic flow of amniotic fluid from the recipient to the donor.
- Selective feticide by cord occlusion is reserved for severe or refractory cases and imminent in utero fetal demise of one twin to improve the survival of the co-twin.

Mosquera C, Miller RS, Simpson LL. Twin-twin transfusion syndrome. Semin Perinatol 2012 Jun;36(3):182–9.

32. What pathophysiologic factors prompt treatment for fetal tachyarrhythmias? What are the possible fetal interventions?

The major concern in fetuses with tachyarrhythmia (e.g., supraventricular tachycardia and atrial flutter) is compromised cardiac output leading to the development of fetal hydrops. When cardiac output is compromised, maternal antiarrhythmic therapy may be initiated. If the fetal arrhythmia remains refractory, direct fetal therapy with antiarrhythmic medications may be considered.

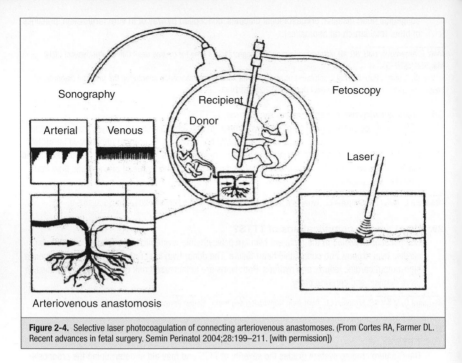

Sonography

Recipient

Donor

Fetoscopy

Arterial

Venous

Laser

Arteriovenous anastomosis

Figure 2-4. Selective laser photocoagulation of connecting arteriovenous anastomoses. (From Cortes RA, Farmer DL. Recent advances in fetal surgery. Semin Perinatol 2004;28:199–211. [with permission])

33. **Describe the pathophysiologic effects of large fetal lung masses.**
   ▪ Esophageal compression interferes with fetal swallowing and results in polyhydramnios.
   ▪ Mediastinal shift causes cardiac compression and obstruction of the great vessels and the development of fetal hydrops.

Cromleholme TM, Coleman B, Hedrick H, et al. Cystic adenomatoid malformation volume ratio predicts outcome in prenatally diagnosed cystic adenomatoid malformation of the lung. J Pediatr Surg 2002;37:331–338.

34. **What is a congenital cystic adenomatoid malformation volume ratio (CVR)?**
   CVR is an ultrasonographic measurement used as a prognostic tool for fetuses with a prenatal diagnosis of congenital cystic adenomatoid malformation (CCAM). CVR is calculated using the formula: [(mass length × height × width) × 0.52] / fetal head circumference; all variables should be in centimeters.

Cromleholme TM, Coleman B, Hedrick H, et al. Cystic adenomatoid malformation volume ratio predicts outcome in prenatally diagnosed cystic adenomatoid malformation of the lung. J Pediatr Surg 2002;37:331–338.

35. **How does the CVR assist the clinician in determining prognosis of infants with CCAM?**
   Neonatal survival approaches 100% in the absence of hydrops. The CVR identifies fetuses at high risk for developing hydrops, and a CVR greater than 1.6 is associated with an 80% risk of developing hydrops; these fetuses may benefit from closer surveillance and possible fetal intervention.

Cromleholme TM, Coleman B, Hedrick H, et al. Cystic adenomatoid malformation volume ratio predicts outcome in prenatally diagnosed cystic adenomatoid malformation of the lung. J Pediatr Surg 2002;37:331–338.

36. **What is the lung-to-head ratio (LHR)?**
   LHR is an ultrasonographic measurement used in fetuses between 24 and 26 weeks of gestation with congenital diaphragmatic hernia. LHR is calculated according to the following

formula: right lung length × right lung length/fetal head circumference; all variables should be in millimeters.

Laudy JAM, Van Gucht M, Van Dooren MF, et al. Congenital diaphragmatic hernia: an evaluation of the prognostic value of the lung-to-head ratio and other prenatal parameters. Prenat Diagn 2003;23:634–639.

37. Does the LHR correlate with neonatal outcome?
In general, LHR greater than or equal to 1.4 is considered a good prognostic indicator, whereas LHR below 0.6 is associated with poor outcomes. Nevertheless, there is a degree of unpredictability in the clinical course despite an accurate LHR measurement.

Laudy JAM, Van Gucht M, Van Dooren MF, et al. Congenital diaphragmatic hernia: An evaluation of the prognostic value of the lung-to-head ratio and other prenatal parameters. Prenat Diagn 2003;23:634–639.

38. Which fetal anomalies may be treated with fetal therapy? What treatment options are available?
The major neonatal diseases that may benefit from fetal intervention are listed in Table 2-2. In utero therapy has been successfully performed for diseases such as primary fetal pleural effusion, lower urinary tract obstruction, neural tube defect, some obstructive heart defects, CCAM, and sacrococcygeal teratoma. Fetal intervention for congenital diaphragmatic hernia is currently investigational.

Adzick NS, Thom EA, Spong CY, et al; MOMS Investigators. A randomized trial of prenatal versus postnatal repair of myelomeningocele. N Engl J Med 2011 Mar 17;364(11):993–1004.
Arzt W, Tulzer G. Fetal surgery for cardiac lesions. Prenat Diagn 2011 Jul;31(7):695–8.
Deprest JA, Nicolaides K, Gratacos E. Fetal surgery for congenital diaphragmatic hernia is back from never gone. Fetal Diagn Ther 2011;29(1):6–17.

39. What are the key principles in determining the potential value of a prenatal therapy for a fetal anomaly?
- The nature and history of the underlying disease should be amenable to fetal intervention.
- Prenatal repair appears to offer advantages above and beyond postnatal correction.
- Failure to intervene is likely to result in permanent injury or death to the fetus.
- Maternal risk is low.

Ville Y. Fetal therapy: practical ethical considerations. Prenat Diagn 2011 Jul;31(7):621–7.

40. What are the major considerations for fetal intervention in cases of congenital cardiac lesions?
- To preserve cardiac structure and function by reversing the pathologic process
- To modify or prevent the development of major postnatal disease

41. Which congenital cardiac lesions show promise for fetal intervention?
Left-sided lesions
- Severe aortic stenosis: Fetal aortic valvuloplasty may reverse left ventricular dysfunction, thereby improving flow through the left side of the heart and left ventricular growth and possibly preventing the development of hypoplastic left heart syndrome (HLHS).
- HLHS and intact/restrictive atrial septum: In utero balloon septostomy may increase in utero pulmonary blood flow, thereby decreasing or preventing pathologic pulmonary parenchymal remodeling and possibly reducing the degree of subsequent postnatal pulmonary hypertension.

Right-sided lesions
- Pulmonary atresia/severe pulmonary valve stenosis with intact ventricular septum: In utero balloon valvuloplasty may preserve cardiac function by decompressing the right ventricular load and ensuring adequate right-sided heart blood flow and right ventricular growth.

Arzt W, Tulzer G. Fetal surgery for cardiac lesions. Prenat Diagn 2011 Jul;31(7):695–8.

TABLE 2-2. AVAILABLE FETAL INTERVENTIONS

FETAL DIAGNOSIS	PEARLS	FETAL INTERVENTION
Myelomeningocele	Incidence: 1:2000 live births	In select cases may reduce need for shunting and improve motor outcomes
	Associated with Arnold–Chiari malformation (ACM) type II	
	70%-85% require ventricular shunt	
	75% have normal intelligence; 50% can live independently	
	Overall mortality: 14%; higher if associated with ACM type II	
Congenital diaphragmatic hernia	Incidence: 1:3000-4000 live births	Fetal intervention is currently not recommended outside of ongoing research trials
	90% are left sided	
	Associated with chromosomal or congenital abnormalities	
	If isolated, morbidity is related to degree of pulmonary hypoplasia	
	Overall mortality: 26%-68%; higher if associated with other defects	
Congenital cystic adenomatoid malformation (CCAM)	Incidence: 1:25,000-1:35,000 pregnancies Multilobar or bilateral lesions are rare	Consider in cases of immature fetus with hydrops Options based on fetal maturity and CCAM type Possible options
	Types:	
	n Macrocystic ≥5 mm (single or multiple cysts)	n Fetal resection for microcystic lesion
	n Microcystic <5 mm ("solid" appearance)	n Thoracoamniotic shunt for macrocystic lesion
	n Mixed	
	10%-15% undergo spontaneous reduction or resolution	
	10%-40% progress to hydrops	
	Morbidity is related to size of defect	
	Mortality: ≈100% if hydrops develops	
Primary fetal pleural effusion	Incidence: 1:15,000 pregnancies	Possible options
	70% are unilateral, usually on the right	Thoracocentesis (in mature fetus)
	Good prognostic indicators: isolated, unilateral, or small volume	Shunt placement (in immature fetus with unilateral lesion)

TABLE 2-2. AVAILABLE FETAL INTERVENTIONS—cont'd		
FETAL DIAGNOSIS	**PEARLS**	**FETAL INTERVENTION**
	Poor prognostic indicators: hydrops, chromosomal abnormalities, or multiple congenital malformations	
	Overall mortality: 15%-20%	
Sacrococcygeal teratoma	Incidence: 1:35,000-40,000 live births	Possible options
	Types: cystic, solid, or mixed	Amnioreduction for polyhydramnios
	High risk: high output cardiac failure, hydrops, or placentomegaly	Cyst aspiration if risk of tumor rupture or mass dystocia
	Malignancy risk increases with delay in excision	Open fetal resection if high output cardiac failure or hydrops
	Morbidity is related to risk of tumor hemorrhage, rupture, or dystocia	
	Overall mortality: 45%-100%	
Lower urinary tract obstruction	Incidence: 1% of pregnancies	Consider in fetus who has poor predicted outcome based on ultrasound and urinary fetal electrolyte findings
	Complications: oligohydramnios, pulmonary hypoplasia, renal dysplasia, and deformational structural anomalies	Possible options
		Vesicoamniotic shunt
	Morbidity is related to timing and duration of obstruction	Open vesicostomy
	Mortality is correlated with the severity of pulmonary hypoplasia	

42. **What is the EXIT procedure**

As shown in Figure 2-5, the ex utero intrapartum treatment (EXIT) is a technique by which a mother undergoes partial cesarean delivery so that placental support to the fetus can be maintained while airway identification, stabilization, and, if necessary, mass resection are performed. The procedure is currently used for the delivery and management of fetal airway compromise resulting from extrinsic mass compression or intrinsic airway defect.

43. **List the congenital malformations that may be indications for the EXIT procedure.**
- Cervical/oral teratoma compressing the airway
- Cervical cystic hygroma compressing the larynx/airway
- Lung mass preventing chest expansion (e.g., CCAM)
- Less common lesions, including fetal goiter, hemangioma, epignathus, neuroblastoma, and congenital high-airway obstruction sequence.

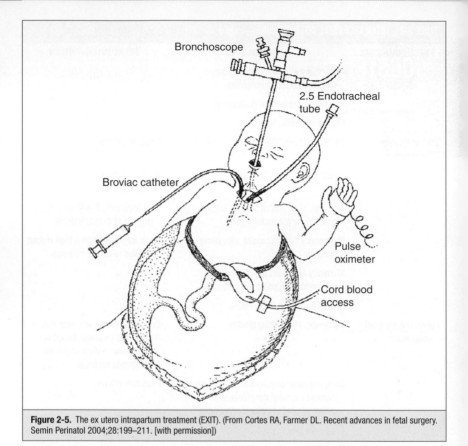

Figure 2-5. The ex utero intrapartum treatment (EXIT). (From Cortes RA, Farmer DL. Recent advances in fetal surgery. Semin Perinatol 2004;28:199–211. [with permission])

44. **What is maternal mirror syndrome?**

    Maternal mirror syndrome is a preeclampsia-like state that occurs in the setting of fetal hydrops; other terms that are used interchangeably are *Ballantyne syndrome* and *pseudotoxemia*. When the syndrome is identified, immediate delivery is generally indicated. Although the symptoms are similar to those of true preeclampsia, mothers with this syndrome typically exhibit anemia caused by hemodilution rather than hemoconcentration and do not commonly develop thrombocytopenia.

CHAPTER 3

OBSTETRIC ISSUES, LABOR, AND DELIVERY

Thomas J. Garite, MD, and C. Andrew Combs, MD, PhD

1. **What is amniocentesis?**

   Amniocentesis is a procedure that involves the aspiration of amniotic fluid from the amniotic sac during pregnancy. It is generally carried out with a spinal needle (20–22 gauge) in a transabdominal approach, using a sterile technique under continuous ultrasound guidance.

   National Institutes of Child Health and Human Development National Registry for Amniocentesis Study Group. Amniocentesis for prenatal diagnosis: safety and accuracy. JAMA 1976;236:1471–1476.

2. **How is amniocentesis classified?**

   Amniocentesis can be classified by the time in the pregnancy when it is done and by its indication. In the second trimester amniocentesis is most often performed for genetic indications. Before 15 weeks' gestation the procedure is called "early" amniocentesis, and 1 milliliter of amniotic fluid per week of gestation is obtained. However, early amniocentesis is gradually being abandoned because it is associated with a high rate of subsequent amniotic fluid leakage (premature rupture of membranes). The majority of amniocenteses for prenatal diagnosis are done between 15 and 20 weeks' gestation.

   In the third trimester amniocentesis is most often performed for fetal lung maturity testing. In the setting of preterm labor or preterm rupture of the membranes, amniocentesis can be used to evaluate possible intraamniotic infection or inflammation. It can also be done for special diagnostic procedures such as polymerase chain reaction for cytomegalovirus in the setting of intrauterine growth restriction (IUGR) or hydrops. Amniocentesis can be helpful in reducing amniotic fluid volume in the setting of polyhydramnios with either premature labor or maternal respiratory difficulty. It is also used for twin-twin transfusion associated with polyhydramnios in one fetus. This type of amniocentesis is often called reduction amniocentesis.

   In Rh and other blood group isoimmunizations, amniocentesis has traditionally been used for bilirubin assessment using ΔOD 450, but it is being done far less frequently now because middle cerebral artery Doppler has been found to be extremely accurate in predicting the degree of fetal anemia. In this setting amniocentesis is used to determine whether the fetus is Rh positive or positive for the sensitized antigen so that testing can be avoided if the fetus is not at risk.

   Canadian Early and Mid-trimester Amniocentesis Trial (CEMAT) Group. Randomised trial to assess safety and fetal outcome of early and mid-trimester amniocentesis. Lancet 1998;351:242–247.

3. **What are the complications of amniocentesis?**

   - Miscarriage and fetal loss (less than 0.1%) above the background rate of spontaneous loss (0.5–1%) in specialized centers with high procedure volumes (Eddleman, Towner). The rate is higher in low-volume centers (Tabor).
   - Transient leakage of amniotic fluid (about 1%)
   - Persistent rupture of membranes (rare)
   - Infection (rare)
   - Fetal trauma (rare)
   - Failure to achieve diagnosis (i.e., cell culture failure, which occurs in 1% of cases)

- Increased Rhesus isoimmunization, especially if the placenta is transversed. In Rh-negative women, Rh immune globulin (e.g., RhoGAM) is given to prevent sensitization.

Eddleman KA, Malone FD, Sullivan L, et al. Pregnancy loss rates after midtrimester amniocentesis. Obstet Gynecol 2006;108:1067–72.

Towner D, Currier RJ, Lorey FW, et al. Miscarriage risk from amniocentesis performed for abnormal maternal serum screening. Am J Obstet Gynecol 2007 Jun;196(6):608.e1–5

Tabor A, Vestergaard CH, Lidegaard ø. Fetal loss rate after chorionic villus sampling and amniocentesis: an 11-year national registry study. Ultrasound Obstet Gynecol 2009 Jul;34(1):19 24.

4. **If genetic studies are indicated, how quickly can the results be obtained?**
   Immediate and preliminary (1- to 3-day) results can be obtained for cytogenetics using fluorescence *in situ* hybridization. Definitive chromosome studies require cultured amniocytes (cells from amniotic fluid) and therefore usually require 10 to 14 days.

5. **What options, aside from amniocentesis, are available for prenatal diagnosis?**
   - Available tests for fetal chromosome evaluation are classified as "diagnostic" (the result is a definitive karyotype) or "screening" (the result quantifies the risk of aneuploidy).
   - Chorionic villus sampling: This is the only alternative to amniocentesis that is considered "diagnostic"; it is performed in the first trimester (9 to 12 weeks). This procedure involves either transvaginal or transabdominal ultrasound-guided needle aspiration of a small amount of placental tissue and can be used for cytogenetic, biochemical, or DNA testing. The procedure-related loss rate is 0.8%.
   - Preimplantation genetic diagnosis: This is an adjunct to *in vitro* fertilization. One or more cells are removed from the developing embryo 2 to 4 days after fertilization and then analyzed. Only normal embryos are selected for implantation. When the parents are carriers of an adverse genetic trait, it may obviate the need for testing during pregnancy. It is not considered "diagnostic" for karyotype, however, because of the high rate of mosaicism.
   - Fetal free DNA screening from maternal blood: This is considered an "advanced screening test" because of very high sensitivity and specificity (>99%) for trisomy 21 and other common aneuploidies. Introduced in late 2011, this testing is currently very expensive and recommended only for women who have one or more risk factors for aneuploidy (based on maternal serum screening, ultrasound screening, advanced maternal age, family history). In women without risk factors, the positive predictive value is not yet known.
   - Second-trimester ultrasound: Many structural fetal defects (e.g., anencephaly, omphalocele) can routinely be seen in patients who undergo ultrasound scanning during the second trimester. Other defects, such as major cardiac defects, can be seen most of the time depending on the sophistication of the center, type of equipment, patient body habitus, and other factors. In addition, many fetuses with chromosome abnormalities including trisomy 13, 18, and 21 syndromes will have findings that will lead to subsequent amniocentesis to confirm the diagnosis.
   - Combinations of first-trimester ultrasound and first-trimester or second-trimester maternal serum screening: These screening tests involve ultrasound evaluation of nuchal translucency at 11 to 14 weeks' gestation, maternal serum levels of human chorionic gonadotropin (hCG) and pregnancy-associated plasma protein A (PAPP-A) at 10 to 14 weeks' gestation, and "triple

✓ KEY POINTS: AMNIOCENTESIS AND GENETIC DIAGNOSIS

1. Before conception: preimplantation diagnosis (in *in vitro* fertilization pregnancies)

2. 9 to 12 weeks: chorionic villus sampling, nuchal translucency, maternal serum hCG, and inhibin

3. <15 weeks: amniocentesis

4. 15 to 20 weeks: α-fetoprotein screening, ultrasound of the fetus

marker" (alpha-fetoprotein (AFP), hCG, estriol) or "quadruple marker" (triple marker plus inhibin-A) at 15 to 20 weeks' gestation. Depending on which combination of tests is performed, detection of Down syndrome is 60% to 95% with a 5% screen positive rate. Reasonable detection rates are also achieved for trisomy 18 and open neural tube defects.

Sundberg K, Bang J, Smidt-Jensen S, et al. Randomised study of risk of fetal loss related to early amniocentesis versus chorionic villus sampling. Lancet 1997;350:697–703.

Goldenberg RL, Andrews WW, Guerrant RL, et al. The preterm prediction study: cervical lactoferrin concentration, other markers of lower genital tract infection, and preterm birth. National Institute of Child Health and Human Development Maternal-Fetal Medicine Units Network. Am J Obstet Gynecol 2000;182:631–635.

Goldenberg RL, Andrews WW, Mercer BM, et al. The preterm prediction study: granulocyte colony-stimulating factor and spontaneous preterm birth. National Institute of Child Health and Human Development Maternal-Fetal Units Network. Am J Obstet Gynecol 2000;182:625–630.

Goldenberg RL, Iams JD, Das A, et al. The preterm prediction study: sequential cervical length and fetal fibronectin testing for the prediction of spontaneous preterm birth. National Institute of Child Health and Human Development Maternal-Fetal Medicine Units Network. Am J Obstet Gynecol 2000;182:636–643.

Iams JD, Goldenberg RL, Mercer BM, et al. National Institute of Child Health and Human Development Maternal-Fetal Medicine Units Network. The preterm prediction study: can low-risk women destined for spontaneous preterm birth be identified? Am J Obstet Gynecol 2001;184:652–5.

Ehrich M, Deciu C, Zwiefelhofer T, et al. Noninvasive detection of fetal trisomy 21 by sequencing of DNA in maternal blood: a study in a clinical setting. Am J Obstet Gynecol 2011;204:205.e1–11.

Palomaki GE, Kloza EM, Lambert-Messerlian GM, et al. DNA sequencing of maternal plasma to detect Down syndrome: an international clinical validation study. Genet Med 2011;13:913–20.

Norton ME, Brar H, Weiss J, et al. Non-Invasive Chromosomal Evaluation (NICE) Study: results of a multicenter prospective cohort study for detection of fetal trisomy 21 and trisomy 18. Am J Obstet Gynecol 2012;207:137.e1–8.

6. **How is third-trimester hemorrhage defined and classified?**
   Third-trimester hemorrhage refers to any bleeding from the genital tract during the third trimester of pregnancy. In practice, it refers to any bleeding that occurs from the time of viability, (i.e., 23 to 24 weeks' gestation). The common causes are classified as placenta previa (7%), placental abruption (13%), and other bleeding (80%), including local lesions of the lower genital tract, vasa previa, early labor, trauma, neoplasia, and marginal placental separation. Such bleeding complicates about 6% of pregnancies.

Konje JC, Walley RJ. Bleeding in late pregnancy. In: James DK, Steer PJ, Weiner CP, Gonik B, editors. High risk pregnancy: management options. Philadelphia: Saunders; 1994. p. 119–136.

7. **How is placenta previa diagnosed?**
   Ultrasound visualization is the method of choice for diagnosis of placenta previa. Multiple reports show a transvaginal approach to be safe and superior in its accuracy compared with transabdominal ultrasound.

Rao KP, Belogolovkin V, Yankowitz J, et al. Abnormal placentation: evidence-based diagnosis and management of placenta previa, placenta accreta, and vasa previa. Obstet Gynecol Surv 2012 Aug;67(8):503–19.

8. **Should a vaginal examination be performed if there is vaginal bleeding?**
   Digital vaginal examination is not recommended when bleeding occurs until placenta previa is excluded by performing an ultrasound examination.

Pearls

If ultrasound is not available in late pregnancy, a useful approach is the double setup examination in which two teams prepared to administer anesthesia are in the operating room. A vaginal examination is performed. If bleeding results from a placenta previa, an emergency cesarean section is performed by the second team.

9. **How is placenta previa classified?**
   - Complete: The placenta symmetrically covers the entire internal os of the cervix.
   - Partial: The placenta lies asymmetrically toward one wall of the uterus and crosses part of the internal os.
   - Marginal: The placental edge just reaches the edge of the internal cervical os.
   - Low-lying placenta: Placental edge is within 2 centimeters of the internal os.

10. **What is the incidence of placenta previa?**
    Placenta previa occurs in 1 in 200 deliveries at term. Complete placenta previa is detected in 5% of second-trimester gestations, with 90% resolving by term; partial placenta previa is seen in 45% of second-trimester gestations and resolves in more than 95% of cases. This apparent resolution is most likely related to the growth of the lower uterine segment in late pregnancy, so the placenta appears to move away from the os.

11. **What are the risk factors for placenta previa?**
    - Previous placenta previa (eightfold risk)
    - Previous uterine surgery (1.5- to fifteenfold risk)
    - Multiparity (1.7-fold risk)
    - Advanced age, older than 35 years (4.7-fold risk)
    - Advanced age, older than 40 years (ninefold risk)
    - Cigarette smoking (1.4- to threefold risk)
    - Multiple-birth pregnancy

12. **What are the complications of placenta previa?**
    - Hemorrhage in third trimester, possibly catastrophic: Uterine contractions, cervical shortening/dilation, and sexual intercourse are common triggers for hemorrhage.
    - Preterm delivery: 50%—the vast majority of increased perinatal mortality with placenta previa is caused by prematurity.
    - Cesarean delivery
    - Placenta accreta: when the placenta infiltrates the uterine wall (1% to 5%; 25% with one previous uterine surgery; 45% if more than one previous surgery)
    - Increased risk of postpartum hemorrhage
    - Fetal growth restriction: Studies are inconsistent, and the majority show no increased rates of IUGR with placenta previa
    - Increased fetal malformations: twofold risk

13. **What is placental abruption? How often does it occur?**
    Placental abruption is the separation of the normally implanted placenta before the birth of the fetus. It results from bleeding from a small arterial vessel into the decidua basalis. It is termed a *revealed abruption* when vaginal bleeding is present (90%) and a *concealed abruption* if no bleeding is visible (10%). It is uniquely dangerous to the fetus and the mother because of its serious pathophysiologic sequelae. The incidence varies but averages about 0.83% or 1 in 120 deliveries. Abruption severe enough to cause fetal death is less common (approximately 1 in 420 deliveries).

Ananth CV, Berkowitz GS, Savitz DA, et al. Placental abruption and adverse perinatal outcome. JAMA 1999;17: 1646–1651.
  Han CS, Schatz F, Lockwood CJ. Abruption-associated prematurity. Clin Perinatol 2011 Sep;38(3):407–21.

14. **What are the main risk factors for a placental abruption? Is placental abruption a recurrent disease?**
    - Maternal hypertension and preeclampsia
    - Increasing maternal age and parity
    - Cigarette smoking
    - Cocaine use

- Trauma
- Uterine anomalies, fibroids
- Premature rupture of the membranes
- Spontaneous or artificial rupture of the membranes
- Prior placental abruption

In subsequent pregnancies the recurrence risk of placental abruption is between 6% and 16%; after two consecutive abruptions the risk is 25%. Women who have a placental abruption severe enough to cause fetal death have a 7% risk of a similar outcome in a subsequent pregnancy.

15. **What maternal and fetal complications occur with placental abruption?**
    Maternal complications
    - Premature labor and delivery
    - Hypovolemic shock
    - Maternal mortality: less than 1%
    - Acute renal failure
    - Disseminated intravascular coagulation
    - Postpartum hemorrhage
    - Severe Rhesus isoimmunization: occurs in Rh-negative mothers unless there is adequate treatment with anti-D immunoglobulin

    Fetal and neonatal complications
    - IUGR: especially in preterm deliveries
    - Increased risk of congenital malformations: 4.4%
    - Neonatal anemia
    - Greater incidence of abnormal neurodevelopment at 2 years
    - Perinatal mortality: 14.4 to 67% higher rates occur at earlier gestations; high rate of stillbirth, fetal distress, and asphyxia. Most mortality is caused by prematurity
    - Fetomaternal hemorrhage with resultant fetal anemia: more common in abruption associated with maternal trauma

16. **What is fetomaternal hemorrhage? What are the complications?**
    Fetomaternal hemorrhage is caused by a disruption of the normal barrier at the placental-decidual interface. It may occur with abruptio placentae; however, it occurs more commonly with abruptio placentae associated with maternal trauma, with maternal trauma without abruptio placentae, or spontaneously without an apparent precipitating event. Approximately 5% of stillbirths without apparent cause are the result of fetomaternal hemorrhage. The diagnosis is made by performing a Kleihauer–Betke test on maternal blood, which allows quantification of fetal cells in maternal serum. In patients with spontaneous fetomaternal hemorrhage, the presenting symptom is decreased fetal movement. If the fetus is still alive and the hemorrhage is severe enough, the diagnosis is often made because of a sinusoidal fetal heart rate (FHR) tracing. Treatment can consist of immediate delivery if the fetus is near term or intrauterine transfusion if the fetus is premature and no abruption is apparent.

Kim YA, Makar RS. Detection of fetomaternal hemorrhage. Am J Hematol 2012;87:417–23.

✓ KEY POINTS: THIRD-TRIMESTER HEMORRHAGE

1. Bleeding at any time during pregnancy is cause for concern and should always be carefully investigated.

2. During the third trimester, however, onset of hemorrhage may be particularly ominous.

3. Some of the diagnoses that should be considered include placenta previa, placental abruption, marginal placental separation, and lesions of the lower genital tract.

4. Approximately 6% of all pregnancies, however, will have some bleeding.

17. **A 32-year-old, G_2P_{1001} woman at term gestation presents in labor. Her membranes are intact, she is afebrile, and the fetal heart tracing is reassuring. Reviewing her prenatal records, you notice that she had a positive Group B streptococcal culture obtained at 34 weeks' gestation. She is allergic to penicillin and "had difficulty breathing and swelled up" when she received it many years ago. What therapy is appropriate?**

The Centers for Disease Control and Prevention (CDC) protocol, as well as the American Academy of Pediatrics (AAP) and American College of Obstetricians and Gynecologists (ACOG) guidelines, recommend prophylactic treatment with penicillin or ampicillin for women in labor who are positive for Group B streptococcus (GBS). There has been a 50% reduction in the rate of neonatal GBS infection in institutions since the CDC protocols were introduced, which underscores the usefulness of appropriate chemoprophylaxis. There is some evidence, however, that part of this reduction in GBS disease has been offset by an increase in gram-negative perinatal infections.

For pencillin-allergic women with high risk of anaphylaxis (as in the present case), the CDC's 2010 guidelines recommend susceptibility testing against both erythromycin and clindamycin. Prophylaxis with erythromycin is no longer recommended, even if sensitivity is documented. Prophylaxis with clindamycin is recommended if GBS is proved sensitive to both clindamycin and erythromycin and if there is no inducible resistance to clindamycin using D-zone testing. If sensitivity is unknown, or if all these requirements are not met, vancomycin is recommended.

Verani JR, McGee L, Schrag SJ. Division of Bacterial Diseases, National Center for Immunization and Respiratory Diseases, Centers for Disease Control and Prevention (CDC). Prevention of perinatal group B streptococcal disease—revised guidelines from CDC, 2010. MMWR Recomm Rep 2010 Nov 19;59(RR-10):1–36.

Byington CL, Polin RA. Policy statement—recommendations for the prevention of perinatal group B streptococcal (GBS) disease. Committee on Infectious Diseases; Committee on Fetus and Newborn. Pediatrics 2011;128:611–6.

Randis TM, Polin RA. Early-onset group B Streptococcal sepsis: new recommendations from the Centres for Disease Control and Prevention. Arch Dis Child Fetal Neonatal Ed 2012;97:F291–4.

18. **What are the major risk factors for preterm labor?**
    - Low socioeconomic status
    - Smoking
    - Chorioamnionitis
    - Prior preterm birth
    - Preterm premature rupture of membranes
    - Maternal age younger than 18 years
    - Urinary tract infection
    - Diethylstilbestrol (DES) exposure
    - Bacterial vaginosis
    - Uterine anomalies
    - Polyhydramnios
    - Hemorrhage
    - Prior cervical surgery

✓ KEY POINTS: PRETERM LABOR

1. One of the most difficult problems with preterm labor is simply making the diagnosis.

2. Many women, believing that they are not yet due to deliver, ignore subtle symptoms of preterm labor until it is too late to intervene.

3. In some women, however, cervical dilation may occur in the absence of contractions, eliminating the possible use of tocolytic agents.

4. One of the most important new therapies for preventing preterm labor appears to be the use of progesterone for women who have previously delivered a preterm infant.

- Congenital anomalies
- Poor nutritional status
- Fetal demise
- Abruptio placentae
- Placenta previa
- Advanced maternal age

McParland PC. Obstetric management of moderate and late preterm labour. Semin Fetal Neonatal Med 2012;17:138–42.

19. **What are absolute contraindications to tocolysis?**
    - Severe pregnancy-induced hypertension/preeclampsia
    - Acute abruptio placentae
    - Chorioamnionitis
    - Fetal death
    - Abnormal FHR tracing indicating need for prompt delivery
    - Fetal anomaly incompatible with life (e.g., anencephaly)

20. **How is the diagnosis of preterm labor made?**
    Preterm labor is defined as regular painful uterine contractions associated with a change in cervical dilation and effacement before 37 weeks of gestation. Often there is concern that by waiting for substantial cervical change before implementing treatment, the delay will result in failed treatment. Furthermore, regular contractions are common in patients who later go on to deliver at term. Thus in randomized series, as many as 50% of episodes of preterm labor do not progress with placebo treatment, and in practice as many as 80% of patients who are treated are not truly in preterm labor.

21. **What is fetal fibronectin?**
    Fetal fibronectin is an extracellular matrix protein, the presence of which in cervicovaginal secretions is a predictor of preterm birth. This predictor has a high negative predictive accuracy (>99% negative predictive value; i.e., the absence of fetal fibronectin indicates <1% chance of delivery within 2 weeks) but only a mediocre positive predictive accuracy.

Joffe GM, Jacques D, Bernis-Heys R, et al. Impact of the fetal fibronectin assay on admissions for preterm labor. Am J Obstet Gynecol 1999;180:581–586.
  Goldenberg RL, Iams JD, Das A, et al. The preterm prediction study: sequential cervical length and fetal fibronectin testing for the prediction of spontaneous preterm birth. National Institute of Child Health and Human Development Maternal-Fetal Medicine Units Network. Am J Obstet Gynecol 2000;182:636–643.

22. **How is fetal fibronectin used?**
    Most commonly, this test is used in patients with preterm contractions in which the diagnosis of preterm labor is uncertain. A negative test result allows greater than 99% reassurance that the patient will not deliver in the next 2 weeks and often prevents unnecessary treatment.

Sanchez-Ramos L, Delke I, Zamora J, et al. Fetal fibronectin as a short-term predictor of preterm birth in symptomatic patients: a meta-analysis. Obstet Gynecol 2009;114:631–40.

23. **What are the common pharmacologic agents used for the inhibition of preterm labor and their mechanisms of action?**
    See Table 3-1.

24. **What are the main adverse effects of tocolytic agents on the fetus and neonate?**
    See Table 3-2.

Conde-Agudelo A, Romero R. Antenatal magnesium sulfate for the prevention of cerebral palsy in preterm infants less than 34 weeks' gestation: a systematic review and metaanalysis. Am J Obstet Gynecol 2009;200:595–609.

TABLE 3-1. COMMON PHARMACOLOGIC AGENTS USED FOR THE INHIBITION OF PRETERM LABOR	
PHARMACOLOGIC AGENT	**MECHANISM OF ACTION**
Beta-adrenergic agonists	Adenylate cyclase inhibitor—sequesters intracellular calcium (e.g., terbutaline, ritodrine)
Magnesium sulfate	Uncertain—magnesium suppresses muscle contraction of myometrial strips *in vitro,* decreases intracellular calcium, and affects acetylcholine release
Prostaglandin synthase inhibitors (indomethacin)	Inhibition of the cyclooxygenase enzyme responsible for prostaglandins that promote uterine contractions
Calcium antagonists (nifedipine)	Inhibition of influx of calcium through the cell membrane

TABLE 3-2. ADVERSE EFFECTS OF TOCOLYTIC AGENTS ON THE FETUS AND NEONATE	
PHARMACOLOGIC AGENT	**ADVERSE EFFECTS**
Beta-adrenergic agonists	Fetal tachycardia, neonatal hypoglycemia, hypocalcemia, and hypotension
Magnesium	Fetal demineralization with prolonged use, neonatal respiratory and motor depression at higher serum levels, ileus
Prostaglandin synthase inhibitors	Constriction of fetal ductus arteriosus leading to pulmonary hypertension, oligohydramnios, decreased fetal urine production, and spontaneous intestinal perforation
Calcium antagonists	No known human effects—decreases fetal arterial PO_2 and pH in animal studies

25. **Is tocolysis effective?**
    There is no question that tocolysis is effective over short-term intervals; however, clinical trials have not consistently demonstrated that gestation can be prolonged significantly or that respiratory distress syndrome can be consistently prevented with tocolysis.

    Abramovici A, Cantu J, Jenkins SM. Tocolytic therapy for acute preterm labor. Obstet Gynecol Clin North Am 2012;39:77–87.

26. **What is premature rupture of membranes (PROM)? Why is it important?**
    The obstetric definition of PROM is rupture of membranes before the onset of labor. "Premature" in this context means only "before onset of labor" and does not imply a preterm gestational age. Thus the term is actually a misnomer. More recently the more accurate term "prelabor rupture of membranes" has been used, especially in the obstetric literature, but it has not been generally adopted in clinical practice. PROM can occur at term or preterm. The latter is commonly abbreviated pPROM. Prolonged PROM (>24 hours) in the term patient is associated with an increased risk of neonatal infection and mortality; however, the duration of membrane rupture does not alter the rate of infection or mortality in the preterm patient. Complications of PROM include the following:
    - Preterm labor: PROM accounts for 25% to 50% of preterm deliveries.
    - Maternal and neonatal infections

KEY POINTS: PREMATURE RUPTURE OF MEMBRANES

1. The factors that lead to premature rupture of membranes may also provoke increased production of cytokines in both the fetus and the mother.

2. Cytokines appear to adversely affect neonatal outcome and to predispose the neonate to both neurologic and pulmonary problems, especially after a preterm birth.

- Increased rates of cord accidents and stillbirth
- Fetal deformation sequence: In the very preterm gestation this includes pulmonary hypoplasia, IUGR, and limb deformities.

27. **A patient makes inquiries regarding multiple courses of steroids to enhance fetal lung maturity. What should you tell her about this approach?**
Multiple courses of antenatal steroids (more than three) are associated with suppression of the fetal adrenal gland and decreased response to stress in a critically ill neonate. In addition, animal and human data suggest less brain growth and developmental delay in childhood after multiple doses of steroids. The benefit of more than one course of antenatal steroids is controversial. A National Institutes of Health consensus conference on antenatal steroids recommended that only a single course of steroids be used and that the use of subsequent courses be limited to patients in research studies that address this question. Several clinical trials tested weekly repeated courses of steroids versus a single course. A Cochrane review concluded that repeated courses may result in a modest reduction in neonatal respiratory distress syndrome. Still, more than three courses can result in other problems, as noted previously. A reasonable compromise is the use of a "rescue course" of steroids—that is, a single repeat course targeted at those most likely to deliver within a week.

NIH Consensus Statement: Effect of Cortiocosteroids for Fetal Maturation on Perinatal Outcomes. NIH Consensus Statement, volume 12. February 28–March 2, 1994.

Garite TJ, Kurtzman J, Maurel K, et al. Obstetrix Collaborative Research Network. Impact of a 'rescue course' of antenatal corticosteroids: a multicenter randomized placebo-controlled trial. Am J Obstet Gynecol 2009;200:248.e1–9. Erratum in: Am J Obstet Gynecol 2009;201:428.

28. **During a review of the perinatal outcomes for premature infants at your hospital, the nurse manager for the intensive care nursery inquires whether there is an effective method to detect women at risk for premature delivery before they present in active preterm labor. What do current data indicate?**
Many strategies have been used to identify patients who are destined to deliver prematurely. Risk assessment scoring using the modified Creasy score (Table 3-3) or other similar systems works well in some populations but not in others. The Creasy score looks at a series of variables in an attempt to define clinical indicators that are likely to result in preterm labor. A major limitation of most clinical risk scoring systems is that they rely heavily on a history of preterm birth in a prior pregnancy, yet the majority of preterm births occur in women without such a history.

Endovaginal ultrasound screening can detect cervical shortening several weeks before the onset of preterm labor in some patients. If a short cervix is found at 18 to 24 weeks, treatment with vaginal progesterone therapy reduces the risk of preterm birth by 40% to 50%.

Fetal fibronectin screening can identify a subgroup of women at high risk for preterm birth, but there is no known therapy that will consistently prevent preterm delivery in women with positive fibronectin screening.

Iams JD, Goldenberg RL, Mercer BM, et al. National Institute of Child Health and Human Development Maternal-Fetal Medicine Units Network. The preterm prediction study: can low-risk women destined for spontaneous preterm birth be identified? Am J Obstet Gynecol 2001 Mar;184:652–5.

TABLE 3-3. RISK FACTORS IN THE PREDICTION OF SPONTANEOUS PRETERM LABOR (MODIFIED CREASY SCORE)	
MAJOR RISK FACTORS	**MINOR RISK FACTORS**
Multiple gestation	Febrile illness
DES exposure	Bleeding after 12 weeks' gestation
Hydramnios	History of pyelonephritis
Uterine anomaly	Cigarette smoking >10 cigarettes/day
Cervix dilated >1 cm at 32 weeks' gestation	One second-trimester abortion
≥ Two second-trimester abortions	More than two first-trimester abortions
Previous preterm delivery	
Previous preterm labor, term delivery	
Abdominal surgery during pregnancy	
History of cone biopsy	
Cervical shortening <1 cm at 32 weeks' gestation	
Uterine irritability	
Cocaine abuse	

29. **Are there any promising therapies to prevent preterm delivery?**

Since 2003, there have been over a dozen trials evaluating prophylactic use of progesterone agents, either vaginal or oral micronized progesterone or intramuscular 17-hydroxyprogesterone caproate (17Pc). In women with prior preterm birth, weekly 17Pc reduced the recurrence of preterm birth by 33% to 45% and vaginal micronized progesterone showed similar benefit in one large trial but not another. In women with short cervix detected by endovaginal ultrasound screening, vaginal micronized progesterone reduced early preterm delivery by 40% to 50% in two large trials. The ACOG has endorsed progesterone therapy in such patients. Several trials showed that these agents are not effective in twin or triplet pregnancies.

Meis PJ, Klebanoff M, Thom E, et al. National Institute of Child Health and Human Development Maternal-Fetal Medicine Units Network. Prevention of recurrent preterm delivery by 17 alpha-hydroxyprogesterone caproate. N Engl J Med 2003;12;348:2379–85. Erratum in: N Engl J Med 2003;25;349:1299.

da Fonseca EB, Bittar RE, Carvalho MH, et al. Prophylactic administration of progesterone by vaginal suppository to reduce the incidence of spontaneous preterm birth in women at increased risk: a randomized placebo-controlled double-blind study. Am J Obstet Gynecol 2003 Feb;188(2):419–24.

da Fonseca EB, Celik E, Parra M, et al. Fetal Medicine Foundation Second Trimester Screening Group. Progesterone and the risk of preterm birth among women with a short cervix. N Engl J Med 2007;2;357:462–9.

Hassan SS, Romero R, Vidyadhari D, et al. PREGNANT Trial. Vaginal progesterone reduces the rate of preterm birth in women with a sonographic short cervix: a multicenter, randomized, double-blind, placebo-controlled trial. Am J Obstet Gynecol 2011;204:221.e1–8.

Combs CA, Garite T, Maurel K, et al. Obstetrix Collaborative Research Network. 17-hydroxyprogesterone caproate for twin pregnancy: a double-blind, randomized clinical trial. Am J Obstet Gynecol 2011;204:221.e1–8.

30. **What are some of the increased risks of twin pregnancies?**
- Preterm birth
- Spontaneous abortion
- IUGR, including discordant growth (which may occur in up to one third of twin pregnancies)
- Fetal malposition
- Placental abnormalities (abruptio placentae, placenta previa)

- Birth asphyxia
- Increased perinatal mortality, especially for preterm, monozygotic, and discordant twins
- Twin-twin transfusion syndrome
- Polyhydramnios

31. **Why are monozygotic twins considered to be at higher risk for complications than dizygotic twins?**

    Monozygotic twins (identical twins) arise from the division of a single fertilized egg. Depending on the timing of the division of the single ovum into separate embryos, the amnionic and chorionic membranes can be shared (if division occurs more than 8 days after fertilization), separate (if it occurs less than 72 hours after fertilization), or mixed (separate amnion, shared chorion if 4 to 8 days after fertilization). Sharing of the chorion, amnion, or both is associated with potential problems of vascular anastomoses (and possible twin-twin transfusion), cord entanglements, and congenital anomalies. These problems increase the risk of IUGR and intrauterine death. They also increase the risk of preterm delivery. Dizygotic twins, however, result from two separately fertilized ova and, as such, usually have a separate amnion and chorion.

32. **What are the varieties of conjoined twins?**

    Conjoined twins are classified according to the degree and nature of their union. These are listed below in order of decreasing frequency:
    - Thoracopagus: joined at the thorax
    - Xiphopagus: joined at the anterior abdominal wall (from the xiphoid to the umbilicus)
    - Pygopagus: joined at the buttocks or rump
    - Ischiopagus: joined at the ischium
    - Craniopagus: joined at the head

✓ KEY POINTS: TWIN PREGNANCIES AND MULTIPLE BIRTHS

1. Multiple births are associated with an increased risk of problems during pregnancy.

2. The higher the number of fetuses, the greater the risk.

3. Preterm labor, twin-twin transfusion, developmental abnormalities, discordant growth, congenital malformations, fetal crowding syndrome, and several other abnormalities are all more common.

4. Monozygotic twins appear to be at greater risk than fraternal twins.

33. **What is perinatal asphyxia?**

    Few terms evoke more trepidation from obstetricians and neonatologists (particularly in a court room, not to mention the delivery room) than perinatal asphyxia. The term *perinatal asphyxia,* however, is so vague and so arbitrarily applied that it is virtually meaningless. In actuality there are two definitions. One is strictly the presence of hypoxia and metabolic acidosis, and the other includes the presence of metabolic acidosis and organ damage. ACOG has suggested that the term not be used, except when all of the following criteria are clearly met:
    - Arterial cord pH sample below 7.0
    - Apgar scores of 4 or less for at least 5 minutes
    - Evidence of altered neurologic status (e.g., obtundation, seizures, altered level of consciousness)
    - Multisystem organ injury or failure

34. **Why has the term *nonreassuring fetal status* been used to replace the term *fetal distress* in practice?**

    In labor electronic FHR monitoring is the primary modality used to determine fetal oxygenation. Although this method is quite reliable when results are normal, when marked abnormalities occur on

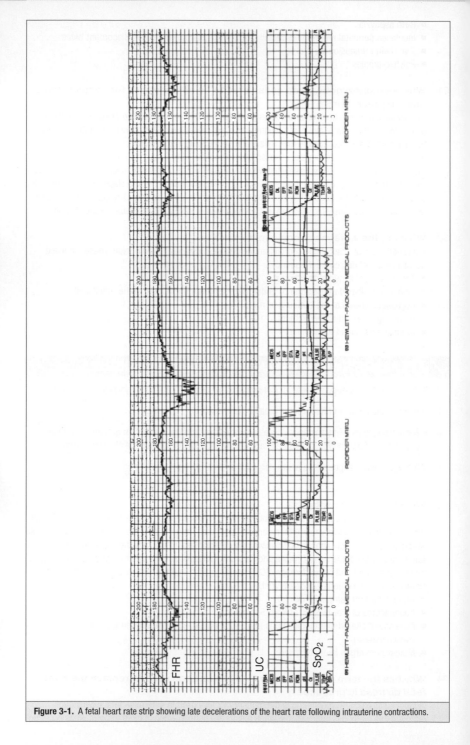

Figure 3-1. A fetal heart rate strip showing late decelerations of the heart rate following intrauterine contractions.

the FHR tracing the infant is more often vigorous and not acidotic at birth. Thus the term *fetal distress* is more often than not inaccurate. A more accurate expression is that the FHR is no longer reassuring and that either other information must be used to establish fetal well-being or, failing that option, the fetus must be delivered (Fig. 3-1).

35. **What is the purpose of antepartum fetal testing?**
Certain fetuses are at risk for antepartum fetal death and asphyxial injury. The purpose of evaluating fetal well-being before labor is to prevent such adverse outcomes by first identifying hypoxia and impending damage or death and then either reversing the process if possible or, failing that, executing delivery in the hope that the baby's condition will improve in the nursery.

✓ KEY POINTS: PERINATAL ASPHYXIA

1. The term *perinatal asphyxia* applies to relatively few pregnancies, yet it commonly makes its way into medical records with some degree of regularity.

2. Delineation of the physiologic abnormalities seen in the fetus and neonate should be used instead of the term *perinatal asphyxia,* which appears to be an exceedingly uncommon event as defined by the ACOG-AAP criteria.

---

36. **What methods of fetal evaluation are in common use in at-risk patients?**
   - Fetal movement counting
   - Nonstress testing (NST)
   - Contraction stress testing (CST)
   - Biophysical profile (BPP) testing
   - Modified BPP
   - Doppler umbilical artery flow analysis

37. **How is fetal movement counting done?**
Many obstetricians teach their patients to assess fetal movement regularly in the latter half of pregnancy. There is no consensus regarding the best method to count fetal movements. However, when fetal movement reaches an alarmingly low level (e.g., fewer than two in an hour), the mother should come in for a test to assess the fetus.

38. **What is NST?**
The FHR accelerates in response to fetal activity. This responsiveness forms the basis of one of the most widely used assessments of fetal well-being, the NST. In the NST the presence of FHR accelerations occur in response to fetal movement. The NST is usually performed in an outpatient setting. The patient is connected to a standard tocodynamometer while the FHR is monitored (by Doppler ultrasound transduction). In general, the clinician looks for at least two accelerations of the FHR of greater than 15 bpm amplitude lasting at least 15 seconds in a 20-minute period of monitoring. If reactivity standards are not met, the tracing is considered nonreactive and a second period of 20 minutes may be observed to eliminate the possibility of fetal sleep. Vibroacoustic stimulation may also be used to rouse the fetus from sleep. If the study is still nonreactive, it should be followed by a CST or a BPP to further assess fetal well-being.

39. **What is a CST?**
A CST was one of the earliest techniques to assess fetal well-being. In this test uterine contractions are induced, either by maternal nipple stimulation or by an intravenous infusion of oxytocin (oxytocin challenge test [OCT]). The former method may be quicker and removes the need to establish an intravenous infusion; the latter is the traditional, time-honored technique. Results are interpreted the same, regardless of the method of inducing contractions. The mother is monitored with a

tocodynamometer and a FHR transducer while uterine contractions are stimulated until adequate, which is defined as three contractions within 10 minutes. In a negative test result, there are no late decelerations of the FHR. In a positive test result, in which there are late decelerations, the risk of mortality and morbidity for the fetus increases, with some reports of mortality as high as 15%. There are, however, many false-positive instances of CST results. In such situations the obstetrician often faces a difficult decision of how aggressively to proceed with delivery of the fetus because the cervix may not be in a favorable condition at that time, and a cesarean section may be required. If the test results are equivocal, it may be reasonable to wait an additional 24 hours to repeat the test.

At present, the CST is primarily used to back up a nonreactive NST. When the NST is persistently nonreactive, and the CST result is positive, the false-positive rate is virtually nil, and delivery is almost always warranted.

40. What is the BPP?

The BPP is a more extensive biophysical assessment of fetal well-being. It includes five parameters that are scored as 2 points each as normal or present, or 0 as abnormal or absent:
- Fetal movement
- Fetal breathing movements
- Fetal tone
- Amniotic fluid volume
- NST assessed by the usual external FHR method

Scores of 8 or 10 are considered normal and reassure the clinician that the fetus will not die or experience damage resulting from a chronic process for the next week. A score of 6 is equivocal and requires repeat testing in 1 day. Scores of 0 to 4 require further evaluation and consideration of delivery.

41. What is the modified BPP?

In large trial it became apparent that the NST alone was associated with a false-negative rate (fetal death within a week of a normal test) that was considerably higher than that of the CST or BPP (1% as opposed to 0.2%). The reason for this is that the loss of fetal movement, and thus reactivity, occurs very late in the process of fetal deterioration and death. Amniotic fluid volume generally declines well before reactivity is lost. Thus the combination of amniotic fluid volume assessment by ultrasound and the NST done weekly has become the test used by many clinicians in testing fetal well-being; the full BPP or the CST is used when the modified BPP result is abnormal.

42. What is the value of measuring umbilical arterial flow?

Waveform analysis of umbilical artery flow using ultrasound-guided Doppler warns the clinician of increased resistance to flow within the placenta. This test is expressed as systolic-to-diastolic ratio. When the situation is severe enough, the flow during diastole either becomes absent or goes in the reverse direction, indicating marked resistance to flow. This form of testing is principally of value in the severely growth-restricted fetus and can give a very early warning of impending fetal demise.

43. What are the indications for obtaining a scalp pH?

A nonreassuring FHR monitoring optimally requires a backup method, except in extreme circumstances where the pattern is clearly indicative of hypoxia and acidosis. Scalp pH has been the gold standard. For various reasons, however (especially the technical difficulties involved in the procedure), recent surveys have indicated that fewer than 5% of clinicians in practice actually use this procedure and choose to err on the side of operative intervention when the FHR pattern is nonreassuring.

44. Who should have umbilical cord blood gas testing? Why not all patients?

Neonatal depression is not always caused by hypoxia and acidosis. Furthermore, given the litigious environment surrounding the issue of perinatal brain damage, the issue of documenting the fetal blood gas status at birth is critical to an objective assessment of the baby's condition. The following are indications for assessing blood gas status at birth:

- Operative intervention for nonreassuring fetal status
- Low Apgar score
- Thick meconium
- Fetuses that had nonreassuring fetal status but did not have operative intervention
- Preterm birth at less than 32 weeks' gestation
- Infants with major congenital anomalies

Although some clinicians believe that all babies should have cord pH determinations, there is little medical value (babies with normal Apgar scores but low pH cord values have normal nursery and follow-up outcome), and it can be argued that a low pH with a normal Apgar could be more harmful than helpful in a medicolegal setting.

✓ KEY POINTS: FETAL EVALUATION

1. The goal of all pregnancies is the preservation of maternal well-being while delivering a healthy neonate.

2. To this end, assessment of the fetus is one of the most important aspects of care during pregnancy.

3. Although techniques for fetal evaluation have greatly contributed to improved outcomes, no technique is infallible and each should be considered only as a single additional piece of information.

4. Reliance on any single test is potentially hazardous to both mother and fetus.

45. **Which drugs that cross the placenta can produce problems in the neonate?**
Virtually all drugs cross the placenta to some degree, but few produce any significant problems for either the fetus or the neonate. Large organic ions such as heparin and insulin do not cross the placenta and are therefore safe. There are some drugs taken by the mother, however, that can be problematic.

- Anticonvulsants: Infants of mothers using anticonvulsants have twice the risk of malformations compared with the general population, especially cleft lip and palate and congenital cardiac defects. Valproic acid may cause neural tube defects, and diphenylhydantoin is associated with fetal hydantoin syndrome (i.e., microcephaly, developmental delay, growth failure, mental retardation, dysmorphic facies, and nail hypoplasia). Carbamazepine may also produce dysmorphism.
- Psychoactive medications: Lithium has been associated with a slightly increased risk of cardiac defects. In addition, lithium can produce polyhydramnios and fetal diabetes insipidus. Hypotonia, lethargy, and feeding problems are also seen in some infants. The effects of other psychotropic agents on the fetus appear minimal, but some cases of teratogenesis have been reported, especially with some benzodiazepines. The critical issue that remains unresolved, however, is whether these drugs alter the development of the maturing fetal central nervous system.
- Anticoagulants: Warfarin is known to produce teratogenic effects in the fetus. Approximately 5% of pregnancies result in fetal warfarin syndrome (i.e., mental retardation, bone stippling, dysmorphic characteristics, ophthalmologic abnormalities). If necessary, warfarin should be replaced by heparin during pregnancy.
- Antihypertensive medications: Angiotensin-converting enzyme inhibitors may cause fetal renal failure In later stages of gestation, leading to oligohydramnios, pulmonary hypoplasia, and fetal deformities.
- Thyroid drugs: Propylthiouracil and methimazole (Tapazole) cross the placenta and can cause a fetal goiter and fetal hypothyroidism. Use of thyroid hormone appears, generally, to be safe. Maternal Graves disease can result in neonatal thyroid storm and hyperthyroidism in rare cases.
- Acne medications: Isotretinoin (Accutane) is a significant human teratogen that should be avoided in women planning to become pregnant. It is associated with a high risk of both structural abnormalities and mental retardation in the newborn. The use of topical tretinoin (Retin-A) appears to be safe.

- Antineoplastic drugs: The anticancer drugs that appear to have the greatest significance for teratogenesis are methotrexate and cyclophosphamide. Both can cause malformations of the skull and bones as well as mental retardation.
- Steroids: The value of steroids for lung maturation is well established. Chronic exposure to steroids has been reported to inhibit neuronal development. Prednisone and prednisolone cross the placenta to a small degree and therefore are the drugs of choice during gestation.
- Antibiotics: Tetracycline is the most notorious drug for producing both skeletal and dental abnormalities in pregnant women. Sulfa drugs may accentuate hyperbilirubinemia during the neonatal period by displacing bilirubin from binding sites. Sulfamethoxazole/trimethoprim has been associated with congenital cardiac defects. Kanamycin and streptomycin (rarely used today) have produced congenital deafness. It is unclear whether gentamicin has the same potential. Careful drug monitoring appears to reduce the likelihood of hearing loss. Some cephalosporins (e.g., cefaclor, cephalexin, cephradine) have been associated with congenital defects, but the association is weak. Most other antibiotics (including acyclovir) appear to be safe for use during pregnancy.
- Prostaglandin synthase inhibitors: Aspirin, ibuprofen, and naproxen may cause *in utero* constriction of the ductus arteriosus in rare cases and probably should be avoided if possible. Indomethacin has been used frequently as a tocolytic agent and is also reported to produce ductal closure, but it appears to be reasonably safe with careful fetal monitoring. These drugs do not appear to be teratogens; however, platelet aggregation is also reduced by many of these agents and may increase the potential for bleeding.
- Alcohol: Fetal alcohol syndrome may occur with even minimal ingestion of alcohol. Symptoms include mental retardation, craniofacial abnormalities, and growth failure.
- Narcotics: The use of narcotics results in significant problems for the neonate, of which the most classic is neonatal drug withdrawal. Withdrawal typically begins in the immediate newborn period and lasts for days to weeks. With some narcotics, such as methadone, withdrawal may not be seen for several days. Babies of mothers who use narcotics appear to have an increased risk of abortion, prematurity, and growth failure.
- Cocaine: Cocaine use appears to result in a higher risk of abortion and stillbirth. Birth weight is generally slightly lower than normal, and there is an increased risk of prematurity. Microcephaly does occur in rare instances with cocaine use during pregnancy. Organ infarction may lead to bowel atresia, porencephaly, and limb maldevelopment.
- Nicotine: Exposure to cigarette smoke *in utero* reduces birth weight by an average of 300 grams if the mother consistently smokes throughout gestation. The risk of apnea and sudden infant death syndrome is increased. The incidence of abruptio placentae also increases.
- Selective serotonin uptake inhibitors: Commonly used as antidepressants, these agents carry a small risk of neonatal pulmonary hypertension. Obstetricians must balance this risk against the serious maternal and fetal risks of untreated depression.

Although this list is relatively complete for many of the drugs known to produce significant fetal problems, the practitioner should always review the most recent medical literature for any updates that might reflect changes in awareness of potential risks of drugs during pregnancy. As was demonstrated by the maternal DES story, the full teratogenic potential of some medications may not be known for many years.

✓ KEY POINTS: MATERNAL DRUGS AND MEDICATIONS DURING PREGNANCY

1. Virtually all drugs cross the placenta to some extent.

2. The same is true of breast milk; most medications enter maternal milk to some degree.

3. Few drugs, however, appear in sufficient concentration to have an adverse effect on the fetus or neonate.

CHAPTER 4

FAMILY-CENTERED AND DEVELOPMENTAL CARE IN THE NEONATAL INTENSIVE CARE UNIT

Karen D. Hendricks-Muñoz, MD, MPH, and Carol C. Prendergast, EdD

1. What is patient-and family-centered care?

Patient- and family-centered care is an approach to planning, delivery, and evaluation of health care that supports partnerships among patients, families, and health care practitioners. It is founded on the principle that the family plays a vital role in ensuring the health and well-being of the infant. Family-centered care provides care to families in a manner that involves respect and empowerment and responds to individual diversity and strengths.

Ahmann E, Abraham MR, Johnson BH. Changing the concept of families as visitors: supporting family presence and participation. Advances: Institute for Family-Centered Care 2002;8:2–15.

2. What are the four guiding principles of patient-and family-centered care?

According to the American Hospital Association and Institute for Family Centered Care 2005, the principles are as follows: (Table 4-1)

3. What are the different approaches to health care delivery?

- **System centered:** The needs of the system drive the delivery of care.
- **Patient centered:** Staff focus on the needs of the infant but do not see the infant within the context of the family.

TABLE 4-1. FOUR GUIDING PRINCIPLES OF PATIENT AND FAMILY-CENTERED CARE

American Hospital Association, Institute for Family-Centered Care: Strategies for leadership: patient- and family-centered care: a resource guide for hospital senior leaders, medical staff and governing boards. Bethesda, MD; 2004. p. 2. Available at http://www.aha.org/aha/key_issues/patient_safety/resources/patientcenteredcare.html

1. Dignity and respect	Health care practitioners listen to and honor patient and family perspectives and choices. Patient and family knowledge, values, beliefs, and cultural backgrounds are included in the planning and delivery of health care.
2. Information sharing	Health care practitioners communicate and share complete and unbiased information with patients and families in ways that are affirming and useful. Patients and families receive timely, complete, and accurate information to effectively participate in care and decision making.
3. Participation	Patients and families are encouraged and supported in participating in care and decision making at the level they choose.
4. Collaboration	Patients, families, health care practitioners, and hospital leaders collaborate in policy and program development, implementation and evaluation, health care facility design, and professional education.

- **Family focused:** The family is the focus or unit of care. Interventions are done to and for them instead of with the patient.
- **Patient-and family-centered:** The priorities and choices of the patient and family are respected. This is a collaborative approach to decision making.

Adapted from Hospitals Moving Forward with Patient- and Family-Centered Care Seminar. Capabilities statement. Bethesda, MD: Institute of Family-Centered Care; 2005. p. 50.

4. **Why is it important to form a partnership in care with a family?**
    See Box 4-1.

BOX 4-1 REASONS TO ENGAGE FAMILIES AS ESSENTIAL PARTNERS IN CARE

1. To foster the parents' confidence as the role of "expert" in relation to their infant
2. To support parent–infant attachment and bonding
3. To help stabilize and strengthen the family unit
4. To equip parents with the necessary skills to be their child's advocate once they leave the neonatal intensive care unit (NICU)
5. To provide the best opportunity for developmentally sound infant and family outcomes, which will yield immeasurable dividends

Hospitals Moving Forward with Patient- and Family-Centered Care Seminar. Bethesda, MD: Institute of Family-Centered Care; 2004. p. 50.

5. **Why is patient- and family-centered care a necessary component of care in the neonatal intensive care unit (NICU)?**
    See Table 4-2.

TABLE 4-2. ADVANTAGES OF PATIENT- AND FAMILY-CENTERED CARE

Johnson BH, Hanson JL, Jeppson ES. Family-centered care: changing practice, changing attitudes. Newborn intensive care: resources for family-centered practice. Bethesda, MD: Institute for Family-Centered Care; 1997. p. 117.

Cisneros KA, Coher K, Dubuisson AB, et al. Implementing potentially better practices for improving family-centered care in neonatal intensive care units: success and challenges. Pediatrics 2003;111:450-60.

Infant and parental advantages	Parent–provider communication and parent satisfaction with care are improved.
	Improves and enhances outcomes for infants by providing appropriate support for families.
	Increases family members' ability to cope with the challenges of caring for their hospitalized premature and critically ill infants.
	Parent–infant attachment is increased.
	Breastfeeding is enhanced.
	It leads to increased parental confidence.
Provider advantages	Medical professionals' satisfaction with their work is increased.
Institutional advantages	There are better health outcomes, hospital economic savings, patient satisfaction with care, and fewer readmissions.

6. What should a patient- and family-centered NICU acknowledge?
See Box 4-2.

BOX 4-2 A FAMILY CENTERED CARE NICU ACKNOWLEDGES THAT:

- Over time, the family has the greatest influence on an infant's health and well-being.
- All families bring important strengths to their infant's health care experiences
- It is important to respond to the individual cultural and linguistic needs of the family
- It is important to nurture the strong bonds that begin between infants and their families at birth and to support those relationships throughout the intensive care experience.
- Innovative facility design and patient- and family-centered environments should be available.

Saunders RP, Abraham MR, Crosby MJ, et al. Evaluation and development of potentially better practices for improving family-centered care in neonatal intensive care units. Pediatrics 2003;111:e437–e449.
Johnson AN. Engaging fathers in the NICU: taking down the barriers to the baby. J Perinat Neonatal Nurs 2008; 22:302–06.

✓ KEY POINTS: FAMILY-CENTERED CARE IN THE NICU

1. Integrates families in the care process

2. Is respectful of family values

3. Supports families' unique differences and diversity

4. Improves parent–infant attachment

5. Enhances breastfeeding

6. Improves parent satisfaction

7. Improves parent–provider communication

8. Improves parents' confidence in the care of their infant

7. How are NICUs changing their approach to health care delivery?
See Box 4-3.

BOX 4-3 PATIENT- AND FAMILY-CENTERED APPROACHES IN THE NICU

- Parents are viewed as *partners* in care.
- Parents are active participants in medical rounds.
- Families are no longer seen as visitors, and there is 24-hour participation in care.
- Parents and families participate in hospital/NICU advisory boards and design committees.
- Parents are involved in unit quality improvement and reseach.
- Parents are part of all design and planning teams for new NICU construction and NICU renovations.
- Parents are provided with opportunities to learn and engage in infant caregiving.
- Parents are encouraged to provide daily kangaroo care/skin-to-skin care.
- Parent-to-parent mentor networks offer support for families.
- Parent information resource centers have been established in the units.

American Academy of Pediatrics Committee on Hosptial Care Policy Statement. Pediatrics 2003;112:691–96.
Sudia-Robinson TM, Freeman SB. Communication patterns and decision-making among parents and health care providers in the neonatal intensive care unit: a case study. Heart Lung 2000;29:143–48.
Van Ripper M. Family provider relationships and well-being in families with preterm infants in the NICU. Heart Lung 2001;30:74–84.
Griffin T. Family-centered care in the NICU. J Perinat Neonatal Nurs 2006;20:98–102.

8. **What are the six key steps used to approach families in the NICU to assess their needs in a family-centered care model?**

   Family assessments in the NICU can be performed in as little as 15 minutes and should be done in a way that supports families and minimizes suffering. The following six key steps can be used as a guideline (Box 4-4):

BOX 4-4 THE SIX KEYS TO FAMILY ASSESSMENT IN THE NICU

- Introduce yourself to all family members.
- Ask about people at the bedside to determine their relationship to the infant, and identify who can receive information other than the parents.
- Know the gender of the infant and, especially, learn the infant's name.
- Stop by frequently to update the parents with changes or other information.
- After any explanation, always ask if there are questions.
- If you do not know an answer, say so and then find out the answer. Do not attempt to "bluff" when you do not know.

Leahey M, Wright L. Maximizing time, minimizing suffering: the 15-minute (or less) family interview. J Fam Nurs 1999;5:259–74.

---

9. **What should be included in a patient-and family-centered neonatal practice?**

   See Box 4-5.

BOX 4-5 EXPECTATIONS OF PATIENT- AND FAMILY-CENTERED NEONATAL PRACTICE

- Privacy is provided for parents at the bedside that is personalized for the infant.
- Health care providers refer to infants and their family members by their names, not with "mommy," "daddy," or "the baby." Such terms are demeaning and disingenuous.
- Information is shared in ways that are useful and affirming of the parents' role.
- Parents, siblings, and families are not visitors and should be encouraged to be with their infants. There is 24-hour access to the NICU.
- Cultural diversity is respected, and family preferences are honored.
- Parents are active participants in medical/nursing rounds by asking questions of and responding to medical providers and are partners in decision making about their infant's care.
- Primary nursing is available. Consistent caregiving is provided.
- Early holding and "kangaroo care" is part of care.
- Infant colostrum care and mother's successful breast milk pumping and feeding is supported through the infant's hospitalization and transistion to home.
- Parents participate in pain care by providing comfort before, during, and after painful procedures.

Lawon G. Facilitation of parenting the premature infant within the newborn intensive care unit. J Perinat Neonatal Nurs 2002;16:71–82.
White RD. Mother's arms—the past and future locus of neonatal care? Clin Perinatol. 2004;Jun 31:83–87.

INFANT DEVELOPMENTAL CARE IN THE NICU

10. **What is developmental care?**

    Developmental care is a method of care that acknowledges that the developing fetus and infant can react favorably or unfavorably to environmental influences. Developmental care is a process that assesses each infant's individual developmental needs and responds to those needs to optimize neurodevelopmental outcome.

Als H. Reading the premature infant. In: Goldson E, editor. Developmental interventions in the neonatal intensive care nursery. New York: Oxford University Press; 1999. p. 18–85.

11. **A premature infant is really a fetus. Is a premature infant capable of reacting or responding to the environment?**
    Absolutely. A premature infant's neurosensory and musculoskeletal development is primed to react to all exposed environments. In the womb, unlike the NICU, a fetus is sheltered from light, sound, and noxious touch.

    Als H, Gilkerson L, Duffy F, et al. A three-center, randomized, controlled trial of individualized developmental care for very low birth weight preterm infants: medical, neurodevelopmental, parenting, and caregiving effects. J Dev Behav Pediatr 2003;24:399–408.

12. **What is the critical biologic aim of developmental care?**
    The aim is to reduce stress and improve or preserve neurodevelopmental outcome. Understanding infant vulnerabilities and responses to stress can lead to a systematic method to support the infant's strengths to alleviate the stress response. Calm infants require less oxygen (and fewer changes in mechanical ventilation), expend less energy, tolerate feeding better, and have a shortened duration of hospitalization.

    Symington A, Pinelli J. Developmental care for promoting development and preventing morbidity in preterm infants. Cochrane Database Syst Rev 2003;4:CD001814.

13. **What are the key components of infant developmental care?**
    Infant developmental care is care responsive to an individual infant's developmental needs. The key components are as follows (Box 4-6):

BOX 4-6 KEY COMPONENTS OF DEVELOPMENTAL CARE

- **Management of the environment:** Decreasing noise and visual stimulation, providing appropriate bedding
- **Collaboration with parents and promotion of infant–parent bonding**
- **Activities that promote self-regulation and state regulation:** Nonnutritive sucking, kangaroo care, cobedding of multiples
- **Fixed midline positioning and containment**
- **Individualizing care and timing of procedures and care provision to promote deep sleep and brain development**

Kenner C, McGrath JM, editors. Developmental care of newborns and infants: a guide for health professionals. St Louis: Mosby; 2004.

✓ **KEY POINTS: GOALS OF DEVELOPMENTAL CARE IN THE NICU**

1. To improve respiratory function

2. To enhance feeding and promote weight gain

3. To support brain and psychological development

4. To prevent muscular skeletal deformities

5. To shorten length of hospitalization

14. **How is developmental care different from the care that is currently provided in the NICU?**
    In current care practices the caregiver has a set treatment plan that is performed regardless of the gestational needs or responses of the infant. In the practice of developmental care,

the caregiver responds to infant behavior to alter or manage the infant's environment before, during, and after the treatment depending on an infant's developmental needs. The caregiver individualizes the treatment process on the basis of the infant's observed behavior and developmental needs.

Als H, Lawhon G, Brown E, et al. Individualized behavioral and environmental care for the very low birth weight preterm infant at high risk for bronchopulmonary dysplasia: neonatal intensive care unit and developmental outcome. Pediatrics 1986;78:1123–32.

Hendricks-Muñoz KD, Prendergast CC. Barriers to provision of developmental care in the neonatal intensive care unit: neonatal nursing perceptions. Am J Perinatol 2007;24:71–77.

Altimier L, Lutes L. Changing units for changing times: the evolution of a NICU. Neonatal Intens Care 2000;3:23–27.

15. **How long have we known that the NICU environment can affect infant outcome?**
    The theory of impact of the environment on infant outcome is not new. As early as 1973, during the "infancy" of neonatal intensive care, environmental effects such as sound, light, and positioning were noted to have a negative impact on infant medical outcomes.

Lotas MJ, Walden M. Individualized developmental care for very low birth-weight infants: a critical review. J Obstet Gynecol Neonat Nurs 1996;25:681–87.

✓ KEY POINTS: COMMON CHARACTERISTICS OF DEVELOPMENTAL CARE

1. An environment supportive of the needs of the child

2. Caregiving staff and families who identify and respond to the needs of the infant

3. Caregiving staff and families who collaborate in care

4. Specific supportive techniques, such as kangaroo care, swaddling, and pacifier use to support development

16. **How is the Newborn Individualized Developmental Care and Assessment Program (NIDCAP) different from other methods of providing developmental care training?**
    NIDCAP is a model of care that emphasizes the behavioral individuality of each infant. Caregivers receive intensive specialized training in neurobehavioral and environmental infant observations that result in a behavioral profile that can be used in the plan of care. This method seeks to diminish the infant's stress experience and enhance the infant's strengths. Wee Care®, another developmental care program, incorporates developmental care training of the entire NICU care team to increase awareness of the importance of the environment and developmental care responses needed to address the needs of high-risk infants.

Als H, Gibes R. Newborn Individualized Developmental Care and Assessment Program (NIDCAP). Training Guide. Boston: Children's Hospital; 1990.

Kenner C, McGrath JM, editors. Developmental care of newborns and infants: a guide for health professionals. St Louis: Mosby; 2004.

17. **Does developmental care for critically ill infants improve outcomes?**
    Yes. Developmental care has been shown to accomplish the following:
    - Facilitate the transition to independent feeding
    - Promote weight gain
    - Shorten hospitalization
    - Reduce hospital charges

- Improve neurobehavioral outcomes
- Reduce parental stress and improve parent perception of the infant

In addition, developmental care methods such as containment, facilitated tuck, and kangaroo care have been shown to reduce infant stress and pain.

Hendricks-Muñoz KD, Prendergast C, Caprio MC, et al. Developmental care: the impact of Wee Care developmental care training on short-term infant outcome and hospital costs. Newborn Infant Nurs Rev 2002;2:39–45.

18. **What neuronal changes occur in the brain of the premature infant in the NICU environment?**

Neuronal changes occurring between 23 and 40 weeks' gestation include the following (Table 4-3):

TABLE 4-3. NEURONAL CHANGES OCCURRING DURING 23 TO 40 WEEKS' GESTATION

Cell migration	Reorientation of cells	Cell proliferation
Cell differentiation	Axonal growth	Formation of dendrites
Myelination	Apoptosis	Formation of synapses

Bourgeois JP. Synaptogenesis in the neocortex of the newborn: the ultimate frontier for individuation? In: Lagercrantz H, Hanson M, Evrard P, et al, editors. The newborn brain. Cambridge: Cambridge University Press; 2002. p. 91–113.

Lagercrantz H, Ringstedt T. Organization of the neuronal circuits in the central nervous system during development. Acta Paediatr 2001;90:707–15.

✓ KEY POINTS: ONGOING NEURONAL CHANGES IN THE NICU

1. Cell migration and proliferation

2. Reorientation and differentiation of cells

3. Axonal growth and formation of dendrites

4. Myelination, apoptosis, and formation of synapses

19. **How critical is the environment for brain development?**

During this critical period of brain development, sensory and environmental influences can regulate wiring of neuronal networks, which can be permanently altered by early abnormal sensory input. In rats pain experienced during the neonatal period is associated with persistent accentuated stress responses, learning deficits, and behavioral changes. In addition, chronic interference with rapid-eye-movement (REM) sleep has been associated with decreased size of the cerebral cortex.

Anand KJ, Coskun V, Thrivikraman KV, et al. Long-term behavioral effects of repetitive pain in neonatal rat pups. Physiol Behav 1999;66:627–37.

Anand KJS, Scalzo FM. Can adverse neonatal experiences alter brain development and subsequent behavior? Biol Neonate 2000;77:69–82.

Gressens P, Rogido M, Paindaveine B, et al. The impact of neonatal intensive care practices on the developing brain. Pediatrics 2002;140:646–53.

Rabinowicz T, de Courten-Myers GM, Petetot JM, et al. Human cortex development: estimates of neuronal numbers indicate major loss late during gestation. J Neuropathol Exp Neurol 1996;55:320–28.

Ruda MA, Ling QD, Hohmann AG, et al. Altered nociceptive neuronal circuits after neonatal peripheral inflammation. Science 2000;289:628–31.

20. **What is the order of development of the fetal senses?**

The senses develop in the following order:

Touch > balance > taste > smell > hearing > and finally sight.

21. What happens when sensory exposure occurs out of sequence?

Animal studies have identified abnormal physiologic and brain development when the senses are stimulated out of order. Quail hatchlings cannot discriminate their mother's cry if exposed to light before hatching. Recent information suggests that premature human infants may be at risk of executive dysfunction and hearing loss when sensory systems have been stimulated out of order.

Graven SN. Sound and the developing infant in the NICU: conclusions and recommendation for care. J Perinatol 2000;20:S88–93.

Turkewitz G, Kenny PA. The role of developmental limitations of sensory input on sensory/perceptual organization. J Dev Behav Pediatr 1985;6:302–08.

TOUCH/TACTILE SYSTEM

22. When does tactile or touch sensation develop in an infant?

Tactile sensory development occurs by 12 to 14 weeks' gestation. It is the first sensory system to develop and plays an important role in overall development. By 14 weeks all sensory connections are present in the fetus.

23. What are the most sensitive areas of the body in a fetus and premature infant?

The areas that are the most sensitive for the fetus and premature infant are the mouth and extremities, especially the hands and feet.

Kenner C, McGrath JM, editors. Developmental care of newborns and infants: a guide for health professionals. St Louis: Mosby; 2004.

MUSCULOSKELETAL SYSTEM

24. What are the physiologic responses to noxious stimuli in premature infants?

Premature infants are very sensitive to what they perceive as noxious touch. When they experience these events, they respond with tachycardia, agitation, hypertension, apnea, a decrease in oxygen saturation, disorganization, and sleep deprivation.

Evans JC. Incidence of hypoxemia associated with caregiving in premature infants. Neonatal Netw 1991;10:17–24.

Liu D, Caldji C, Sharma S, et al. Influence of neonatal rearing conditions on stress-induced adrenocorticotropin responses and norepinephrine release in the hypothalamic paraventricular nucleus. J Neuroendocrinol 2000;12:5–12.

25. What is the normal position of an infant in the womb?

In the buoyant conditions of the womb, the infant remains in a flexed, contained, and midline position at all times. The head, back, and feet are contained by the uterine boundaries. This position allows for soothing and self-regulation by touching of the face and sucking on fingers.

26. How does the loss of the uterine environment affect muscular development in an infant?

Muscular development in the womb is critically dependent on the buoyancy and contained uterine space. The constant give-and-take of the uterine push against the fetal body fosters proper development of flexion and extension muscular tone in the infant.

Mouradian LE, Als H. The influence of neonatal intensive care unit caregiving practices on motor functioning of preterm infants. Am J Occup Ther 1994;48:527–33.

27. In the NICU, why is it important to provide boundaries for muscular development in a premature infant?

Synaptic connections are stimulated with repeated use, and they weaken with disuse. Once the infant is outside the womb, the loss of uterine containment cannot support muscular development.

A weak, premature infant is unable to counteract the effects of gravity and assumes a flattened posture with extremity extension, abduction, and external rotation on the bed surface. Over time, this position will lead to abnormal developmental tone and positional deformities.

Grenier IR, Bigsby R, Vergara ER, et al. Comparison of motor self-regulatory and stress behaviors of preterm infants across body positions. Am J Occup Ther 2003;57:289–97.

28. Why is it important to turn a premature infant every few hours?

Premature infants in the womb are buoyant and turn easily, equalizing pressure stimuli. In the NICU the impact of gravity inhibits any movement by the infant, who must rely on caregivers for proper positioning. Infants who are not turned are fixed in one position for prolonged periods and are at risk for development of muscular skeletal deformities that negatively affect the infant's future motor development and the ability to eat, explore, play, and develop social and other skills.

Downs JA, Edwards AD, McCormick DC, et al. Effect of intervention on the development of hip posture in very preterm babies. Arch Dis Child 1991;66:197–201.

Sweeney JK, Gutierrez P. Musculoskeletal implications of preterm infant positioning in the NICU. J Perinat Neonat Nurs 2002;16:58–70.

29. Premature infants often have misshapen heads. Why does this happen?

A progressive lateral flattening of the skull, called scaphocephaly or dolichocephaly, results in a narrow and elongated infant head. This occurs because the skull of the premature infant is thinner, softer, and at greater risk for postural deformities. Although this deformity appears to have no effect on brain development, lateral flattening may affect facial jaw and orbital alignment. Additionally, infant attractiveness has been identified as a factor that may affect parental social attachment. With good care, these changes in appearance can be significantly minimized.

Cartilidge PHT, Rutter N. Reduction of head flattening in preterm infants. Archives Dis Child 1988;63:755–757.

✓ KEY POINTS: WHAT PROPER INFANT POSITIONING CAN PREVENT

1. Cranial flattening (scaphocephaly)

2. Torso deformities

3. Scapular deformities

4. Frog-leg pelvic deformities

5. Facial deformities from endotracheal tubes

VESTIBULAR SYSTEM

30. When is the vestibular system developed in a premature infant?

By 14 to 16 weeks' gestation the vestibular system, situated in the nonauditory labyrinth of the inner ear, is in place, allowing the fetus and infant to maintain balance in the womb. The vestibular system is important for movement, gravity, and directional balance.

Lai CH, Chan YS. Development of the vestibular system. Neuroembryology 2002;1:61–71.

31. How should an infant be turned to support the vestibular system?

The infant should be turned slowly and gradually, maintaining a midline flexed position.

Long JG, Philip AGS, Lucey JF. Excessive handling as a cause of hypoxemia. Pediatrics 1980;65:203–08.

SMELL AND TASTE

32. When is taste developed in an infant?
The chemoreceptors for taste are developed in a fetus by 16 to 18 weeks' gestation. Taste buds appear early, at 8 to 9 weeks' gestation, with receptors fully present by 16 weeks.

Mennella JA, Beauchamp GK. Early flavor experiences: research update. Nutr Rev 1998;56:205–11.

33. What kinds of tastes do infants prefer?
Infants prefer sweet tastes and withdraw from bitter tastes.

Tatzer E, Schubert MT, Timischl W, et al. Discrimination of taste and preference for sweet in premature babies. Early Hum Dev 1985;12:23–30.

34. When is smell developed in infants?
The olfactory system develops early and is thought to be functioning in a fetus at 16 to 18 weeks' gestation.

Schaal B, Orgeur P, Rognon C. Odor sensing in the human fetus: anatomical, functional, and chemeo-ecological bases. In: Lecanuet J-P, Fifer WP, Krasnegor NA, Smotherman WP, editors. Fetal development: a psychobiological perspective. Hillsdale, NJ: Lawrence Erlbaum Associates; 1995. p. 205–37.

35. What is the rationale for non-nutritive sucking (e.g., pacifier)?
Non-nutritive sucking facilitates the development of sucking behavior and improves digestion of enteral feeds. Controlled studies have demonstrated that non-nutritive sucking resulted in improved gavage tube-to-bottle transition, improved behavior (including improvement in sleep states), decreased stress behavior, and decreased length of hospital stay.

Pinelli J, Symington A. Non-nutritive sucking for the promotion of physiologic stability and nutrition in preterm infant. Cochrane Database Syst Rev 2001;3:CD001071.

HEARING

36. When is an infant capable of responding to sound?
A fetus is capable of responding to sound by 25 weeks' gestation. All major auditory structures are in place at this time. Both cortical and brainstem auditory-evoked responses can be elicited at 24 to 28 weeks' gestation, although the morphology and latency is different than in the term infant.

Birnholz JC, Benacerraf BR. The development of human fetal hearing. Science 1983;222:516–18.

37. Is noise associated with permanent long-term sequelae for a premature infant?
Yes. Preterm infants are at risk for sensorineural hearing loss, which occurs at a rate of 10% compared with 0.5% for term infants. Noise may interfere with the development of auditory pathways necessary for communication and language skills. Premature infants are at risk for auditory processing deficits such as speech sound discrimination and other disorders of syntax, semantics, and auditory memory.

Lary S, Briassoulis G, de Vries L, et al. Hearing threshold in preterm and term infants by auditory brainstem response. J Pediatr 1985;107:593–99.
Gerhardt KJ, Abrams RM. Fetal exposures to sound and vibroacoustic stimulation. J Perinatol 2000;20:S21–S30.

✓ KEY POINTS: PREDETERMINED ORDER FOR DEVELOPMENT OF SENSES

1. Tactile/touch

2. Vestibular/balance

3. Gustatory/taste

4. Olfactory/smell

5. Auditory/hearing

6. Vision/sight

VISION

38. When is vision fully functioning in a fetus?
Vision is the last sensory system to develop in a fetus. All major structures and visual pathways for vision are complete by 24 weeks' gestation. Visual-evoked responses (VERs) have been elicited (but with prolonged latency) as early as 24 weeks' gestation. By 36 weeks' gestation, the VER is similar to that of an infant carried to term.

Penn AA, Shatz CJ. Principles of endogenous and sensory activity-dependent brain development: the visual system. In: Lagercrantz H, Hanson M, Evrard P, et al, editors. The newborn brain. Cambridge: Cambridge University Press; 2002. p. 204–25.

39. Are closed eyelids enough to shield infants from light exposure in the NICU?
No. A premature infant is unable to guard against light exposure and requires shielding from the common sources of light in the NICU. At least 38% of white light can penetrate the eyelids and disturb an infant. There is also concern that excessive light exposure at 32 to 40 weeks' gestational age may lead to sensory interference. Sensory interference may occur when immature sensory systems are stimulated out of order or are bombarded with inappropriate stimuli.

Graven SN, Browne J. Visual development in the human fetus, infant, and your child. Newborn and Infant Nursing Reviews 2008;8(4);194–201.

PAIN AND STRESS

40. How are infant stress and provision of developmental care linked?
Provision of developmental care is a method of care that provides a soothing, supportive, and responsive environment. This type of care decreases infant stress because caregivers and families, instructed in developmental care practices, can identify and provide therapy to relieve stress in infants.

Field T. Alleviating stress in newborn infants in the intensive care unit. Clin Perinatol 1990;17:1–9.
  Milette IH, Richard L, Martel MJ. Evaluation of a developmental care training program for neonatal nurses. J Child Health Care 2005;9:94–109.

41. Why is stress management so important in the NICU?
Research suggests that stress from the environment can prolong hospitalization and worsen medical conditions such as chronic lung disease. Stress may have long-term consequences on brain development and organization. Use of developmental care is a proactive approach to identify and reduce stress for infants in the NICU.

Peters KL. Neonatal stress reactivity and cortisol. J Perinat Neonat Nurs 1998;11:45–49.
  Peters KL. Does routine nursing care complicate the physiologic status of the premature neonate with respiratory distress syndrome? J Perinat Neonat Nurs 1992;6:67–84.

42. **How is environmental stress and pain identified in a fetus or premature infant?**

Pain and stress in a fetus are identified by physiologic (e.g., vital sign changes) and behavioral responses (e.g., tremors, crying). Understanding infant states of behavioral organization can assist in identifying pain and stress in infants. The states of organization are as follows (Box 4-7):

BOX 4-7 STATES OF INFANT ORGANIZATION

- State 1: deep sleep
- State 2: light sleep
- State 3: dozing
- State 4: quiet awake
- State 5: active awake
- State 6: crying

Gorski PA, Davison ME, Brazleton TB. Stages of behavioral organization in the high risk neonate: theoretical and clinical considerations. Semin Perinatol 1979;3:61–73.

Ingersoll EW, Thoman EB. Sleep/wake states of preterm infants: stability, developmental change, diurnal variation, and relation with caregiving activity. Child Dev. 1999 Jan-Feb;70(1):1-10.

43. **What are common daily stressful factors that an infant in the NICU encounters?**

In addition to light and sound, NICU medical and nursing procedures necessary to ensure the infant's survival are by nature stressful. Suctioning, chest physical therapy, gavage tube insertion and feeding, intravenous line placements, chest radiographs, ultrasound studies, ophthalmologic examinations, daily physical examinations, frequent assessments of vital signs, bathing, and weighing have all been shown to cause significant stress in preterm or critically ill infants.

Murdock D. Handling during neonatal intensive care. Arch Dis Child 1984;59:957–61.

44. **Are apnea and decreased oxygen saturation common infant stress responses?**

Yes. In one study three of four hypoxic or oxygen-desaturation episodes in preterm infants were associated with caregiving procedures. Similarly, increased concentrations of stress hormones have been observed in association with routine nursing procedures.

Evans J. Incidence of hypoxia associated with care giving in premature infants. Neonatal Netw 1991;10:17–24.

Blickman JG, Brown ER, Als H, et al. Imaging procedures and developmental outcomes in the neonatal intensive care unit. J Perinatol 1990;10:304–06.

45. **What are the pain-reducing interventions recommended by the international evidence-based group for neonatal pain?**

Nonpharmacologic treatments to reduce pain and stress in infants include behavioral and environmental strategies such as non-nutritive sucking, administration of sucrose, swaddling and containment, attention to sound and light, limiting environmental stressors (e.g., by individualizing care times), and allowing for rest periods.

Anand KJS and the International Evidence-Based Group for Neonatal Pain. Consensus statement for the prevention and management of pain in the newborn. Arch Pediatr Adolesc Med 2001;155:173–80.

Pickler RH, Frankel HB, Walsh KM, et al. Effects of nonnutritive sucking on behavioral organization and feeding performance in preterm infants. Nurs Res 1995;45:132–135.

Pinelli J: Nonnutritive sucking in high-risk infants: benign intervention or legitimate therapy? J Obstet Gynecol Neonatal Nurs 2002;31:582–591.

Pinelli J, Symington A. How rewarding can a pacifier be? A systematic review of nonnutritive sucking in preterm infants. Neonatal Netw 2000;19:41–48.

46. **How is a premature infant different from a term infant in the expression of pain and stress?**

A premature infant is unable to sustain physiologic and behavioral responses to pain for prolonged periods. Infant pain scales may not be as clinically useful because the responses may be dampened or may not be identified by caregivers.

Johnston CC, Steven BJ, Yang F, et al. Differential response to pain by very premature neonates. Pain 1995;61:471–479.

47. **What are examples of stress cues that infants use to communicate with caregivers or parents?**

Autonomic stress cues can be divided into three categories:
1. Color change: Cyanosis, pallor, mottling, flushing
2. Cardiorespiratory signs: Irregular respirations, apnea, retractions, nasal flaring, tachycardia, oxygen desaturation, bradycardia
3. Gastrointestinal signs: Hiccups, emesis, feeding intolerance

Franck LS, Lawhon G. Environmental and behavioral strategies to prevent and manage neonatal pain. In: Anand KJS, Stevens BJ, McGrath PJ, editors: Pain research and clinical management. Amsterdam: Elsevier Science; 2000. p. 203–16.

THE NICU ENVIRONMENT

48. **What are the common components of the NICU environment that can be altered by implementation of developmental care?**

The NICU environment includes sound, light, touch, handling, caregivers, facilities, bedding, positioning, and parents (Table 4-4).

TABLE 4-4. COMMON SOUNDS IN THE NICU	
American Academy of Pediatrics, Committee on Environmental Health: Noise. A hazard for the fetus and newborn. Pediatrics 1997;100:724–27.	
COMMON ACTIVITIES	**SOUND INTENSITY**
Intravenous pump alarms	61-78 dB
Writing on tops of incubators	59-64 dB
Vacuum sounds	70 dB
Teams rounding in the NICU	75-85 dB
Bottles being placed on top of incubators	96 dB
Metal door cabinet of incubator opening and closing	96 dB
Telephones ringing	80 dB

Latas M. Effects of light and sound in the neonatal intensive care unit environment on the low-birth-weight infant. NAACOG Clin Iss 1992;3:3444.
   Korones SB. Disturbances and infant rest. In: Moore TD, editor. Iatrogenic problems in neonatal intensive care. Report of the 69th Ross Conference on Pediatric Research. Columbus, OH: Ross Laboratories; 1976.

49. **What are the sound levels in the NICU?**

Sound levels in the NICU are often greater than 90 dB.

Chang YJ, Lin CH, Lin LH. Noise and related events in a neonatal intensive care unit. Acta Paediatr Taiwan 2001;42:212S–217S.
   Graven SN: Sound and the developing infant in the NICU: Conclusions and recommendation for care. J Perinatol 2000;20:S88–S93.

50. **How is sound measured?**
Sound is a function of frequency and intensity. Intensity of sound is measured in decibels. The decibel (dB) is a unit that logarithmically expresses the pressure of the power of sound. Frequency is measured in hertz (Hz). The adult hearing frequency range is 30 to 20,000 Hz. Preterm infants generally have a restricted frequency range of 500 to 1000 Hz compared with term infants, who have a frequency range that is similar to the speech range of 500 to 4000 Hz.

51. **What level of sound is a fetus exposed to in the womb?**
In the womb the intensity of sound recorded in the amniotic fluid has been of low frequency—less than 1000 Hz, although it can reach 70 to 85 dB. There are no peaks in intensity or frequency in the womb. In the NICU the intensity increases to greater than 90 dB, and the frequency ranges from 500 to 10,000 Hz.

Bremmer T. Noise and the premature infant: physiological effects and practice implications. J Obstet Gynecol Neonatal Nurs 2003;32:447–54.

52. **How does the sound stimulus create stress in an infant?**
Sound exposure can increase infant agitation, increase intracranial pressure, decrease oxygen saturations, and affect sensorineural development.

Chang YJ, Lin CH, Lin LH. Noise and related events in a neonatal intensive care unit. Acta Paediatr Taiwan 2001;42:212S–217S.
    Long JG, Lucey JF, Philip AGS. Noise and hypoxemia in the intensive care nursery. Pediatrics 1980;65:143–145.

53. **What levels of sound wake infants?**
Sound levels above 70 dB are incompatible with sleep in term infants, whereas sound levels greater than 55 dB arouse an infant from light sleep.

Graven SN: Sound and the developing infant in the NICU: Conclusions and recommendation for care. J Perinatol 2000;20:S88–S93.

54. **What are the American Academy of Pediatrics' (AAP) recommendations for sound in the NICU?**
Current recommendations from the AAP call for a sound level of less than 45 dB and a minimization of sound levels that are greater than 80 dB to less than 10-minute durations.

American Academy of Pediatrics, Committee on Environmental Health: Noise. A hazard for the fetus and newborn. Pediatrics 1997;100:724–727.

55. **What is the easiest and most cost-effective way to decrease sound in the NICU?**
See Box 4-8.

BOX 4-8 METHODS TO DECREASE SOUND IN THE NICU

- Use a sound meter with unit-based guidelines for sound to alert staff to high sound intensity.
- Use incubator covers to decrease noise levels inside the incubator.
- Use soft ear plugs/covers during routine procedures. These have been found to increase oxygen saturation, decrease behavioral state changes, and increase quiet sleep time.

Zahr LK, de Traversay J. Premature infant responses to noise reduction by earmuffs: effects on behavioral and physiologic measures. J Perinatol 1995;15:448–55.

---

56. **What are other staff interventions that can be used to decrease sound in the NICU?**
See Box 4-9.

BOX 4-9   STAFF INTERVENTIONS TO DECREASE SOUND IN THE NICU

- Taking medical rounds away from the bedside
- Limiting and altering conversation at the bedside
- Setting beepers to vibration mode while in the NICU
- Placing signs to remind staff and family members to be quiet
- Using incubators early in the infant's postnatal course
- Removing radios from the NICU care and treatment areas
- Padding garbage cans
- Setting phones on low ring tones or vibration/light signals

Bremmer T. Noise and the premature infant: physiological effects and practice implications. J Obstet Gynecol Neonatal Nurs 2003;32:447–54.

57. Is it true that children may experience hearing loss if their mothers have been exposed to high levels of sound?

Yes. Increased hearing loss has been reported in school-aged children whose mothers were exposed to noise levels of 65 to 85 dB during working environments 8 hours daily during pregnancy.

Luke B, Mamelle N, Keith L. The association between occupational factors and preterm birth: a United States nurses' study. Am J Obstet Gynecol 1995;173:849–62.

Lalande NM, Hetu R, Lambert J. Is occupational noise exposure during pregnancy a risk factor of damage to the auditory system of the fetus? Am J Intern Med 1986;10:427–435.

58. How can light cause stress and pain in the NICU?

Bright lights are stressful for neonates and have been shown to increase infant agitation, interfere with weight gain, and cause lower oxygen desaturation. The intrauterine environment is dim with minimal light. The NICU environment has been designed to require light to perform procedures. The NICU overhead light (80 to 90 footcandle [fc]) is much brighter than the intrauterine environment or light at home, which approaches 50 to 60 fc.

Graven SN, Browne J. Visual development in the human fetus, infant and your child. Newborn & Infant Nursing Reviews 2008;8(4);104-201.

59. Should light in the NICU be cycled?

Yes. Cycled light (cycled dim light with near darkness) before 32 weeks' gestation has a positive effect on the infant, creating the circadian rhythm (a biological process that recurs naturally on a 24-hour basis). The circadian clock located in the anterior hypothalamus is present early, by 18 weeks' gestation, and influences the rhythmic production of several hormones, such as melatonin, cortisol, and growth hormone. Circadian rhythms are also important for respiratory and cardiac function as well as infant sleep–wake state, the level of alertness, and body temperature. The constant high-intensity light usually found in the NICU can interfere with the natural circadian rhythms and eye development. Cycling dark (0.5 to 1 fc) and dim light levels (20 to 30 fc) in the NICU every 12 hours is one way to support the development of normal day and night rhythms. This type of care has been associated with trends for lower heart and respiratory rates, increased behavioral organization, faster weight gain, and decreased length of hospitalization and ventilator days in infants.

Mirmiran M, Ariagno R. Influence of light in the NICU on the development of circadian rhythms in preterm infants. Sem Perinat 2000;24:247–57.

Brandon DH, Holditch-Davis D, Belyea M. Preterm infants born at less than 31 weeks' gestation have improved growth in cycled light compared with continuous near darkness. J Pediatrics 2002;140:192–99.

Mirmiran M, Kok JH: Circadian rhythms in early human development. Early Hum Dev 1991;26:121–24.

60. **How is light intensity measured?**
    Light intensity is measured in fc or lux. A foot candle is a unit of illumination that is produced by a standard candle at the distance of 1 foot. One fc is approximately equal to 10 lux. The lux is the international unit of illumination. A lux is the illumination on the surface at a distance of 1 meter from a light source.

61. **What are the current AAP hospital recommendations for light intensity in the NICU?**
    Recent recommendations for preterm infants are to maintain light levels at 1 to 30 fc by day and 0.5 fc at night. General hospital recommendations restrict light to 60 fc.

Kenner C, McGrath JM, editors. Developmental care of newborns and infants: a guide for health professionals. St Louis: Mosby; 2004.

62. **What is the easiest and most cost-effective way to decrease light in the NICU?**
    See Box 4-10.

BOX 4-10 EFFECTIVE METHODS TO DECREASE LIGHT IN THE NICU

- Use a light meter with unit-based guidelines to achieve light-intensity standards.
- Educate staff regarding the impact of light on infant outcome.
- Decrease light intensity by covering the infant's eyes with protective covers during examination.
- Reposition incubators or cover incubators to avoid direct natural light that may come from windows.
- Minimize overhead light intensity, and individualize light exposure for each child by using individual light source controls and dimmers.
- Realize that windows and overhead light are the two most common sources of increased light intensity, and evaluate their impact.

Mirmiran M, Ariagno R. Influence of light in the NICU on the development of circadian rhythms in preterm infants. Sem Perinat 2000;24:247–57.
Latas M. Effects of light and sound in the neonatal intensive care unit environment on the low-birth-weight infant. NAACOG Clin Iss 1992;3:3444.

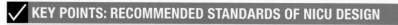 **KEY POINTS: RECOMMENDED STANDARDS OF NICU DESIGN**

1. Adjustable ambient lighting levels through a range of 10 to 600 lux (1 to 60 fc)

2. Separate procedural lighting available at each infant's care area

3. At least one source of daylight (60 fc) with shading devices

4. A combination of continuous background sound and transient sound not exceeding an hourly mean of 50 dB, with maximum transient sound not exceeding 70 dB

---

63. **How often are infants touched during a routine day in the NICU?**
    It has been estimated that a critically ill infant is handled or manipulated for monitoring or other therapeutic procedures more than 150 times per day with less than 10 minutes of uninterrupted rest.

Zahr LK, Balia S. Responses of premature infants to routine nursing interventions and noise in the NICU. Nurs Res 1995;44:179–185.

64. **What does containment mean, and why is it useful?**
    Containment and facilitated tuck are methods to decrease the stress response in infants undergoing a procedure. During containment the infant is gathered and flexed midline to decrease stress.

Harrison LL, Williams AK, Berbaum ML, et al. Physiologic and behavioral effects of gentle human touch on preterm infants. Res Nurs Health 2000;23:435–46.

65. **What is clustering of care, and is it important?**

Clustering of care, in which care is grouped during a care session, has been replaced with individualizing care. This individualized method is used to provide a group of caregiving activities during a time period that provides and allows for infant rest between procedures.

Appleton SM. "Handle with care": an investigation of the handling received by preterm infants in intensive care. J Neo Nurs 1997;3:23–27.

Holditch-Davis D, Torres C, O'Hale A, et al. Standardized rest periods affect the incidence of apnea and rate of weight gain in convalescent preterm infants. Neonatal Netw 1996;15:87.

KANGAROO CARE: SKIN-TO-SKIN TECHNIQUE

66. **What is kangaroo care?**

Kangaroo care, defined as skin-to-skin contact, originally consisted of placing a diapered infant in an upright position on the mother's bare chest. In Bogota, Columbia, where kangaroo care was initiated, the practice decreased infant mortality. Kangaroo Care has been endorsed by the World Health Organization (WHO) to improve infant survival and enhance breastfeeding in developing countries. Families become an intricate part of Kangaroo Care; fathers and other family members can be encouraged to participate in this care technique to allow maternal rest and support the infant.

Moore ER, Anderson GC, Bergman N. Early skin-to-skin contact for mothers and their healthy newborn infants. Cochrane Database Syst Rev 2007;3:CD003519.

Conde-Agudelo A, Belizan JM, Diaz-Rossello J. Kangaroo mother care to reduce morbidity and mortality in low birthweight infants. Cochrane Database Syst Rev 2011:CD002771.

67. **What are the benefits of kangaroo care for the infant?**

Infants who receive kangaroo care and mothers who provide it exhibit many benefits (Table 4-5).

TABLE 4-5. BENEFITS OF KANGAROO CARE	
Infant	Improved growth
	Physiologic stability of heart and respiratory rate
	Fewer respiratory illnesses
	Reduced incidence of nosocomial infections
	Enhanced survival
Maternal	Enhanced breast feeding
	Decreased postpartum depression
	Greater satisfaction in care providers

Weiss SJ, Wilson P, Morrison D. Maternal tactile stimulation and the neurodevelopment of low birth weight infants. Infancy 2004;5:85–107.

Chow M., Anderson, GC, Good M, et al. A randomized controlled trial of early kangaroo care for preterm infants: effects on temperature, weight, behavior, and acuity. J Nur Res 2002;10:129–42.

de Alencar AE, Arraes LC, de Albuquerque EC, et al. Effect of Kangaroo mother care on postpartum depression. J Trop Pediatr. 2009;55:36–8.

Lawn JE, Mwansa-Kambafwile J, Horta BL, et al. 'Kangaroo mother care' to prevent neonatal deaths due to preterm birth complications. Int J Epidemiol 2010;39(Suppl 1):i144–54.

Charpak N, Ruiz-Pelaez JG, Figueroa de CZ, et al: A randomized, controlled trial of kangaroo mother care: results of follow-up at 1 year of corrected age. Pediatrics 2001;108:1072.

68. How should kangaroo care be implemented in the NICU?

Kangaroo care should be implemented with detailed competency and written guidelines that are agreed on by all caregivers and families. Guidelines generally include the following:

- Eligibility of the infant for kangaroo care: multidisciplinary agreement
- Preparation of provider: education of role of this technical carer and competency training of providers in the provision of kangaroo care transfer and ongoing infant evaluation.
- Preparation of the parents: education related to the procedure, expectations
- Monitors needed: temperature, cardiorespiratory, and saturation monitors
- Methods to maintain temperature: infant cap and blanket over parent and infant
- Evaluation and recording of the infant's responses during the procedure

Gayle G, Franck L, Lund C. Skin to skin (kangaroo) holding of the intubated premature infant. Neonat Netw 1993;12:49–57.
Gayle G, VandenBerg KA. Kangaroo care. Neonat Network 1998;17:69–71.

69. Is kangaroo care widely practiced in NICUs in the United States?

Yes. A survey in 2002 found that 82% of NICUs were practicing kangaroo care. Some barriers to its use still exist that can be improved using provider and parent competency training and development of strategies for infants with certain illnesses.

Engler AJ, Ludington-Hoe SM, Cusson RM, et al. Kangaroo care: national survey of practice, knowledge, barriers and perceptions. Am J Matern Child Nur 2002;27:146–53.

✓ KEY POINTS: KANGAROO CARE

1. Benefits infant and mother

2. Endorsed by WHO to enhance infant survival and promote breastfeeding

3. Use is enhanced by competency training and education

CHAPTER 5

NICU ENVIRONMENT AND PRINCIPLES OF INFECTION CONTROL

Saima Aftab, MD, and Jacquelyn R. Evans, MD

1. **What are some general measures that can reduce or minimize the risk of nosocomial infections?**

   Nosocomial infections are a serious concern in the NICU setting. The extremely small and immunologically compromised status of the patients makes them particularly vulnerable. Success in preventing nosocomial infections depends largely on a team approach, with the full commitment of frontline staff. The most effective measures are strict hand-washing and hand hygiene. Elimination of overcrowding and understaffing, strict adherence to central line maintenance and removal guidelines, careful preparation and storage of infant formulas, increasing breastfeeding rates, decreasing the number of heel sticks and attempts at venipuncture, using single-dose administration of medications when possible, avoiding drugs associated with an increased risk of nosocomial infection (histamine$_2$ blockers and corticosteroids), and use of sterile suctioning techniques have all been shown to be important factors in reducing nosocomial infection rates.

2. **What are best practices for hand hygiene?**

   Hand-washing and "degerming" remain the simplest and most effective methods of preventing transmission of infectious agents from clinicians to infants and from infants to infants. The Centers for Disease Control and Prevention (CDC) recommend the following practices in health care settings:

   - A 15-second wash with soap and water before initial patient care or when hands are visibly dirty or contaminated with blood or body fluids
   - Degerming (using an alcohol-based hand rub with emollient) immediately before and after all direct patient contact. This approach is effective in reducing the number of bacterial, fungal, and viral pathogens.

   In addition, the American Academy of Pediatrics (AAP) Guidelines for Perinatal Care, 4th edition, has the following recommendations for all staff members coming in contact with neonates:

   - Personnel should remove rings, watches, and bracelets before entering nursery or obstetric areas.
   - Fingernails should be trimmed short, and no artificial fingernails or nail polish should be permitted.

3. **What is a CLABSI?**

   A CLABSI or a central line–associated blood stream infection is a primary bloodstream infection in a patient who had a central line within a 48-hour period of developing the infection.

4. **Is there a minimum time duration in which the central line must be in place before an infection can be categorized as a CLABSI?**

   No, according to the CDC, there is no minimum time duration that a central line needs to be in place before an infection is categorized as a CLABSI.

5. **How can ventilator-associated pneumonias be prevented?**

   A ventilator-associated pneumonia (VAP) is a pneumonia that develops in a ventilated patient starting at 48 hours after the initiation of mechanical ventilation. Very-low and extremely-low-birth-weight babies who are intubated are at particularly high risk. Preventive strategies include strict hand hygiene, elevating the head of the bed 30 to 60 degrees, in-line suctioning, oral hygiene, and the use of non-invasive ventilation when possible.

Foglia E, Meier MD, Elward A. Ventilator-associated pneumonia in neonatal and pediatric intensive care unit patients. Clin Microbiol Rev 2007;20:409–25.

6. **What are some of the multidrug-resistant organisms encountered in a NICU?**
Table 5-1 lists some of the multidrug-resistant organisms found in the NICU.

NICU ENVIRONMENT: PARENTAL RESPONSES TO THE NICU

7. **What are some of the stresses experienced by parents whose infant is being cared for in the NICU?**
Parental reactions to a severe, life-altering event run the entire gamut of emotional response, including shock, denial, grief, fear, sadness, anger, and guilt. The following are typical parental concerns:
- Infant appearance, comfort, health, course of hospitalization
- Separation from infant; not feeling like a parent
- Disruption of family life, family routines, time, household tasks, spousal communication
- Concerns for siblings
- Own health and well-being
- Difficulties with breastfeeding and pumping
- Communications with or actions of medical staff
- Postdischarge expectations
- NICU environment

It is important to remember that mothers and fathers may prioritize these concerns differently, and this discordance alone may be a source of severe family distress. As one family member put it, "There is no such thing as a good NICU experience." The physician and nurse, however, can have a positive impact on a family's NICU experience simply by acknowledging and assisting the family in dealing with these stresses.

TABLE 5-1. MULTIDRUG RESISTANT ORGANISMS ENCOUNTERED IN AN NICU

Modified from Cipolla D, Giuffrè M, Mammina C, Corsello G: Prevention of nosocomial infections and surveillance of emerging resistances in NICU. J Mater Fetal Neonatal Med 2011;24; 23–26.

Methicillin-resistant *Staphylococcus aureus* (MRSA)	Frequent colonization and outbreaks. Frequent involvement of colonized health care workers (HCWs) in the transmission chains. High frequency of MRSA late-onset infections. Efficacy of decolonization and active surveillance.
Vancomycin-resistant enterococci (VRE)	Very different prevalence rates depending on geographical area and antibiotic policy. Enteric reservoir. Episodic but dangerous spread. Long-term survival on environmental surfaces.
Multidrug-resistant gram-negatives (MDRGN) (*Enterobacteriaceae*, glucose nonfermenting gram negatives, resistant *Pseudomonas* strains)	Selected by broad spectrum antibiotics (mostly by third-generation cephalosporins). Enteric reservoir, but for some species possible environmental reservoir. Epidemic spread driven by cross-transmission via caregiver's hands. Production of extended spectrum beta-lactamases (ESBLs).
Carbapenem-resistant microorganisms (*Enterobacteriaceae*, *Acinetobacter baumannii*)	Only sporadically reported in NICU. Extensively drug-resistant strains. The most serious threat to the available antimicrobial therapeutic options from both the clinical and public health points of view.

8. **What are some of the stresses experienced by the family of a preterm infant after hospital discharge?**

The stresses are more dramatic for families of infants with ongoing medical issues and home care needs than for families of healthy preterm infants. The following are some common stresses:
- Insecurity about parenting abilities
- Marital stress and possible discord
- Bonding and attachment issues caused by prolonged hospitalization
- Financial stress, especially when there is a loss of income because one parent needs to remain home with the infant
- Inadequate or lack of insurance coverage for home care needs (e.g., nursing, equipment, special formulas and therapies)
- Isolation, reduced contact with family and friends owing to concerns about exposure to infection (especially during winter months)
- Resentment felt by siblings because of parents' attention and time spent with new infant

Hughes MA, McCollum J, Sheftel D, et al. How parents cope with the experience of neonatal intensive care. Child Health Care 1994;23:1–14.

NICU ENVIRONMENTAL CONDITION

9. **What is the optimal intensity and pattern of ambient light exposure for a preterm infant?**

Although the answer is not definitively known, current data suggest that relatively dim ambient light (180 to 200 lux, or typical indoor lighting), cycled to an even dimmer level at night, may be preferable to lighting of unvaried intensity or chaotically varied lighting. The evidence for this is as follows:
- Cycled dim light entrains circadian rhythm in newborn primates.
- Day/night differences in activity are observed during the first 10 days after discharge in preterm infants exposed to diurnal-cycled dim ambient light (i.e., the babies are more likely to sleep at night and be awake during the day). These characteristics develop later in infants exposed to continuous dim lighting.
- Day/night light cycling in the NICU may improve postdischarge weight gain compared with chaotic light cycling.
- There is little evidence that neonates born before 35 weeks' gestation establish circadian variations in behavior, temperature, and activity in response to day/night light variation. However, such effects are well documented at term and thereafter.

Rivkees S. Emergence and influences of circadian rhythmicity in infants. Clin Perinatol 2004;31:217–28.

10. **What are the effects of high noise levels on preterm babies in a neonatal ICU?**

By 26 to 28 weeks gestational age, the preterm infant's auditory system is sufficiently mature for loud noise to produce changes in heart rate, blood pressure, respiration, and oxygenation. The possible impact of high noise exposure on the long-term neurodevelopmental outcomes of these high-risk preterm neonates is also a concern. The NICU can be an unpredictably noisy place as a result of the alarms, ventilators, phones, and staff conversations. Also, the baby's own crying can be a significant source of noise because loud sounds tend to be amplified within the incubator. In 1997 the AAP determined that safe sound levels in the NICU should not exceed an hourly level of 45 decibels on an A-weighted scale (dBA). It is well established that noise levels in the NICU often exceed these recommended levels.

Wachman EM, Lahav A. The effects of noise on preterm infants in the NICU. Arch Dis Child Fetal Neonatal Ed 2011;96:F305–F309.

11. **What are the major etiologies of deafness in the newborn?**

Hearing loss is the most common congenital condition in the United States. Universal newborn hearing screening has been endorsed by multiple organizations, including the AAP, National Institutes of

Health (NIH), and the CDC and is now mandatory in most states. Early intervention can be critical and assists in the development of speech and improved learning. Infants with the following risk factors have higher rates of hearing deficits:

- Low birth weight
- Congenital infections (e.g., rubella, toxoplasmosis, cytomegalovirus, syphilis, herpes)
- Exposure to toxins (including ototoxic antibiotics and loop diuretics)
- Exposure to assisted ventilation
- Exposure to extracorporeal membrane oxygenation
- Hyperbilirubinemia requiring exchange transfusion
- Hypoxic-ischemic encephalopathy
- Craniofacial anomalies
- Family history of deafness

Graziani LJ, Desai S, Baumgart S, et al. Clinical antecedents of neurologic and audiologic abnormalities in survivors of neonatal ECMO—a group comparison study. J Child Neurol 1997;12:415–22.

12. **What is the estimate of visual acuity of a term infant? When does color vision develop?**
At birth the newborn has at least 20/150 vision, and color vision develops at 2 months of age.

13. **What are the four modes of heat loss in a neonate?**
Table 5-2 lists the four modes of heat loss.

THE NEONATE: BIRTH INJURIES

14. **What are the different patterns of brachial plexus injury?**
See Table 5-3.

15. **What are the risk factors associated with shoulder dystocia?**
Shoulder dystocia occurs in as many as 2% of vaginal deliveries. It is caused by entrapment of the shoulders between the pubic symphysis anteriorly and the sacral promontory posteriorly. Risk factors include fetal macrosomia, maternal diabetes and obesity, history of dystocia in a prior birth, and prolonged second stage of labor. In half the cases, there is no identifiable risk factor. The most common

TABLE 5–2. MODES OF HEAT LOSS IN A NEONATE

Modified from Allen F. Heat loss prevention in neonates. J Perinatol 2008;28:S57–S59.

Conduction	Heat loss that occurs from contact of the baby's skin with a colder object. This loss can be prevented by placing the baby on warmed blankets or mattress and ensuring that the provider's hands are warm.
Convection	Heat loss that takes place when heat is transferred to the cooler air surrounding the infant. This phenomenon can be prevented by increasing the room temperature in delivery rooms and closing doors and windows to minimize drafts.
Evaporation	Heat loss that occurs when water molecules move to the air from wet skin. Evaporative loss can be prevented by promptly drying the baby after birth, and, in the case of very-low-birth-weight babies, covering them with a plastic wrap.
Radiation	Heat loss caused by heat transfer to cooler objects that are not in direct contact with the neonate. This can be prevented by having double-walled incubators and placing incubators far from walls and windows.

serious consequence of shoulder dystocia is brachial plexus injury, which occurs in as many as 20% of infants at risk. In most cases, injury results from downward traction and lateral extension of the fetal head and neck when delivering the anterior shoulder. Brachial plexus injury, however, has been reported in infants experiencing no known dystocia and injury before the onset of labor has been documented, supporting *in utero* nerve compression as a possible cause.

16. **What is a caput?**
    A caput succedaneum is a common subcutaneous fluid collection on the scalp of newborn infants that is occasionally hemorrhagic but rarely is associated with major blood loss. A caput typically crosses suture lines, has poorly defined margins, and is usually found on the presenting part of the head (Fig. 5-1).

TABLE 5-3. PATTERNS OF BRACHIAL PLEXUS INJURY

DEFECT	SPINAL LEVEL	CLINICAL FINDING
Erb palsy	C5, C6	Arm is adducted internally rotated with extension of the elbow, pronation of the forearm. Waiter tip hand, asymmetric Moro reflexes.
Klumpke paralysis	C8, T1	Absent grasp reflex, weakness of the intrinsic muscles of the hand and the long flexors of the wrist and fingers. Claw-hand deformity.
Complete brachial plexus disruption	C5, C6, C7, C8, T1	Complete arm is paralyzed; it hangs motionless, flaccid, and powerless. Absent reflexes.
Phrenic nerve paralysis	C3, C4, C5	Irregular, labored respirations with tachypnea and cyanosis or apnea
Horner syndrome	T1 injury to the sympathetic nerves	Unilateral ptosis, miosis, anhydrosis, and enophthalmosis

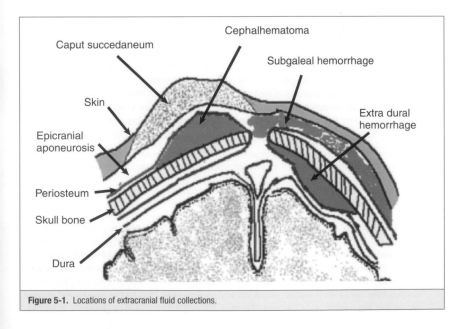

Figure 5-1. Locations of extracranial fluid collections.

17. **What is the clinical presentation of a subgaleal hemorrhage?**

A subgaleal hemorrhage is a hemorrhage beneath the aponeurosis covering the scalp and connecting the frontal and occipital components of the occipitofrontalis muscle. Blood may spread beneath the entire scalp and into the subcutaneous tissue of the posterior neck (see Fig. 5-1). A subgaleal hematoma typically presents as a fluctuant ballotable mass that initially increases in size in the first 24 to 48 hours after birth and resolves over 2 to 3 weeks. This injury, however, is often extremely serious and may be life-threatening in 10% to 20% of cases. The hemorrhage is associated with vacuum extraction and is attributed to linear skull fracture, suture diastasis, or parietal bone fragmentation that often accompanies the hemorrhage. Insofar as the subaponeurotic space serves as a large potential space, the infant can lose a substantial part of his blood volume, leading to shock in the most severe cases. Management includes close observation of the infant for blood loss and consumption coagulopathy, particularly in the first 24 hours after birth and a slowly rising hyperbilirubinemia.

Schierholz E, Walker S. Responding to traumatic birth: subgaleal hemorrhage, assessment, and management during transport. Adv Neonatal Care 2010;10:311–15.

18. **What is the clinical presentation of a cephalohematoma?**

A cephalohematoma is a hemorrhage in the plane between the bone and the periosteum on the outer surface of the skull (see Fig. 5-1). A cephalohematoma typically presents as a well-circumscribed, firm mass overlying the skull that is confined by cranial sutures. The mass usually increases in size after birth before resolving over a few weeks. Calcification within the hematoma may result in a hard skull protuberance that may require months of skull growth and remodeling for resolution. Most cephalohematomas are unilateral and located over the parietal bone. The hemorrhage is often associated with forceps extraction and is attributed to shearing forces that separate the periosteum from the bone. The volume of blood lost is not usually life-threatening because of the small size of the subperiosteal space. An underlying linear skull fracture is detected in 10% to 25% of cephalohematomas.

THE NEONATE: PERINATAL FINDINGS, EXPOSURES AND TERATOGENS

19. **What is the risk of perinatal transmission of human immunodeficiency virus (HIV) in an infected mother?**

Mother-to-child transmission (MTCT) of HIV type 1 (HIV-1) can take place *in utero,* during labor and delivery, or postnatally by way of breastfeeding. Knowledge of the timing of transmission is essential for the design of potential strategies. In infants who are not breastfed, approximately one third of transmissions occur during gestation; the remaining two thirds occur during delivery. In the breastfed infant, however, as much as one third to one half of overall transmissions may occur after delivery and during lactation. Rates of MTCT vary from 10% to 30% among nonbreastfeeding HIV-1–infected women in more developed countries to 25% to 45% among breastfeeding populations in Africa.

Fowler M, Simonds R, Roongpisuthipong A. Update on perinatal HIV transmission. Pediatr Clin North Am 2000;47:21–38.

Fowler M, Newell M. Breastfeeding and HIV-1 transmission in resource-limited settings. J Acquir Immune Defic Syndr 2002;30:230–39

Shetty AK, Maldonado M. Preventing mother-to-child transmission of human immunodeficiency virus type 1 in resource-poor countries. Pediatr Infect Dis J 2003;22:553–555.

20. **What measures can reduce the risk of perinatal transmission of HIV?**

The PACTG 076 trial showed that in nonbreastfed infants a three-part complex regimen of zidovudine (ZDV) given orally to pregnant HIV-1–infected women starting between 14 and 34 weeks' gestation, intravenously during labor, and orally to the infant for the first 6 weeks after birth dramatically reduced the risk of transmission by 68%. This protective effect of ZDV on risk of perinatal transmission has been seen even in mothers with a low viral load of below 1000 copies, independent of cesarean section, birth weight, and CD4 count. Therefore ZDV prophylaxis should be given even to women with very low or undetectable viral load levels. Mothers with a higher viral load or recent infection in pregnancy should undergo a consultation with an infectious disease specialist, and the baby may need to be started on a multidrug regimen shortly after birth to minimize the risk of infection.

Mofenson LM, Lambert JS, Stiehm ER, et al. Risk factors for perinatal transmission of human immunodeficiency virus type 1 in women treated with zidovudine. N Engl J Med 1999;341:385–393.

21. **What are the fetal and neonatal effects of infection with varicella virus?**
    Maternal varicella has varied effects on the fetus and newborn depending on the timing of the infection. Infection early in pregnancy (i.e., between 8 weeks and 20 weeks) can result in congenital varicella syndrome with skin lesions; ocular defects; hypoplasia of limb, bone, and muscle; and central nervous system lesions. The risk is greatest between 13 weeks and 20 weeks, when a 7% risk of congenital varicella is reported. Of note, herpes zoster during pregnancy is not associated with the varicella syndrome. During midpregnancy varicella may be more severe in the pregnant woman, with an increased risk of varicella pneumonitis. Fetal varicella may occur, but stigmata of the congenital varicella syndrome would not be expected. Varicella-zoster immune globulin (VZIG) should be given to infants born to mothers whose symptoms presented in the interval from 5 days before to 2 days after delivery. Approximately 24% to 50% of infants so exposed will develop clinical disease, and of these 20% to 30% may die. This treatment will not prevent the infant from developing varicella, but it will lessen the severity of the disease. Nevertheless, 15% of treated infants may develop severe infection. VZIG lengthens the incubation period to 28 days from 21 days after exposure. VZIG also is indicated for hospitalized premature infants older than 28 weeks' gestation who were exposed to varicella and whose mothers have not had varicella disease or vaccine, as well as to all exposed preterm infants younger than 28 weeks' gestational age.

22. **What measures can minimize the risk of perinatal hepatitis B virus (HBV) infection?**
    Transmission to infants is usually through contact with infected blood or body fluids and rarely from an infected placenta or from contaminated fomites. HBV is not transmitted by the fecal/oral route or through breast milk. Perinatal transmission is most likely (70% to 90%) for infants born to mothers who are positive for both HBsAg and hepatitis E (HBeAg) antigens; the risk is 5% to 20% for infants born to HBsAg-positive mothers who are HBeAg negative. Although the overall risk for perinatal transmission is relatively low in the United States, HBV infection remains an important preventable cause for chronic liver failure and hepatocellular carcinoma during adult life.
    HBV immunoprophylaxis for infants:
    - HBV vaccine is recommended for all infants, with the first dose to be given before hospital discharge. The first dose of HBV vaccine *may* be given at 2 months with other vaccines, but it should be delayed only in infants whose mothers are known to be HBsAg negative.
    - For infants whose mothers are HBsAg positive, hepatitis B immune globulin (HBIG) and HPV vaccine should be given as soon as possible after birth. Although immunoprophylaxis of perinatal infection is most effective if given within 12 hours of birth, data regarding the efficacy of HBIG beyond 12 hours after perinatal exposure are insufficient. It is generally recommended that HBIG be provided up to 7 days in these infants.
    - HBIG should also be strongly considered for infants whose maternal HBsAg status is not available within 12 hours of birth, particularly if there are concerns that the mother is at risk or the infant has a birth weight of less than 2 kilograms.
    - All infants born to HBsAg-positive women should be tested for HBsAg and anti-HBs after completion of the immunization series and after loss of antibodies received from HBIG administered during infancy

23. **What are the clinical manifestations of fetal alcohol syndrome (FAS)?**
    Alcohol is one of the most common teratogens; FAS occurs in 0.5 to 2 per 1000 live births. Physical findings of FAS include short palpebral fissures, smooth vermillion border of upper lip, cardiac malformations such as ventricular septal defect and tetralogy of Fallot with pulmonary stenosis. FAS is also associated with an increased risk of neurodevelopmental impairment and growth failure.

24. **What are the fetal risks of maternal angiotensin-converting enzyme (ACE) inhibitor use during pregnancy?**
    ACE inhibitors are used in the treatment of hypertension and the management of heart failure. The use of ACE inhibitors throughout pregnancy or during the second and third trimesters has been associated with a number of complications, including fetal oligohydramnios and neonatal anuria resulting from persistent inhibition of the renin-angiotensin system, as well as fetal hypotension with subsequent poor perfusion of tissues. Patent ductus arteriosus also has been reported and has been hypothesized to result from the effect of these agents on kinase II, which increases production of prostaglandin. Hypoplasia of the skull, spontaneous abortion, and intrauterine demise has also been reported. Thus ACE inhibitors should not be used during pregnancy.

Bullo M, Tschumi S, Bucher BS, et al. Pregnancy outcome following exposure to angiotensin-converting enzyme inhibitors or angiotensin receptor antagonists: a systematic review. Hypertension 2012;60:444–50.

25. **What are the teratogenic effects of prenatal exposure to retinoic acid?**
    Isotretinoin is a vitamin A derivative that is prescribed for the treatment of cystic acne. Isotretinoin embryopathy, also known as retinoic acid embryopathy, is associated with embryonic exposure to isotretinoin beyond the 15th day after conception.
    Isotretinoin impedes normal neural crest migration in the developing embryo, resulting in defects of central nervous system development, severe ear anomalies, conotruncal heart defects, and thymic abnormalities. A prospective study of 31 5-year-old children who were exposed to isotretinoin during the critical period showed that 19% had intelligence quotients (IQs) less than 70, and 28% had IQs ranging from 71 to 85. The prevalence of isotretinoin embryopathy is 30% to 35% for babies who are exposed during the critical period.

26. **What are the fetal and neonatal implications of uncontrolled maternal phenylketonuria (PKU)?**
    Teratogenic risk in mothers suffering from PKU is caused by the degree and duration of elevated phenylalanine concentrations during pregnancy. Phenylalanine crosses the placenta by active transport during pregnancy resulting in 70% to 80% increased fetal concentration of phenylalanine compared to maternal levels.
    Phenylalanine embryopathy includes intrauterine growth restriction, mental retardation, microcephaly, and cardiac malformations. Among infants born to mothers with untreated PKU whose blood phenylalanine concentrations exceeded 20 mg/dL (1200 μmol/L), 73% to 92% exhibited microcephaly and mental retardation, and 12% had congenital heart disease.
    To best protect the fetus, maternal phenylalanine concentrations should be controlled to less than 6 mg/dL (less than 360 mmol/L) in the preconceptional period and during pregnancy.

27. **What are the neonatal presentations of perinatally acquired chlamydia infection?**
    Chlamydia trachomatis infection of neonates results from perinatal exposure to the mother's infected cervical secretions. Initial *C. trachomatis* perinatal infection involves mucous membranes of the eye, oropharynx, urogenital tract, and rectum. *C. trachomatis* infection in neonates is most often recognized by conjunctivitis that develops 5 to 12 days after birth. Neonatal ocular prophylaxis with silver nitrate solution or antibiotic ointment does not prevent perinatal transmission of *C. trachomatis* from mother to infant. *C. trachomatis* is also a common cause of subacute, afebrile pneumonia with onset at 1 to 3 months of age. *C. trachomatis* pneumonia, although often mild, may cause severe symptoms that require hospitalization. Asymptomatic infections also can occur in the oropharynx, genital tract, and rectum of neonates. The current recommendation is for watchful waiting and treating with erythromycin only those infants who develop symptoms of a *C. trachomatis* infection.

28. **What are the different clinical presentations of amniotic band syndrome?**
    Rupture of the amnion is associated with a number of structural defects that result from mechanical compression of the developing fetus. Specifically, strands of ruptured amnion can entrap developing

limbs, leading to intrauterine amputations and syndactyly, which typically are asymmetric. The amniotic bands also can act as tethers that restrict fetal movement and result in lower limb deformities, such as clubfoot. If there is associated oligohydramnios from amniotic fluid leakage there may be some degree of pulmonary hypoplasia. The diagnosis can be confirmed by examination of the placenta.

THE NEONATE: FEEDING AND GENERAL ASPECTS OF CARE

29. What are the immunologic properties of breast milk?

Human milk is protective against enteropathogenic *Escherichia coli* and other gastrointestinal pathogens. This protection is greatest during an infant's first 3 months of life and declines with increasing age. Breastfeeding confers protection through active components of human milk, which include cells, antibodies, carrier proteins, enzymes, and hormones. The process of breastfeeding itself may decrease exposure to bacteria that could be present in contaminated bottles, milk, or water. Finally, administration of human milk initiates and maintains the growth of *Lactobacillus bifidus* in the gut; this decreases luminal pH, which inhibits the growth of *E. coli* and other gram-negative pathogens. For these and other reasons, breastfeeding should be encouraged.

30. What is the importance of skin-to-skin contact or "kangaroo care?"

Skin-to-skin contact, or kangaroo care, has an important role in establishing parent–infant bonding in the NICU. Some observational data suggest that during kangaroo care the premature infant has long periods of deep sleep. There is also an increase of delta brush electroencephalogram waves during kangaroo care, which signifies increased synapse formation. Additionally, skin-to-skin contact has been associated with increased milk supply production and success of lactation. There are also long-term positive effects in maturation of the infant's emotional and cognitive regulatory capacities.

Vidyasagar D, Narang A. Perinatal and neonatal care in developing countries. In: Martin RJ, Fanaroff AA, Walsh MC, editors. Fanaroff and Martin's neonatal perinatal medicine. Philadelphia: Mosby Elsevier; 2006. p. 96–7.

31. What are the risk factors for the development of cerebral palsy (CP)?

Most cases of birth asphyxia are not followed by the development of CP, and most cases of CP are not associated with birth asphyxia. One multivariate analysis of antecedents of CP suggests that only about 9% of all cases of CP can be attributed solely to birth asphyxia. The clinical surrogates of birth asphyxia, such as Apgar score, fetal heart rate abnormalities, and umbilical blood pH, correlate poorly with subsequent neurodevelopmental outcome. Among pregnancy complications, maternal preeclampsia is associated with a decreased risk of CP.

Although twins are at an increased risk of CP relative to singletons, much of this increase in risk can be attributed to the lower mean gestational age at delivery of twins. Prematurity and low birth weight are significant risk factors for CP. The incidence of CP is estimated at 1 per 1000 live births among infants whose birth weights are greater than 2500 g, 15 per 1000 live births among low-birth-weight (<2500 g) infants, and 78 per 1000 live births among extremely-low-birthweight (<1000 g) infants. Gestational age–specific rates of CP, however, are not increased in twin gestation.

32. What are the contraindications to breastfeeding?

- An infant diagnosed with galactosemia, a rare genetic metabolic disorder
- The infant whose mother:
  - Has been infected with the human immunodeficiency virus (HIV)
  - Is taking antiretroviral medications
  - Has untreated, active tuberculosis
  - Is infected with human T-cell lymphotropic virus type I or type II
  - Is using or is dependent on an illicit drug

- Is taking prescribed cancer chemotherapy agents, such as antimetabolites that interfere with DNA replication and cell division
- Is undergoing radiation therapies (however, such nuclear medicine therapies require only a temporary interruption in breastfeeding)

American Academy of Pediatrics Work Group on Breastfeeding. Breastfeeding and the use of human milk. Pediatr 1997;100(6):1035–39.

33. **How long can expressed breast milk be stored and used?**
It is not necessary to freeze milk that is not used immediately; mother's milk can be stored in the refrigerator for up to 48 hours before bacterial contamination increases. It can be stored from 3 weeks to 6 months in the refrigerator freezer. Up to 12 months of storage is allowed in a deep freezer (−4° F). The milk should be thawed under running water, with care taken to avoid overheating and causing thermal injury to the infant. Microwave ovens should not be used to thaw human milk because microwaves destroy immunoglobulins and may overheat the milk. Once thawed, the milk may be refrigerated for up to 24 hours.

34. **When does the rooting reflex develop?**
The rooting reflex is elicited by stroking with a finger the upper or lower lip or either corner of the infant's mouth, which results in the infant turning the head, searching for the finger, and attempting to suck. Sucking tends to reinforce the rooting; a recent feeding tends to suppress it. The rooting reflex tests the integrity of the sensory pathways of the trigeminal nerve and of the motor pathways of the trigeminal, facial, and hypoglossal nerves. This reflex is absent at 26 weeks' gestational age, can be elicited with long patency at 30 weeks, and is fully developed at 34 weeks. The reflex disappears by 4 months of age.

35. **How is the tonic neck reflex elicited?**
To elicit the tonic neck reflex, the infant is placed in a supine position with the head in the midline, and the head is turned slowly to one side. This maneuver results in extension of the arm on the side to which the head is turned and flexion of the arm on the opposite side. The lower limbs respond similarly, but less strikingly. Ultimately, the infant assumes a "fencing" posture. The tonic neck reflex is one of the last primitive neonatal reflexes to appear during human gestation. It appears at 35 weeks of gestational age, is most prominent at 2 months after birth, and disappears by 6 months of age.

36. **When does the palmar grasp reflex develop?**
The palmar grasp reflex is one of the earliest primitive neonatal reflexes to appear during human gestation. The reflex is elicited by stroking with a finger the palmar surface of the infant's hand, which results in flexion of the fingers in a grasping motion. This reflex can be elicited, albeit weakly, as early as at 26 weeks' gestational age, is stronger at 32 weeks, and is strong enough to allow the examiner to lift the infant from the bed at 37 weeks. The palmar grasp reflex begins to fade at 2 months of age and disappears by 4 months with the development of a voluntary grasp.

37. **How is the crossed extension reflex elicited?**
To elicit the crossed extension reflex, one leg is held firmly in extension and the sole of the foot is rubbed. The reflex is observed in the opposite (free) leg in three successive phases: initial flexion (withdrawal); subsequent extension and fanning of the toes; and, in its fully developed form, adduction of the free leg toward the stimulated side, as if to push away the stimulus. This reflex is absent at 26 weeks' gestational age, can be elicited in its partial form (only flexion) at 30 weeks, and is complete at 34 weeks. The crossed extension reflex disappears by approximately 2 months of age.

38. **What are the possible implications for a delay in the passage of meconium?**
Failure to pass meconium can be a sign of intestinal obstruction. Meconium normally is passed within 24 hours of birth in 95% of term infants and within 48 hours in the remainder. Preterm infants

may take even longer to pass meconium. Failure to pass meconium within the first 24 to 48 hours after birth is a classic finding for meconium ileus, meconium plug, anorectal malformations, and Hirschsprung disease.

Bekkali N, Hamers SL, Schipperus MR, et al. Duration of meconium passage in preterm and term infants. Arch Dis Child Fetal Neonatal Ed 2008;93:F376-79.

39. When should concern arise if a neonate has not voided?
Approximately 13% of term and 21% of preterm newborns will void in the delivery room. More than 98% of term infants will have voided by 30 hours after birth; failure to do so should prompt a thorough examination of the baby for a palpable bladder or an abdominal mass. If a baby fails to void by 48 hours after birth, further investigation is warranted to rule out renal impairment.

Clark DA. Times of first void and first stool in 500 newborns. Pediatrics 1977;60:457-59.

40. What is considered a normal weight loss for a newborn?
Healthy term neonates may lose up to 10% of their weight in the first few days after birth. In low-birth-weight and extremely-low-birth-weight neonates, this weight loss may reach as much as 15% of birth weight. Breastfed babies and babies with a lower birth weight are particularly at risk for excessive weight loss. It is important to monitor weight change after birth because excessive weight loss may lead to dehydration and electrolyte disturbances and may be associated with delayed bilirubin clearance and increase the risk of jaundice, requiring phototherapy.

Check DB, Wishart J, MacLennan A, et al. Cell hydration in the normally grown, premature and the low weight for gestational age infant. Early Hum Dev 1984;10:75-6.

41. What is the significance of polydactyly in a newborn?
The term *polydactyly* refers to partial or complete supernumerary digits, one of the most common limb malformations. *Postaxial polydactyly* refers to an extra postaxial digit (i.e., little finger or toe), whereas *preaxial polydactyly* refers to an extra preaxial digit (i.e., thumb or great toe). Postaxial polydactyly is far more common than preaxial. As an isolated anomaly, polydactyly may be inherited as an autosomal dominant trait, with a racial preponderance in African-American subjects. It may also be a manifestation of multiple malformation sequence (Table 5-4).

42. What is the significance of preauricular skin tags and ear pits in a newborn?
The reported incidence of such preauricular anomalies (tags and pits) ranges from 0.3% to 5%. These preauricular malformations usually appear in isolation and are usually considered to be of minor clinical importance. Preauricular anomalies, however, may be associated with other major craniofacial anomalies, including auricle and ear canal malformations and genetic syndromes (e.g., Treacher Collins, Goldenhar, or branchio-oto-renal syndromes). There is a higher incidence of hearing

---

TABLE 5-4. SYNDROMES COMMONLY ASSOCIATED WITH POLYDACTYLY

Modified from Hudgins L, Cassidy SB. Congenital anomalies. In: Martin RJ, Fanaroff AA, Walsh MC, editors. Fanaroff and Martin's neonatal perinatal medicine. 9th ed. Philadelphia: Mosby Elsevier; 2011. p. 544-48

Postaxial polydactyly	Trisomy 13
	Meckel–Gruber syndrome
	Chondroectodermal dysplasia
	Bardet–Biedl syndrome
	McKusick–Kaufman syndrome
Preaxial polydactyly	Carpenter syndrome
	Majewski short rib–polydactyly syndrome

impairment in infants with preauricular anomalies; however, the routine transient-evoked otoacoustic emissions test is an effective screening tool even in this population. Routine renal imaging to evaluate for renal or urologic anomalies is not warranted in infants with isolated minor external ear anomalies unless accompanied by other systemic malformations or a strong family history.

Roth DA, Hildesheimer M, Bardenstein S, et al. Preauricular skin tags and ear pits are associated with permanent hearing impairment in newborns. Pediatrics 2008;122:e884–90.
Deshpande SA, Watson H. Renal ultrasonography not required in babies with isolated minor ear anomalies. Arch Dis Child Fetal Neonatal Ed 2006;91:F29–30.

43. What are the morbidities seen in a late preterm infant?
Infants born at 34–0/7 to 36–6/7 weeks' gestation have been defined as "late preterm." This population of infants has been a focus of attention because of their large and growing contribution to the incidence of preterm births (70%) and the recognition that these infants have identified short- and long-term complications that differentiate them from their full-term counterparts. Common complications are listed in Table 5-5.

44. What is the significance of increased nuchal translucency on prenatal ultrasound?
Nuchal translucency (NT) has been well studied, and gestational age–specific norms have been established. Between 10 and 14 weeks' gestation, increased NT detects a greater proportion (77%) of fetuses with Down syndrome than the proportion detected by maternal age alone (30%) or by the use of triple analyte screening (alpha-fetoprotein, human chorionic gonadotropin, and estriol) (60%).

Factors in the pathogenesis in the NT increase include abnormalities involving abnormal development of the lymphatic system, as in Noonan syndrome or congenital lymphedema, or impaired lymphatic drainage associated with reduced fetal movements, as in fetal congenital neuromuscular disorders. Fetal cardiac dysfunction associated with abnormal diastolic function, as measured by decreased ductus venosus flow, may result in increased NT.

If increased NT is followed by normal karyotype analysis, normal cardiac and structural examinations on serial ultrasounds, and if the NT has resolved by 20 to 22 weeks' gestation, prognosis reverts to that of the general population.

Senat MV, Frydman R. Increased nuchal translucency with normal karyotype. Gynecol Obstet Fertil 2007;35:507–15.

45. What is the natural history of congenital torticollis?
The incidence of congenital muscular torticollis is 3 per 1000 live births and is associated with breech presentation, difficult forceps delivery, and primiparous mothers. Occasionally, a round or fusiform mass is palpable in the sternocleidomastoid muscle (SCM). This mass usually disappears by 8 months of age. Stretching exercises of the SCM will relieve the contracture in most cases. Parents

TABLE 5-5. COMPLICATIONS ASSOCIATED WITH LATE PRETERM INFANTS	
Short-term complications	Hypothermia
	Hypoglycemia
	Respiratory distress
	Apnea
	Jaundice
	Feeding difficulties
Long-term complications	School failure
	Behavioral and developmental problems
	Social difficulties
	Increased mortality rate

are instructed to extend and rotate the infant's head and neck several times a day. If neglected, congenital torticollis will cause flattening of the face and ear and plagiocephaly. If full range of motion is not successful by 18 months of age, surgical correction involving release or lengthening of the SCM can be considered.

46. What is the etiology of ophthalmia neonatorium?
Neonatal conjunctivitis may be caused by a variety of pyogenic organisms, but sexually transmitted organisms are frequent in the neonatal period. In developed countries where screening for prevention of gonorrhea is conducted during pregnancy, chlamydia is by far the most common organism responsible for ophthalmia. Noninfectious causes of ophthalmia include chemical irritation, primarily from silver nitrate prophylaxis (Table 5-6).

47. What are the adverse fetal effects of maternal smoking?
Tobacco smoking is associated with an increased risk for fetal loss, with an estimated increase by a factor of 1.2 for every 10 cigarettes smoked per day. In addition to the risk of fetal loss, smoking in pregnancy increases the risk for fetal undernutrition and preterm delivery. Maternal smoking also has been associated with an increased risk for sudden infant death syndrome.

48. What is the significance of a choroid plexus cyst on prenatal ultrasound?
Choroid plexus cysts are seen in the fetus in approximately 1% of all pregnancies. These cysts are usually smaller than 1 cm and are located in the body of the plexus, although they may protrude into the ventricular cavity.

TABLE 5-6. CAUSES OF OPTHALMIA NEONATORIUM	
Chemical conjunctivitis	Chemical irritation following eye prophylaxis with silver nitrate or antibiotic drops may occur in up to 90% of treated infants. Chemical conjunctivitis usually is noted within hours after instillation of the offending drops and resolves by 48 hours in most cases. Irritation is typically bilateral. Examination of the exudate shows epithelial desquamation and polymorphonuclear leukocytes. The culture is negative or may show normal flora.
Gonococcal conjunctivitis	Conjunctivitis caused by *Neisseria gonorrhea* produces an acute purulent conjunctivitis that appears 2 to 5 days after birth. Infants typically develop severe edema of the eyelids, chemosis, and progressive profuse purulent conjunctival exudates. Progressive disease causes corneal ulceration and may cause perforation and loss of vision or loss of the globe. The infection can spread systemically and result in death. Diagnosis is confirmed by culture of the exudate. Gram stain shows the presence of gram-negative diplococci and polymorphonuclear leukocytes.
Chlamydial conjunctivitis	Conjunctivitis develops in 25% to 50% of exposed infants. Chlamydial conjunctivitis often starts as a watery discharge, progressing rapidly to purulent exudate with marked swelling of the eyelids. Although it may occur as early as 24 hours after birth, conjunctivitis generally develops between 10 and 14 days of life. Inflammation may be mild or severe, with primary involvement of the tarsal conjunctiva. The exudate is a mixed polymorphonuclear and mononuclear leukocytic infiltrate. The follicular nature of the infection is absent in neonates because of their lack of lymphoid tissue, but pseudomembranes may be evident. The inclusion bodies that are diagnostic of chlamydia are located within the epithelial cells of the conjunctival surface.

These cysts are most often asymptomatic and almost all resolve spontaneously by the 26th to 28th week of gestation, but large cysts can cause hydrocephalus. Choroid plexus cysts are more prevalent in fetuses with trisomy 18, trisomy 21, and Aicardi syndrome. Chromosomal abnormalities should be considered if the cysts are large (>1 cm), bilateral, or irregular, or if the mother is 32 years of age or older. An increased prevalence of choroid plexus cysts has also been reported in the presence of other structural anomalies and when the maternal serum screening markers are abnormal.

Herini F, Tsuneishi S, Takada S, et al. Clinical features of infants with subependymal germinolysis and choroid plexus cysts. Pediatr Int 2003;45:692–96.

Epelman M, Daneman A, Blaser SI, et al. Differential diagnosis of intracranial cystic lesions at head US: correlation with CT and MR imaging. Radiographics 2006;26:173–96.

CARE OF THE NEONATE: CORD CARE, IMMUNIZATIONS, AND CIRCUMCISIONS

49. Are routine circumcisions recommended in all male neonates?

Although there is some evidence of the potential medical benefits of newborn male circumcision, according to the AAP policy statement on circumcisions, these data are not sufficient to recommend routine neonatal circumcision. Generally, for healthy term neonates with no other underlying problem, parents should determine what is in the best interest of the child. To make an informed choice, parents of all male infants should be given accurate and unbiased information and be provided the opportunity to discuss this decision. If a decision for circumcision is made, procedural analgesia should be provided.

American Academy of Pediatrics. Circumcision policy statement. Task Force on Circumcision. Pediatrics 1993;103:686–93.

50. What are the recommended practices for umbilical cord care?

Current practices for umbilical cord care vary across centers and range from application of triple dye or alcohol to natural drying, but the data regarding these practices and their impact on cord separation, complications, and health care use are limited. There is no evidence that any one of the above methods is superior to the other in preventing infection and preventing complications. In developed countries the most important aspect of cord care is hand-washing and ensuring that the cord site remains clean and dry. In poorer countries a topical antiseptic may be of benefit.

Zupan J, Garner P, Omari AA. Topical umbilical cord care at birth. Cochrane Database Syst Rev 2004;3:CD001057.

Mullany LC, Darmstadt GL, Tielsch JM. Role of antimicrobial applications to the umbilical cord in neonates to prevent bacterial colonization and infection: a review of the evidence. Pediatr Infect Dis J 2003;11:996–1002.

51. Who should receive respiratory syncytial virus (RSV) immunoprophylaxis with palivizumab?

RSV is one of the most common childhood respiratory illnesses. Patients at particularly high risk of severe RSV respiratory infections are former preterm infants with chronic lung disease (CLD) and infants with cyanotic or complicated congenital heart disease. In these patients RSV bronchiolitis may be associated with short- or long-term complications that include recurrent wheezing, reactive airway disease, and abnormalities in pulmonary function leading to hospitalization.

Palivizumab is a monoclonal immunoglobulin with neutralizing activity against RSV. In clinical trials immunoprophylaxis with palivizumab has been shown to decrease the risk of hospitalization resulting from RSV in high-risk patients.

In general, palivizumab prophylaxis may be considered for infants and children younger than 24 months with CLD who receive medical therapy (supplemental oxygen, bronchodilator, diuretic, or chronic corticosteroid therapy) for CLD within 6 months before the start of the RSV season. These infants and young children should receive a maximum of 5 doses during RSV season. Patients with the most severe CLD who continue to require medical therapy may benefit from prophylaxis during a second RSV season. In addition, babies born before 32 weeks' gestation who do not have CLD may benefit from palivizumab. Finally, for infants born between 32 and 35 weeks' gestation, environmental risk factors such as day-care attendance, younger siblings, and whether the parents smoke should be taken into account. It is also important to take into consideration the gestational age at birth and the chronologic age at the peak of RSV season. Updates on regional RSV outbreaks are available at www.cdc.gov.

American Academy Of Pediatrics Committee on Infectious Diseases modified recommendations for use of palivizumab for prevention of respiratory syncytial virus infections. Pediatrics 2009;124:1694–1701.

52. Can rotavirus vaccine be administered to former preterm babies?
Yes, absolutely.

Premature infants are at increased risk for hospitalization caused by viral gastroenteritis during their first year of life. The amount of time to administer all 3 doses of rotavirus vaccine is limited (only up to 32 weeks' chronologic age). Because adequate immunity does not develop until after the second dose, aggressive strategies are needed in the outpatient setting to administer all three doses to premature infants, who often are delayed in their immunizations.

The potential for horizontal transmission of vaccine virus was not assessed through epidemiologic studies, and thus the risk of horizontal transmission remains a theoretical possibility. The CDC Advisory Committee on Immunization Practices (ACIP) considers the benefits of rotavirus vaccine vaccination of premature infants to outweigh these theoretical risks. Given these data, it is appropriate to routinely administer oral rotavirus vaccine to all preterm neonates on the day of NICU discharge if they are between 6 and 14 6/7 weeks' chronologic age. Primary physicians need to be aware of the inpatient dose schedule and must pursue immunization every 4 weeks (the minimum dose interval) for infants whose immunizations have been delayed to ensure that all doses be received by the upper limit of 32 weeks' chronologic age.

Gad A, Shah S. Special immunization considerations of the preterm infant. J Pediatr Health Care 2007;21:385–91.
Advisory Committee on Immunization Practices. Prevention of rotavirus gastroenteritis among infants and children. MMWR 2009;58(RR-2):1–25.

53. When should a parent begin to worry if an umbilical cord has not fallen off?
The umbilical cord generally dries up and sloughs off by 2 weeks of life. Delayed separation (i.e., up to 45 days) can be normal. However, persistence of the cord beyond 30 days should prompt consideration of the following:
- An underlying functional abnormality of neutrophils (leukocyte adhesion deficiency) or neutropenia, because these cells are involved in cord autolysis
- Factor XIII deficiency (see Chapter 12).
- Presence of a persistant omphalomesenteric duct or persistant urachus.

Kemp AS, Lubitz L. Delayed cord separation in alloimmune neutropenia. Arch Dis Child 1993;68:52–3.

PROCEDURES

54. What are some common complications of peripheral intravenous (IV) access?
- Infiltrates, burns, and sloughs: Nearly every IV line is removed because of an infiltrate; the point is not to let a small one progress to a major burn or slough. Careful assessment of indwelling catheters, especially the ease with which the line flushes, will often prevent serious extravasations. The most common sites of serious infiltrates are on the dorsum of hands and feet. Hypertonic solutions, especially those containing bicarbonate or calcium, appear to cause the worst IV burns.
- Inadvertent arterial cannulation: This may cause severe downstream necrosis when medications or hypertonic fluids are infused. Arteries may sometimes be mistaken for veins in the groin, antecubital fossa, ventral wrist, and scalp.
- Infection: Infection control procedures must be strictly followed when cannulating a peripheral vein (especially when inserting a percutaneous central venous line). The ideal of sterile insertion

seems to wane as the IV line gets more difficult to insert, and the goal may disappear altogether with multiple attempts. The rate of nosocomial sepsis approaches 40% among very-low-birth-weight infants in some nurseries. Recent efforts to reduce catheter-related line infections, however, have demonstrated that infection rates can be held below 5 per 1000 line days in the NICU.

Butler-O'Hara M, D'Angio CT, Hoey H, et al. An evidence-based catheter bundle alters central venous catheter strategy in newborn infants. J Pediatr 2012;160:972–7.

55. **How do you estimate the insertion distance necessary for umbilical catheters?**
    Measuring the distance from the umbilicus to the shoulder (lateral end of clavicle) allows an estimation of the desired length (Table 5-7).

56. **What are the risks of umbilical catheters?**
    The short-term risks are as follows:
    - Perforation and development of retroperitoneal hemorrhage (umbilical artery [UA] catheter)
    - Decreased femoral pulses and blanching of limbs and/or buttocks (UA catheter)
    - Accidental hemorrhage (both UA and umbilical vein [UV] catheters)
    - Infection (both UA and UV catheters)
    - Cardiac rhythm disturbances (usually UV catheters, if catheter enters the right atrium)
    - Hemopericardium (extremely rare, usually right atrial perforation from UV catheter)
    - Air embolus (both UA and UV catheters). In a spontaneously breathing baby, *never* open a UV catheter to the air if the tip is above the diaphragm.

    The long-term risks are as follows:
    - Embolization and infarcts (both UA and UV catheters)
    - Thrombosis of hepatic vein (UV catheter)
    - Liver necrosis (UV catheter)
    - Aortic thrombi and hypertension (UA catheter)
    - Renal artery thrombosis (UA catheter)
    - Mesenteric thrombosis and necrotizing enterocolitis (UA catheter)
    - Infection (both UA and UV catheters)

TABLE 5-7.   INSERTION DISTANCE FOR UMBILICAL CATHETERS

Adapted from Dunn PM. Localization of umbilical catheters by post mortem measurement. Arch Dis Child 1966;41:69.

SHOULDER TO UMBILICUS (cm)	AORTIC CATHETER TO DIAPHRAGM (cm)	AORTIC CATHETER TO AORTIC BIFURCATION (cm)	VENOUS CATHETER TO RIGHT ATRIUM (cm)
9	11	5	6
10	12	5	6-7
11	13	6	7
12	14	7	8
13	15	8	8-9
14	16	9	9
15	17	10	10
16	18	10-11	11
17	20	11-12	11-12

57. **How do you determine the appropriate length for nasotracheal tube insertion?**
    See Table 5-8 for detailed instructions on nasotracheal tube insertion.

58. **How do you determine the appropriate length for an orotracheal tube insertion?**
    Measuring from the lip of the baby to the tip of the endotracheal (ET) tube, the baby's weight in kilograms plus 6 is a useful memory tool.

    Of course, it is always necessary to verify ET tube position by auscultation and x-ray. Furthermore, if a tube must be adjusted more than a small amount, a repeat chest radiograph should be considered. Remember also that depending on how an oral ET tube is taped, there will be some degree of movement in the trachea when the head is turned from one side to the other.

NEONATAL HYPERBILIRUBINEMIA

59. **How common is hyperbilirubinemia? How do we define its severity?**
    For infants in the first week of life:
    - 90% of healthy term newborns have total serum bilirubin (TSB) levels above 2 mg/dL
    - 50% have levels greater than 6 mg/dL
    - 5% have levels above 13 mg/dL

    Bhutani et al. (see chapter on well infant care) constructed a percentile nomogram of TSB values plotted against age in hours, based on serial predischarge and postdischarge blood samples collected from 2840 normal newborns at 36 weeks' gestation in the first week of life (Fig. 5-2). By the fourth day of life, approximately 95% of TSB values were at or below 17 mg/dL, a value the authors considered indicative of severe neonatal hyperbilirubinemia.

TABLE 5-8.	DETERMINATION OF APPROPRIATE LENGTH FOR NASOTRACHEAL TUBE INSERTION

Adapted from Coldiron JS. Estimation of nasotracheal tube length in neonates. Pediatrics 1968;41:823-828.

CROWN HEEL LENGTH (cm)	NASOTRACHEAL LENGTH (cm)
30	6.50
32	7.00
34	7.50
36	8.00
38	8.25
40	8.75
42	9.25
44	9.50
46	10.00
48	10.25
50	10.50
52	11.00
54	11.50
56	12.00
58	12.50

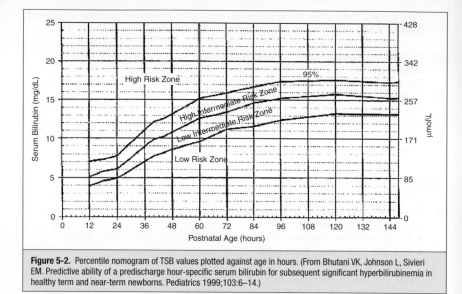

Figure 5-2. Percentile nomogram of TSB values plotted against age in hours. (From Bhutani VK, Johnson L, Sivieri EM. Predictive ability of a predischarge hour-specific serum bilirubin for subsequent significant hyperbilirubinemia in healthy term and near-term newborns. Pediatrics 1999;103:6–14.)

60. **What are the primary causes of neonatal hyperbilirubinemia?**
   - Increased bilirubin production resulting from enhanced red cell turnover
   - Decreased bilirubin clearance caused by decreased hepatic clearance or increased enterohepatic circulation

61. **What are the usual causes of increased bilirubin production?**
   Bilirubin is the end product of heme catabolism. In newborns bilirubin production is distributed as follows:
   - 75% from normal destruction of senescent red blood cells (RBCs)
   - 25% from the breakdown products of ineffective erythropoiesis and from nonhemoglobin sources such as cytochromes and catalyses
   The following factors are among those associated with increased bilirubin production:
   - Normally elevated hemoglobin levels (15 to 20 gm/dL)
   - Prematurity
   - Blood group incompatibility
   - Breakdown of extravascular blood
   - Maternal diabetes
   - Ethnicity, especially East Asian
   - RBC enzyme defects (e.g., glucose-6-phosphate dehydrogenase [G6PD] deficiency)
   - RBC membrane defects (e.g., hereditary spherocytosis)
   - Hemoglobinopathies
   - Other hemolytic processes, such as sepsis
   - Extensive bruising or large hematomas

62. **What are the common causes of delayed clearance of bilirubin?**
   Bilirubin clearance from the body requires hepatic processing (conjugation), biliary excretion, and fecal or urinary elimination of intestinally metabolized bilirubin products. The following conditions may interfere with or delay this process:
   - Diminished uptake of bilirubin by the hepatocyte
   - Decreased glucuronyl transferase enzyme conjugating activity
   - Familial disorders of bilirubin excretion

- Sluggish or obstructed biliary excretion, which causes an increase in serum direct bilirubin
- Active enterohepatic circulation (e.g., antibiotic treatment, prolonged gut transit time, delayed passage of meconium, and inadequate enteral intake), which can increase the level of unconjugated bilirubin
- Prematurity (because all of the systems noted are even less mature)

63. **What are the hematologic manifestations of neonatal hemolysis?**
    - Decrease in hemoglobin concentration
    - Reticulocytosis: greater than 8% at birth, greater than 5% in first 2 to 3 days, and greater than 2% after first week
    - Changes in the peripheral smear: microspherocytosis, anisocytosis, target cells
    - Elevated carboxyhemoglobin levels

64. **How does carbon monoxide (CO) relate to bilirubin production?**
    - The degradation of heme to biliverdin by heme oxygenase releases equimolar amounts of CO and ferrous iron.
    - Between 80% and 90% of endogenous CO results from heme degradation.
    - Although CO binds tightly to hemoglobin, producing carboxyhemoglobin, it is liberated by the mass action effect of oxygen and expelled in expired breath. Thus end-tidal CO can be used as a measure of bilirubin production.

Stevenson DK, Vreman HJ. Carbon monoxide and bilirubin production in neonates. Pediatrics 1997;100:252–254.

65. **Do transcutaneous bilirubin (TCB) measurements correlate with TSB measurements regardless of variations in skin pigmentation in newborns?**
    Yes. At TSB levels below 15 mg/dL, the correlation coefficient between TCB and TSB is 0.90 or greater, regardless of gestational age and racial or ethnic group, with the following provisions:
    - The device uses multiwavelength spectral reflectance.
    - Measurements are not useful after phototherapy, which bleaches the skin.

Bhutani V, Gourley GR, Adler S, et al. Noninvasive measurement of total serum bilirubin in a multiracial predischarge newborn population to assess the risk of severe hyperbilirubinemia. Pediatrics 2000;106:E17.

66. **What are the potential mechanisms of bilirubin neurotoxicity?**
    The exact mechanism of bilirubin neurotoxicity remains unknown. Hypotheses include the following:
    - Bilirubin disruption of cellular enzyme and regulatory function by inhibition of protein/peptide phosphorylation
    - Interference with the phosphorylation of synapsin I, inhibiting neurotransmitter release
    - Interference with protein and DNA synthesis
    - Direct inhibition of exocytic release and synaptic storage of brain catecholamines
    Bilirubin transmission across the blood–brain barrier is probably a dynamic, potentially reversible process rather than an all-or-none phenomenon leading inevitably to toxic cellular disruption. For example, hypercapnia, by increasing cerebral blood flow and altering pH, increases both the influx and efflux of bilirubin across the blood–brain barrier, resulting in high-level, short-term exposure. In hyperosmolality, on the other hand, the cell entry of bilirubin is slower, but efflux is compromised and the level of exposure is lower but of longer duration. It is not clear which of these processes is more likely to result in lasting neurotoxicity.

Hansen TWR. Bilirubin brain toxicity. J Perinatol 2001;21:S48–S51.

67. **Which areas of the brain are stained by bilirubin during acute bilirubin encephalopathy?**
    The following areas are most commonly affected:
    - Basal ganglia: particularly the globus pallidus and subthalamic nuclei
    - Hippocampus

- Substantia nigra
- Cranial nerve nuclei: oculomotor, vestibular, cochlear, and facial
- Reticular formation of the pons
- Inferior olivary nuclei
- Cerebellar nuclei: especially the dentate
- Anterior horn cells of the spinal cord

The yellow staining may last 7 to 10 days. The distribution of bilirubin staining often corresponds to the distribution of neuronal injury. However, damage to the basal ganglia and brainstem nuclei (oculomotor and cochlear) are most evident clinically. Involvement of cerebral cortical nuclei is not a prominent feature of kernicterus.

68. **Why do certain parts of the brain have a predilection for bilirubin-related neuronal injury?**
    - Neurons are more easily injured than glial cells.
    - Neurons have selective regional susceptibility to bilirubin injury.
    - The neuronal surface has abundant gangliosides that readily bind to bilirubin.
    - Glial cells may be preferentially protected by increased activity of a mitochondrial bilirubin oxidase.

69. **What are the clinical manifestations of acute bilirubin encephalopathy?**
    Clinical manifestations of acute bilirubin encephalopathy can be insidious and progress rapidly to severe and life-threatening illness. The signs of bilirubin-induced neurologic dysfunction (BIND) can be grouped as in Table 5-9.

70. **What is the tetrad of clinical signs of kernicterus?**
    The term *kernicterus* should be reserved for the chronic sequelae of acute bilirubin encephalopathy. Clinical signs include the following:
    - Motor: choreoathetoid cerebral palsy, motor delay
    - Cochlear: sensorineural deafness (auditory aphasia)
    - Oculomotor: gaze abnormalities, upward gaze paresis
    - Dental enamel dysplasia

    In kernicterus, intellectual impairment and cognitive dysfunction are variable. Note that preterm infants may not always manifest these classic signs even when the neuropathologic findings are consistent with kernicterus.

TABLE 5-9.	CLINICAL FEATURES OF BILIRUBIN-INDUCED NEUROLOGIC DYSFUNCTION (BIND)		
SIGNS	**MILD**	**MODERATE**	**SEVERE**
Behavior	Too sleepy Decreased feeding Decreased vigor	Lethargic and/or irritable (state-dependent); very poor feeding	Semi-coma Apnea Seizures Fever
Muscle tone	Slight but persistent decrease in tone	Mild to moderate hypertonicity Mild nuchal/truncal arching	Severe hypotonia or hypertonia Atonia Opisthotonus, posturing, bicycling
Cry pattern	High-pitched	Shrill and piercing (especially when stimulated)	Inconsolable, very weak; cries only with stimulation

71. What factors potentiate bilirubin deposition in the brain?

- Increased free bilirubin caused by (1) elevated bilirubin–albumin ratio or hypoalbuminemia, (2) competitive displacement of unconjugated bilirubin bound to albumin by small molecules such as sulfa drugs or benzoate (a preservative in several drugs), or (3) impaired bilirubin–albumin binding
- Increased proportion of bilirubin as bilirubin acid (in acidosis)
- Increased transport of bilirubin across the blood–brain barrier (in hypercarbia)
- Injury to the blood–brain barrier with asphyxia/hypoxia, hyperosmolarity (with use of hypertonic solutions), seizures, meningitis, sepsis with shock, and hypercapnia
- Loss of cerebral blood flow autoregulation
- Increased neuronal susceptibility (in hypoxemia/ischemia)
- Increased susceptibility to excitotoxic amino acids and reperfusion injury
- Illness (in respiratory distress syndrome, infection, shock)

72. What serum albumin value should lead to concerns regarding bilirubin neurotoxicity?

The bilirubin-to-albumin (B:A) ratio has been shown by Japanese investigators to predict bilirubin-related abnormalities in auditory brainstem-evoked responses. In an ideal situation, one molecule of albumin is capable of tightly bonding with one molecule of bilirubin, giving a potential equimolar B:A ratio. However, because some of the binding sites on albumin may be unavailable for bilirubin, free bilirubin is anticipated when the molar B:A ratio exceeds 0.80. This observation translates to 7 mg of bilirubin for 1 g of albumin. A molar ratio of less than 0.65 (5.5 mg of bilirubin per gram of albumin) could be considered safe in term and near-term babies. Thus for a baby with a serum albumin level of 3 g/dL, a TSB value greater than 21 mg/dL is likely to exceed the albumin-binding sites available for bilirubin. In preterm and sick babies the B:A ratio may underestimate the risk of irreversible injury because the binding affinity of albumin for bilirubin is compromised.

73. What are the common drugs that displace bilirubin from the albumin-binding sites?

Common drugs that displace bilirubin from the binding sites on albumin, in descending order of effect, include the following:

- Ceftriaxone
- Sulfisoxazole
- Cefmetazole
- Sulfamethoxazole
- Cefonicid
- Cefotetan
- Moxalactam
- Salicylates
- Carbenicillin
- Ethacrynic acid
- Aminophylline
- Ibuprofen

Ampicillin, cefotaxime, and vancomycin can be safely given to an infant with jaundice.

74. At what level of bilirubin should a premature baby receive phototherapy?

The empiric approach has been to apply phototherapy early at relatively low TSB values. Aggressive use of phototherapy in preterm babies (especially those with birth weights below 1000 g) has been associated with near elimination of low-bilirubin kernicterus. The following are two approaches:

- In an at-risk or bruised very-low-birth-weight baby, initiate phototherapy by 24 hours of age.
- Initiate phototherapy at 0.5% of body weight. For example, in a baby with a birth weight of 800 gm, phototherapy might be started when the TSB is 4 mg/dL or greater.

It should be noted, however, that strong scientific evidence for these recommendations is not available. These approaches are based primarily on empiric observation and common practice.

TABLE 5-10. MANAGEMENT OF HYPERBILIRUBINEMIA IN THE HEALTHY TERM NEWBORN TSB LEVEL (mg/dL [R [b/L])

AGE (hr)	CONSIDER PHOTOTHERAPY*	PHOTOTHERAPY	EXCHANGE TRANSFUSION IF INTENSIVE PHOTOTHERAPY FAILS[†]	EXCHANGE TRANSFUSION AND EXTENSIVE PHOTOTHERAPY
≤24[‡] (see below)				
25–48	≥12 (200)	≥15 (260)	≥20 (340)	≥25 (430)
49–72	≥15 (260)	≥18 (310)	≥25 (430)	≥30 (510)
>72	≥17 (290)	≥20 (340)	≥25 (430)	≥30 (510)

TSB, Total serum bilirubin.
*Phototherapy at these TSB levels is a clinical option, meaning that the intervention is available and may be used on the basis of individual clinical judgment.
[†]Intensive phototherapy should produce a decrease of TSB of 1 to 2 mg/dL within 4 to 6 hours, and the TSB level should continue to fall and remain below the threshold level for exchange transfusion. If this does not occur, it is considered a failure of phototherapy.
[‡]Term infants who are clinically jaundiced at ≤24 hours of age are not considered healthy and require further evaluation.

75. **At what level is bilirubin neurotoxic in the term newborn?**
    There are no precise data to correlate a specific bilirubin value with neurotoxicity. The decision to treat hyperbilirubinemia is based on the infant's history, course, physical findings (especially neurologic signs), and increasing levels of bilirubin, as well as a risk-to-benefit analysis of the disease process and the intervention. The AAP proposes the algorithm in Table 5-10 for healthy term newborns who do not have hemolytic jaundice. An alternative paradigm for applying phototherapy in term or near-term newborns (35 to 37 6/7 weeks' gestation) is shown in Figure 5-3.

American Academy of Pediatrics, Subcommittee on Hyperbilirubinemia. Management of hyperbilirubinemia in the newborn infant 35 or more weeks' gestation. Pediatrics 2004;114:297–316.

76. **What are the major risk factors for severe hyperbilirubinemia in term newborns?**
    - Jaundice within first 24 hours after birth
    - A sibling who had jaundice as a neonate
    - Unrecognized hemolysis such as ABO blood type incompatibility or Rh incompatibility
    - Nonoptimal sucking/nursing
    - Deficiency in G6PD
    - Infection
    - Cephalohematomas or bruising
    - East Asian or Mediterranean descent
    - Maternal diabetes

Centers for Disease Control and Prevention. Kernicterus in full-term infants—United States, 1994–1998. MMWR 2001;50:491–494.

77. **Which newborns require a systematic assessment for the risk of severe hyperbilirubinemia before hospital discharge?**
    All newborns should have this assessment. Assessment strategies include the following:
    - Universal predischarge TSB or transcutaneous assessment.
    - TSB estimate based on a combination of risk factor assessment and visual assessment. Note that visual assessment alone is inadequate.

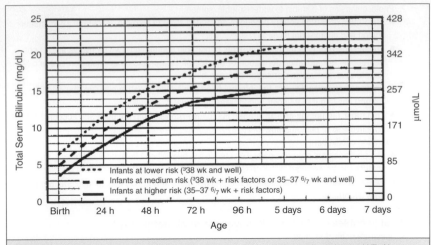

Figure 5-3. Alternative paradigm for applying phototherapy in term or near-term newborns. Use total bilirubin. Do not subtract direct reading or conjugated bilirubin. Risk factors include isoimmune hemolytic disease, G6PD deficiency, asphyxia, significant lethargy, temperature instability, sepsis, acidosis, or albumin level below 3.0 g/dL (if measured). For infants 35 to 37⁶/₇ weeks, you can adjust TSB levels for intervention around the median risk line. It is an option to intervene at lower TSB levels closer to 35 weeks and at higher TSB levels for infants closer to 37⁶/₇ weeks. It is an option to provide conventional phototherapy in hospital or at home at TSB levels 2 to 3 mg/dL (30 to 50 mmol/L) below those shown, but home phototherapy should not be used with any infant who has risk factors.

78. **Why is a near-term newborn more likely to have excessive hyperbilirubinemia than the term newborn?**
    Near-term infants weighing more than 2000 g are generally cared for in "well-baby" nurseries. However, because of their biologic immaturity, these babies are more likely to exhibit the following:
    - They accept feedings more slowly.
    - They exhibit slower maturation of hepatic glucuronyl transferase enzyme activity
    - They have delayed passage of meconium
    - They have prolonged enterohepatic circulation

    Late preterm babies are often discharged by 48 hours of age (like term babies) and are more likely to be readmitted with dehydration, excessive hyperbilirubinemia, and even kernicterus. In some instances near-term neonates may be at even greater risk than more premature infants who do enter the NICU, not only for bilirubin problems but also for infection and pulmonary disease. The following is important to remember: *Near-term infants are not term infants.* Predischarge evaluation, risk assessment, nutritional support, diligent plans for follow-up, and mandatory revisits are crucial to ensure the well-being of these babies.

79. **How does phototherapy work?**
    The mechanism of phototherapy involves the following steps:
    1. Light absorption by the bilirubin molecule
        - *In vitro,* the unconjugated bilirubin molecule absorbs light maximally in the blue portion of the visible spectrum, at a wavelength of 450 nm.
        - *In vivo,* because of bilirubin binding to albumin and tissue proteins as well as improved skin penetration at longer wavelengths, incident light in the blue-green spectrum may be more effective.

2. Photoconversion of bilirubin to water-soluble isomers
   - Absorption of photon energy produces an excited state of bilirubin, leading to photoisomerization and photooxidation.
   - Photoisomerization is the main pathway of bilirubin elimination. Two pathways are (1) configurational isomerization (formation of the 4Z,15E isomer and other photoisomers) and (2) structural isomerization (formation of lumirubin).
   - Photoisomerization disrupts the internal hydrogen bonds of native bilirubin (the 4Z,15Z isomer), making it more polar and increasing its water solubility.
   - Lumirubin, but not the 4Z,15E isomer, is rapidly excreted from the body and accounts for the effectiveness of phototherapy.
3. Excretion of bilirubin
   - The photoisomers are principally excreted in the bile. When cholestasis is present, the photoisomers can be excreted in the urine.
   - Excessive serum concentrations of the photoisomers (lumirubin) may manifest as bronze baby syndrome.

80. **What variables control the effectiveness of phototherapy?**
    - Spectrum of incident light
    - Irradiance of the phototherapy unit
    - Exposed surface area of the infant
    - Distance of the infant from the light source

81. **What is the irradiance of phototherapy?**
    Irradiance is the dosage of light ($mwatts/cm^2/nm$) at the skin surface. The rate of bilirubin decline is proportional to the dose of phototherapy. Devices that measure irradiance accurately are easy to operate. The maximal achievable irradiance is generally between 30 and 40 $mwatts/cm^2/nm$. The minimally effective irradiance is approximately 5 $mwatts/cm^2/nm$.

82. **What is "intensive" phototherapy?**
    Maximization of irradiance in the blue-green spectrum by use of high levels of irradiance (usually 30 [mu] $W/cm^2/nm$ or higher) and by optimizing the surface area exposed, usually by the following means:
    - Spectrum-specific bulbs
    - "Double" or "triple" light sources
    - Close light–infant distances
    - Undressing the baby
    If not given with care, intensive phototherapy may generate large amounts of heat, increase insensible water loss, overheat the baby, or burn the baby's skin. Heat-generating phototherapy lamps should not be placed closer to the infant than is recommended by the manufacturer.

Maisels MJ. Phototherapy—traditional and nontraditional. J Perinatol 2001;21:S93–S97.

83. **By how much should phototherapy reduce bilirubin levels in the first 24 hours of treatment?**
    - Intensive phototherapy: up to 30% to 50% decline from initial TSB in term infants with nonhemolytic jaundice
    - Standard phototherapy: approximately 6% to 20% decline

84. **What are the side effects of phototherapy?**
    Side effects are generally mild and manageable and include the following:
    - Increased insensible water loss, especially in preterm neonates and those cared for under radiant warmers. Different light sources have variable effects on insensible water loss.
    - Reduced gut transit time, probably related to increased bilirubin and photoproducts in the gut

- Decreased platelet counts to less than 150,000/mm^3 (controversial)
- Transient riboflavin deficiency that usually resolves within 24 hours of the discontinuation of phototherapy

85. **Do events during labor and delivery influence the severity of hyperbilirubinemia?**
Absolutely not. The following events have *not* been shown to affect the severity or incidence of hyperbilirubinemia:
- Pitocin induction
- Epidural anesthesia and maternal anesthetic agents
- Maternal vitamin K levels
- Tocolytic agents
- Mode of delivery: no known effect unless associated with bruising or cephalohematoma

86. **When should phototherapy be stopped in term and late preterm babies?**
When phototherapy is discontinued in a term or late preterm baby with nonhemolytic disease, the "rebound hyperbilirubinemia" is generally modest. Some arbitrary recommendations for discontinuing phototherapy include the following:
- Stop phototherapy when bilirubin values are below 12 to 15 mg/dL.
- Alternatively, continue phototherapy until bilirubin values are lower than 40th percentile track for the hour-specific bilirubin level.
- Similar recommendations for hemolytic and nonhemolytic jaundice apply.
- Rebound levels in hemolytic jaundice may be higher; recheck bilirubin at 6 to 12 hours after phototherapy.
- With intensive phototherapy, consider step-wise weaning to avoid a significant rebound effect.

87. **When do bilirubin levels peak in term and preterm neonates?**
In full-term newborns bilirubin levels peak at 5 to 6 mg/dL between 48 and 120 hours of age in Caucasian and African-American babies and 10 to 14 mg/dL and 72 to 120 hours of age in Asian-American babies. In preterm neonates peak levels are much higher (10 to 12 mg/dL) and occur later between the 5th and 7th days of life.

Wong RJ, DeSandre GH, Sibley E, et al. Neonatal jaundice and liver disease. In Martin RJ, Fanaroff AA, Walsh MC, editors. Fanaroff and Martin's neonatal perinatal medicine. Philadelphia: Mosby Elsevier; 2006. p. 1425-26.

88. **When should phototherapy be stopped in preterm infants?**
There is no consensus or adequate clinical data to address this issue. Phototherapy may be discontinued at the level at which it was considered appropriate to initiate the intervention, generally at or below 5 mg/dL for infants weighing less than 1 kg. It is important to monitor bilirubin levels serially after discontinuing phototherapy to ensure that they continue to trend downward.

89. **When should term and near-term infants receive an exchange transfusion for hyperbilirubinemia?**
See Figure 5-4.

90. **Should intravenous immunoglobulin (IVIG) administration be considered in babies with severe Rh hemolytic disease?**
Yes. Maternal administration of IVIG lessens the severity of fetal hemolysis. Administration of IVIG to neonates with severe Rh hemolytic disease accomplishes the following:
- Reduces hemolysis (as measured by carboxyhemoglobin levels)
- Lowers bilirubin levels
- Reduces need for exchange transfusion
- Shortens hospital stays

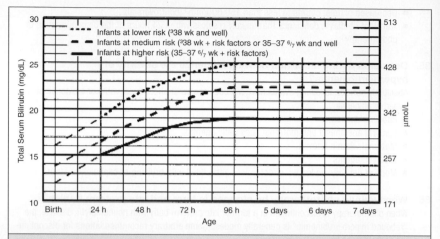

Figure 5-4. Exchange transfusion for hyperbilirubinemia. The *dashed lines* for the first 24 hours indicate uncertainty owing to a wide range of clinical circumstances and a range of responses to phototherapy. Immediate exchange transfusion is recommended if the infant shows signs of acute bilirubin encephalopathy (e.g., hypertonia, arching, retrocollis, opisthotonos, fever, high-pitched cry) or if the TSB level is equal to or greater than 5 mg/dL [85 micro M/L above these lines]. Risk factors isoimmune hemolytic disease, G6PD deficiency asplyxia, significant lethargy, temperature instability, sepsis, acidosis. Use total bilirubin. Do not subtract direct reading or conjugated bilirubin. If the infant is well and at 35 to 37⁵⁄ weeks (median risk), you can individualize TSB levels for exchange on the basis of actual gestational age. (From American Academy of Pediatrics Subcommittee on Hyperbilirubinemia. Management of hyperbilirubinemia in the newborn infant 35 or more weeks of gestation. Pediatrics 2004;114:297–316; and Johnson LH, Bhutani VK, Brown AK. System-based approach to management of neonatal jaundice and prevention of kernicterus. J Pediatr 2002;140:396–403.)

91. **Why has double-volume exchange transfusion been recommended instead of a single-volume or triple-volume exchange transfusion?**

An effective double-volume exchange transfusion (160 mL/kg) reduces the serum bilirubin levels by two time constants (84.5% reduction). With a one-volume exchange transfusion (80 mL/kg), bilirubin is reduced one time constant (63%), and with a three-volume exchange it is reduced by 95%. The three-volume exchange transfusion is not used because it prolongs the procedure and increases the risk of a complication without substantially improving the clearance compared with a two-volume exchange.

92. **What are some potential severe complications of an exchange transfusion?**

Cardiac/vascular
- Arrhythmia
- Vascular perforation by catheter
- Acute hemorrhage
- Thrombus
- Acute volume overload
- Massive air embolism (Note: *Never* open the umbilical venous catheter to the atmosphere.)

Metabolic (especially in preterm infants)
- Severe acidosis
- Hyperkalemia
- Hypocalcemia

93. **Is there any reason to discontinue breastfeeding in an excessively jaundiced baby?**

No. At times, however, it may be helpful to interrupt breastfeeding for approximately 24 hours to diagnose breast milk jaundice. In such cases the bilirubin levels usually drop precipitously but may rebound when breastfeeding resumes.

94. **What advice should be given to a mother who is breastfeeding her jaundiced baby?**
   - Continue breastfeeding. Evaluate for adequate latching and audible swallowing of milk by the baby, and assess whether the infant seems to be consoled after feeding.
   - Use an electric breast pump to facilitate "let-down of milk" and to collect expressed breast milk for extra supplementation.
   - Avoid maternal use of opioid analgesics (e.g., Percocet, Tylenol III, and other codeine preparations) that could have an impact on the newborn's feeding and stooling.
   - Identify ways to reduce maternal stress and anxiety to promote lactation.

Johnson LH, Bhutani VK, Brown AK. System-based approach to management of neonatal jaundice and prevention of kernicterus. J Pediatr 2002;140:396–403.

CHAPTER 6

CARDIOLOGY SECRETS

Mitchell I. Cohen, MD, FACC, FHRS, and Christopher L. Lindblade, MD

HISTORY OF PEDIATRIC CARDIOLOGY

1. **When was the first report of a successful ligation of a patent ductus arteriosus (PDA)?**
   The first successful ligation of a PDA was by Gross and Hubbard in 1938.

2. **Who was responsible for the first successful palliation of cyanotic congenital heart disease?**
   Dr. Alfred Blalock (Professor of Surgery at Johns Hopkins), Dr. Helen Taussig (Director of the Pediatric Cardiology Clinic at Johns Hopkins), and Mr. Vivien Thomas (Research Assistant for Dr. Blalock at Johns Hopkins). Their tireless work contributed to the successful research and techniques behind the Blalock–Taussig shunt. The first successful operation occurred in November 1944.

3. **When was the first neonatal heart transplant?**
   Christiaan Barnard performed the first cardiac transplantation in South Africa in 1967. Infant heart transplantation was attempted unsuccessfully 3 days later by Adrian Kantrowitz in New York City. Neonatal heart transplantation would not be achieved, however, until November 15, 1985, by Leonard Bailey at Loma Linda Medical Center.

Neill CA, Clark EB. The developing heart: a history of pediatric cardiology. London: Kluwer Academic Associates; 1995.
   Bailey LL. Origins of neonatal heart transplantation: an historical perspective. Semin Thorac Cardiovasc Surg Pediatr Card Surg Annu 2011;14(1):98–100.

FETAL ECHOCARDIOGRAPHY AND PRENATAL CONDITIONS THAT CAN CONTRIBUTE TO NEONATAL HEART DISEASE

4. **What are the indications for a fetal echocardiogram?**
   Maternal indications:
   - Family history of congenital heart disease
   - Metabolic disorders (diabetes, phenylketonuria)
   - Exposure to teratogens
   - Exposure to prostaglandin synthase inhibitors (ibuprofen, salicylic acid)
   - Rubella infection
   - Autoimmune disease (systemic lupus erythematosus, Sjögren syndrome)
   - Familial inherited disorders (e.g., Marfan syndrome, Noonan syndrome)
   - *In vitro* fertilization
   Fetal indications:
   - Abnormal obstetric ultrasound screen
   - Extracardiac abnormality
   - Chromosomal abnormality
   - Arrhythmia
   - Hydrops fetalis

- Increased first trimester nuchal translucency
- Multiple gestation and suspicion of twin-twin transfusion
- Genetic syndromes

5. **What is the incidence of congenital heart disease? What is the recurrence risk if a previous child has congenital heart disease?**
   The incidence of congenital heart disease is 0.8%. The recurrence risk with a prior sibling with a cardiovascular anomaly is between 1% and 4%.

6. **What are the common genetic and chromosomal syndromes associated with congenital heart disease?**
   Table 6-1 lists common genetic and chromosomal syndromes associated with congenital heart disease.

TABLE 6-1. COMMON GENETIC OR CHROMOSOMAL SYNDROMES ASSOCIATED WITH CONGENITAL HEART DISEASE

Adapted from Drose J. Fetal echocardiography. 1st ed. Philadelphia: Saunders; 1988.

GENETIC OR CHROMOSOMAL SYNDROME	COMMON CARDIAC ANATOMIC LESION
Apert syndrome	Ventricular septal defect, coarctation of the aorta, tetralogy of Fallot
Beckwith–Wiedemann syndrome	Atrial septal defect, ventricular septal defect, hypertrophic cardiomyopathy
CHARGE syndrome	Endocardial cushion defect, ventricular septal defect, double outlet right ventricle, tetralogy of Fallot
DiGeorge syndrome	Interrupted aortic arch, truncus arteriosus, tetralogy of Fallot, right aortic arch, ventricular septal defect, aberrant right subclavian artery
Ellis–van Creveld syndrome	Atrial septal defect, single/common atrium
Holt–Oram syndrome	Atrial septal defect, ventricular septal defect
Kartagener syndrome	Mirror image dextrocardia
Marfan syndrome	Dilated aortic root, mitral valve prolapse, tricuspid valve prolapse
Neurofibromatosis	Atrial septal defect, coarctation of the aorta, interrupted aortic arch, pulmonic stenosis, ventricular septal defect, complete heart block, hypertrophic cardiomyopathy
Noonan syndrome	Pulmonary stenosis, hypertrophic cardiomyopathy, tetralogy of Fallot
Pentalogy of Cantrell	Atrial septal defect, ventricular septal defect, total anomalous pulmonary venous drainage, tetralogy of Fallot, ectopia cordis
Pierre Robin syndrome	Pulmonary stenosis, atrial septal defect
Thrombocytopenia absent radius (TAR) syndrome	Atrial septal defect, tetralogy of Fallot
Treacher Collins syndrome	Ventricular septal defect, atrial septal defect
Tuberous sclerosis	Rhabdomyoma, angioma, coarctation of the aorta, interrupted aortic arch
Trisomy 13	Ventricular septal defect, atrial septal defect, endocardial cushion defect, tetralogy of Fallot

TABLE 6-1. COMMON GENETIC OR CHROMOSOMAL SYNDROMES ASSOCIATED WITH CONGENITAL HEART DISEASE —Cont'd

GENETIC OR CHROMOSOMAL SYNDROME	COMMON CARDIAC ANATOMIC LESION
Trisomy 18	Bicuspid aortic valve, pulmonic stenosis, ventricular septal defect, atrial septal defect, endocardial cushion defect, polyvalvular thickening
Trisomy 21	Endocardial cushion defect, ventricular septal defect, atrial septal defect, tetralogy of Fallot, coarctation of the aorta
Turner syndrome	Bicuspid aortic valve, coarctation of the aorta, aortic stenosis, ventricular septal defect, atrial septal defect
VACTERL syndrome	Ventricular septal defect, atrial septal defect, tetralogy of Fallot
Williams syndrome	Supravalvular aortic or pulmonic stenosis
Wolf–Hirschhorn syndrome	Atrial septal defect, ventricular septal defect

7. **What teratogens are known to cause congenital heart disease?**
Table 6-2 lists teratogens known to cause congenital heart disease.

Rychik J, Ayres N, Cuneo B, et al. American Society of Echocardiography guidelines and standards for performance of the fetal echocardiogram. J Am Soc Echocardiogr 2004;17:803–10.
Drose J. Fetal echocardiography. 1st ed. Philadelphia: Saunders; 1988.
Gelb B. Genetic basis of congenital heart disease. Curr Opin Cardiol 2004;19:110–115.

TABLE 6-2. TERATOGENS THAT CAUSE CONGENITAL HEART DISEASE

Table adapted from Drose J. Fetal echocardiography. 1st ed. Philadelphia: Saunders; 1988.

TERATOGEN	COMMON CARDIAC ANATOMIC LESION
Fetal alcohol syndrome	Ventricular septal defect, atrial septal defect, tetralogy of Fallot, coarctation of the aorta
Fetal hydantoin (Dilantin) syndrome	Ventricular septal defect, tetralogy of Fallot, pulmonic stenosis, patent ductus arteriosus, atrial septal defect, coarctation of the aorta
Fetal trimethadione syndrome	Ventricular septal defect, d-transposition of the great vessels, tetralogy of Fallot, hypoplastic left heart syndrome, double outlet right ventricle, pulmonary atresia, atrial septal defect, aortic stenosis, pulmonic stenosis
Fetal carbamazepine syndrome	Ventricular septal defect, tetralogy of Fallot
Valproic acid	Ventricular septal defect, coarctation of the aorta, interrupted aortic arch, tetralogy of Fallot, hypoplastic left heart syndrome, aortic stenosis, atrial septal defect, pulmonary atresia
Retinoic acid embryopathy	Conotruncal malformations
Thalidomide embryopathy	Conotruncal malformations
Maternal phenylketonuria (PKU) (fetal effects)	Tetralogy of Fallot, ventricular septal defect, coarctation of the aorta

TABLE 6-2. TERATOGENS THAT CAUSE CONGENITAL HEART DISEASE —Cont'd	
TERATOGEN	**COMMON CARDIAC ANATOMIC LESION**
Maternal systemic lupus erythematosus/Sjögren syndrome (fetal effects)	Complete congenital heart block, dilated cardiomyopathy
Fetal rubella syndrome	Patent ductus arteriosus, peripheral pulmonary artery stenosis
Maternal diabetes	Hypertrophic cardiomyopathy, conotruncal abnormalities

✓ KEY POINTS: PHYSIOLOGIC VARIABLES IN FETAL AND PERINATAL LIFE

1. The pulmonary vascular resistance begins to fall after birth and reaches a nadir by 6 to 8 weeks of age.

2. Oxygen is a potent vasodilator and contributes to the fall in the pulmonary vascular resistance after birth.

8. **What four shunts are present in the fetal circulation?**
   - Ductus venosus: allows placental blood flow to bypass the liver; becomes the ligamentum venosum after birth
   - Fossa ovalis: allows the umbilical venous return to bypass the right ventricle and pulmonary circulation; foraminal flap composed of septum primum closes the fossa ovalis after birth
   - PDA: allows right ventricular blood to bypass the pulmonary circulation; becomes the ligamentum arteriosum after birth
   - Placenta: organ with the lowest resistance in the placental–fetal circulation; therefore receives the greatest combined ventricular output (Fig. 6-1).

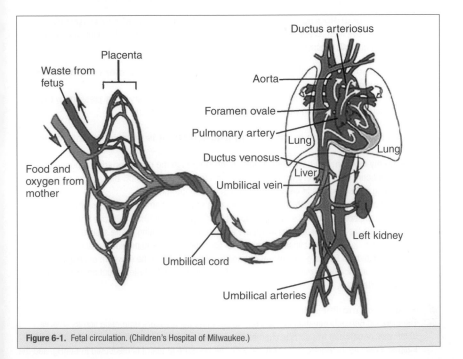

Figure 6-1. Fetal circulation. (Children's Hospital of Milwaukee.)

9. **Why does the fossa ovalis close shortly after birth?**
The fossa ovalis is composed of the septum primum overlying the septum secundum in the left atrium. In fetal life the right atrial pressure is greater than the left atrial pressure, causing the fossa ovalis to remain patent. After birth, with the increase in pulmonary blood flow and pulmonary venous return to the left atrium, the left atrial pressure increases and causes the septum primum to close against the septum secundum, thereby closing the fossa ovalis. This functional closure of the fossa ovalis occurs within the first few days after birth. This change is followed by complete obliteration of the fossa ovalis shunt at approximately 4 months after birth.

10. **What are the determinants of pulmonary vascular resistance (PVR)?**
Pulmonary vascular resistance = pulmonary artery pressure/pulmonary blood flow

11. **How does PVR change after birth?**
The very high PVR in the fetus results in low pulmonary blood flow, with diversion of the right ventricular blood away from the pulmonary vascular bed and towards the systemic vascular bed through the ductus arteriosus. This dynamic results in increased thickness of the muscular medial layer of the pulmonary arteries. As a newborn's lungs expand, they inspire oxygen, which is a potent vasodilator that causes the pulmonary vascular resistance to fall. The rise in the PaO_2 causes the smooth muscle in the pulmonary circulation to relax, and vasodilation occurs. The PVR falls dramatically during the first week of life. As the smooth muscle of the pulmonary arteries continues to thin, the PVR continues to fall, reaching a nadir at 6 to 8 weeks after delivery.

Park MK. Pediatric cardiology for the practitioners. 3rd ed. St Louis: Mosby; 1996.

✓ KEY POINTS: ECHOCARDIOGRAPHIC ASSESSMENT OF VENTRICULAR FUNCTION AND PULMONARY HYPERTENSION

1. Echocardiography can be used to noninvasively assess right ventricular/pulmonary artery pressure.

12. **Why is echocardiography useful in the assessment of ventricular function?**
It is a noninvasive method that qualitatively and quantitatively assesses right and left ventricular systolic and diastolic function.

13. **Why is echocardiography particularly useful in the assessment of pulmonary hypertension?**
It can be used for noninvasive assessment of right ventricular/pulmonary artery pressure by evaluating the tricuspid regurgitation velocity and the ventricular septal contour.

14. **Name three scenarios in which a right-to-left shunt is seen in the infant with a PDA.**
   - A healthy newborn can have right-to-left shunting through the ductus arteriosus during the first 24 hours after delivery with the transitional circulation. If this flow occurs, the right-to-left shunting usually occurs in early systole and is brief in duration.
   - A newborn with left-sided obstructive lesions (such as coarctation of the aorta, interrupted aortic arch, severe aortic stenosis, or hypoplastic left heart syndrome [HLHS]) will have right-to-left shunting through the ductus arteriosus in systole and left-to-right shunting in late systole and in diastole. The right-to-left shunting bypasses the level of flow obstruction and provides systemic blood flow.
   - Infants with high PVR (e.g., persistent pulmonary hypertension of the newborn or congenital heart disease complicated by marked elevation of PVR) may have right-to-left shunting through the ductus arteriosus.

15. **What is the modified Bernoulli equation?**
The modified Bernoulli equation enables one to calculate the pressure difference across an area of stenosis or between two cardiac chambers using the velocity of blood flow across the areas of interest. *Pressure 1− Pressure 2 = 4 (V_2 − $V_1{}^2$).* The pressure gradient is measured in mmHg, and the

velocity is measured in meters/sec. Because V_1 is assumed to be of low velocity (< 1 m/sec), it can be ignored and the formula can be approximated as Pressure 1– Pressure 2 = 4 ($Vmax^2$).

16. **How can the modified Bernoulli equation be useful in interpreting pulmonary artery pressures in a neonate?**
   This formula allows the pulmonary artery pressure to be estimated. Two examples are as follows:
   - If the velocity across a tricuspid regurgitant jet is 4 m/sec, the calculated right ventricular pressure will be 64 mmHg [P = 4 × (V max^2) which is 4 × (4^2)= 64 mmHg]. By adding an estimation of right atrial pressure (usually use 5 mmHg), the estimated right ventricular pressure (as well as a pulmonary artery pressure in the absence of pulmonary stenosis) would be 69 mmHg. Therefore this patient has pulmonary hypertension.
   - If the jet velocity across a ventricular septal defect (VSD) is 4 m/sec, the calculated pressure difference between the right and left ventricles would be 64 mmHg [P = 4 x (4^2)= 64 mmHg). In a patient with a systolic blood pressure of 80 mmHg, the right ventricular pressure can be estimated by subtracting the calculated pressure difference between the ventricles from the systolic blood pressure (systolic arm blood pressure 80 mmHg – 64 mmHg = 16 mmHg (right ventricular pressure). In this patient the right ventricular pressure and the pulmonary artery pressure would be normal.

17. **What is the definition of the echocardiographic term shortening fraction?**
   Shortening fraction is the percentage change in the internal diameter of the left ventricle dimension from end-diastole to end-systole. It is a measure of cardiac function. Preload, contractility, and afterload all influence the shortening fraction.

18. **How is shortening fraction measured?**
   The formula to measure shortening fraction is as follows:

   $$\% \text{ Shortening Fractions (SF)} = (\text{LV diastolic diameter} - \text{LV systolic diameter} / \text{LV diastolic diameter}) \times 100$$

   $$\text{LV} = \text{Left Ventricle}$$

   Shortening fraction is typically measured by M-mode assessment of the left ventricular dimension in the parasternal short-axis or long-axis views. Shortening fraction less than 28% is consistent with reduced left ventricular systolic function. Shortening fraction greater than 38% is consistent with hyperdynamic left ventricular systolic function. The normal range for shortening fraction is 28% to 38%.

19. **What is the definition of the echocardiographic term ejection fraction?**
   Ejection fraction is the percentage change in the left ventricular volume from end-diastole to end-systole.

20. **How is ejection fraction measured by echocardiography?**
   Left ventricular ejection fraction can be calculated by M-mode measurements. However, the method recommended by the American Society of Echocardiography to measure ejection fraction is Simpson's biplane method, which measures end-diastolic and end-systolic volumes in two orthogonal views. The formula is as follows:

   $$\% \text{ EF} = (\text{LV diastolic volume} - \text{LV systolic Volume} / \text{LV diastolic volume}) \times 100$$

   EF = Ejection fraction. LV = Left ventricular. The normal range for left ventricular ejection fraction is 55% to 70%.

21. **How does ejection fraction differ from shortening fraction?**
   Shortening fraction will be inaccurate when there are regional wall motion abnormalities or septal wall flattening in the presence of right ventricular volume or pressure overload. Ejection fraction, when measured by Simpson's biplane method, accounts for wall motion abnormalities, although it can be more time consuming to measure.

22. During postnatal life, as PVR falls, what changes can be expected in the magnitude of a left-to-right shunt of a large VSD?

With a large-pressure nonrestrictive VSD, the right ventricular and pulmonary artery pressures remain high. The right and left ventricular pressures remain equal with a nonrestrictive VSD. As the pressure across the pulmonary vascular bed will not change and the PVR falls, the pulmonary blood flow (PBF) will increase because there is an inverse relationship between PBF and PVR. PBF = Δ Pressure across the pulmonary vascular bed/PVR. Therefore the magnitude of the left-to-right shunt will increase.

Snider AR, Serwer GA, Ritter SB. Echocardiography in pediatric heart disease. 2nd ed. St Louis: Mosby; 1997.

Lai WW, Mertens LL, Cohen MS, et al. Echocardiography in pediatric and congenital heart disease from fetus to adult. West Sussex: Wiley-Blackwell; 2009.

✓ KEY POINTS: INNOCENT MURMURS

1. All innocent murmurs should have normal electrocardiographic readings and normal cardiac silhouettes on chest x-ray.

23. What are the common innocent murmurs heard in the newborn period?
- Peripheral pulmonary stenosis (PPS): This murmur is a soft, grade 1-2/6 systolic ejection murmur, heard best at the left upper sternal border, with radiation to both axillae and the back. It will usually disappear or be much softer at 6 to 8 weeks after delivery in normal infants and completely disappear by 6 months after delivery.
- Transient systolic murmur of a closing PDA. This murmur is a 1-2/6 systolic ejection murmur, best heard at the left upper sternal border and also in the left infraclavicular area. The murmur usually disappears by day 2 of life in term infants.

24. What causes the murmur in an infant with PPS?
Two theories exist regarding the origin of a PPS murmur. First, the branch pulmonary arteries are relatively small in diameter shortly after birth. Second, the branch pulmonary arteries bifurcate at an acute angle from the main pulmonary artery, creating mild flow turbulence. As the neonate grows, this angle becomes less acute.

✓ KEY POINTS: PHYSIOLOGY OF THE CYANOTIC NEONATE

1. The hyperoxia test does not rule out some common mixing congenital heart lesions.

2. Reversed differential cyanosis can be seen when the postductal saturations are higher than the preductal saturations. This sign can be seen in d-transposition of the great arteries with a coarctation of the aorta, d-transposition of the great arteries with interrupted aortic arch, and d-transposition of the great arteries with pulmonary hypertension.

25. What is central cyanosis and what are some of the causes in the newborn?
Central cyanosis occurs when deoxygenated blood enters the systemic circulation, creating the appearance of cyanosis of the oral mucosa, lips, tongue, and trunk. Cyanotic heart disease with right-to-left cardiac shunting, inadequate ventilation (central nervous system depression or airway obstruction), ventilation/perfusion problems (V/Q mismatch), and pulmonary arteriovenous fistulae are causes of central cyanosis.

26. At what level of desaturation is cyanosis detectable at physical examination in most neonates?
Cyanosis may be perceived when there is 5 g of reduced (deoxygenated) hemoglobin in the capillaries. In a neonate cyanosis is observed when the oxygen saturation is below 70%. Neonates have a

higher hematocrit level than infants that results in a lower oxygen saturation needed to detect clinical central cyanosis. An experienced observer can sometimes detect cyanosis when the saturation falls between 80% and 85%.

27. What is peripheral cyanosis?

Peripheral cyanosis can occur in states of low cardiac output, even when the arterial saturation is normal. When the cardiac output is low, the arteriovenous oxygen difference widens, leading to an increased amount of reduced hemoglobin in the capillaries. Low output cyanosis is commonly referred to as *acrocyanosis*. Polycythemia can also cause cyanosis because of the increased levels of reduced hemoglobin in the circulation.

28. What is differential cyanosis, and what are the implications *(pink upper body and blue lower body)*?

Measuring oxygen saturation at both preductal and postductal sites is part of the initial evaluation in a patient with suspected heart disease. If the preductal oxygen saturation is higher than the postductal oxygen saturation, there is differential cyanosis. This sign occurs when the great arteries are normally related and deoxygenated blood from the pulmonary circulation enters the descending aorta through a PDA (right-to-left shunting). This pattern of cyanosis is seen with persistent pulmonary hypertension of the newborn (PPHN) and with left ventricular outflow obstruction (aortic arch hypoplasia, interrupted aortic arch, critical coarctation, and critical aortic stenosis).

29. What is reversed differential cyanosis *(blue upper body and pink lower body)*?

Reversed differential cyanosis occurs when the postductal saturation is higher than the preductal saturation. The classic clinical scenario for reversed differential cyanosis occurs with transposition of the great arteries with preductal aortic arch obstruction or pulmonary hypertension when oxygenated blood from the pulmonary artery enters the descending aorta by right-to-left shunting through the ductus arteriosus. Reversed differential cyanosis also occurs with total anomalous pulmonary venous connection above the diaphragm. It is seen less frequently when there is an anomalous right subclavian artery connected by the ductus to the right pulmonary artery.

30. What is oxygen capacity and oxygen saturation?

Oxygen capacity refers to the maximal amount of oxygen that can be bound to each gram of hemoglobin in blood. (i.e., oxygen capacity = 1.36 mL × hemoglobin level; as each gram of hemoglobin takes up 1.36 mL of oxygen). The total oxygen-carrying capacity is specific to each patient. Oxygen saturation is the amount of oxygen actually bound to hemoglobin compared with the oxygen capacity. It is expressed as a percentage. Oxygen saturation can tell how much oxygen is being carried only if the amount of hemoglobin is known.

31. What is the oxygen dissociation curve, and what influences it?

The oxygen dissociation curve shows the relationship between oxygen saturation (%) and the partial pressure of oxygen, Po_2, in mmHg. This relationship is a sigmoid-shaped curve, with it being fairly flat in the upper range of oxygen saturation (above 85%). Blood pH, temperature, Pco_2, 2,3-diphosphoblycerate, and the type of hemoglobin influence the relationship between oxygen saturation and the partial pressure of oxygen (Fig. 6-2).

32. What is a hyperoxia test, and how is it used in differentiating pulmonary and cardiac causes of cyanosis?

A hyperoxia test attempts to differentiate between pulmonary disease with V/Q mismatch and cyanotic congenital heart disease. Initially, one measures the oxygen saturation in room air. If the oxygen saturation is low, the patient should be placed in 100% Fio_2. The patient with pulmonary disease will show an increase in Po_2 (to a variable degree). In the patient with a fixed intracardiac mixing lesion, the Po_2 does not change significantly. A preductal and postductal arterial blood gas result should be obtained. A preductal arterial blood gas result can be obtained from the right radial artery. A postductal arterial blood gas can be obtained either from an umbilical artery or from a lower extremity artery. In pulmonary

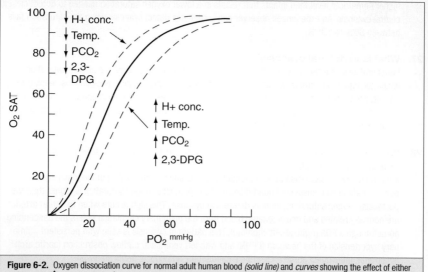

Figure 6-2. Oxygen dissociation curve for normal adult human blood *(solid line)* and *curves* showing the effect of either an increase (↑) or a decrease (↓) in hydrogen ion concentration, body temperature, Pco_2, and 2,3-DPG level *(dotted lines)*. (From Gessner I, Vitorica B: Pediatric cardiology: a problem-oriented approach. Philadelphia: Saunders; 1993. p. 98.)

disease the preductal arterial Po_2 in 100% Fio_2 usually exceeds 150 mmHg. If the ductus arteriosus is patent and a right-to-left ductal shunt occurs because of high PVR, the postductal Po_2 will be lower than the preductal Po_2. In addition, the arterial Pco_2 is elevated relative to the patient's respiratory effort.

In cyanotic congenital heart disease (CHD), the Po_2 in room air is below 70 mmHg (usually <50 mmHg) and does not change significantly in 100% oxygen. Typically, the arterial Pco_2 is normal or low. This finding is the result of hyperventilation that occurs as a response to the hypoxia. Acidosis is typically of a metabolic nature because of abnormal systemic perfusion, tissue hypoxia, or both. In some cases the hyperoxia test must be done with the administration of positive pressure ventilation to expand atelectatic lung adequately to exchange gas.

33. **Which critical cyanotic lesions may not be excluded if the hyperoxia test yields a Po_2 after 10 minutes greater than 150 torr?**
   Common mixing lesions may not be excluded. Examples are total anomalous pulmonary venous return, tetralogy of Fallot with a predominant left-to-right shunt, and HLHS.

34. **What are the current guidelines for pulse oximetry screening of newborns to detect critical cyanotic congenital heart disease?**
   As published in *Pediatrics* in 2011, pulse oximetry assessment of the right hand and a foot is recommended before discharge of all newborns from the hospital. If the oxygen saturation is less than 90% in the right hand or foot, the test is positive and further evaluation is needed. If the oxygen saturation is 95% or greater in the right hand or foot and the difference is 3% or less between the two sites, then the test is negative. If the oxygen saturation is 90% to 95% or greater than 3% difference between the two sites is found, then the test should be repeated in 1 hour up to two times. It is considered a positive screen if these findings are reproduced twice.

Rudolph A. Congenital diseases of the heart: clinical-physiological considerations. Armonk, New York: Futura; 2001. p. 81–5.

Yap SH, Anania N, Alboliras ET, et al. Reversed differential cyanosis in the newborn: a clinical finding in the supracardiac total anomalous pulmonary venous connection. Pediatr Cardiol 2009;30:359–362.

Kemper AR, Mahle WT, Martin GR, et al. Strategies for implementing screening for critical congenital heart disease. Pediatrics 2011;128:1259–67.

✓ KEY POINTS: CONGESTIVE HEART FAILURE

1. Different cardiac lesions present with congestive heart failure (CHF) at different times postnatally.

35. What are the major causes of heart failure in a fetus?

Severe anemia, bradyarrhythmia, tachyarrhythmia, infection, large systemic arteriovenous (AV) fistula (e.g., vein of Galen AV malformation), and severe atrioventricular valve insufficiency.

36. What are the signs and symptoms of heart failure in the newborn infant?

Heart failure in infants manifests as signs and symptoms of increased pulmonary blood flow (PBF) or inadequate systemic blood flow. Signs of excessive PBF include tachypnea, sweating, poor feeding, failure to thrive, gallop rhythm, and hepatomegaly. Congenital heart disease may present as shock or catastrophic heart failure in an infant with obstructive left-sided lesions and decreased systemic blood flow. Symptoms may include a loud S_2 and decreased peripheral pulses. Assessment of pre-ductal and postductal saturations should be sought.

37. What are some heart conditions that can present in the first week of life and result in CHF?

Ductal-dependent abnormalities:
- HLHS
- Tetralogy of Fallot with pulmonary atresia
- Interrupted aortic arch type B (interruption of the aorta between the left common carotid artery and the left subclavian artery)
- Pulmonary atresia with intact ventricular septum
- Coarctation of the aorta
- Critical aortic stenosis

Non–ductal-dependent abnormalities:
- Total anomalous pulmonary venous return
- Truncus arteriosus
- AV septal defect (endocardial cushion defect)
- Myocardial dysfunction (cardiomyopathy)
  - Myocarditis
  - Inborn errors of metabolism
- Supraventricular tachycardia/arrhythmia
- Single ventricle complex
- Congenital AV block

38. What are some heart lesions that can cause heart failure in the infant beyond the newborn period?

Obstruction to systemic blood flow:
- Coarctation of the aorta
- Severe aortic stenosis

Left-to-right shunt:
- VSD
- AV septal defect
- PDA

Mixing lesions:
- Total anomalous pulmonary venous return, without obstruction
- Single ventricle with excessive PBF
- D-transposition of the great arteries
- Large VSD
- Truncus arteriosus

Myocardial dysfunction/pericardial disease:
- Anomalous left coronary artery
- Myocarditis
- Arrhythmia (supraventricular tachycardia [SVT])
  - Accessory pathway
  - Ectopic atrial tachycardia
  - Permanent junctional reciprocating tachycardia
  - Atrial flutter with 1:1 AV conduction
- Endocarditis/pericarditis
- Dilated cardiomyopathy
  - Hereditary
  - Metabolic
  - X-linked
  - Other (e.g., Pompe disease)

39. **Why does the newborn heart have a reduced ability to adapt to stress?**
The newborn heart has fewer myofilaments with which to generate the force of contraction. The newborn ventricle has decreased compliance compared with an adult ventricle. Therefore the newborn heart generates less augmentation in stroke volume for a given increase in diastolic volume. The oxygen consumption and cardiac output/m^2 are much higher in the newborn, and there is very little systolic reserve. Tachycardia is therefore the usual neonatal response to stress, because any increase in stroke volume is limited.

40. **What medications are used for CHF in the neonate?**
The goals of treating the neonate depend on the etiology of the CHF. Is the CHF a result of an arrhythmia, myopathic process, decreased systemic blood flow, or increased PBF? The main drugs used to treat CHF in the newborn are inotropic agents, diuretics, and afterload reduction agents. PGE is indicated when ductal-dependent cardiac lesions are diagnosed. Supraventricular arrhythmias with significant heart failure require prompt pharmacologic or electrical cardioversion. CHF secondary to a myopathy should be treated with inotropic agents, diuretics, afterload reduction agents, or a combination thereof.

41. **What are compensatory mechanisms during heart failure?**
Compensatory mechanisms include increased heart rate, enhanced stroke volume (Frank–Starling mechanism), sympathetic nerve activation (increased sympathetic tone, renin-angiotensin system activation), increased 2,3-diphosphoglycerate, increased atrial natriuretic peptides, and myocardial hypertrophy.

Silberbach M, Hannon D. Presentation of congenital heart disease in the neonate and young infant. Pediatr Rev 2007;28(4):123–31.
Anderson RH, Baker EJ, Penny DJ, et al. Paediatric cardiology. 3rd ed. Philadelphia: Churchill Livingstone Elsevier; 2010.

✓ KEY POINTS: TREATMENT OF HYPOTENSION ON THE NEONATE

1. Dopamine and dobutamine have different physiologic effects in the newborn.

2. Dopamine is a good inotrope to use (depending on dose) if there is a risk of renal ischemia, low cardiac output, or hypotension with decreased systemic vascular resistance.

3. Dobutamine is a good inotrope to use for low cardiac output in patients at risk for myocardial ischemia, pulmonary hypertension, and left ventricular diastolic dysfunction.

42. **What is the most frequent primary cause of hypotension in the preterm neonate in the immediate postnatal period?**

In the preterm infant the immature cardiovascular system is poorly equipped to handle the transitional circulation from a low vascular resistance circulation, when the placenta is removed, to the sudden presence of a high systemic circulation. The immature myocardium, residual fetal circulatory shunts, cytokine release mediated hypotension, and the impact of positive pressure ventilation on venous return and cardiac output all contribute to inadequate systemic perfusion. However, the primary mechanism of hypotension in a preterm infant is inadequate peripheral vasomotor regulation. Although hypovolemia is a common cause of hypotension in the pediatric population, hypovolemia in sick preterm infants is infrequently the cause of hypotension during the immediate postnatal period.

43. **Why are the deleterious effects of hypotension of greater concern in preterm neonates?**

Preterm neonates have a relative inability to regulate cerebral blood flow compared with those born at term. Hypotension is associated with decreased cerebral blood flow. Hypotension and rapid wide swings in blood pressure have been shown to be predictive of both germinal matrix-intraventricular hemorrhage and periventricular leukomalacia.

44. **What are the mechanisms of action of the cardiovascular effects of dopamine in the preterm neonate?**

In preterm neonates dopamine increases blood pressure primarily through vasoconstriction (increased afterload) as the immature cardiovascular system has an enhanced alpha-adrenergic sensitivity. Dopamine also increases preload by decreasing the venous capacitance, which may also contribute to the beneficial cardiovascular effects of dopamine. Low-dose dopamine (2 to 5 μg/kg/min) has this primary alpha-adrenergic effect. Higher-dose dopamine will have a beta$_1$-adrenergic effect on the myocardium. Dopamine has a renal but not mesenteric or cerebral vascular effect in preterm infants.

45. **What are the pros and cons of dopamine and dobutamine in the treatment of hypotension in a preterm neonate?**

Dopamine may be the preferred inotrope in the treatment of hypotension secondary to neonatal sepsis because it increases peripheral vascular contractility. However, dobutamine may be preferred in treatment of hypotension secondary to cardiomyopathy, which frequently occurs with perinatal asphyxia. Whereas dopamine has a greater increase in arterial blood pressure than dobutamine, dobutamine has been shown to increase superior vena cava blood flow and may improve end-organ perfusion to a great extent.

Nichols DG, Cameron DE, Greeley WJ, et al. Critical heart disease in infants and children. 1st ed. St Louis: Mosby; 1995.
    Short BL, Meurs KV, Evans JR, et al. Summary Proceedings from the Cardiology Group on Cardiovascular Instability in Preterm Infants. Pediatrics 2006;117:S34–39.
    Engle WD, LeFlore JL. Hypotension in the neonate. Neoreviews 2002;3:e137.

✓ **KEY POINTS: CYANOTIC CONGENITAL HEART DISEASE**

1. An unrestrictive atrial communication is crucial in certain cyanotic congenital heart lesions to provide mixing (right-to-left) and/or cardiac output.

2. The most common cyanotic lesion presenting in the newborn period is d-transposition of the great arteries.

3. An electrocardiogram with a left axis shift in a cyanotic newborn baby may be consistent with tricuspid atresia.

4. Cyanotic CHD does not include cyanosis secondary to intrapulmonary right-to-left shunting.

46. **What is the most common cyanotic lesion presenting in the newborn period?**
D-transposition of the great arteries is the most common form of cyanotic congenital heart disease in the neonate, and accounts for between 6% and 10% of infants with congenital heart disease. In children "outside" the newborn period, tetralogy of Fallot is the most common, representing 7% to 9% of cardiac cases of cyanosis.

47. **What are the five Ts of cyanotic congenital heart disease? What are other principal cyanotic heart lesions that do not begin with a T?**
The five Ts
- Transposition of the great arteries
- Tetralogy of Fallot
- Truncus arteriosus
- Total anomalous pulmonary venous return
- Tricuspid atresia
The Non-Ts
- Ebstein anomaly of the tricuspid valve
- HLHS
- Pulmonary atresia

48. **Why is neonatal pulse oximetry screening performed?**
The screening is performed for the following reasons:
- Prenatal screening depicts less than 50% of all CHD.
- Routine newborn examination misses more than 50% of all infants with CHD.
- Of CHD-related deaths in the first week of life, 25% of cases do not have a diagnosis of CHD.

49. **What is d-transposition of the great arteries?**
In d-transposition of the great arteries, the aorta arises from the morphologic right ventricle and the pulmonary artery arises from the morphologic left ventricle. Variation in the origin and course of the right and left coronary arteries may occur and can generally be determined by echocardiography before surgery.

50. **What is the pathophysiology of d-transposition of the great arteries?**
The circulation is in parallel instead of a normal in-series circulation. (right atrium→right ventricle→aorta)(pulmonary vein→left atrium→pulmonary artery). The systemic venous blood does not get oxygenated. Survival depends on intercirculatory shunts (atrial septal defect [ASD], VSD, PDA).

51. **What are the symptoms in patients with d-transposition of the great arteries?**
Patients with d-transposition of the great arteries may have an intact ventricular septum and exhibit cyanosis in the first hours to days of life. They will develop tachypnea, respiratory distress, and acidosis and die if not treated. Patients with d-transposition of the great arteries with a reasonable VSD may have minimal cyanosis and present with CHF in the first 4 to 8 weeks of life. A smaller group of patients may have transposition of the great arteries, VSD, and pulmonary stenosis and have a more variable presentation.

52. **How do prostaglandins work in d-transposition of the great arteries?**
Prostaglandins keep the ductus arteriosus patent and help assist with the mixing of the circulations, thereby improving oxygenation.

53. **In infants with d-transposition of the great arteries, how does a balloon atrial septostomy improve systemic oxygen saturation?**
Progressive hypoxemia from poor intercirculatory mixing is a medical emergency. An atrial septostomy may be necessary to improve hypoxemia even after Prostaglandin E1 (PGE) has maintained

ductal patency. The balloon atrial septostomy permits unrestricted bidirectional mixing of fully saturated blood in the left atrium with desaturated blood in the right atrium to achieve a higher net saturation of blood in the systemic circulation. After this procedure, patency of the ductus is generally no
longer essential. Variations in oxygen saturation can be expected, although mixing is usually excellent.

54. **What is tetralogy of Fallot?**
Tetralogy of Fallot is the most common CHD-related cause of cyanosis beyond 1 year of age. The constellation of anatomic features consists of a VSD, pulmonary stenosis, right ventricular hypertrophy, and over-
riding of the aorta over the ventricular septum. A right-sided aortic arch may be present in 25% of cases.

55. **What are the clinical manifestations of tetralogy of Fallot at birth?**
The most common clinical manifestation is a murmur secondary to obstruction across the right
ventricular outflow tract. The murmur is not caused by the VSD (large defect, equal pressures in both
ventricles). Cyanosis depends on the severity of the right ventricular outflow tract obstruction along
with the presence or absence of a PDA.

56. **What is total anomalous pulmonary venous return (TAPVR)?**
In TAPVR all the pulmonary veins drain into the systemic veins. TAPVR is rare, occurring in 2% to 3% of
all cases of congenital heart disease. The different types of total anomalous pulmonary venous return
depend on their drainage sites. There is a marked predominance of males for the infracardiac type.

57. **What are the different types of TAPVR?**
- *Supracardiac*: represents 50% of all total anomalous pulmonary venous return. The pulmonary
  veins usually drain into the right superior vena cava via a left vertical vein. Although generally
  nonobstructive, they can be obstructed in some cases (the vertical vein is "pinched" between
  the left pulmonary artery and the left bronchus, or at superior vena cava insertion).
- *Cardiac*: represents 20% of all total anomalous pulmonary venous return. The pulmonary veins
  drain into the coronary sinus or directly into the right atrium. They can be obstructed (obstruction can occur at the site of the obligate right-to-left atrial shunt) or non-obstructed.
- *Infra cardiac*: represents 20% of all total anomalous pulmonary venous return. The common
  pulmonary vein drains below the diaphragm into the portal venous system, ductus venosus,
  inferior vena cava, or hepatic veins. These veins are almost always obstructed.
- *Mixed*: represents 10% of all total anomalous pulmonary venous return. It represents a combination of the other types of TAPVR (Fig. 6-3).

58. **What accounts for the varying clinical manifestations of TAPVR in a neonate?**
The different presentations of TAPVR depend on whether or not the pulmonary veins are obstructed.
Neonates with obstructed TAPVR present within the first few hours of life with severe pulmonary
venous congestion, tachypnea, tachycardia, and cyanosis. The clinical picture of obstructed TAPVR
may be indistinguishable from that of severe respiratory distress syndrome (RDS). In infants with
nonobstructed total anomalous pulmonary veins, tachypnea develops gradually, with a typical presentation occurring in approximately 4 to 6 weeks.

59. **Why is an atrial communication important in TAPVR?**
In the absence of an atrial communication in TAPVR, blood cannot get to the left atrium or left
ventricle and out the aorta to provide any cardiac output. An ASD is necessary for survival with this
lesion. An echocardiogram should demonstrate right ventricular hypertrophy and a right-to-left shunt
via a patent foramen ovale (PFO).

60. **What is the management of TAPVR?**
In patients with obstructed TAPVR, cardiac surgery is an emergency and involves anastamosis of the
common pulmonary vein to the left atrium. Nonobstructive TAPVR can be managed semi-electively,
with the key factor being initial control of CHF.

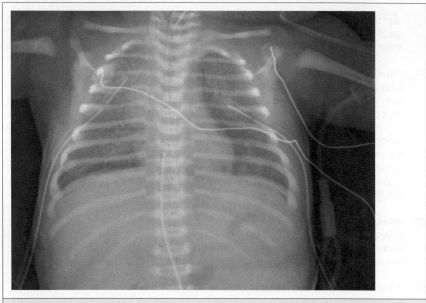

Figure 6-3. AP chest radiograph in a neonate with obstructed supracardiac total anomalous pulmonary venous return. Bilateral chest tubes present. Note the striking obstructed interstitial pulmonary pattern.

61. **What is scimitar syndrome?**

Scimitar syndrome has the following components: right lung hypoplasia, anomalous connection of the right pulmonary veins to the inferior vena cava, right pulmonary artery hypoplasia, anomalous systemic arterial supply to the right lung, bronchial anomalies, and dextroposition of the heart, reflecting the hypoplastic right lung. The term *scimitar syndrome* derives from a feature on the chest x-ray: the right pulmonary veins cast a shadow resembling the handle of a scimitar in the right lower zone as they drain anomalously into the inferior vena cava.

62. **What is the pathology and pathophysiology of truncus arteriosus?**

In truncus arteriosus one large vessel arises from the heart. The coronary arteries, pulmonary arteries, and systemic arteries arise from a single common trunk. A VSD is always present. The truncal valve may be stenotic or regurgitant.

63. **What are clinical manifestations of truncus arteriosus in a neonate?**

Cyanosis may or may not be seen immediately after birth. Signs of CHF develop days to several weeks after birth as the PVR falls, increasing PBF. Cyanosis may be minimal secondary to high PBF. Tachypnea or difficulty feeding can be a sign of CHF. With truncal stenosis there can be a systolic ejection murmur. There is a single second heart sound. The pulses are bounding, and significant truncal regurgitation will generally produce a widened pulse pressure with a prominent diastolic murmur.

64. **What syndrome can be associated with truncus arteriosus?**

DiGeorge syndrome with hypocalcemia is present in approximately one third of cases with truncus arteriosus. Attention to the presence of a thymic shadow should be sought on the chest radiograph.

65. **What are the clinical manifestations of a neonate with HLHS?**

Infants with HLHS can present within the first few hours to days of life. Clinical symptoms depend on the status of the inter-atrial communication, patency of the ductus, PVR, and potentially the degree

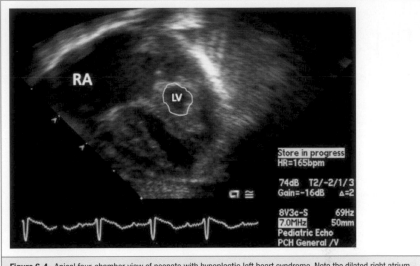

Figure 6-4. Apical four-chamber view of neonate with hypoplastic left heart syndrome. Note the dilated right atrium (RA) and ventricle with severely hypoplastic, non–apex-forming left ventricle (LV; outlined).

of AV valve competency. Common clinical signs are tachypnea, hepatomegaly, pulmonary rales, and a single second heart sound (S_2). Cyanosis may be minimal. Closure of the ductus will result in decreased peripheral pulses and a "shock-like" picture (Fig. 6-4).

66. **What is the management of HLHS?**

Management of HLHS requires correction of acidosis; prostaglandins; avoidance of hyperventilation; and most important, maintenance of adequate systemic perfusion. Generally, supplemental oxygen is unnecessary. Echocardiography should assess the ventricular function, patency of the ductus, and adequacy of the inter-atrial communication.

67. **Under what circumstances can information from an electrocardiogram in a cyanotic neonate help indicate the presence of congenital heart disease?**

The key is an abnormal frontal plane axis. A *leftward* axis for a newborn (i.e., left superior axis −90 to 0 [see Fig. 6-5]) strongly implies a structural anomaly of the heart. Dominant left ventricular forces often accompany this anomaly. The differential diagnosis includes tricuspid atresia, pulmonary valve atresia with intact ventricular septum, critical pulmonary stenosis, or complex single left ventricle.

A *rightward superior/northwest* axis (i.e. −90 to −180 degrees) suggests an AV canal defect. *Note: A normal electrocardiographic reading does not rule out CHD.*

68. **What are some common chest x-ray findings in infants with cyanotic congenital heart lesions?**

- *d-transposition of the great arteries with an intact ventricular septum:* Cardiomegaly with increased pulmonary vascular markings. Egg-shaped cardiac silhouette, with a narrow, superior mediastinum.

- *Tetralogy of Fallot :* Normal heart size or smaller than normal. Decreased pulmonary vascular markings, concave main pulmonary artery segment with an upturned apex (boot-shaped heart). This can have a right-sided aortic arch.

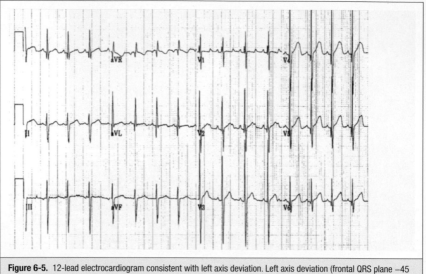

Figure 6-5. 12-lead electrocardiogram consistent with left axis deviation. Left axis deviation (frontal QRS plane −45 degrees) may be seen with tricuspid atresia.

- *Total anomalous pulmonary venous return*: Cardiomegaly with right atrial and ventricular enlargement. Increased pulmonary vascular markings. "Snowman" heart can be seen with supracardiac, unobstructed veins (usually seen after several months). With pulmonary venous obstruction there is radiographic evidence of pulmonary edema (diffuse reticular pattern).
- *Tricuspid atresia*: Normal size, or mild cardiomegaly. Straight right heart border. Decreased pulmonary vascular markings.
- *Pulmonary atresia*: Normal size, or mild cardiomegaly. Right atrial enlargement. Decreased pulmonary vascular markings.
- *Ebstein anomaly of the tricuspid valve*: In severe cases the heart is enormous, balloon shaped, and occupies almost the entire cardiothoracic area (Figs. 6-6 and 6-7).
- *Truncus arteriosus*: Cardiomegaly, with increased pulmonary vascular markings. Right-sided aortic arch may be seen (30% of cases).
- *Single ventricle*: Depends on presence or absence of pulmonary stenosis. Can have cardiomegaly with increased pulmonary vascular markings, or a relatively normal-sized heart with decreased pulmonary vascular markings.

69. **What cardiac lesions should one consider when the radiologist says the infant has a right-sided aortic arch?**
    - Truncus arteriosus (36%)
    - Tetralogy of Fallot (13% to 34%)
    - Double outlet right ventricle (20%)
    - Tricuspid atresia (5% to 8%)
    - Transposition of the great vessels (3%)
    - VSD (2% to 6%)

Silberbach M, Hannon D. Presentation of congenital heart disease in the neonate and young infant. Pediatr Rev 2007;28(4):123–31.

Rao PS. Diagnosis and management of cyanotic congenital heart disease: Part I. Indian J Pediatr 2009;76(1):57–70.

Rao PS. Diagnosis and management of cyanotic congenital heart disease: Part II. Indian J Pediatr 2009;76(3):297–308

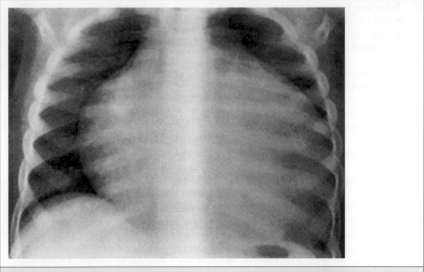

Figure 6-6. AP chest radiograph revealing significant cardiomegaly ("wall-to-wall heart") consistent with Ebstein's anomaly of the tricuspid valve.

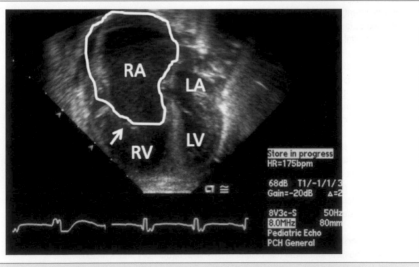

Figure 6-7. Ebstein's malformation of the tricuspid valve. Four-chamber echocardiogram demonstrating an inferiorly displaced tricuspid valve (arrow). The right atrium (RA) is enlarged (outlined). The tricuspid valve is well below the level of the mitral valve. LA, left atrium; LV, left ventricle; RV, right ventricle.

✓ KEY POINTS: ACYANOTIC AND OBSTRUCTIVE CONGENITAL HEART LESIONS

1. Neonates with a large left-to-right shunt typically develop CHF at 3 to 6 weeks of age, when the PVR drops and the left-to-right shunting increases with increased flow into the pulmonary arteries. This increase in PBF will result in increased flow across the mitral valve and enlarge the left ventricle.

70. **What are the common causes of left-to-right shunts in the newborn infant?**
    - VSD
    - PDA
    - AV septal defect (AV canal; endocardial cushion defect)

71. **What acyanotic heart defects are typically seen in children with Down syndrome?**
    AV septal defects (also commonly called endocardial cushion defects or AV canal defects) are common in children with Down syndrome. Endocardial cushion defects can be complete with large ventricular and atrial components or incomplete with just a defect in the septum primum and a smaller VSD. AV canal defects of any variety have a cleft in the mitral valve. Competency of the AV valve should be assessed by echocardiography.

72. **Why do infants with large VSDs escape detection in the newborn period?**
    Infants with a VSD are usually identified after they leave the hospital because both the heart murmur of a VSD and the symptoms of heart failure do not appear during the first few days of life. In the immediate postnatal period, the PVR is still elevated, thereby limiting the shunting of blood from the left ventricle into the right ventricle and across the pulmonary bed. As the PVR falls (PVR↓), an increased volume of blood flows through the defect, which increases the intensity of the murmur and the amount of PBF (↑PBF).

73. **Name three conditions associated with persistent patency of the ductus arteriosus.**
    - Prematurity
    - Hypoxia (pulmonary disease/high altitude)
    - Congenital rubella syndrome

74. **What are three common obstructive heart lesions that can present in the newborn period?**
    - Severe/critical pulmonary stenosis
    - Severe/critical aortic stenosis
    - Coarctation of the aorta

75. **What is critical pulmonary stenosis?**
    Pulmonary stenosis in a neonate that is sufficiently severe to cause cyanosis and acidosis (rare) with signs of right-sided heart failure (rare) is defined as critical pulmonary stenosis. Ductal patency is *essential* for maintaining PBF. The degree of pulmonary stenosis can be measured by echocardiography. Pulmonary balloon valvuloplasty, in the cardiac catheterization laboratory, is undertaken to relieve the stenosis after stabilization of the infant.

76. **What is critical aortic stenosis?**
    Aortic stenosis in a neonate that results in CHF with circulatory shock (acidosis and poor peripheral pulses) is termed *critical aortic stenosis.* In affected infants the systemic circulation depends on the patency of the ductus arteriosus with flow from the pulmonary artery into the descending aorta. *These infants are ductal dependent to provide cardiac output.* In some infants inotropic support, ventilation, and correction of acidosis may be required. The aortic valve can be tricuspid, bicuspid, or unicuspid. Aortic stenosis may be a component of other left-sided anomalies. Echocardiography should assess not only the architecture of the aortic valve but also the mitral valve architecture and the degree, if any, of left ventricular hypoplasia. Most infants are palliated by an aortic balloon valvuloplasty; however, long-term follow-up is mandatory.

77. **What is a neonatal coarctation, and how does it present?**

Neonatal coarctation of the aorta is obstruction in the thoracic aorta or the transverse aortic arch and requires patency of the ductus arteriosus to maintain cardiac output. Typically, these infants become symptomatic when the ductus arteriosus closes. A murmur may be present. Four-extremity blood pressure measurements should be obtained, with careful attention to the right arm and lower extremities. In extreme cases affected infants have signs and symptoms of acute circulatory shock, with decreased or absent femoral pulses. Neonates with circulatory collapse should be fully resuscitated before surgery with correction of acidosis. Prostaglandins should be administered to reestablish ductal patency, because there is an obligate right-to-left ductal shunt. In neonates with critical coarctation (ductal dependent), surgery is required and can generally be performed by a left thoracotomy.

78. **If the apex of the heart is on the opposite side of the patient from the stomach, what is the likelihood that the patient has congenital heart disease?**

The likelihood of congenital heart disease is between 90% and 95%. This condition is referred to as *dextrocardia*.

79. **What are the different types of interrupted aortic arch?**

- Type A: Interruption is distal to the left subclavian artery
- Type B: Interruption is between the left carotid artery and the left subclavian artery. An aberrant right subclavian artery can also be seen in this condition (most common; approximately 40% of all cases)
- Type C: Interruption is between the innominate artery and the left carotid artery

80. **What other lesions are commonly seen with interrupted aortic arch?**

VSD and PDA are commonly present.

81. **What genetic abnormality and clinical features are associated with interrupted aortic arch?**

DiGeorge syndrome (22q11 Deletion Syndrome) is a constellation of clinical symptoms that includes a lack of thymus gland and a lack of parathyroid (hypocalcemia), with certain common conotruncal heart defects. A similar syndrome (velocardiofacial syndrome) may have associated midline facial defects (i.e., cleft palate) with a lower proclivity for thymic deficiency.

Anderson RH, Baker EJ, Penny DJ, et al. Paediatric cardiology. 3rd ed. Philadelphia: Churchill Livingstone Elsevier; 2010.

Rosenthal E. Coarctation of the aorta from fetus to adult: curable condition or life-long process? Heart 2005;91:1495–1502.

Greenberg F. DiGeorge syndrome: an historical review of clinical and cytogenic features. J Med Genet 1993;30(3):803–806.

✓ KEY POINTS: VASCULAR RINGS

1. Vascular rings should be suspected based on respiratory symptoms or dysphagia.

2. Either computed tomography angiography or magnetic resonance imaging is typically considered the preferred definitive imaging modality in the diagnosis of a vascular ring.

82. **What is the difference between a complete and an incomplete vascular ring?**

A complete vascular ring is formed by abnormal vascular structures completely encircling the trachea and esophagus (e.g., double aortic arch and a right aortic arch with a left-sided ligamentum arteriosum). An incomplete vascular ring occurs when there is vascular compression of the trachea and esophagus without completely encircling these structures (e.g., innominate artery compression and pulmonary sling).

	Anatomy	Esophagogram	Other Radiographic Findings	Symptoms	Treatment
Double aortic arch	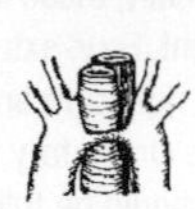	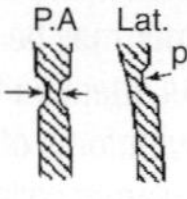 P.A Lat. post→	Anterior compression of trachea	Respiratory difficulty (onset <3 mos.) Swallowing dysfunction	Surgical division of a smaller arch
Right aortic arch with left ligamentum arteriosum	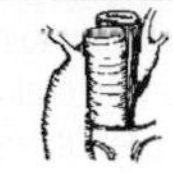	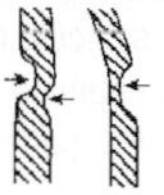		Mild respiratory difficulty (onset >1 year) Swallowing dysfunction	Surgical division of the ligamentum arteriosum
Anomalous innominate artery	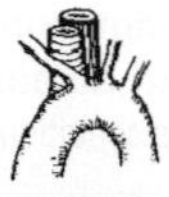	Normal	Anterior compression of trachea	Stridor and/or cough in infancy	Conservative management, or surgical suturing of the artery to the sternum
Aberrant right subclavian artery	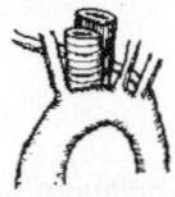	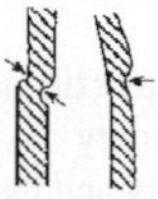		Occasional swallowing dysfunction	Usually no treatment is necessary
"Vascular sling"	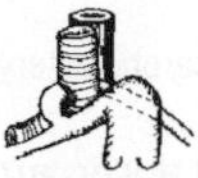	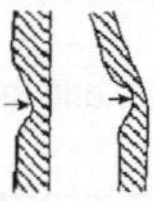	Right-sided emphysema or atelectasis. Posterior compression of trachea or right main stem bronchus	Wheezing and cyanotic episodes since birth	Surgical division of the anomalous LPA (from the RPA) and anastomosis to the MPA

Figure 6-8. Different types of vascular rings. LPA, Left pulmonary artery; RPA, right pulmonary artery; MPA, main pulmonary artery. (From Park MK: Pediatric cardiology for practitioners. 3rd ed. St Louis: Mosby; 1996. p. 246.)

83. **What is the clinical presentation of a vascular ring?**

    Most infants with vascular rings present with symptoms within the first several weeks to months of life, with a double aortic arch and pulmonary sling being symptomatic earlier than the other rings. Infants may hold their heads hyperextended to alleviate the symptoms of airway obstruction. Symptoms of respiratory distress, stridor, "seal bark" cough, apnea, dysphagia, and recurrent respiratory infections may occur. Dysphagia may first be detected when infants transition from liquid formula to solid food (Fig. 6-8).

84. **What is the most common vascular ring?**

    Double aortic arch is the most common vascular ring (40%). A right-sided aortic arch with a left ligamentum is the second most common vascular ring (30%).

85. **What are the indications for surgical intervention?**

    Surgical intervention is indicated in all symptomatic patients with vascular rings. Symptoms include respiratory distress, recurrent respiratory infections, dysphagia, and apneic spells.

86. **What imaging modalities are used for assessing vascular rings?**

    Initial evaluation for a vascular ring should be a chest x-ray. Additional imaging, including a barium swallow and echocardiogram, is helpful in this diagnosis of a vascular ring. However, computed tomography angiography, which can now be done rapidly and therefore does not require general anesthesia, is considered by most institutions to be the single best diagnostic test when a vascular ring is suspected. Magnetic resonance imaging is the preferred diagnostic test at other centers. Bronchoscopy is extremely helpful in assessing the airway compromise.

87. **How does a surgeon repair some of the more common forms of vascular rings?**
    - Double aortic arch: A thoracotomy is performed on the side opposite the dominant aortic arch (typically a left thoracotomy). The lesser arch is clamped, divided, and oversewn. The ligamentum arteriosum is always ligated and divided. Dissection around the esophagus and trachea to lyse any residual adhesive bands is performed.
    - Right aortic arch and left ligamentum arteriosum: A left thoracotomy is performed with dissection and lysis of any residual adhesive bands around the esophagus and trachea.
    - Pulmonary artery sling: Transection of the left pulmonary artery with translocation of the left pulmonary artery anterior to the trachea to its normal position arising from the main pulmonary artery. A barium swallow will reveal an anterior indentation of the esophagous on the lateral projection.

Moes CAF, Freedom RM. Rings, slings and other things: vascular structures contributing to a neonatal noose. In: Freedom RM, Benson LN, Smallhorn JF, editors. Neonatal heart disease. New York: Springer-Verlag; 1992. p.731–49.

Woods RK, Sharp RJ, Holcomb GW 3rd, et al. Vascular anomalies and tracheoesophageal compression: a single institution's 25 year experience. Ann Thorac Surg 2001;72(2):434–8 [discussion 438–9].

Russell HM, Backer CL. Pediatric thoracic problems: patent ductus arteriosus, vascular rings, congenital tracheal stenosis, and pectus deformities. Surg Clin N Am 2010;90:1091–1113.

✓ **KEY POINTS: SEGMENTAL CARDIAC AND CARDIAC MALPOSITION ANALYSIS**

1. When using a chest x-ray to evaluate a patient with congenital heart disease, identification of the stomach bubble and liver shadow will help assess abdominal situs.

2. Although electrocardiography may define the location of the sinoatrial node and ventricular mass, echocardiography is the diagnostic test of choice to define the cardiac segments.

88. **How are segmental relationships expressed in congenital heart disease?**
    The segmental approach to the classification of congenital heart disease was originally proposed by Dr. Richard Van Praagh and colleagues in the 1960s and early 1970s. The three main cardiac segments are (1) atria, (2) ventricles, and (3) great arteries. Therefore congenital heart disease is expressed in these three segments.
    - Atrial sidedness: S (solitus), I (inversus), and A (ambiguus)
    - Ventricular looping: D loop, L loop, and X (indeterminate loop)
    - Great artery relationship: S (solitus), I (inversus or mirror image of normal), D (d-transposition), and L (l-transposition)
    Normal cardiac segmental anatomy is {S, D, S}.

89. **How can electrocardiography localize where the anatomic right and left ventricles are located?**
    Because depolarization occurs in the left ventricle before the right ventricle, the presence/location of the Q waves over the precordium can assist in the anatomic location of the left ventricle and right ventricle. If Q waves are seen in V_5 and V_6, and lead 1, the left ventricle is D-looped and on the left side. If Q waves are seen in V_4R, V_1 and V_2, but not seen in V_5 and V_6, it is likely that the ventricles are L-looped (Figs. 6-9 and 6-10).

90. **What are three noninvasive modalities used to assess atrial location?**
    The chest x-ray, electrocardiography, and echocardiogram are three modalities that can help locate the position of the atria.

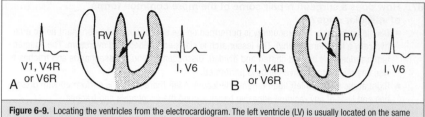

Figure 6-9. Locating the ventricles from the electrocardiogram. The left ventricle (LV) is usually located on the same side as the precordial leads that show Q waves. If V_6 shows a Q wave, the LV is on the left side. If V_4R and V_1 show a Q wave, the LV is to the right of the anatomic right ventricle (RV). Note that SQ waves are also present in V1 in severe right ventricular hypertrophy (RVH). (From Park MK, Guntheroth WG. How to read: pediatric ECGs. 3rd ed. St Louis: Mosby; 1992. p. 253.)

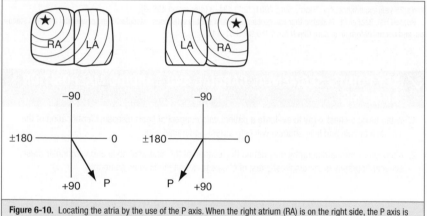

Figure 6-10. Locating the atria by the use of the P axis. When the right atrium (RA) is on the right side, the P axis is in the left lower quadrant (0 to 90 degrees). When the RA is on the left side, the P axis is in the right lower quadrant (90 to −180 degrees). LA, Left atrium. (From Park MK, Guntheroth WG. How to read: pediatric ECGs. 3rd ed. St Louis: Mosby; 1992. p. 252.)

91. How does the abdominal x-ray help determine right atrial position?

The atrial sidedness follows the visceral organ arrangement.

- If abdominal situs is present (liver on the right and stomach on the left), then the right atrium is on the right.
- If abdominal inversus is present (liver on the left and stomach on the right), then the right atrium in on the left.
- If abdominal situs ambiguus is present (liver is midline), then there are typically two right atria or two left atria.

92. What is heterotaxy syndrome?

The word *heterotaxy* means "different arrangement." There is abnormal relationship and arrangement of the cardiac atria and the thoracoabdominal organs, including the spleen, lungs and intestines. Polysplenia (associated with left atrial isomerism) or asplenia (right atrial isomerism) is present. These patients are at high risk for malrotation of the intestines, which should be investigated with ultrasound or barium study. The cardiac malformations are complex typically, with abnormal venoatrial connections (Fig. 6-11).

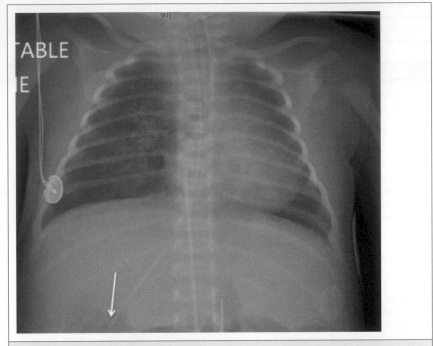

Figure 6-11. AP chest radiograph in a neonate with complex heart disease with heterotaxy. Note the stomach bubble (NG tube; arrow) is on the right side. The umbilical arterial catheter and aortic knob likely confirm a right-sided aortic arch. There is mild interstitial edema.

93. How does electrocardiography help determine atrial position?

The sinoatrial node (the pacemaker of the heart) is located in the right atrium. The p wave axis on the electrocardiogram will determine from where the sinoatrial node pulse is originating and therefore where the sinoatrial node and right atrium are located.

94. What determines the "right atrium" on echocardiogram?

The coronary sinus and the suprahepatic portion of the inferior vena cava drain to the right atrium. In atrial situs solitus the systemic veins (superior and inferior vena cavae) drain to the right atrium, and the pulmonary veins drain to the left atrium. However, the most reliable echocardiographic marker of the right atrium is the drainage of the coronary sinus and the suprahepatic inferior vena cava.

95. What is dextrocardia?

Dextrocardia is a condition in which the heart lies in the right side of the chest. It may occur with dextroposition, when the heart is pushed into the right side of the chest (e.g., left-sided diaphragmatic hernia or hypoplastic right lung). It also may occur when the cardiac apex is directed to the right side of the patient. This term does not define the segmental atrioventricular or ventriculoarterial relationships.

96. What is mesocardia?

Mesocardia occurs when the heart occupies the midline of the thorax.

Van Praagh R, Weinberg PM, Foran RB, et al. Malposition of the heart. In: Adams FH, Emmanoulides GC, RT Reimenschneider TH, editors. Moss' heart disease in infants, children and adolescents. 5th ed. Baltimore: Williams and Wilkins; 1994.

Jacobs JP, Anderson RH, Weinberg PM, et al. The nomenclature, definition and classification of cardiac structure in the setting of heterotaxy. Cardiol Young 2007;17(Suppl. 2):1–28.

Cohen MS, Anderson RH, Cohen MI, et al. Controversies, genetics, diagnostic assessment, and outcomes relating to the heterotaxy syndrome. Cardiol Young 2007;17(2):29–43.

✓ KEY POINTS: FEEDING NEONATES WITH CHD

1. Close clinical assessment is needed when feeding neonates with ductal-dependent congenital heart disease.

2. Complexity of congenital heart defect and time of intubation are two predictors of postoperative feeding dysfunction.

---

97. **What are modalities used to determine feeding readiness in neonates with ductal-dependent CHD?**

There are noticeable variations in strategies for preoperative feeding management between providers. Approximately 56% of clinicians will provide enteral feedings to neonates with ductal-dependent CHD. Clinicians practicing outside the United States are eight times more likely to enterally feed ductal-dependent neonates than clinicians practicing in the United States. Clinical assessment, arterial blood gas assessment, blood lactate level, diastolic blood pressure, echocardiogram, abdominal x-ray, and abdominal near-infrared spectroscopy may be helpful in making this decision.

98. **What is the most common reason that enteral feedings are withheld from neonates with ductal-dependent CHD?**

The most commonly reported reason for exercising caution when feeding neonates with ductal-dependent CHD is the theoretical risk of intestinal hypoperfusion, which may lead to necrotizing enterocolitis. The two most common findings seen in neonates with CHD and necrotizing enterocolits are widened pulse pressure and low diastolic blood pressure, which are seen in patients with retrograde diastolic flow in the descending aorta.

Howley LW, Kaufman J, Wymore E, et al. Enteral feeding in neonates with prostaglandin-dependent congenital cardiac disease: international survey on current trends and variations in practice. Cardiol Young 2012;22:121–127.

Medoff-Cooper B, Naim M, Torowicz D, et al. Feeding, growth, and nutrition in children with congenitally malformed hearts. Cardiol Young 2010;20(Suppl. 3):149–153.

Kogon BE, Ramaswamy V, Todd K, et al. Feeding difficulty in newborns following congenital heart surgery. Congenit Heart Dis 2007;2:332–37.

CARDIAC SURGERY

99. **What congenital heart lesions are treated with placement of a shunt in the newborn period?**

The modified Blalock–Taussig shunt is a Gore-Tex interposition shunt placed between the subclavian artery (right or left) and the right or left pulmonary artery. It is used for congenital heart lesions that require increased PBF in the neonatal and infancy periods. Examples include lesions with a hypoplastic pulmonary annulus, atretic pulmonary valve annulus, or severely hypoplastic main and branch pulmonary arteries. The cardiac malformations in such instances would include severe tetralogy of Fallot, tetralogy of Fallot with pulmonary atresia, tricuspid atresia, pulmonary atresia with VSD, and pulmonary atresia with intact ventricular septum. A modified Blalock–Taussig shunt is used in the first stage of HLHS repair (modified Norwood operation) (Fig. 6-12).

100. **What are the major shunts used in heart surgery?**

The modified Blalock–Taussig, the bidirectional Glenn procedure, and the Sano modification of the Norwood operation are the most common types of shunts used today. The Waterston shunt

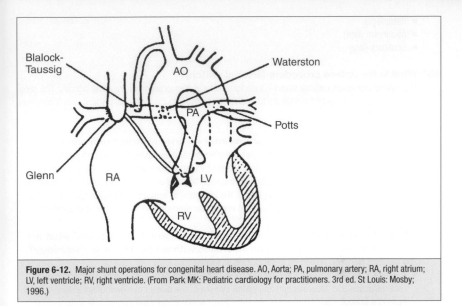

Figure 6-12. Major shunt operations for congenital heart disease. AO, Aorta; PA, pulmonary artery; RA, right atrium; LV, left ventricle; RV, right ventricle. (From Park MK: Pediatric cardiology for practitioners. 3rd ed. St Louis: Mosby; 1996.)

(anastomosis from the ascending aorta to the right pulmonary artery) and the Potts shunt (anastomosis from the descending aorta to the left pulmonary artery) shunts are no longer used.

101. **What is a Glenn procedure, and in what kinds of congenital heart disease is it used?**
   A bidirectional Glenn anastomosis is a connection from the right superior vena cava to the right pulmonary artery, or the left superior vena cava to the left pulmonary artery, or both (bicaval bidirectional Glenn anastomosis). The pulmonary arteries are in continuity, so a right bidirectional Glenn anastomosis connection will send blood flow into the right and the left pulmonary arteries. This anastomosis is usually the intermediate step to a Fontan procedure. Lesions for which a bidirectional Glenn procedure is used include those with single ventricle anatomy (HLHS, hypoplastic right heart syndrome, tricuspid atresia, and pulmonary atresia).

102. **How is coarctation of the aorta approached?**
   In neonates coarctation of the aorta is generally approached through a left thoracotomy. In older children a primary catheter balloon intervention may be considered. The three standard surgical approaches involve resection and end-to-end anastamosis (most common), subclavian flap repair (ligation of distal subclavian artery to use the proximal portion to overlay patch the coarctation segment), or patching with foreign material (Dacron).

103. **What are the potential complications after repair of coarctation of the aorta?**
   - Residual obstruction
   - Bleeding
   - Hemothorax
   - Chylothorax
   - Recurrent laryngeal nerve injury
   - Phrenic nerve injury
   - Hoarseness
   - Paradoxical hypertension (rare in neonate)

- Paraplegia
- Aneurysm (late)
- Scoliosis (late)

104. What is the Jatene procedure (arterial switch)?
The Jatene procedure (arterial switch) is performed for d-transposition of the great arteries. The coronary arteries are removed from the aorta and re-implanted into the pulmonary artery, which becomes the new aorta.

105. What are the potential complications after an arterial switch procedure?
Left ventricular dysfunction, supraventricular arrhythmias, and supravalvar aortic and pulmonary stenosis are all potential complications. Both left ventricular dysfunction and arrhythmias may be a sign of coronary insufficiency. In patients with transposition of the great arteries and a VSD, a residual VSD should be ruled out by echocardiography. The presence of ventricular arrhythmias should also elicit questions regarding the adequacy of the ventricular function and coronary re-implantation.

106. What is the Norwood procedure (or modified Norwood, stage I), and what are the two additional procedures for neonates with single-ventricle physiology?
The modified Norwood procedure is performed as follows:
- A. Stage 1: Anastomosis of the proximal main pulmonary artery to the aorta, with aortic arch reconstruction and trans-section and patch closure of the distal main pulmonary artery; a modified right Blalock–Taussig shunt (right subclavian artery to right pulmonary artery) to provide PBF, and lastly, atrial septectomy to allow for adequate left-to-right atrial communication.
- A. Stage 1 (alternate approach): In some centers a Norwood–Sano operation is performed as a first stage. In this operation the modified Blalock–Taussig shunt is replaced with a right ventricle to main pulmonary artery connection (Sano modification) to provide PBF.
- B. Stage 2: Bidirectional Glenn anastomosis (approximately 4 to 6 months)
- C. Stage 3: Completion of a Fontan operation (approximately 1 to 2 years)

107. What are some of the warning signs of postoperative cardiac tamponade?
Tachycardia, decrease in oxygen saturation, increase in cardiac filling pressures, abrupt decrease in chest tube drainage, increasing cardiac size on chest x-ray, and poor perfusion are all warning signs of postoperative cardiac tamponade. Abrupt resolution of postoperative bleeding should prompt consideration for development of a pericardial effusion. Pulsus paradoxus may not be evident in mechanically ventilated patients unless they are spontaneously breathing.

108. What are some of the concerns in a neonate with an "open chest" after heart surgery?
The infant should be kept deeply sedated and generally paralyzed. The wound should be covered. Lung tidal volume should be adjusted appropriately so that the lung does not herniate. Monitored cardiac pressures are usually low. These patients require broad-spectrum antibiotic coverage. Before the chest is closed, vigorous diuresis is usually required. When the chest is eventually closed, all of the intravascular pressures will increase, airway compliance will increase, and tidal volume should be adjusted downward.

109. Why is junctional ectopic tachycardia important to recognize in the postoperative period?
Junctional ectopic tachycardia (JET) is a common arrhythmia after surgery. The rhythm generally occurs in the first 24 to 48 hours following surgery. Typical electrocardiographic findings include AV dissociation and narrow QRS morphology with a rapid QRS rate (170 to 210 bpm). Treatment for JET involves slowing the ectopic rate to allow restoration of AV synchrony. Core temperature cooling (i.e., 35 to 36° C) has been effective. Amiodarone has also been used to slow the junctional rate so as to allow temporary pacing to restore AV synchrony. Typically, as the infant recovers from surgery with less need for intravenous inotropic support, the JET resolves.

110. **If the infant cannot be taken off cardiopulmonary bypass after surgery, what are the options?**
Extracorporeal membrane organization (ECMO) can provide a means to assist the heart and lungs (or both) temporarily. Venoarterial ECMO is used in neonatal patients with either life-threatening pulmonary disease (congenital diaphragmatic hernia, or persistent fetal circulation) or neonates with postoperative ventricular failure.

Chang AC, Hanley FL, Wernovsky G, et al. Pediatric cardiac intensive care. Baltimore: Williams & Wilkins; 1998.
Anderson RH, Baker EJ, Penny DJ, et al. Paediatric cardiology. 3rd ed. Philadelphia: Churchill Livingstone Elsevier; 2010.
Gazit AZ, Huddleston CB, Checcia PA, et al. Care of the pediatric cardiac surgery patient part I. Curr Probl Surg 2010;47:185–250.
Gazit AZ, Huddleston CB, Checcia PA, et al. Care of the pediatric cardiac surgery patient part I. Curr Probl Surg 2010;47:261–376.

✓ KEY POINTS: PREOPERATIVE STABILIZATION

1. There are a variety of presentations in an infant with congenital heart disease.

2. The starting dose of prostaglandin E_1 (PGE1) is 0.05 to 0.10 µg/kg/min.

3. To maintain patency of the ductus arteriosus, prostaglandin E1 (PGE1) is used in both right- and left-sided heart obstructive lesions; often the dose can be lowered to 0.01 to 0.02 µg/kg/min.

---

111. **What are the principles of preoperative management in the neonate with critical congenital heart disease?**
In critical congenital heart lesions the ultimate outcome depends on timely and accurate assessment of the structural anomaly and on evaluation and resuscitation of secondary organ damage. The principles of preoperative management are as follows:
- Initial stabilization: airway management, vascular access, and maintaining patency of a ductus arteriosus with PGE1. Delineation of the anatomic defect should be performed by echocardiography.
- Evaluation and treatment of additional organ system dysfunction, particularly of the pulmonary, renal, hepatic, and central nervous system
- Evaluation of other congenital heart defects
- Genetic evaluation
- Cardiac catheterization if indicated
- Surgical management if indicated, when all other systems are optimized

112. **How should PGE1 be administered?**
The starting dose of PGE1 is 0.05 to 0.1 µg/kg/min. This drug should be administered using a continuous intravenous drip, preferentially through an umbilical venous line, or a well-functioning intravenous line. Once the effects of PGE1 are seen (improved oxygen saturations, decreased acidemia), the dose can be slowly reduced to 0.01 µg/kg/min.

113. **What are the neonatal presentations of CHD?**
- Persistent cyanosis
- Differential diagnosis: CHD, lung parenchyma disease, primary pulmonary hypertension, ductal=dependent pulmonary CHD.
- Low cardiac output
- Differential diagnosis: CHD, septic shock, ductal-dependent systemic CHD
- CHF
- Differential diagnosis: CHD with left→right shunt, viral respiratory infections superimposed on mild CHD, lung parenchyma disease, primary pulmonary hypertension, ductal-dependent pulmonary CHD.

114. In which patients should PGE1 be used?
- Neonates who fail a hyperoxia test: This procedure indicates an infant who is highly likely to have congenital heart disease that is ductal dependent.
- Neonates with a confirmed congenital heart defect (by echocardiography) that is ductal dependent for pulmonary or systemic blood flow, or a lesion that requires a PDA for inter-circulatory mixing
- The neonate who presents with circulatory shock in weeks 1 to 2 of life

115. What are some of the side effects of PGE1?
Side effects of PGE1 include the following:
- Apnea
- Peripheral vasodilation
- Hypotension
- Temperature elevation
- Diarrhea

Side effects may be more complex in infants weighing less than 2 kg.

116. In what lesions does keeping the ductus open help improve PBF, and in what lesions does keeping the ductus open help improve cardiac output?
In lesions with right ventricular outflow obstruction, the ductus arteriosus helps improve PBF by shunting blood into the pulmonary arteries, (e.g., tetralogy of Fallot with severe pulmonary valvar or subvalvar obstruction, tricuspid atresia, pulmonary atresia). In lesions with left ventricular outflow obstruction (e.g., HLHS, critical aortic stenosis, neonatal coarctation of the aorta), the ductus arteriosus maintains cardiac output to the systemic bed, optimizing myocardial perfusion.

117. Will a hyperoxia test always increase the PaO_2 in PPHN?
Patients with PPHN may fail to demonstrate a significant rise in PaO_2 secondary to right→left shunting. Patients with PPHN have oligemic lung fields on chest radiograph. Approximately 10% of neonates on venoarterial ECMO for respiratory distress and PPHN will have unsuspected CHD.

118. What testing should generally be performed before CHD surgery in a neonate?
Genetic testing with fluorescence in situ hybridization (FISH) analysis should be considered, especially if a conotruncal abnormality is present. Abdominal ultrasound should be considered if there is any association of known renal, splenic, or situs concerns. Laboratory studies including renal and hepatic function should be evaluated to look for end-organ dysfunction. A head ultrasound or other central nervous system imaging modality may be considered, especially if there were any *in utero* concerns.

119. How are unsuspected CHD and sepsis related?
Neonates with sepsis will demonstrate similar clinical findings to those of neonates with ductal-dependent systemic CHD. Antibiotic delivery will have little impact in this cohort. Patency of the ductus is critical in the group with CHD to maintain coronary perfusion and prevent myocardial ischemia.

Chang AC, Hanley FL, Wernovsky G, et al. Pediatric cardiac intensive care. Baltimore: Williams & Wilkins; 1998.
Brooks PA, Penny DJ. Management of the sick neonate with suspected heart disease. Early Hum Dev 2008;84:155–159.

✓ KEY POINTS: POSTOPERATIVE MANAGEMENT

1. During the care of postoperative patients, it is important to assess the patient, not just the laboratory values and the numbers.

120. **What information is needed to care for the neonate with congenital heart disease after cardiothoracic surgery?**
- The underlying anatomic defect and the expectations of surgical repair
- The clinical/physiologic status of the infant in the preoperative period
- The anesthetic regimen used during surgery
- The duration of the cardiopulmonary bypass, aortic cross clamp time, and circulatory arrest time
- The details of the operative procedure
- The data available from monitoring catheters, physical examination, radiographs, echocardiography, and electrocardiography
- Intraoperative monitors:
  - Pulse oximetry
  - Heart rate, blood pressure, end-tidal CO_2
  - Bradyarrhythmias, if any
  - Tachyarrhythmias, if any
  - ST segment changes

121. **What is the purpose of the postoperative echocardiogram?**
The postoperative echocardiogram, most commonly transesophageal, should assess for the following:
- Residual lesions
- Ventricular function (both right ventricular and left ventricular)
- Adequacy of the semilunar and AV valves
- Diastolic function
- General assessment of the preload (volume) of the ventricular chambers

122. **What are the most common noncardiac causes of respiratory compromise after cardiothoracic surgery?**
See Table 6-3.

123. **What cardiac surgical procedures are associated with phrenic nerve palsy?**
Procedures associated with phrenic nerve injury:
- Aortic arch reconstruction
- Interrupted aortic arch repair or coarctation repair
- Arterial switch operation
- Tetralogy of Fallot:
  - Tetralogy of Fallot/absent pulmonary valve repair: pulmonary artery plication
  - Tetralogy of Fallot/pulmonary atresia: unifocalization
- Truncus arteriosus repair
- PDA ligation
- Systemic-to-pulmonary shunt

Adapted from Marino BS, Wernovsky G. Preoperative and postoperative care of the infant with critical congenital heart disease. In: Avery GB, Fletcher MA, MacDonald MG, editors. Neonatology: athophysiology and management of the newborn. Philadelphia: Lippincott Williams and Wilkins; 1999. p. 664.

124. **What are the common reasons a chylothorax occurs after cardiac surgery?**
Chylothorax is a rare complication of cardiac surgery with an incidence of approximately 0.85% to 3.8%. Chylothorax may occur as a direct injury to the thoracic duct in surgeries such as coarctation of the aorta repair or PDA ligation. Second, it may occur with thrombosis of the superior vena cava, leading to increased hydrostatic pressure in the superior vena cava and thoracic duct. Third, high central venous pressures after a surgery such as a Glenn palliation for HLHS may cause chylothorax. Most common surgeries that are complicated by chylothoraces are tetralogy of Fallot, Glenn and Fontan palliation, and orthotopic heart transplantation.

TABLE 6-3. NONCARDIAC CAUSES OF RESPIRATORY COMPROMISE AFTER CARDIOTHORACIC SURGERY[2]

(Adapted from Newth CJL, Hammer J. Pulmonary issues. In: Chang AC, Hanley FL, Wernovsky G, Wessel DL, editors. Pediatric cardiac intensive care. Baltimore: Williams & Wilkins; 1998. p 352.)

CENTRAL NERVOUS SYSTEM	NEUROMUSCULAR
1. General anesthesia	1. Residual neuromuscular blockade
2. Administration of analgesics or sedative/hypnotics	2. Respiratory muscle weakness—from disuse and/or malnutrition
3. Hypoxic-ischemic encephalopathy	**Alveolar disease**
4. Apnea of prematurity	1. Acute lung injury from cardiopulmonary bypass
Isolated neuropathies	2. Increased lung fluid from left-to-right shunt lesions
1. Hemidiaphragmatic paresis or paralysis - phrenic nerve injury	3. Atelectasis
2. Vocal cord paralysis - recurrent	4. Pneumonia
Airway abnormalities proximal to the alveoli	5. Pulmonary hemorrhage
1. Tracheostomy or endotracheal tube obstruction	6. Pulmonary hypoplasia
2. Post-extubation subglottic edema	**Extrinsic lung compression**
3. Laryngotracheomalacia	1. Pleural effusion (transudate vs. exudate)
4. Left mainstem bronchomalacia from long-standing left atrial or left pulmonary artery enlargement	2. Pneumothorax, hemothorax, chylothorax
	Chest Wall
	1. Midsternal
	2. Thoracotomy
	3. Clam-shell incisions

125. **What is a recommended strategy to treat a chylothorax postoperatively?**
Placement of a chest tube with the initiation of a medium-chain triglyceride diet is the initial management. Total parenteral nutrition with enteric rest (nothing by mouth) may be needed if conservative management fails. Adjuvant therapy includes diuretics, albumin infusions, immuno-globulin replacement, electrolyte replacement, and fresh frozen plasma and antithrombin replacement. Anticoagulation with heparin or enoxaparin should be considered. Corticosteroids have been shown to have some benefit after the Fontan operation. Octreotide infusion followed by thoracic duct ligation may be needed in cases not amenable to other measures. Caution should be used with octreotide, and it is generally recommended that the patient receive nothing by mouth during octreotide infusion.

126. **What are the major risk factors for postoperative feeding dysfunction?**
Increased risk adjusted congenital heart surgery score, prolonged intubation time, low birth weight, and neurological co-morbidities.

127. **How can cardiac output be assessed after cardiothoracic surgery?**
- Physical examination
  - Pulses
  - Peripheral perfusion

- Vital signs
  - Heart rate
  - Blood pressure
- Monitoring
  - Urine output
  - Somatic and cerebral near-infrared spectroscopy (NIRS)
- Laboratory studies/images
  - Blood gas (absence of acidosis)
  - Absence of lactate
  - Echocardiogram
  - Normal end-organ function

128. What is near-infrared spectroscopy (NIRS)?
NIRS is a noninvasive method that is used to monitor hemoglobin oxygen saturation using nonpulsatile oximetry. A fair correlation exists between superior vena cava venous oxygen saturation and cerebral NIRS. Somatic NIRS (renal) may be helpful to show regional perfusion. NIRS in conjunction with pulse oximetry may yield an estimate of cardiac output.

129. What consideration should be given to the neonate after surgery for oral or nasogastric feeding?
Although there is no correct answer, the clinician should consider whether the infant was fed before surgery, length of bypass and circulatory arrest times, adequacy of the cardiac output, presence of bowel sounds, minimization of vasoconstrictive agents, and the absence of lactic acidosis. Local systemic monitoring with NIRS may be helpful.

Marino BS, Wernovsky G. Preoperative and postoperative care of the infant with critical congenital heart disease. In: Avery GB, Fletcher MA, MacDonald MG, editors. Neonatology: pathophysiology and management of the newborn. Philadelphia: Lippincott: Williams and Wilkins; 1999. p. 664.

Newth CJL, Hammer J. Pulmonary issues. In: Chang AC, Hanley FL, Wernovsky G, Wessel DL, editors. Pediatric cardiac intensive care. Baltimore: Williams and Wilkins; 1998. p. 352.

Ricci Z, Garisto C, Favia I, et al. Cerebral NIRS as a marker of superior vena cava oxygen saturation in neonate with congenital heart disease. Paediatr Anaesth 2010;20:1040–45.

Hirsch JC, Charpie JR, Ohye R, et al. Near-infrared spectroscopy: what we know and we need to know—a systematic review of congenital heart disease literature. J Thorac Cardiovasc Surg 2009;137:154–59.

CARDIAC TRANSPLANTATION

130. What are signs of rejection in a neonate who had undergone a cardiac transplant?
Most rejection episodes in the era of cyclosporine immunosuppression are relatively asymptomatic, especially in the older child. The neonatal recipient, however, can often have the nonspecific findings of fever, irritability, tachycardia, loss of appetite, and an S_3 gallop on physical examination.

131. What are major long-term complications that can occur after heart transplantation?
Rejection, infection, coronary artery disease, hypertension, renal dysfunction, and tumors may occur.

132. Can a heart that is rejecting have preserved systolic function on echocardiogram?
Yes.

133. What are the important hemodynamic considerations in the post-transplanted heart?

During cardiac transplantation all nerves to the heart are severed so that there is no direct sympathetic or parasympathetic control of heart rate. Concomitantly, during the first few postoperative days the stroke volume of the transplanted heart is relatively fixed, and the contractility of the heart is diminished secondary to the ischemia that occurred during harvest and implantation. Cardiac output is directly proportional to changes in the heart rate in the early postoperative period. Therefore many surgeons try to maintain cardiac output by pacing the heart with temporary pacing wires.

134. Are neonates at an advantage compared with older children with regard to heart transplantation?

Some evidence suggests that infants who receive transplants when younger than 6 months of age have improved survival 10 years after the transplant compared with older children. Newborn infants do not have a mature complement system and do not produce a typical isohemagglutinin response to blood groups. As such, it is possible to perform ABO-incompatible heart transplantation during infancy.

Canter CE, Shaddy RE, Bernstein D, et al. Indications for heart transplantation in pediatric heart disease. Circulation 2007;115:658–676.

Anderson RH, Baker EJ, Penny DJ, et al. Paediatric cardiology. 3rd ed. Philadelphia: Churchill Livingstone Elsevier; 2010.

Bernstein D. Heart transplantation in neonates: achievements, challenges, and controversies for the future. Neo Rev 2000;8:e152–8.

Saczkowski R, Dacey C, Bernier P. Does ABO-incompatible and ABO-compatible neonatal heart transplant have equivalent survival? Interact Cardiovasc Thorac Surg 2010;10:1026–33.

✓ KEY POINTS: INTERVENTIONAL CARDIOLOGY

1. After cardiac catheterization in a neonate, it is crucial to assess vital signs, femoral and dorsalis pedis pulses, and hematocrit levels.

135. Which kinds of congenital heart disease may benefit from a cardiac catheterization interventional procedure?

See Table 6-4.

TABLE 6-4. CONGENITAL HEART DISEASES THAT MAY BENEFIT FROM CARDIAC CATHETERIZATION INTERVENTIONAL PROCEDURES

CONGENITAL HEART DISEASE	CARDIAC INTERVENTIONAL PROCEDURE
Transposition of the great arteries/intact ventricular septum	Rashkind balloon atrial septostomy
Critical aortic stenosis	Aortic balloon valvuloplasty
Critical pulmonic stenosis	Pulmonary balloon valvuloplasty
Restrictive atrial septum • Tricuspid atresia • Pulmonary atresia with intact ventricular septum • Restrictive atrial septum • Total anomalous pulmonary venous return • Hypoplastic left heart syndrome	Balloon or blade atrial septostomy
Pulmonary atresia/intact ventricular septum	Pulmonary valve perforation (radiofrequency)

136. **Which anomaly of the systemic veins may prevent access to the right side of the heart from the femoral veins?**
An interrupted inferior vena cava prevents access to the right side of the heart from the femoral veins. This interruption, however, is usually below the level of the hepatic veins. Therefore the umbilical vein remains an alternative way to gain access to the right side of the heart.

137. **How is a balloon atrial septostomy performed?**
Although originally developed using fluoroscopy, a balloon atrial septostomy may be performed at the bedside using transthoracic echocardiography guidance.

Kutty S, Zahn E. Interventional therapy for neonates with critical congenital heart disease. Catheterization and cardiovascular interventions. 2008;72:663–74.
Freedom RM, Mawson JB, Yoo SJ, et al. Congenital heart disease: textbook of angiography. Armonk, NY: Futura; 1997.

✓ **KEY POINTS: INTERPRETING NORMAL AND ABNORMAL ELECTROCARDIOGRAMS IN THE NEWBORN PERIOD**

1. Left axis deviation in a newborn electrocardiography is abnormal.

2. T waves should be inverted in V_1 by 3 days of age.

138. **What is characteristic of a full-term normal newborn electrocardiographic reading?**
Compared with the electrocardiographic reading of an older infant or child, the newborn electrocardiographic reading is remarkable for the following reasons:
- Right axis deviation +55-200 degrees (premature infants are generally 65-174 degrees)
- Right ventricular dominance, tall R wave in V_1, and deep S wave in V_6
- Positive T wave in the right precordial leads V_3r, V_4r, and V_1
- Longer QTc interval up to 0.46 sec
- QRS duration less than 80 msec
- Right ventricular forces decrease over the first 6 months of life.

139. **What electrocardiographic findings are always abnormal in a newborn?**
The normal electrocardiogram in a newborn shows a preponderance of right ventricular forces because the right and left ventricles are of equal mass at birth. The mean QRS axis for a newborn is 110 degrees. Left axis deviation (<30 degrees) is always abnormal. Downward forces in the QRS in lead AVF and upward forces in lead 1 indicate a left axis deviation. This appearance is typically associated with tricuspid atresia. Patients with AV septal defects typically have a superiorly oriented frontal QRS loop manifested by dominant S waves in the inferior leads (III and aVF) and a prominent R wave in aVR. This finding is in contradistinction to tricuspid atresia in which the RV precordial leads lack RV dominance.

140. **What is the definition and differential diagnosis of sinus tachycardia in a newborn?**
The upper limit of normal for a quiet awake newborn in 166 bpm. Healthy newborn infants may transiently reach 230 bpm. The differential diagnoses should include fever, infection, anemia, pain, hypovolemia, hyperthyroidsim, myocarditis, and drug interaction.

141. **What is the definition and differential diagnosis of sinus bradycardia in a newborn?**
Sinus bracycardia is defined as sinus rhythm with a heart rate (awake) below the lower normal limit (91 bpm first week of life and 107 bpm first month of life). Symptoms of severe bradycardia may

include poor growth, feeding intolerance, and dyspnea. The differential diagnoses include central nervous system abnormalities, hypothermia, hypopituitarism, increased intracranial pressure, maternal drugs, hypothyroidism, long QTc, and a transient form related to maternal anti Ro/SSA+ mothers. Blocked premature atrial beats are common, often having a pause that may average out the heart rate on the monitor to a lower than clinically relevant number, but rarely cause symptoms.

142. **What is the most common tachyarrhythmia in the newborn, and how is it treated?**
SVT is the most common tachycardia in the term newborn and premature infant and manifests as a narrow complex tachycardia at rates of 250 to 300 bpm. The mechanism is usually a re-entrant type of tachycardia. It can be treated with adenosine (100 to 250 μg/kg) given as a rapid push. Adenosine blocks conduction through the AV node, resulting in a transient bradycardia and interruption of the re-entrant circuit. Once the heart rate has been converted to normal sinus rhythm, the infant should have a 12-lead electrocardiogram to rule out a delta wave and the presence of a Wolff–Parkinson–White type of SVT.

143. **What are the electrocardiographic signs of abnormal right ventricular hypertrophy in a newborn?**
- A Q wave in V_1 (qR or qRs pattern) suggests right ventricular hypertrophy.
- An upright T wave in V_1 after the third day of life also is consistent with right ventricular hypertrophy.
- Increased R wave in V_1
- Increased S wave in V_6

144. **How is the diagnosis of ventricular tachycardia made?**
Ventricular tachycardia typically has a broad QRS complex (>120 msec). Ventricular-atrial dissociation may be present. A 12-lead electrocardiogram may reveal a QRS axis different than the sinus QRS axis. Fusion (sinus capture beats and a tachycardia beat) affirms the diagnosis.

145. **What are the electrocardiographic abnormalities observed in infants with hyperkalemia?**
- The earliest change seen in a patient with hyperkalemia is the development of tall, peaked T waves in the precordial leads.
- With further elevation of the serum potassium concentration, there is a reduction in the R wave, a widening of the QRS complex, ST-segment elevation or depression, and PR prolongation.
- Ultimately, there is further widening of the QRS complex and cardiac arrest (Fig. 6-13).

146. **What are the electrocardiographic abnormalities observed in infants with hypokalemia?**
- Depressions of the ST segment with flattening of the T wave
- Development of prominent U waves with QTU prolongation
- Development of ventricular arrhythmias

147. **What other electrolyte disturbance mimics hypokalemia?**
Hypomagnesemia may mimic hypokalemia.

148. **What electrocardiographic disturbances are seen in infants with hypocalcemia?**
Prolongation of the QT interval may be evident.

149. **What electrocardiographic changes are associated with digitalis?**
- *Digitalis effect*: Shortening of QTc, sagging of the ST segment, decreased T wave amplitude, and slowing of heart rate. Digitalis effects are usually seen during ventricular repolarization.

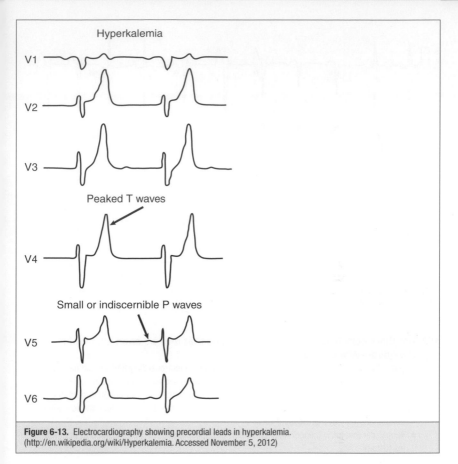

Figure 6-13. Electrocardiography showing precordial leads in hyperkalemia. (http://en.wikipedia.org/wiki/Hyperkalemia. Accessed November 5, 2012)

- *Digitalis toxicity:* Prolongation of PR interval, sinus bradycardia, heart block (second degree), arrhythmias—supraventricular and ventricular. Toxic effects of digoxin are usually seen in the formation and conduction of the impulse.

150. What is a delta wave?
A delta wave is a slurring in the upstroke of the QRS complex; it generally occurs in association with a short PR interval. The delta wave signifies that some or all of the atrial depolarization to the ventricle is by way of a bypass tract rather than solely antegrade through the AV node. This finding is associated with a Wolff–Parkinson–White pattern on the electrocardiogram. Patients with a Wolff–Parkinson–White pattern may develop SVT (also called Wolff–Parkinson–White syndrome) (Fig. 6-14).

151. What is the Wolff–Parkinson–White syndrome?
Anatomic substrate results in a direct electrical communication between the atria and the ventricles rather than through the AV node. Conduction becomes a fusion between AV nodal conduction and antegrade conduction via the bypass tract. Patients with an electrocardiogram having a Wolff–Parkinson–White pattern may have SVT and be considered as having Wolff–Parkinson–White syndrome.

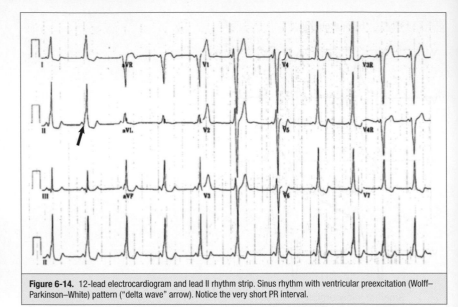

Figure 6-14. 12-lead electrocardiogram and lead II rhythm strip. Sinus rhythm with ventricular preexcitation (Wolff–Parkinson–White) pattern ("delta wave" arrow). Notice the very short PR interval.

152. **Are there certain congenital heart lesions that may be seen with Wolff–Parkinson–White syndrome?**

   All patients with a Wolff–Parkinson–White pattern on their electrocardiograms should have an echocardiogram to rule out structural heart disease. Digoxin should not be used in patients with Wolff–Parkinson–White syndrome because of its effect on increasing conduction through the accessory pathway rather than through the normal AV node. Associated lesions include the following:
   - Ebstein anomaly of the tricuspid valve
   - Ventricular inversion (congenitally corrected transpositions; levo-transposition of the great arteries [l-tga])
   - Hypertrophic cardiomyopathy
   - Cardiac tumors

153. **What is a normal QTc interval in a newborn infant?**

   The upper limit of normal (2SD) is 440 msec on the fourth day of life (2.5% of normal neonates will have a prolonged QTc). Newborns with a prolonged QTc on the first day of life should have a repeat electrocardiogram performed in 1 or 2 days. Prolonged QTc has been associated with an increased risk of sudden infant death syndrome. Newborns with a QTc greater than 440 msec should have a very detailed family history obtained for early sudden cardiac death, seizures, syncope, and unexplained car accidents.

154. **What other conditions may be included in the differential diagnosis of a prolonged QT interval on an electrocardiogram?**
   - Hypocalcemia
   - Hypokalemia
   - Central nervous system abnormalities
   - Macrolide antibiotics
   - Prokinetics (Fig. 6-15)

Schwartz PJ, Garson A Jr., Paul T, et al. Guidelines for the interpretation of the neonatal electrocardiogram. Eur Heart J. 2002;23:1329–44.

Taeusch HW, Ballard RA, Gleason CA. Avery's disease of the newborn. 8th ed. Philadelphia: Elsevier Saunders; 2005.

KEY POINTS: ARRHYTHMIAS

1. Maternal connective tissue diseases (systemic lupus erythematosus and Sjögren syndrome) can cause complete congenital heart block or dilated cardiomyopathy (or both) in the fetus and infant.

2. Atrial premature contractions are benign arrhythmias. On rare occasions and if sufficiently frequent, they can trigger SVT.

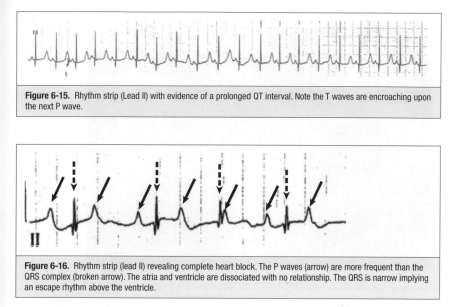

Figure 6-15. Rhythm strip (Lead II) with evidence of a prolonged QT interval. Note the T waves are encroaching upon the next P wave.

Figure 6-16. Rhythm strip (lead II) revealing complete heart block. The P waves (arrow) are more frequent than the QRS complex (broken arrow). The atria and ventricle are dissociated with no relationship. The QRS is narrow implying an escape rhythm above the ventricle.

155. **What are congenital anatomic and nonanatomic causes of congenital complete heart block in the fetus?**

    Congenital complete heart block in the fetus can occur as a result of structural congenital heart disease (L-TGA, left atrial isomerism, or maternal collagen vascular disease). Heart block occurs in women with a variety of connective tissue diseases (e.g., systemic lupus erythematosus, Sjögren syndrome). The incidence is 1/15,000 to 1/20,000 infants. Anti-RO (SSA) and La (SSB) antibodies are found in many of these women, but only a minority of fetuses are affected. Most cases are identified between 18 and 24 weeks' gestation (Fig. 6-16).

156. **What are common benign arrhythmias seen in the fetus?**

    The most common benign arrhythmia in the fetus is a premature atrial contraction. This benign dysrhythmia is commonly detected during fetal monitoring. Blocked premature atrial contractions often cause what appears to be a pause on the monitoring strips, and they occur when the ventricle is refractory and not conducted (Fig. 6-17).

157. **What type of arrhythmias can be diagnosed in the fetus?**

    All types of tachyarrhythmias and bradyarrhythmias can be detected. Premature beats account for 80% to 90% of fetal arrhythmias but are generally benign. Re-entrant supraventricular tachyarrhythmias account for 5% of fetal arrhythmias, complete heart block 2.5%, and atrial flutter 1% to 2%. Ventricular arrhythmias are rare (Fig. 6-18).

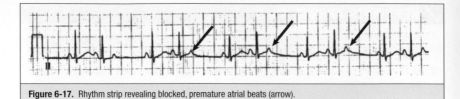

Figure 6-17. Rhythm strip revealing blocked, premature atrial beats (arrow).

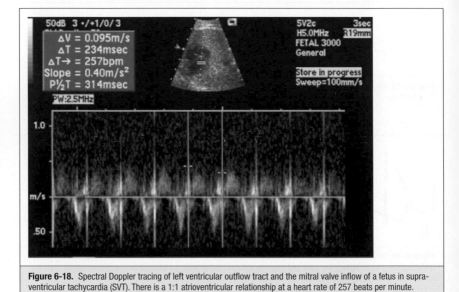

Figure 6-18. Spectral Doppler tracing of left ventricular outflow tract and the mitral valve inflow of a fetus in supraventricular tachycardia (SVT). There is a 1:1 atrioventricular relationship at a heart rate of 257 beats per minute.

158. What is the most common form of SVT in a neonate?

The most common SVT in a neonate relates to an accessory pathway. In this form of SVT conduction tends to proceed antegrade via the AV node and retrograde through the bypass tract. The electrocardiogram tends to have a narrow QRS complex with a short repolarization interval and rates greater than 220 bpm. A rare form of SVT (permanent junctional reciprocating tachycardia) may have a long repolarization with a more incessant course and slower rates (180 to 200 bpm).

159. What is the natural history of SVT presenting in the neonatal period?

Spontaneous resolution of SVT will occur in the first year of life in nearly 50% of patients. Most (60% to 90%) of infants with Wolff–Parkinson–White syndrome undergo spontaneous resolution by 1 year of age.

160. What drugs should be considered for maintenance therapy in neonates with SVT?

Antiarrhythmic preference is often based on the severity of the symptoms. For straightforward SVT that terminated with intravenous adenosine, beta blockers tend to be relatively safe and effective. In infants with beta-blocker refractory SVT, alternative drugs to consider are flecainide, sotalol, and amiodarone. All three of these drugs have potential pro-arrhythmic side effects and institution of such antiarrhythmics should occur in a hospital (monitor/telemetry) setting. In general flecainide should

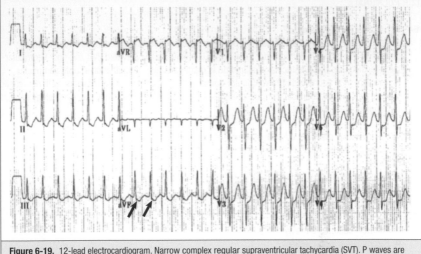

Figure 6-19. 12-lead electrocardiogram. Narrow complex regular supraventricular tachycardia (SVT). P waves are visible at the tail of the QRS (arrow).

not be administered to patients with significant structural heart disease. The QTc should be closely followed in patients on either sotalol or amiodarone (Fig. 6-19).

161. How is atrial flutter managed in a neonate?

Atrial flutter is a relatively uncommon arrhythmia in newborns and infants. Presenting symptoms typically occur within the first 2 days of life, and there does not tend to be an association with structural heart defects. The ventricular rate depends on the degree of AV nodal conduction. Spontaneous termination is rare. Direct cardioversion or overdrive esophageal atrial pacing therapies are effective in more than half of the cases. Symptoms of CHF relate to the duration of the tachycardia. Approximately 20% of infants may have a second supraventricular arrhythmia, which will typically manifest within 48 hours.

162. What is the long QT (LQT) syndrome?

LQT syndrome is a genetic mutation of several genes encoding ionic (Na+/K+) currents responsible for ventricular repolarization. The incidence is 1 in 3000 to 1 in 5000. A detailed family history is critical and should assess for early sudden death, fainting, seizures, and unexplained car accidents. There is a low penetrance, and gene carriers may not always show the phenotype at a young age. Beta blockers are the first choice of therapy and should be instituted in patients with the diagnosis regardless of symptoms.

163. Which LQT patients are at highest risk?

- QTc greater than 600 msec
- T wave alternans
- 2:1 AV block
- Sensorineural hearing loss

Fischbach PS, Frias PA, Strieper MJ, et al. Natural history and current therapy for complete heart block in children and patients with congenital heart disease. Congenit Heart Dis 2007;4:224–234.

Kothari DS, Skinner JR. Neonatal tachycardias: an update. Arch Dis Child Fetal Neonatol 2006;91:F136–F144.

Perry JC, Garson A. Supraventricular tachycardia due to Wolff-Parkinson-White syndrome I children: early disappearance and late recurrence. J Am Coll Cardiol 1991;16:1215–20.

Texter KM, Kertesz NJ, Friedman RA, et al. Atrial flutter in infants. J Am Coll Cardiol 2006;48:1040–6.

COR PULMONALE

164. What is cor pulmonale?
Cor pulmonale is a severe abnormality in right ventricular function that occurs as a result of lung pathology. The common denominator in all cases is a significantly elevated PVR and right ventricular hypertension. The right ventricular dysfunction is manifested as a combination of right ventricular hypertrophy with decreased right ventricular compliance, and right ventricular dilation with decreased systolic function. By definition, cor pulmonale excludes all cases of right ventricular pathology caused by congenital heart disease.

165. What are the causes of cor pulmonale in a newborn infant?
Cor pulmonale may result from any chronic pathology that causes PVR to remain elevated after birth.
- Bronchopulmonary dysplasia (BPD)
- Upper airway obstruction
- Cystic fibrosis
- Neuromuscular disease
- Thoracic cage abnormality
- Parenchymal lung disease
- Restrictive lung disease
- Vascular diseases

166. What is the clinical presentation of cor pulmonale?
- Poor feeding
- Exercise intolerance
- Tachypnea
- Prominent right ventricular impulse and loud P_2
- Right-sided heart failure and hepatic enlargement

167. What is the chronic management of cor pulmonale?
The chronic management of cor pulmonale depends on the underlying etiology. Factors that worsen PVR, such as hypoxia and acidosis, should be avoided. Intralipid administration as part of hyperalimentation may also increase pulmonary artery pressure and should be used only with great caution. Diuretics are commonly used in infants with BPD, although the evidence for their long-term benefit is not well established. A variety of pulmonary vasodilators are available with different actions and side effect profiles.

Nichols DG, Cameron DE, Greeley WJ, et al. Critical heart disease in infants and children. St Louis: Mosby; 1995.

✓ KEY POINTS: ENDOCARDITIS

1. Neonates with congenital heart disease and neonates with structurally normal hearts who have an indwelling central venous catheter are at risk for developing endocarditis.

168. What are the most common pathogens that cause endocarditis in neonates?
Staphylococcus spp., Group B *Streptococcus, Escherichia coli, Listeria monocytogenes, Candida* spp., and gram-negative organisms such as *Acinetobacter* spp., *Serratia* spp., *Enterobacter* spp., and *Klebsiella* spp.

169. Which neonates are at risk for developing endocarditis?

Infants with underlying congenital heart disease, infants with normal cardiac anatomy and a PDA, and infants with an indwelling central venous catheter are at risk for developing endocarditis.

170. What are signs of endocarditis in the neonate?

Early signs of endocarditis in neonates may be very subtle; heart murmurs, skin abscesses, and hepatomegaly are the most common signs found in neonatal patients. The findings that one sees in children with subacute bacterial endocarditis—splenomegaly, petechiae, and splinter hemorrhages— are not usually seen in the newborn infant.

Pearlman SA, Higgins S, Eppes S, et al. Infective endocarditis in the premature infant. Clin Pediatr 1998;37(12):741–6.

✓ **KEY POINTS: CARDIOMYOPATHY IN THE NEONATE**

1. The diagnosis of a cardiomyopathy in a newborn infant warrants a full genetic, metabolic, and infectious disease evaluation.

171. What are the three types of cardiomyopathy in the neonate and the echocardiographic finding with each type?

Table 6-5 lists these three types of cardiomyopathy.

172. Which metabolic disease is associated with hypertrophic cardiomyopathy, short PR interval, and huge QRS voltage?

Pompe disease (glycogen storage disease type II or acid maltase deficiency).

173. What are the symptoms commonly observed in infants with dilated cardiomyopathy?

CHF, feeding intolerance, tachypnea, tachycardia, arrhythmias, and sudden cardiac death.

174. What common syndrome is associated with hypertrtophic cardiomyopapthy?

Noonan syndrome (10%).

TABLE 6-5. ECHOCARDIOGRAPHIC FINDINGS IN THE THREE TYPES OF NEONATAL CARDIOMYOPATHY		
TYPE OF CARDIOMYOPATHY	**FUNCTION SEEN ON ECHO**	**OTHER ECHO FINDINGS**
Dilated cardiomyopathy	Globular left ventricle Globular and poorly contracting right ventricular size, and contractility possibly normal or similarly depressed	Endocardial fibroelastosis
Hypertrophic cardiomyopathy	Marked left or biventricular hypertrophy with normal/hyperdynamic systolic function	+/– Presence of asymmetric septal hypertrophy (left ventricle) The left ventricular cavity smaller than normal Ventricular filling impaired by diastolic relaxation abnormalities
Restrictive cardiomyopathy	Normal ventricular size and contractility	Abnormal diastolic filling Markedly decreased ventricular compliance

175. What are the common causes of dilated cardiomyopathy (DCM)?

The annual incidence of DCM (<1 year of age) is 4.4 in 100,000 children. The most common causes are myocarditis and neuromuscular disorders. Forms of DCM may be familial, autosomal dominant, autosomal recessive, or X-linked. Inborn errors of metabolism, including Barth syndrome, carnitine deficiency, and mitochondrial disorders, should be sought. Genetic and metabolic consultation should be considered early in the diagnosis of neonatal DCM.

176. What is the clinical outcome of DCM?

The natural history of DCM in infants and children relates to the diverse nature of the disorder and the age at presentation. For all children the median age at diagnosis is 1.5 years with a 1-year and 5-year survival rate at 87% and 77%, respectively. Transplantation is generally not offered for patients with neuromuscular disorders or inborn errors of metabolism.

Keren A, Popp RL. Assignment of patients into the classification of cardiomyopathies. Circulation 1992;86:1622–1633.

Gilbert-Barness E. Review: metabolic cardiomyopathy and conduction system defects in children. Ann Clin Lab Sci 2004;34:15–34.

Towbin J, Lowe AM, Colan SD, et al. Incidence, causes, and outcomes of dilated cardiomyopathy in children. JAMA 2006;296:1867–76.

Daubney PEF, Nugent AW, Chondros P, et al. Clinical features and outcomes of childhood dilated cardiomyopathy. Results from a national population based study. Circulation 2006;114:2671–78.

CARDIAC TUMORS

177. What are the most frequent histologic types of primary cardiac tumors in infants and newborns?

Rhabdomyoma is the most common cardiac tumor seen in newborns and infants (approximately 50%). Rhabdomyomas are considered hamartomas, overgrowth of normal tissue at the site of origin, rather than true neoplasms. Rhabdomyomas seldom cause obstruction and usually regress. Symptoms in neonates are variable but if present relate to intracardiac obstruction, myocardial involvement, or arrhythmias.

Fibroma is the second most common primary cardiac tumor in infants and young children, accounting for approximately 25% of such tumors. These are benign connective tissue tumors arising from fibroblasts and myofibroblasts. They are usually single and intramural; they may involve the left ventricular posterior wall and septum. Fibromas are often located in the left ventricle and may cause left ventricular outflow tract obstruction and CHF. Surgical excision is required for cure insofar as spontaneous regression is rare.

178. What are other types of cardiac tumors?

- Intrapericardial teratomas (commonly present with pericardial effusion)
- Atrial myxomas (frequent in older children and adolescents; benign)
- Mesothelioma localized to the AV node (can produce heart block or sudden death in adolescents)
- Sarcoma or angiosarcoma (seen primarily in right atrium; metastasizes to lung, lymph nodes, mediastinum, liver, kidneys, adrenal glands)

179. What is the most frequent disease associated with primary rhabdomyoma?

Approximately 50% to 75% of patients with cardiac rhabdomyomas have tuberous sclerosis. Multiple rhabdomyomas are more consistent with the diagnosis of tuberous sclerosis than a solitary tumor. Classically, tuberous sclerosis is associated with the triad of epilepsy, mental retardation, and facial angiofibromas.

180. What arrhythmias may be associated with rhabdomyomas?

Bradycardia, SVT, Wolff–Parkinson–White syndrome, and ventricular tachycardia.

181. How do intracardiac tumors cause perinatal or neonatal death?

Depending on size and location, cardiac tumors have been demonstrated to cause death from the following:

- Severe intractable dysrhythmia
- Non-immune hydrops
- Decreased cardiac output secondary to inflow or outflow obstruction

Becker AE. Primary heart tumors in the pediatric age group: a review of salient pathologic features relevant for clinicians. Pediatr Cardiol 2000;21:317–23.

Isaacs H Jr. Fetal and neonatal cardiac tumors. Pediatr Cardiol 2004;25:252–73.

CHAPTER 7

DERMATOLOGY

Victoria R. Barrio, MD, FAAD, FAAP, Kimberly D. Morel, MD, FAAD, FAAP, and Lawrence F. Eichenfield, MD, FAAD, FAAP

1. **List five ways that newborn skin is different than adult skin.**
   Newborn skin is thinner, it is less hairy, it has less pigment, it has a weaker attachment of the epidermis to the dermis, and newborns may have brown fat.

   Eichenfield LF, Frieden IJ, Esterly NB. Textbook of neonatal dermatology. 2nd ed. Philadelphia: Saunders; 2008.

2. **An infant is born at 29 weeks' gestation. What are some clinical problems that may be related to immature skin barrier function in this baby?**
   The skin of premature infants is immature and has compromised barrier function (Fig. 7-1). Clinical consequences include increased transepidermal water loss; fluid and electrolyte disturbances; temperature instability; infection (cutaneous and systemic); absorption of substances applied to the skin; and susceptibility to mechanical, chemical, and thermal stresses.

3. **Approximately when will an infant born at 30 weeks' gestation develop an intact barrier function?**
   Most premature infants exhibit rapid maturation of skin barrier function over the first 2 to 3 weeks of life. In infants born before 25 weeks' gestation, skin barrier function may require 8 weeks or longer after birth to mature.

4. **Infants (especially premature infants) are at increased risk of side effects from absorption of substances from topical application (see the following Key**

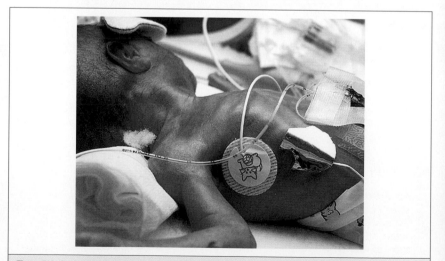

Figure 7-1. Premature infant skin. The skin appears very translucent, and blood vessels are readily apparent.

Points box). **Which topical medications can lead to methemoglobinemia if too much absorption occurs?**
Prilocaine, resorcinol, aniline dyes, and methylene blue can lead to methemoglobinemia.

Mohorovic L, Materljan E, Brumini G. Consequences of methemoglobinemia in pregnancy in newborns, children, and adults: issues raised by new findings on methemoglobin catabolism. J Matern Fetal Neonatal Med 2010;23:956–9.

5. **Which endocrine side effect has been reported after topical application of povidone-iodine on newborn, especially preterm, skin?**
Hypothyroxinemia and goiter have been reported.

Mancini AJ. Skin. Pediatrics 2004;113:1114–1119.

6. **Two weeks into a neonatal intensive care unit course, an infant born at 27 weeks' gestation develops two superficial erosions on the anterior trunk. Subsequently, these heal with a brownish, wrinkled appearance. What is the diagnosis? What is the cause?**
Skin injury may accompany routine care of very premature infants. Anetoderma of prematurity is the term for focal depressions or outpouchings, which are presumed to be a response to mechanical or thermal injury to the skin.

 KEY POINTS: RISK FACTORS FOR PERCUTANEOUS ABSORPTION AND TOXICITY OF TOPICALLY APPLIED SUBSTANCES

1. Immaturity of the epidermal barrier in preterm infants

2. Increased body surface area–to–weight ratio in infants

3. Immature hepatic drug metabolism systems

4. Immature renal excretion systems

5. Less adipose tissue present

6. Decreased serum binding proteins (albumin)

7. **What infection should be considered in a premature infant who develops pustules around a tape site (e.g., around an armboard for stabilization of an intravenous tube)?**
Although bacteria, especially *Staphylococcus* and *Streptococcus* species, should always be considered as a cause of cutaneous pustules, tape sites have been associated with opportunistic fungal infections of the skin, especially involving *Aspergillus* species. Other fungi and yeast, including *Rhizopus* and *Candida* organisms, should also be considered. Performing a biopsy and culture is a standard approach to diagnosis.

Smolinski KN, Shah SS, Honig PJ, et al. Neonatal cutaneous fungal infections. Curr Opin Pediatr 2005;17(4):486–93.

8. **An infant in the newborn nursery required repeated heel sticks for blood chemistries. What possible side effect could show up after discharge, and when would you expect to see it?**
Infants that receive numerous heel sticks may develop calcinosis cutis over the heel. This seldom shows up until several months after discharge. The presenting symptoms are small yellow or white papules that can be mistaken for warts. They are generally not symptomatic and will often resolve by 30 months of age. If they become problematic, they can be treated with curettage.

9. **What is subcutaneous fat necrosis of the newborn?**

Subcutaneous fat necrosis of the newborn usually appears within the first weeks of life with red to violaceous mobile plaques, especially on the back, thighs, and cheeks. The cause of subcutaneous fat necrosis is not definitively known.

10. **In which clinical situations may subcutaneous fat necrosis of the newborn occur?**

Subcutaneous fat necrosis may occur in cases of fetal distress, birth trauma, infection, or cold stress. It is increasingly being seen after the use of whole body cooling for the treatment of hypoxic-ischemic birth injury.

Zifman E, Mouler M, Eliakim A, et al. Subcutaneous fat necrosis and hypercalcemia following therapeutic hypothermia—a patient report and review of the literature. J Pediatr Endocrinol Metab 2010;23(11):1185–8.

11. **How should newborns with subcutaneous fat necrosis be monitored?**

Although the disorder is most often benign and self-limited, in some cases subcutaneous fat necrosis of the newborn may be associated with hypercalcemia and death. Therefore serum calcium levels must be monitored, and caregivers must be vigilant for clinical signs and symptoms of hypercalcemia.

12. **What is the clinical presentation of sclerema neonatorum?**

Findings of sclerema usually appear in the first 2 weeks of life but can begin as late as 4 months. Infants who are poorly nourished, dehydrated, hypothermic, or septic are most commonly affected. Sclerema neonatorum begins in the lower extremities with the appearance of hard, cool skin and decreased mobility and subsequently ascends to involve the trunk and face. Palms, soles, and genitalia are usually not involved. Joints become immobile, and the face appears masklike. Sclerema may be associated with necrotizing enterocolitis, pneumonia, intracranial hemorrhage, hypoglycemia, and electrolyte disturbances.

Zeb A, Darmstadt GL. Sclerema neonatorum: a review of nomenclature, clinical presentation, histological features, differential diagnoses and management. J Perinatol 2008;28:453–60.

13. **What is the cause of sclerema? Why is it more common in infants with infection, hypothermia, or other stressors?**

Sclerema is likely a result of lipoenzyme dysfunction and occurs in infants who are stressed with severe illnesses. More specifically, dysfunction of enzymes regulating the conversion of saturated fatty acids to unsaturated fatty acids results in an excess of saturated fatty acids. This dysfunction promotes fat solidification. The incidence of sclerema has decreased significantly in recent years because events such as malnutrition, dehydration, and hypothermia occur less commonly in modern nurseries. Treating the underlying condition can result in resolution of sclerema. Some authors also propose systemic steroids or therapy with exchange transfusions.

14. **What is cutis marmorata, and which infants have it?**

Cutis marmorata is a reticulated (i.e., netlike) mottling of the skin seen in most infants. It is seen most often when the environment is cooler and will usually improve if the infant is warmed. It usually improves in childhood, but can be persistent in patients with Down syndrome, trisomy 18, and Cornelia de Lange syndrome.

15. **What is harlequin color change?**

Harlequin color change is a demarcated erythema forming on the dependent half of the body of newborns. In some cases the baby appears as if a line were drawn right down the midline. The more superior half of the body appears pale. This appearance can occur in any position and commonly lasts from seconds up to 20 minutes. It is rarely seen after 10 days of life. Harlequin color change is explained by immature autonomic vasomotor control because it is more common in premature infants and is reversible. If the baby is flipped over during an episode, the newly dependent portion will become erythematous.

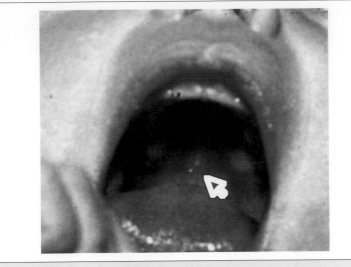

Figure 7-2. Epstein pearls.

16. **Name three forms of epidermal inclusion cysts that are commonly found in neonates.**
    - Milia: Tiny cysts, usually found on the face, occurring in up to 40% of newborns
    - Epstein pearls (Fig. 7-2): Cysts found on the palate of approximately 64% of newborns
    - Bohn nodules: Alveolar cysts found along the lingual gum margins and the lateral palate

    All three forms represent cystic retention of keratin, appear and resolve in the first month, and can be present at birth. They are white, 1- to 2-mm papules that can be found singularly or in clusters.

17. **What is aplasia cutis congenita?**
    Aplasia cutis congenita results from failure of the development of the normal layers of skin. It occurs most often on the scalp and may present clinically as an ulcer, healed erosion, or well-formed scar. Therefore it is often mistaken for trauma caused by a scalp pH probe. In cases of large lesions or lesions overlying the midline neurocranial axis, imaging should be considered because aplasia cutis congenita may be associated with underlying malformations of bone or may extend deeply to the meninges. Large and irregular lesions can also be associated with Adams–Oliver syndrome and chromosomal abnormalities.

18. **What is a dermoid cyst?**
    Dermoid cysts form along embryonic fusion lines. They are congenital but may not be seen until childhood, when they begin to enlarge. They commonly occur along the orbital ridge. Surgical removal is recommended because they can become infected. When they are located along the lateral eyebrow, they do not require specific imaging. Other locations, especially midline, can have a connection to the central nervous system and should be imaged before surgery.

19. **What is the best treatment for a small bump or hole with a hair growing in it present on the midline nose at birth?**
    This description fits a dermoid sinus. Midline lesions should always raise the possibility of a developmental defect. The presence of a hair coming out of the sinus is especially significant because it is considered a marker for a connection with the central nervous system. The baby should be imaged before the defect is repaired.

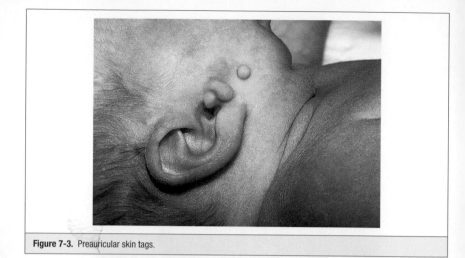

Figure 7-3. Preauricular skin tags.

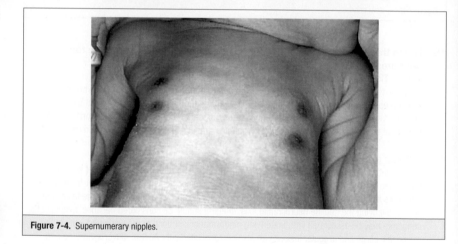

Figure 7-4. Supernumerary nipples.

20. **What is the significance of preauricular skin tags?**

Preauricular skin tags, also called accessory tragi, are embryonic remnants of the first branchial arch (Fig. 7-3). The formation of the first branchial arch occurs during the fourth week of fetal development. Because this may be associated with hearing abnormalities, patients should have their hearing screened before they are discharged from the hospital. The evidence for associated renal problems in patients with no other associated abnormalities is controversial. Renal ultrasound should be considered for patients with additional dysmorphic features or a family history of deafness or renal malformations.

Roth DA, Hildesheimer M, Bardenstein S, et al. Preauricular skin tags and ear pits are associated with permanent hearing impairment in newborns. Pediatrics 2008;122(4):e884–90.

21. **What are accessory nipples? Where are they located?**

Accessory nipples, also called supernumerary nipples (Fig. 7-4), are embryonic remnants of the mammary line that extend from the axilla to the inner thigh. They appear as pink or brown papules, with or without surrounding areola, anywhere along the mammary line. There have been conflicting reports about an association with urinary tract abnormalities. Current studies, however, have not found an association in patients who have no other anomalies.

22. **What is a congenital melanocytic nevus (CMN)?**
A CMN is usually defined as a melanocytic lesion that is present at birth. The incidence is reported to be 0.5% to 2%.

23. **What are some complications of CMNs?**
Most CMNs do not have any associated complications. CMNs are often subdivided according to their size. A common classification is that a CMN greater than 20 cm in adulthood is considered to be large. Melanoma has been reported to arise within congenital lesions, but the exact risk for this complication is unclear. It is known that large lesions carry the greatest risk and that melanoma, when it occurs, does so earlier in life. Leptomeningeal melanosis is a rare complication that may occur in association with a giant congenital nevus with numerous satellite nevi.

Slutsky JB, Barr JM, Femia AN, et al. Large congenital melanocytic nevi: associated risks and management considerations. Semin Cutan Med Surg 2010;29(2):79–84.

24. **What are neonatal acne and transient cephalic neonatal pustulosis (TCNP)? How do these entities differ from infantile acne?**
The cause and nomenclature of these conditions remain somewhat controversial. Some neonatal outbreaks, although commonly called *neonatal acne,* are not composed of distinct pimples (i.e., comedones) but rather superficial pustules.
- Neonatal acne usually begins at a few weeks of life and resolves over several months. Affected infants exhibit multiple inflammatory erythematous papules and pustules. Treatment is rarely needed.
- TCNP has been proposed as a subset of what has been called neonatal acne, which is caused by *Malassezia* species rather than by an elevation in androgen levels (which is present in infantile or classic acne). Others have proposed that there is no true neonatal acne and that the term *TCNP* (or *neonatal cephalic pustulosis*) should be used as a substitute. Like neonatal acne, TCNP usually begins at a few weeks of life and resolves in several months. Affected infants demonstrate multiple inflammatory erythematous papules and pustules. Comedonal lesions are rare, and treatment is rarely needed, although some experts believe that topical antiyeast agents speed resolution.
- Infantile acne is truly an acneiform condition, with open and closed comedones as well as papules and pustules. It usually presents later, usually beyond the age of 2 to 3 months, and generally resolves between the ages of 6 and 12 months. That time sequence parallels decreases in fetal adrenal pubertal androgen levels and male testosterone levels (one possible reason males are more commonly affected). Unlike neonatal acne or TCNP, infantile acne may persist and cause scarring. For this reason, like adolescent acne, it is treated with topical antibiotics and occasionally with retinoids or systemic agents.

Niamba P, Weill FX, Sarlangue J, et al. Is neonatal cephalic pustulosis (neonatal acne) triggered by Malassezia sympodialis? Arch Dermatol 1998;134:995–998.
Friedlander SF, Baldwin HE, Mancini AJ, et al. The acne continuum: an age-based approach to therapy. Semin Cutan Med Surg 2011;30:S6–11.

25. **Is erythema toxicum toxic? In which kind of infant is it seen?**
Erythema toxicum is a benign condition (Fig. 7-5). Erythema toxicum is no alien to the nursery; it is present in 50% of term newborns. It is much less prevalent in premature infants, however, occurring in only approximately 5%.

26. **When do the lesions of erythema toxicum occur? What do they look like?**
Erythema toxicum usually begins between 24 and 48 hours of life and spontaneously resolves in 4 to 5 days; however, new lesions can occur up to day 10 of life. Exacerbations and remissions may occur

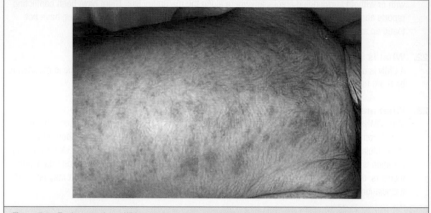

Figure 7-5. Erythema toxicum. White papules on an erythematous base are evident.

in the first 2 weeks of life. Erythema toxicum lesions are irregularly bordered, erythematous macules, 2 to 3 cm in diameter, with central yellowish vesicopustules. They are mostly discrete, but some erythematous macules become confluent. Lesions do not involve the palms or soles.

27. **Which type of cells is seen on microscopic examination of pustules scraped from erythema toxicum lesions?**
Wright-Giemsa stains of pustule scrapings show mostly eosinophils. Up to 15% of affected infants demonstrate peripheral eosinophilia as well.

28. **What is the standard treatment for milia, sebaceous gland hyperplasia (Fig. 7-6), transient neonatal pustular melanosis, erythema toxicum, and sucking blisters?**
"Nothing works." In other words, it is not necessary to do anything other than reassure the family that the condition will resolve over time (Table 7-1).

29. **How are miliaria crystallina (also known as prickly heat) and miliaria rubra differentiated? How are they treated?**
Miliaria is found in up to 15% of neonates. Both forms are caused by eccrine duct obstruction and resultant sweat leakage to different levels of skin (crystallina if the leakage occurs under the stratum corneum; rubra if it takes place at the upper dermis). Miliaria is more common in hot, humid environments and is distributed to the forehead, upper trunk, and other covered surfaces. The best method of treatment is to try to keep the baby from becoming overheated. Removing excessive layers or putting the baby in an air-conditioned room may also be helpful. Topical ointments may aggravate the condition and are therefore not recommended.

30. **Why is the presence of pruritus a poor way to differentiate atopic dermatitis from seborrheic dermatitis in infants?**
Although atopic dermatitis classically includes pruritus, infants (especially newborns) may not have the coordination to scratch. However, occipital alopecia can result from excessive rubbing of the back of the head against the bedsheets. In this situation hair may fall out or break off as a result of friction.

31. **Describe the usual distribution of the rash caused by atopic dermatitis and that caused by seborrheic dermatitis in neonates.**
If dermatitis involves the axillae or groin, it is more likely to be seborrheic dermatitis. If extensor surfaces such as forearms and shins are involved, atopic dermatitis is more likely. Both atopic dermatitis

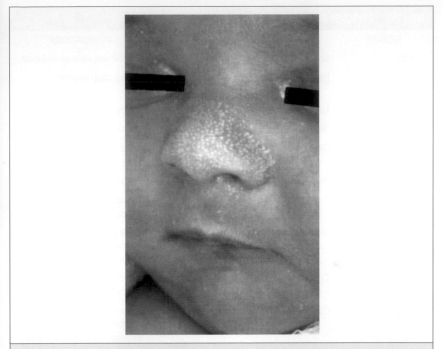

Figure 7-6. An infant with sebaceous hyperplasia.

TABLE 7-1. NEONATAL SKIN LESIONS

CONDITION	ONSET	RESOLUTION	TREATMENT
Milia	Can be at birth, <1 month old	Usually <1 month	None
Sebaceous gland hyperplasia	Can be at birth, <1 month old	Usually <1 month	None
Transient neonatal pustular melanosis	Usually present at birth	Vesicopustules <5 days; pigment macules <3 month	None
Erythema toxicum	24-48 hours, new lesions <10 days old	Each lesion <5 days; all lesions, <2 weeks	None
Sucking blisters	Present at birth	Days	None

and seborrheic dermatitis involve scalp and posterior auricular areas, although seborrheic dermatitis has large, yellowish scale and, when severe, characteristically extends down to the forehead and eyebrow areas (Table 7-2).

32. **What is intertrigo, and what are some possible causes?**
   Intertrigo literally means an erythematous rash on opposing skin surfaces or skin folds. The common causes of intertrigo include seborrheic dermatitis or infections (e.g., *Candida* spp.) Other infections

TABLE 7-2.   CAUSES OF DIAPER DERMATITIS

DISEASE	DIAPER RASH	ASSOCIATIONS
Candida	Bright red satellites, involves the creases	Antibiotic use, concurrent thrush
Irritant	Involves the exposed surfaces, spares creases, can have perianal erosions	Diarrhea, cloth diapers
Impetigo	Flaccid bullae and superficial erosions	Often no associations
Streptococcal	Tender beefy red erythema perinanal area	Often no association
Seborrheic dermatitis	Shiny pink patches involving entire diaper area	Scalp and face involvement
Psoriasis	Involves entire diaper area and beyond	Often patches on the face and trunk
Allergic contact	Areas well demarcated to places of contact with allergen	Disposable diapers and diaper wipes
Zinc deficiency	Crusted eczematous involvement of entire diaper area	Irritable baby, perioral involvement, failure to thrive, can be seen in cystic fibrosis
Langerhans cell histiocytosis	Crusted papules or erosions, often in the creases	Crusted papules on the scalp and body
Hemangioma	Can present with nonhealing ulceration	Often single hemangioma; if segmental, look for associated developmental abnormalities
Kawasaki disease	Many presentations, but often perineal erythema with desquamation	Fever, lymphadenopathy, irritability, conjunctivitis, fissured liips

include *Staphylococcus aureus* or Streptococcal infections. Psoriasis, nutritional deficiency, and histiocytosis may also present as intertrigo. Clues to the diagnosis of histiocytosis include the presence of petechial or red-brown macules and papules, which are recalcitrant to topical therapy and occasionally associated with an enlarged lymph node or nodes.

33. **What is scalded skin syndrome?**

    Staphylococcal scalded skin syndrome (SSSS) is caused by toxins released by *S. aureus* that lead to blistering and desquamation of the skin. The Nikolsky sign is positive; simply rubbing the skin causes denudation of skin or formation of a blister. Clustered outbreaks of SSSS have been reported in newborn nurseries. Remember, however, that scalding thermal burns caused by bathing the newborn in overly hot water are also possible.

34. **What is a "blueberry muffin baby?"**

    This term is used to describe neonates whose skin resembles a blueberry muffin (i.e., the skin shows diffuse, dark blue to violaceous purpuric macules and papules). The spots represent dermal hematopoiesis and are a sign of serious systemic disease, most often congenital infection. The congenital infection most commonly associated with this appearance is congenital rubella, although the condition may be caused by other microorganisms and diseases as well.

35. **Which diseases can cause blueberry muffin syndrome?**

    - Hemolytic disease of the newborn
    - Toxoplasmosis

- Neoplastic disease
- Rubella
- Leukemia
- Cytomegalovirus
- Neuroblastoma
- Herpes
- Langerhans cell histiocytosis
- Coxsackie B2 virus
- Congenital rhabdomyosarcoma with cutaneous metastases
- Parvovirus B19
- Aicardi–Goutières syndrome

36. **What are the risk factors for development of hemangiomas?**
   Infantile hemangiomas are common vascular tumors that arise during the neonatal period. They are often not visible at birth but are noticed within the first weeks of life. One study found that 10% of Caucasian children had hemangiomas when examined at 1 year of age. Hemangiomas occur more frequently in female children, with a female-to-male incidence of 2 to 5:1. In addition, they arise more commonly in premature infants, low-birth-weight infants, and infants born to older mothers and those with placenta previa and preeclampsia.

37. **What do strawberries and caverns have to do with hemangiomas?**
   In older medical books and the lay literature, superficial hemangiomas were called strawberry birthmarks because the color and texture of affected skin is somewhat reminiscent of a strawberry. Deep hemangiomas have been called cavernous hemangiomas, but the term is particularly confusing because it has also been used to describe venous malformations, which are a completely different kind of vascular birthmark. Therefore it is prudent to avoid both terms and to use instead the terms *superficial, deep,* or *mixed hemangiomas* to describe the particular type of hemangioma.

38. **When does the proliferation "clock" start for infantile hemangiomas?**
   This is one "clock" that does not get corrected for gestational age. Although hemangiomas are more common in preterm infants, and the female-to-male ratio is less pronounced, the chronologic age at which hemangiomas are noted to begin proliferation is the same as for full-term infants.

   Garzon MC, Drolet BA, Baselga E, et al. Comparison of infantile hemangiomas in preterm and term infants: a prospective study. Arch Dermatol 2008;144(9):1231–2.

39. **What are the differences between hemangiomas and vascular malformations?**
   The classification of vascular birthmarks has historically been problematic. The most commonly accepted classification was introduced by the International Society for the Study of Vascular Anomalies in the 1990s. It divides vascular birthmarks into two broad categories:
   - Vascular tumors: These include the most common birthmark, the hemangioma of infancy, and other rare childhood-onset vascular tumors. The lesions are proliferating lesions composed of blood vessels. Hemangiomas have a characteristic natural history. Although not usually noticed

✓ KEY POINTS: DIFFERENTIAL DIAGNOSIS OF CONGENITAL VASCULAR-APPEARING NODULE

1. Vascular tumor (e.g., congenital hemangioma)

2. Vascular malformation (e.g., arterial, venous, lymphatic, capillary malformation)

3. Congenital malignancy (e.g., neuroblastoma, rhabdomyosarcoma, fibrosarcoma, primitive neuroectodermal tumor, lipoblastoma, liposarcoma)

at birth, they are commonly observed in the first few weeks of life, undergo rapid proliferation that may last for several months, and then slowly regress over several years. At the end of the period of spontaneous regression, they may be undetectable or leave a residual mass or textural changes. Hemangiomas are distinct histologically and show increased endothelial turnover.

- Vascular malformations: These include various lesions (e.g., capillary malformations [port-wine stains], venous, lymphatic, arteriovenous, and mixed malformations). They are classified according to the type of vessels that compose them. They are often noted in the immediate newborn period. Vascular malformations grow with the child, although they may become more prominent as the child matures. They do not show a marked increase in proliferation and differ histologically from tumors. Most important, they do not regress spontaneously, and they persist throughout the patient's lifetime. Therefore management is significantly different from that undertaken for a hemangioma.

40. **In which situations should you worry about coexistent internal hemangiomas?**
Infants who present with more than five cutaneous hemangiomas are more likely to have underlying internal hemangiomas. The liver and gastrointestinal tract are the most common sites of extracutaneous involvement. It is important to remember that normal liver sonogram results in the neonatal period do not rule out subsequent hepatic hemangiomatosis because symptoms may develop during the proliferative phase of the hemangioma.

Not all children with multiple skin hemangiomas have underlying systemic involvement; conversely, children with visceral hemangiomas may have no skin lesions. Children with hemangiomas located on the lower face in a "beard" pattern may have laryngeal hemangiomas that may not become detectable until they compromise breathing. Therefore a pediatric otolaryngologist should evaluate these children early in life, and early treatment is often required.

Drolet BA, Chamlin SL, Garzon MC, et al. Prospective study of spinal anomalies in children with infantile hemangiomas of the lumbosacral skin. J Pediatr 2010;157(5):789–94.

41. **What are some of the complications that can occur with a hemangioma?**
Even smaller lesions in problematic locations can lead to complications. Hemangiomas located around the eye may obstruct the visual axis or lead to astigmatism by deforming the shape of the globe, which leads to visual impairment. Lesions on the tip of the nose can cause deformation of the cartilage and permanent disfigurement. Large lesions with high flow may cause congestive heart failure. Ulceration may complicate large or small hemangiomas. Ulceration is most common in the diaper area and in high-friction areas.

42. **What is the significance of segmental hemangiomas?**
Segmental hemangiomas are flatter hemangiomas that seem to involve a whole facial segment (>5 cm) or a large area on the pelvis. They are often markers of other developemental abnormalities. Large facial hemangiomas are associated with PHACE syndrome (Posterior fossa malformation, Hemangioma, Arterial abnormalities, Cardiac abnormalities, Eye abnormalities). Segmental hemangiomas that involve the sacrum and perineum can be associated with genitourinary anomalies and tethered spinal cord.

Metry D, Heyer G, Hess C, et al. Consensus statement on diagnostic criteria for PHACE syndrome. Pediatrics 2009;124(5):1447–56.

43. **What endocrine study should be considered for an infant with a liver hemangioma?**
Thyroid function testing should be considered. Hemangioma tissue may exhibit enzyme activity (type 3 iodothyronine deiodinase), which inactivates thyroid hormone. Laboratory testing should be performed even if the newborn screen results were within normal limits because enzyme activity can increase during the proliferative phase of the hemangioma.

Huang SA, Tu HM, Harney JW, et al. Severe hypothyroidism caused by type 3 iodothyronine deiodinase in infantile hemangiomas. N Engl J Med 2000;343:185–189.

44. What is a RICH?

RICH is an acronym for a rapidly involuting congenital hemangioma.

45. What is the difference between hemangioma of infancy and RICH?

Hemangiomas of infancy can have precursor lesions present at birth but usually do not begin to proliferate until after 2 weeks of age. They proliferate for several months and slowly involute over years. Congenital hemangiomas are present more fully formed at birth. They undergo rapid involution, usually within 1 or 2 years, and are thus named *rapidly involuting congenital hemangiomas*. There is also a subtype of congenital hemangiomas that do not involute and are therefore named noninvoluting congenital hemangiomas (NICHs).

46. Which malignancies can mimic the appearance of a congenital hemangioma?

Neuroblastoma, rhabdomyosarcoma, fibrosarcoma, primitive neuroectodermal tumor, liposarcoma, and lipoblastoma are among the lesions that may mimic the appearance of a hemangioma.

47. What treatments have been used for problematic hemangiomas?

Although smaller hemangiomas that are not problematic do not require treatment, other types do require treatment to prevent problems. Problematic hemangiomas include those that compromise vital functions, cause significant distortion or disfigurement of normal underlying structures, and have ulcerated or become infected. Treatment strategy varies depending on the clinical situation. The recent use of propranolol to treat hemangiomas has led to significant improvement in care. However, this is a relatively new indication for this medication, and considerations with its use are appropriate.

Leaute-Labreze C, Dumas de la Roque E, Hubiche T, et al. Propranolol for severe hemangiomas of infancy. N Engl J Med 2008;358(24):2649–51.

48. What are the potential side effects of treating infantile hemangiomas with propranolol?

Propranolol is a nonselective beta blocker. Side effects include hypotension, bradycardia, hypoglycemia (especially when fasting), bronchospasm, and sleep disturbance. Underlying heart disease or arrhythmias should be ruled out before starting off-label use of this medication to treat infantile hemangiomas.

49. How should a child with a hemangioma located over the lumbosacral spine be evaluated?

Hemangiomas in this location may be associated with underlying spinal cord anomalies (e.g., a tethered spinal cord), underlying bony defects, and anomalies of the genitourinary and gastrointestinal systems. For detection of a tethered cord, magnetic resonance imaging is the study of choice. (See the following Key Points box for additional cutaneous clues to underlying spinal cord abnormalities and Fig. 7-7 for a striking example of multiple congenital anomalies overlying the midline lumbosacral spine).

50. What is Kasabach–Merritt phenomenon? With which tumors is it associated?

Kasabach–Merritt phenomenon (or syndrome) is a rare complication that occurs in infants with large vascular tumors. Patients usually exhibit symptoms in the first few months of life with a rapidly enlarging vascular mass associated with profound thrombocytopenia and coagulopathy. It is a life-threatening condition. In the past this phenomenon was thought to be a complication of garden-variety hemangiomas, but recent evidence indicates an association with rare vascular tumors such as kaposiform hemangioendothelioma and tufted angioma.

Kelly M. Kasabach-Merritt phenomenon. Pediatr Clin North Am 2010;57:1085–9.

51. What is a lymphangioma?

A lymphangioma, also known as a lymphatic malformation, is a vascular malformation composed of lymphatic tissue. These lesions are sometimes noted in the immediate newborn period or may

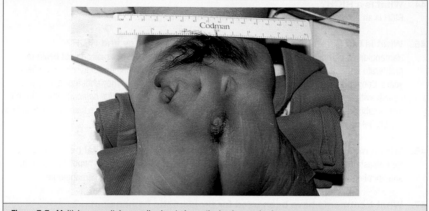

Figure 7-7. Multiple congenital anomalies located over the lumbosacral spine.

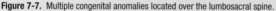

become more prominent as a child grows. They do not regress spontaneously. A cystic hygroma is one type of lymphatic malformation that is composed of larger cystic spaces, also called a macrocystic lymphatic malformation. It usually is apparent in the immediate newborn period and is located on the head and neck. Some patients with cystic hygroma have underlying genetic abnormalities such as Turner syndrome.

✓ KEY POINTS: MIDLINE LUMBOSACRAL CUTANEOUS CLUES TO AN UNDERLYING TETHERED CORD OR OCCULT SPINA BIFIDA

1. Sacral pits (particularly with lateral deviation of the gluteal cleft, if they are large, or more than 2.5 cm from the anal verge)

2. Hairy patches

3. Appendages (skin tag or tail)

4. Sacral lipoma

5. Vascular lesions (hemangioma, port-wine stain)

6. Dermoid sinus

7. Aplasia cutis congenita or scar

8. Two or more markers together is particularly concerning

52. How is a port-wine stain treated?

A port-wine stain is a malformation composed of small capillary and venular-size vessels. As a child matures, the lesion may darken, thicken, and develop blebs. Pulsed dye laser therapy is the preferred method of treatment and may lead to significant lightening in many patients. Multiple treatments are usually required. These lesions differ from the "stork bite" and "angel kiss" nevus simplex, which do not progress and do not need to be treated.

Bencini PL, Tourlaki A, De Giorgi V, et al. Laser use for cutaneous vascular alterations of cosmetic interest. Dermatol Ther 2012;25:340–51.

53. **When should Sturge–Weber syndrome be considered in a child with facial port-wine stain? What are the characteristic findings in Sturge–Weber syndrome?**
Approximately 10% of children with a port-wine stain in the distribution of the ophthalmic branch of the trigeminal nerve have findings of Sturge–Weber syndrome. Sturge–Weber syndrome is characterized by seizures (onset usually occurs in patients younger than 2 years old), hemiplegia, mental retardation, and glaucoma. In infancy, however, many of these findings may not be present or may be difficult to discern. Similarly, a computed tomography or magnetic resonance imaging scan in infancy may not show the characteristic calcification, cerebral atrophy, or abnormalities of the cortex and white matter. An enlarged choroid plexus or increased myelination, though, may be present early in the course of Sturge–Weber syndrome. Neonates with a port-wine stain in that distribution should have an urgent eye examination to assess for possible glaucoma.

54. **What are the modes of inheritance of neurofibromatosis types 1 and 2? What protein mutations are involved in these genetic diseases?**
Both diseases are autosomal dominant, but spontaneous mutations account for approximately half of cases. The incidence of neurofibromatosis type 1 is 1 in 2500; the mutated gene product is neurofibromin, a protein involved in tumor suppression. Neurofibromatosis type 2 has a reported incidence of 1 in 33,000; the involved gene product is merlin, which mediates cytoskeleton and extracellular movement.

Williams VC, Lucas J, Babcock MA, et al. Neurofibromatosis type 1 revisited. Pediatrics. 2009;123:124–33.

55. **When should neurofibromatosis type 1 be suspected in a newborn?**
Neurofibromatosis type 1 should be suspected in any infant with multiple café-au-lait spots, congenital glaucoma, a plexiform neurofibroma, or pseudoarthrosis. Without a positive family history, however, it can be difficult to diagnose neurofibromatosis in the first months of life. The diagnosis requires two or more of the following criteria: at least six café-au-lait macules of at least 0.5 cm before puberty (1.5 cm postpuberty), at least two neurofibromas, one plexiform neurofibroma, axillary freckles or inguinal freckles, at least two Lisch nodules (iris hamartomas), osseous lesions, or a first-degree relative with neurofibromatosis type 1. Other features that are associated with neurofibromatosis in older children include learning disability, macrocephaly, short stature, scoliosis, juvenile xanthogranulomas, angiomas, mental retardation, impaired coordination, seizures, cerebral tumors (i.e., optic gliomas), increased risk of malignancy, and hypertension.

56. **What is the most common cutaneous finding in neonates with tuberous sclerosis?**
Hypopigmented macules, known as ash leaf spots, are the most common skin findings of tuberous sclerosis in infants. Connective tissue nevi, known as shagreen patches, may also be present at birth. Adenoma sebaceum (facial angiofibromas) generally appear at 3 years of age and older; periungual or gum fibromas appear in early adulthood. During the first months of life hypopigmented macules may be recognizable only with a Wood's lamp because of the general lack of pigmentation in the skin. Another manifestation of tuberous sclerosis during the neonatal period that is of concern is a rhabdomyoma within the heart. Infants diagnosed with tuberous sclerosis should have a cardiac echocardiography examination performed. Cardiac lesions that are asymptomatic often regress by the first year of life.

57. **Are hypopigmented macules always a sign of tuberous sclerosis?**
Absolutely not. Most hypopigmented macules are a variant of normal conditions. However, multiple ash leaf–like macules, a family history of tuberous sclerosis, neonatal seizures, cardiac rhabdomyomas, or renal cysts should alert the clinician to the possible diagnosis of tuberous sclerosis.

58. **Tuberous sclerosis is inherited in an autosomal dominant fashion. What is peculiar about the genetic abnormalities associated with the tuberous sclerosis phenotype?**
Two distinct chromosomal complexes on two different chromosomes are implicated as areas of mutation that result in tuberous sclerosis. Tuberous sclerosis complex 1 results from mutations in

the gene hamartin on chromosome 9, located at 9q34.3. Tuberous sclerosis complex 2 is caused by mutations in the tuberin gene on chromosome 16 at 16p13.3.

59. What is a collodion baby?

Collodion baby is a term used to describe a neonate born with a yellow, shiny membrane that resembles collodion. It is often associated with ichthyosis. The word *ichthyosis* comes from the greek word *ichthys*, meaning "fish." Patients with these conditions can have thickened, scaly or flaky skin.

60. Which type of ichthyosis is most commonly associated with a collodion baby?

Of newborns with collodion membrane, the most common ichthyosis that develops is nonbullous ichthyosiform erythroderma, also called congenital ichthyosiform erythroderma. Lamellar ichthyosis is another rare form of ichthyosis that may present initially with collodion membrane. Both are classified as autosomal recessive congenital ichthyoses. Approximately 5% of babies with collodion membrane do not go on to have clinically significant skin disease. Furthermore, not all patients with ichthyotic skin disease have a collodion membrane at birth.

Oji V, Tadini G, Akiyama M, et al. Revised nomenclature and classification of inherited ichthyoses: results of the First Ichthyosis Consensus Conference in Sorèze 2009. J Am Acad Dermatol 2010;63:607–41.

61. What tests may be considered helpful in a newborn with a collodion membrane?

Starting from the top, a microscopic examination of the hair can be performed, because patients with the rare condition trichothiodystrophy will have a distinctive "tiger tail" appearance under polarized light. An ophthalmology examination may show signs of "glistening dots," which is pathognomonic for Sjögren–Larsson syndrome. A peripheral blood smear is useful to evaluate for lipid inclusions within white blood cells, which may be present in neutral lipid storage disease (Chanarin–Dorfman syndrome). In neonates with an ichthyosis syndrome a skin biopsy may not be helpful in the neonatal period because the cutaneous phenotype takes time to develop.

62. How should one care for a baby with collodion membrane?

Supportive care is important until the collodion membrane sheds. Affected newborns experience difficulty with temperature regulation, are prone to sepsis, and have increased fluid and nutritional requirements. Therefore temperature should be controlled in an incubator, and any signs of infection should be promptly investigated and treated. Ectropion occurs as a result of taut skin everting eyelid margins, which leaves patients at risk for corneal ulceration. Topical ocular lubricants should be instituted early. Eclabium occurs by a similar mechanism of taut skin everting the lips. Nasogastric tube feedings may be required for poor suck and feeding difficulties.

63. What is a harlequin baby?

The term *harlequin baby* is used to describe neonates born with massive shiny plates of stratum corneum with deep, red fissures that form geometric patterns resembling a harlequin costume. This entity is quite different from a harlequin color change, which is benign. As in neonates with collodion membrane, temperature regulation is defective, fluid requirements are increased, and risk of infection is high. The skin defect is usually restrictive, and respiratory insufficiency results. Harlequin babies rarely survive beyond the neonatal period.

64. What ichthyotic skin disease is associated with failure to progress during maternal labor?

The X-linked ichthyosis steroid sulfatase deficiency is associated with failure to progress during labor. Mothers have difficulty with cervical dilation and fail to adequately respond to intravenous oxytocin often necessitating a forceps delivery or cesearean section.

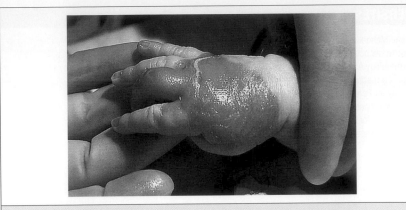

Figure 7-8. Epidermolysis bullosa.

65. What is keratitis–ichthyosis–deafness (KID) syndrome? How does it manifest in children?

KID syndrome is a rare disorder characterized by keratitis, ichthyosis, and congenital neurosensory deafness. Newborns have erythematous, thickened skin that eventually peels. The face and extremities then become ichthyotic; scaly keratoconjunctivitis usually develops during infancy.

66. Are newborns with epidermolytic hyperkeratosis hyperkeratotic?

Epidermolytic hyperkeratosis is also called bullous congenital ichthyosiform erythroderma, and under the updated classification it is called epidermolytic ichthyosis. Newborns most often demonstrate blisters or bullae along with denuded skin. Although subtle hyperkeratosis appears in some newborns, it usually develops over time as the blistering subsides.

67. What is epidermolysis bullosa?

Epidermolysis bullosa is a heterogeneous group of inherited disorders characterized by skin fragility and blistering (Fig. 7-8). Most patients develop symptoms in the newborn period. The most common types are epidermolysis bullosa simplex, junctional epidermolysis bullosa, and dystrophic epidermolysis bullosa. Within each subset there are different clinical phenotypes. It is now understood that these diseases are caused by an inability to synthesize proteins that play an important role in maintaining the skin's integrity. Epidermolysis bullosa simplex is caused by mutations in keratins located in the basal layer of the epidermis; junctional epidermolysis bullosa is caused by defects in the protein laminin 5 and other proteins at the dermal–epidermal junction, and dystrophic epidermolysis bullosa is caused by a defect in collagen VII. There is no cure for these conditions, and treatment is supportive, although trials of bone marrow transplant and gene transfer are ongoing.

Fine JD, Eady RA, Bauer EA, et al. The classification of inherited epidermolysis bullosa (EB): Report of the Third International Concensus Meeting on Diagnosis and Classification of EB. J Am Acad Dermatol 2008;58(6):931–50.

68. What are the basic principles of skin care for children with epidermolysis bullosa?

Skin trauma (e.g., rubbing, chafing) is strongly discouraged, because the skin will likely blister or erode at the site. Tape should not be applied directly to the skin. New blisters should be ruptured with a sterile needle or lancet (to prevent them from enlarging), with the blister roof left in place, and dressed with a topical antibiotic and nonadherent dressing (e.g., plain petrolatum and gauze). The blisters should be monitored closely because superinfection may be a complication. Infants with severe forms of epidermolysis bullosa are at risk for nutritional deficiencies, poor weight gain, and anemia.

WEBSITES

Online Mendelian Inheritance in Man (OMIM)
http://www.ncbi.nlm.nih.gov/entrez/query.fcgi?db=OMIM
Dermatology Atlas
http://dermatlas.med.jhmi.edu/derm
Society for Pediatric Dermatology
http://www.pedsderm.net
Foundation for Ichthyosis and Related Skin Types (FIRST)
http://www.scalyskin.org

CHAPTER 8

ENDOCRINOLOGY AND METABOLISM

Marisa Censani, MD, Mary Pat Gallagher, MD, Wendy K. Chung, MD, PhD, and Sharon E. Oberfield, MD

HYPOCALCEMIA

1. **What perinatal factors are associated with hypocalcemia in the immediate newborn period?**
   - Prematurity
   - Asphyxia
   - Maternal diabetes
   - Maternal hyperparathyroidism
   - Transient congenital hypoparathyroidism
   - Congenital absence or hypoplasia of the parathyroid glands (sporadic or as part of DiGeorge syndrome)

2. **How are calcium levels expected to change in premature infants during the first few days of life?**
   In newborn infants there is a physiologic decline in serum total and ionized calcium during the first 48 hours of life. This decline is exaggerated in preterm infants compared with term infants, with a direct correlation between serum calcium and gestational age (Fig. 8-1). Because no symptoms are specific for early hypocalcemia in preterm infants, the diagnosis is made by demonstrating a serum calcium level below 7 mg/dL (1.75 mmol/L).

3. **Is treatment of hypocalcemia necessary in premature infants?**
   Calcium therapy may block the normal physiologic adaptation to hypocalcemia, which includes increasing serum levels of parathyroid hormone (PTH) and 1,25(OH)$_2$ vitamin D in the first few days of life.
   Further arguments against the need for the treatment of incidentally noted hypocalcemia in the preterm infant are the following:
   - Hypocalcemia of prematurity is usually asymptomatic.
   - It resolves spontaneously.
   - Long-term follow-up studies have shown no benefit with treatment.
   - Total serum calcium level is a poor predictor of ionized serum calcium in premature infants.
   - Intravenous (IV) calcium is associated with complications such as cardiac arrhythmias and ulcerations as a result of soft-tissue infiltration of the infusate.

Loughead JL, Tsang RC. Neonatal calcium and phosphorus metabolism. In: Cowett RM, editor. Principles of perinatal-neonatal medicine. New York: Springer-Verlag; 1998. p. 879–908.
   Moya, FR, Laughon, M. Common problems of the newborn. In: Reece EA, Hobbins JC, editors. Clinical obstetrics: the fetus and mother. 3rd ed. Massachusetts: Blackwell; 2008. p. 1247.

4. **When is treatment of hypocalcemia recommended in premature infants?**
   In the absence of additional data, it is conventional to treat all serum calcium levels below 6 mg/dL, even in asymptomatic neonates. The addition of 200 mg/kg/day of 10% calcium gluconate to standard IV solutions provides 20 mg/kg/day of elemental calcium. If symptoms are present (especially cardiac arrhythmia or seizures), a bolus of 100 mg/kg of 10% calcium gluconate (10 mg/kg elemental

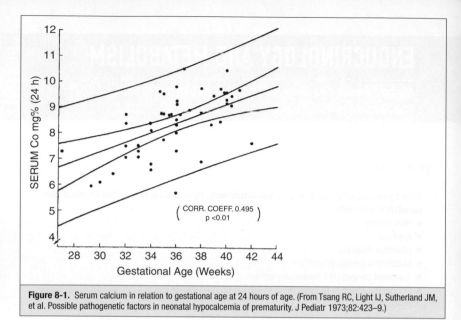

Figure 8-1. Serum calcium in relation to gestational age at 24 hours of age. (From Tsang RC, Light IJ, Sutherland JM, et al. Possible pathogenetic factors in neonatal hypocalcemia of prematurity. J Pediatr 1973;82:423–9.)

calcium) may be given intravenously over 10 minutes with careful cardiac monitoring. One should be cautious using a peripheral IV means to administer calcium because calcium can be very irritating to tissues.

✓ KEY POINTS: HYPOCALCEMIA

1. Neonatal hypocalcemia is associated with prematurity, asphyxia, maternal diabetes, transient hypoparathyroidism, permanent congenital hypothyroidism, and (rarely) maternal hyperparathyroidism.

2. The most common reason for hypocalcemia in the newborn period is prematurity.

3. Breast milk rickets is seen in premature infants because of the relatively low mineral (e.g., calcium and phosphorus) content of breast milk.

4. Serum calcium levels are frequently elevated in patients with Williams syndrome.

5. Normal magnesium levels are needed for optimal functioning of the parathyroid glands.

5. **How can the calcium requirements for premature infants be met by oral feedings?**
Recent studies in premature infants using stable isotopes of calcium showed a true calcium absorption rate of 50% to 90%. Thus to meet an accretion rate of 100 mg/kg/day with an absorption rate of 75% and an assumed retention rate of 75% (which may be on the high side), oral intake of calcium for growing premature infants should be about 200 mg/kg/day. This large intake in infants with very low birth weight can be achieved only with special formulas for low-birth-weight infants or mineral fortifiers for breast milk–fed preterm infants.

Tsang RC, Lucas A, Uauy R, et al., editors. Nutritional needs of the preterm infant. Baltimore: Williams & Wilkins; 1993.

6. **How can the calcium requirements for premature infants be met by hyperalimentation solutions?**

This problem is much more difficult to address, although intestinal absorption is not a factor. In the early weeks of life with fluid intakes of 150 mg/kg/day, it is difficult to exceed an IV calcium intake of 60 mg/kg/day in the smallest premature infants (weight <1000 g) with standard total parenteral nutrition (TPN) solutions. When the concentration of calcium exceeds 60 mg/dL (3 mEq/dL) in TPN solutions, precipitation with phosphate may occur, depending on variables such as temperature, pH, amino acid content, and even the method by which the nutrients are added to the solution.

7. **What is the pathophysiology of "breast milk rickets" in premature infants?**

Clinical rickets develops in preterm infants with very low birth weight who are fed human milk not fortified with minerals and vitamins. Typically, the disease presents after 8 weeks of life with severe hypophosphatemia, "relative hypercalcemia," and hypercalciuria. The x-ray findings mimic those of rickets resulting from vitamin D deficiency. The biochemical findings are the result of low mineral intake. Because human milk is low in both calcium and phosphorus, the very low phosphorus intake (about 50% of calcium intake) severely limits deposition of calcium in bone.

Caution: Because treatment with phosphorus alone can result in severe hypocalcemia, supplements of both minerals are imperative.

8. **What is the differential diagnosis of the etiology of a hypocalcemic seizure in a 14-day-old term infant?**

Seizures secondary to hypocalcemia are very unlikely in a previously healthy term infant at 2 weeks of age. The differential diagnosis includes late infantile tetany associated with high phosphate load (e.g., feedings with cow milk), acid–base disturbances caused by diarrhea treated with alkali therapy, and congenital hypomagnesemia (rare).

9. **What is the appropriate therapy for a hypocalcemic seizure in a 14-day-old term infant?**

Treatment of hypocalcemic seizures is the same for both premature and term infants. In general, 10% calcium gluconate containing 9.4 mg/mL of elemental calcium is the drug of choice. The usual dose of 2 mL/kg body weight (18 mg/kg of elemental calcium). Infusion should occur slowly over the course of 10 minutes with heart rate monitoring. Make sure the line is patent before infusing calcium.

HYPERCALCEMIA

10. **How many fractions of calcium are found in the serum? Which can be measured in the clinical laboratory?**

There are three fractions of calcium in serum: ionized calcium (50%), calcium bound to serum proteins (40%), and calcium complexed to serum anions (10%). Ionized calcium and total calcium can be measured in most hospital laboratories.

11. **What are the normal serum calcium values in term infants?**

Normal values (in milligrams per deciliter, expressed as mean± standard deviation and range) depend on chronologic age and laboratory variation (to a lesser degree):

- Cord: 10.2 +/− 0.6 (9.3–11.7)
- 2 hours: 9.7 +/− 0.6 (8.8–11.3)
- 24 hours: 9 +/−0.6 (7.8–10)

Loughead JL, Mimouni F, Tsang RC. Serum ionized calcium concentrations in normal neonates. Am J Dis Child 1988;142:516–18.

12. **What are the normal serum values in preterm infants?**
    Normal values (in milligrams per deciliter, expressed as mean ± standard deviation and range) depend on gestational age:
    - 23–27 weeks: 10.0 +/−1.0 (8.1–11.9)
    - 28–31 weeks: 10.2 +/−1.2 (8–12.5)
    - 32–34 weeks: 10.5 +/−1 (8.6–12.4)
    - 35–36 weeks:10.4 +/−1.1 (8.3–12.5)
    - >36 weeks: 10.9 +/−0.5 (9.8–11.9)

    Fenton TR, Lyon AW, Rose MS. Cord blood calcium, phosphate, magnesium, and alkaline phosphatase gestational age-specific reference intervals for preterm infants. BMC Pediatr 2011;11:76.

13. **List the manifestations of hypercalcemia in neonates.**
    - Lethargy
    - Irritability
    - Polyuria
    - Vomiting
    - Constipation
    - Failure to thrive

14. **What values "define" hypercalcemia in newborn infants?**
    Total serum calcium above 10.8 mg/dL or ionized serum calcium above 5.4 mg/dL.

15. **What are some of the causes of hypercalcemia in neonates?**
    - Iatrogenic hypercalcemia
    - Subcutaneous fat necrosis
    - Idiopathic infantile hypercalcemia
    - Williams syndrome
    - Hyperparathyroidism (primary and secondary)
    - PTH-related peptide tumor
    - Hyperprostaglandin E syndrome
    - Hypophosphatasia
    - Familial hypercalciuric hypercalcemia
    - Blue diaper syndrome
    - Thyrotoxicosis
    - Vitamin A intoxication
    - Chronic thiazide toxicity
    - Excessive maternal intake of vitamin D

16. **How is acute hypercalcemia managed in newborn infants?**
    - Promote diuresis by administering IV fluids (normal saline).
    - Administer furosemide, and monitor serum electrolytes carefully only after adequate hydration is given.
    - Hydrocortisone (1 mg/kg every 6 hours) is of value only in chronic situations to reduce intestinal absorption of calcium.
    - In severe cases dialysis may be required to lower calcium levels while the patient is awaiting definitive treatment of the underlying cause.

    Bachrach LK, Lum CK. Etidronate in subcutaneous fat necrosis of the newborn. J Pediatr 1999;135:530–1.

17. **A 3-day-old infant born small for gestational age at term has a total serum calcium level of 13.2 mg/dL. She was delivered by emergency cesarean**

section and was diagnosed with supravalvular aortic stenosis. What is the likely diagnosis?

Williams syndrome is the likely diagnosis in an infant with hypercalcemia and supravalvular stenosis who was born small for gestational age. It results from a deletion of the elastin gene on 7q11.23. Affected infants are often described as having "elfin" faces.

Pohlenz J, Van Vliet G. Developmental abnormalities of the thyroid. In: Weiss RE, Refetoff S, editors. Genetic diagnosis of endocrine disorders. Amsterdam: Academic Press/Elsevier; 2010. p.101.

18. **A term infant is incidentally noted to have a calcium level of 12.2 mg/dL at 4 days of age. Family history reveals that the father has also been evaluated for elevated calcium levels. What would you expect to find on measurement of the infant's urinary calcium level? What is the most likely diagnosis? What is the appropriate therapy?**

The most likely diagnosis is an autosomal dominant mutation of the calcium-sensing receptor, or "hypocalciuric hypercalcemia." The infant's urinary calcium level will be inappropriately low for the serum calcium. In the heterozygous state this is generally thought to be a benign condition, and treatment is not indicated. Rare cases of homozygous mutations result in severe neonatal hyperparathyroidism, which is a life-threatening disorder.

Hsu SC, Levine MA. Perinatal calcium metabolism: physiology and pathophysiology. Semin Neonatol 2004;9:23–36.

19. **Why is the diaper blue in blue diaper syndrome?**

A defect in the intestinal transport of tryptophan causes excretion of blue, water-insoluble tryptophan metabolites. The reason that these children have high calcium levels is not well understood.

HYPOMAGNESEMIA AND HYPERMAGNESEMIA

20. **How are millimoles (mmol) of magnesium converted to milliequivalents (mEq) and milligrams (mg)?**

   1 mmol = 2 mEq = 24 mg. Therefore, 1 mEq of magnesium = 12 mg.

21. **What two types of magnesium reactions are important in human physiology?**

   Intracellular and extracellular types of magnesium reactions are important.

22. **What is the role of magnesium in intracellular reactions?**

   Magnesium is the second most abundant intracellular cation after potassium and helps to regulate cellular metabolism. As part of the magnesium-adenosine triphosphate complex, it is essential for all biosynthetic processes, including glycolysis, formation of cyclic adenosine monophosphate, and transmission of the genetic code. In addition, any reaction that uses or produces energy requires magnesium.

23. **What are the extracellular reactions that involve magnesium?**

   Only 1% of magnesium is contained in extracellular fluid. However, extracellular concentrations are critical for maintenance of electric potentials of nerve and muscle membranes and for the transmission of impulses across the neuromuscular junction. Magnesium and calcium may act synergistically or antagonistically in many of these processes.

24. **What causes magnesium depletion in neonates?**

   - Maternal diabetes
   - Maternal magnesium deficiency
   - Renal losses of magnesium in acidotic states

- Use of nutrient solutions containing insufficient amounts of magnesium
- Renal tubular defects
- Intestinal wasting of magnesium (rare X-linked condition)
- Gastrointestinal losses (through emesis, nasogastric suctioning, and diarrhea)
- Prematurity, which increases the risk for magnesium deficiency
- Intrauterine growth retardation

Rubin LP. Neonatal disorders of serum magnesium. In: Taeusch HW, Ballard RA, editors. Avery's diseases of the newborn. 7th ed. Philadelphia: Saunders; 1998. p. 1189–1206.

25. What are the signs and symptoms of magnesium deficiency in neonates?
Most infants are asymptomatic. On rare occasions the following signs and symptoms may be seen:
- Color: pallor, cyanosis, or duskiness
- Affect: out of touch with surroundings, apathetic, irritable when disturbed, restless
- Eyes: staring with infrequent blinking, oculogyric crises
- Heart: tachycardia (bradycardia during apneic episodes)
- Respiration: brief apnea, sometimes followed by tachypnea
- Neuromuscular system: motor weakness, transient spasticity, abnormal reflexes; if hypocalcemia develops (discussed later), the infant may show signs associated with calcium deficiency, including seizures

26. What are the effects of hypomagnesemia on calcium homeostasis?
Hypomagnesemia usually increases the secretion of PTH, thereby increasing calcium levels. In chronic magnesium-deficient states, however, secretion of PTH is reduced. In such circumstances hypomagnesemia may induce hypocalcemia.

Spiegel, DM. Normal and abnormal magnesium metabolism. In: Schrier RW, editor. Renal and electrolyte disorders. 7th ed. Philadelphia: Lippincott Williams & Wilkins; 2010. p. 240.

27. What causes hypermagnesemia in neonates?
- Maternal treatment with magnesium (for preeclampsia or tocolysis)
- Excessive magnesium administration to neonate (e.g., TPN, antacids, treatment of pulmonary hypertension)

28. How should hypomagnesemia be treated parenterally?
- Hypomagnesemia usually is treated intravenously or intramuscularly with a 50% solution of magnesium sulfate.
- One milliliter of a 50% solution contains 4 mEq of elemental magnesium. The usual dose is 0.1 to 0.25 mL/kg/day.
- Serum magnesium levels should be monitored every 12 hours.

29. What are the signs of hypermagnesemia in neonates?
- Flaccidity
- Unresponsiveness
- Respiratory insufficiency
- Apnea (especially when aminoglycoside antibiotics are used concurrently)
- Ileus
- Delayed passage of meconium
In extreme cases cardiorespiratory function ceases, and death ensues.

30. How is hypermagnesemia treated?
- Stop the administration of magnesium.
- Make sure the infant is well hydrated.
- Consider diuretic therapy.

- In severe cases exchange transfusion (with acid-citrate-dextrose solution) is effective.
- The effects of calcium salts are equivocal.

THYROID DISORDERS

31. What is the incidence of congenital hypothyroidism?
Congenital hypothyroidism occurs in 1 in 4000 liveborn infants.

32. What are the embryonic stages of development of the fetal hypothalamic–pituitary–thyroid axis?
- Thyroid tissue is first identified at the base of the tongue 16 to 17 days after conception.
- By 7 weeks' gestation the gland has migrated to its final position in the anterior neck and has developed its characteristic bilobed structure.
- By 10 weeks' gestation the fetal thyroid gland is trapping iodine and synthesizing thyroxine (T_4).
- By 10 weeks' gestation, the fetal hypothalamus is synthesizing thyrotropin-releasing hormone (TRH). Most fetal TRH, however, is made in extrahypothalamic tissues (e.g., placenta, pancreas). Hypothalamic TRH production does not mature fully until the perinatal period.
- By 10 to 12 weeks' gestation, the fetal pituitary gland is synthesizing thyroid-stimulating hormone (TSH).

Fisher DA, Dussault JH, Sack J, et al. Ontogenesis of hypothalamic-pituitary-thyroid function and metabolism in man, sheep and rat. Rec Prog Hormone Res 1977;33:59–116.

33. When does the fetal hypothalamic–pituitary–thyroid axis begin to function?
The hypothalamic–pituitary–thyroid axis is in place by the end of the first trimester. The thyroid and pituitary glands reach mature secretory capacity by 30 to 35 weeks of gestation. The feedback inter-relationship among the units is fully established when hypothalamic TRH maturation is completed by 1 to 2 months after birth.

Fisher DA, Klein AH. Thyroid development and disorders of thyroid function in the newborn. N Engl J Med 1981;304:706.

34. Describe the pattern of secretion of T_4 during gestation.
The amount of T_4 secreted by the fetal thyroid gland increases slowly until midgestation (20 to 24 weeks) when, stimulated by increasing amounts of TSH from the fetal pituitary, T_4 levels begin to increase more rapidly, reaching a normal adult level by approximately 30 weeks' gestation. Thereafter T_4 increases slowly to high normal levels at term gestation.

Fisher DA. Fetal thyroid function: diagnosis and management of fetal thyroid disorders. Clin Obstet Gynecol 1997;40:16–31.

35. Describe the pattern of TSH secretion during gestation.
The amount of circulating TSH begins to increase in midgestation (20 weeks) and reaches a peak level of approximately 15 μU/mL by 30 weeks' gestation. The TSH level then declines gradually to about 10 μU/mL at term.

36. Do maternal TSH and maternal iodine cross the placenta?
Maternal TSH does not cross the placenta, but maternal iodine crosses the placenta freely and is essential for the synthesis of thyroid hormones by the fetus.

37. Do maternal T_3 and T_4 levels have any effect on the fetus?
The placenta is a barrier to the passages of thyroid hormones and contains enzymes that break down maternal T_4 and T_3 into inactive metabolites. Only a small percentage of circulating maternal T_4 and very little (if any) T_3 reaches the fetus. However, the amount of maternal T_4 that does cross the placenta is significant. During the first 10 to 12 weeks of gestation, all of the circulating T_4 in the fetus is from maternal sources; thus early brain development depends on maternal hormone. Even after the fetus synthesizes its own T_4 in the second and third trimesters, maternal T_4 is essential for normal

TABLE 8-1. SERUM THYROXINE (µg/dL) AT DIFFERENT GESTATIONAL AGES*

Adapted from Cuestas RA. Thyroid function in healthy premature infants. J Pediatr 1978;92:963–7.

TIME	30 to 31	31 to 33	34 to 35	36 to 37	TERM
Cord	6.5 (1)	7.5 (2.1)	6.7 (1.2)	7.5 (2.8)	8.2 (1.8)
3 to 10 days	7.7 (1.8)	8.5 (1.9)	10 (2.4)	12.7 (2.5)	15.9 (3)
11 to 20 days	7.5 (1.8)	8.3 (1.6)	10.5 (1.8)	11.2 (2.9)	12.2 (2)
*Mean (standard deviation).					

neurologic development, including neuronal proliferation and maturation, dendritic arborization, and synapse formation. It accounts for approximately 30% of fetal T_4 levels at term.

Lazarus JH, Bestwick JP, Channon S, et al. Antenatal thyroid screening and childhood cognitive function. N Engl J Med 2012;366:493–501.
    Gyamfi C, Wapner RJ, D'Alton ME. Thyroid dysfunction in pregnancy: the basic science and clinical evidence surrounding the controversy in management. Obstet Gynecol 2009;113(3):702–7.

38. **What happens to TSH levels at parturition?**
    Within 15 to 20 minutes after birth, the fetal pituitary releases a surge of TSH, probably in response to cooling. TSH reaches a peak of about 80 µU/mL in approximately 30 minutes, decreases rapidly over the first 24 hours of life, and then drops more gradually to levels comparable to normal adult levels by the end of the first 1 to 2 weeks of life.

39. **How does the TSH surge affect T_4 levels?**
    Serum T_4 levels increase rapidly, reaching a peak level of about 17 µg/dL at 24 hours. T_4 then gradually decreases to levels at the upper limit of normal adult values over the first 4 to 5 weeks of life. Free T_4 levels follow the same pattern, reaching a peak of 3.5 ng/dL at 24 to 36 hours.

40. **How do levels of thyroid hormone differ in premature and term infants?**
    The levels of TRH, TSH, T4, free T_4, and T_3 are lower in premature infants than in term infants, and the postnatal surges of TSH and T_4, although qualitatively similar, are blunted. These differences are related directly to gestational age: the lower the gestational age, the lower the levels and responses of thyroid-related hormones (Table 8-1).

41. **What is hypothyroxinemia of prematurity?**
    The term refers to infants with low birth weight (30 to 35 weeks' gestation) or very low birth weight (<30 weeks' gestation), who have an even more attenuated rise in T_4, after which T_4 levels drop below cord levels in the first week of life. Then they rise gradually over 3 to 6 weeks to approach levels of term infants (Table 8-2).

42. **Should hypothyroxinemia of prematurity be treated?**
    The premature infant with low T_4 and persistently elevated TSH has either transient or permanent hypothyroidism and should be treated with T_4 until the nature of the condition becomes clear. However, whether premature infants with low T_4 and normal TSH levels should be treated remains controversial.

Fisher DA. Thyroid function and dysfunction in premature infants. Pediatr Endocrinol Rev 2007;4(4):317–28.
    Rapaport R, Rose SR, Freemark M. Hypothyroxinemia in the preterm infant: the benefits and risks of thyroxine treatment. J Pediatr 2001;139(2):182–8.

43. **Does breastfeeding provide needed T_4 to premature infants with an immature hypothalamic–pituitary–thyroid axis?**
    This question has not yet been answered. There are some case reports in the literature suggesting that breastfeeding delays the onset of hypothyroidism, but others argue against that finding.

TABLE 8-2. THYROID FUNCTION IN PRETERM AND TERM INFANTS*

http://www.uptodate.com/contents/image?imageKey=PEDS%2F72215&topicKey=PEDS%2F5840&rank=4~150&source=
see_link&search=thyroid+function&utdPopup=true

Adapted from Williams FL, Simpson J, Delahunty C, et al. Developmental trends in cord and postpartum serum thyroid hormones in preterm infants. J Clin Endocrinol Metab 2004;89:5314.

GESTATION (WEEKS)	AGE OF SPECIMEN	FREE T_4 (ng/dL)	T_4 (µg/dL)	T_3 (ng/dL)	TSH (µU/mL)
23 to 27 weeks	Cord	1.28 (0.4)	5.4 (2.0)	20 (15)	6.8 (2.9)
	7 d	1.47 (0.6)	4 (1.8)	33 (20)	3.5 (2.6)
	14 d	1.45 (0.5)	4.7 (2.6)	41 (25)	3.9 (2.7)
	28 d	1.50 (0.4)	6.1 (2.3)	63 (27)	3.8 (4.7)
28 to 30 weeks	Cord	1.45 (0.4)	6.3 (2)	29 (21)	7.0 (3.7)
	7 d	1.82 (0.7)	6.3 (2.1)	56 (24)	3.6 (2.5)
	14 d	1.65 (0.4)	6.6 (2.3)	72 (28)	4.9 (11.2)
	28 d	1.71 (0.4)	7.5 (2.3)	87 (31)	3.6 (2.5)
31 to 34 weeks	Cord	1.49 (0.3)	7.6 (2.3)	35 (23)	7.9 (5.2)
	7 d	2.14 (0.6)	9.4 (3.4)	92 (36)	3.6 (4.8)
	14 d	1.98 (0.4)	9.1 (3.6)	110 (41)	3.8 (9.3)
	28 d	1.88 (0.5)	8.9 (3.0)	120 (40)	3.5 (3.4)
>37 weeks	Cord	1.41 (0.3)	9.2 (1.9)	60 (35)	6.7 (4.8)
	7 d	2.70 (0.6)	12.7 (2.9)	148 (50)	2.6 (1.8)
	14 d	2.03 (0.3)	10.7 (1.4)	167 (31)	2.5 (2.0)
	28 d	1.65 (0.3)	9.7 (2.2)	176 (32)	1.8 (0.9)

T_4, Thyroxine; T_3, triiodothyronine; TSH, thyroid-stimulating hormone; free T_4, free thyroxine.
*Mean (standard deviation).

44. **Why do we screen for congenital hypothyroidism?**
    Signs and symptoms of hypothyroidism are subtle at birth, and the characteristic appearance of cretinism may not be apparent for 3 to 4 months. The brain requires thyroid hormone for normal development until approximately 2 to 3 years of age, and deficiency of thyroid hormone during this period causes irreversible brain damage to an extent related directly to the length of time of the hypothyroidism. Thus it is of vital importance to identify a hypothyroid infant as quickly as possible, even before clinical signs appear.

45. **When and how is thyroid screening done?**
    A heel-stick blood sample is taken at discharge or 3 days of life, whichever is earlier. In most parts of the United States, T_4 is measured first, then TSH is measured in samples with the lowest 10% to 29% of T_4 results.

LaFranchi SH. Approach to the diagnosis and treatment of neonatal hypothyroidism. J Clin Endocrinol Metab 2011;96(10):2959–67.
American Academy of Pediatrics. Update of newborn screening and therapy for congenital hypothyroidism. Pediatrics. 2006;117(6):2290–303.

46. **What are the causes of congenital hypothyroidism and the incidence of each type?**
    See Table 8-3.

47. **How does maternal Graves disease affect the fetus and neonate?**
    The thyroid-stimulating immunoglobulins (TSIs) cross the placenta and may cause fetal thyrotoxicosis, resulting in goiter, tachycardia, rapid skeletal maturation, premature birth, and congestive heart failure. Long-term neurologic deficits may result because excessive T_4 reduces neuronal proliferation.
    Only approximately 1 in 70 neonates born to thyrotoxic mothers exhibit clinical thyrotoxicosis. Such infants may show a phase of transient hypothyroidism caused by antithyroid drugs (half-life, 2 to 3 days), then thyrotoxicosis resulting from maternal TSIs. Transient congenital hypothyroidism can result from transplacental transfer of maternal thyrotopin-blocking antibodies.

    Feingold SB, Brown RS. Neonatal thyroid function. NeoReviews 2010;11;e640–e646.

48. **How may treatment of maternal Graves disease affect the fetus and neonate?**
    - Antithyroid drugs (e.g., propylthiouracil [PTU], methimazole) cross the placenta and may block the fetal thyroid, leading to fetal hypothyroidism.
    - Radioactive iodine crosses the placenta and ablates the fetal thyroid.
    - Beta-adrenergic agents (e.g., propranolol) cross the placenta and have been associated with intrauterine growth retardation, bradycardia, respiratory distress, and hypoglycemia.

    Downing S, Halpern L, Carswell J, et al. Severe maternal hypothyroidism corrected prior to the third trimester is associated with normal cognitive outcome in the offspring thyroid. 2012;22(6):625–30.

49. **Is breastfeeding contraindicated in mothers with Graves disease?**
    Methimazole and carbamazole are excreted into breast milk in quantities that may affect the infant adversely. If breastfeeding cannot be avoided, the infant should undergo thyroid function tests at weekly intervals to avoid potential hypothyroidism. PTU is not a contraindication to breastfeeding because only approximately 0.1% is excreted in breast milk.

50. **What are the signs of neonatal thyrotoxicosis?**
    - Goiter
    - Low birth weight with normal length
    - Proptosis
    - Periorbital edema

TABLE 8-3. CAUSES OF CONGENITAL HYPOTHYROIDISM AND INCIDENCE OF EACH

From Fisher FA. Disorders of the thyroid in the newborn and infant. In: Sperling MA, editor. Pediatric endocrinology. Philadelphia: Saunders; 1996. p. 57.

CAUSE	INCIDENCE	PERCENTAGE OF CASES
Thyroid dysgenesis (aplasia, hypoplasia, ectopy)	1:4000	75%
Thyroid dyshormonogenesis	1:30,000	10%
Hypothalamic–pituitary hypothyroidism	1:100,000	5%
Transient hypothyroidism (secondary to drugs or maternal antibodies, idiopathic)	1:40,000	10%

- Hyperactivity, hyperirritability
- Poor weight gain despite ravenous feeding
- Frequent stooling

✓ KEY POINTS: THYROID-RELATED DISORDERS

1. Hypothyroxinemia of prematurity is associated with a developmental immaturity of the hypothalamic–pituitary–thyroid axis and therefore should never be used as an explanation for low thyroid levels in the presence of an elevated TSH level.

2. Hypopituitarism in a neonate most often presents with hypoglycemia and may also cause hyponatremia, jaundice, micropenis, and undescended testes.

3. The most common cause of virilized external genitalia in a 46,XX infant is 21-hydroxylase deficiency.

4. The fetal hypothalamic–pituitary–thyroid axis is in place by the end of the first trimester but is not fully mature until 2 months postpartum (term).

5. Maternal T_4 does cross the placenta and is essential for the normal neurologic development of the fetus.

6. TSH and T_4 levels rise in both premature and term infants immediately after birth; however, the rise in premature infants is blunted.

7. Infants with neonatal thyrotoxicosis are at an increased risk for congestive heart failure and learning disorders.

51. Does neonatal thyrotoxicosis require treatment?
Neonatal thyrotoxicosis normally is a self-limited disease that subsides by about 3 months of age when maternal TSIs are metabolized. However, tachycardia, irritability, and poor weight gain require treatment with methimazole with or without propranolol. The danger of treatment is oversuppression of the neonatal thyroid and consequent hypothyroidism.

52. How do iodide-containing medicines affect the fetal thyroid state?
The mature thyroid stops synthesis of T_4 in the presence of excessive iodine (i.e., Wolff–Chaikoff effect) but escapes from this inhibition when intrathyroidal iodine pools are depleted. The fetal thyroid cannot escape the inhibition and develops into a goiter that can be large enough to require emergency transection at birth. In addition, the continued blockade of T_4 production by iodine leads to fetal hypothyroidism.

Note: Premature infants are also unable to escape from the inhibitory effect of iodine and may become hypothyroid when subjected to multiple povidone-iodine washings or iodinated contrast agents, associated with an elevation of TSH. This is particularly important in infants who have required repeated procedures.

Allemand D, Grüters A, Beyer P, et al. Iodine in contrast agents and skin disinfectants is the major cause for hypothyroidism in premature infants during intensive care. Hormone Res 1987;28:42–9.

ADRENAL DISORDERS

53. Which disorders of adrenal steroidogenesis should be suspected as a possible cause for virilization of a 46,XX fetus?
- 21-hydroxylase deficiency: This disorder results in virilization in females, salt wasting (aldosterone deficient, 75%), and signs of cortisol deficiency (e.g., hypoglycemia, shock).
- 11-hydroxylase deficiency: Salt retention and hypertension are seen in 50% to 80% of cases, and virilization is seen in females.

54. **Which disorders of adrenal steroidogenesis should be suspected as a possible cause for undervirilization of a 46,XY fetus?**
    - Steroidogenic acute regulatory (StAR) protein deficiency (i.e., congenital adrenal lipoid hyperplasia) leads to salt wasting and ambiguous genitalia in males.
    - 3-α-hydroxysteroid dehydrogenase deficiency results in salt wasting, mild virilization in females, and ambiguous genitalia in males.
    - 17-β-hydroxylase deficiency results in hypertension and ambiguous genitalia in males.

55. **In infants with congenital adrenal hyperplasia (CAH) caused by 21-hydroxylase deficiency, which of the following is abnormal: (1) genetic sex, (2) gonadal differentiation, (3) internal genital formation and structure, or (4) external genitalia in females?**
    The answer is (4). In female infants with CAH, the karyotype (genetic sex) is normal (46XX). The müllerian ducts develop normally into a uterus and fallopian tubes without secretion of antimüllerian hormone. No wolffian duct derivatives are formed because no fetal testis is present. The elevated adrenal androgen levels cause virilization of the external genitalia.

Speiser PW, White PC. Congenital adrenal hyperplasia. N Engl J Med. 2003;349(8):776–788.

56. **List the sources of maternal androgens that cause masculinization.**
    - Androgen-secreting tumors
    - Ingestion of synthetic progestins, androgens, or danazol (a derivative of testosterone)

57. **A male fetus is exposed to maternal progestin at 10 weeks of gestation. What is the possible manifestation?**
    Exposure of male fetuses to progestin at 8 to 14 weeks of gestation may result in hypospadias.

Carmichael SL, Shaw GM, Laurent C, et al. Maternal progestin intake and risk of hypospadias. Arch Pediatr Adolesc Med 2005;159(10):957–62.

58. **What causes adrenal hemorrhage in neonates?**
    Adrenal hemorrhage occurs more frequently after breech delivery, with eventual calcification in some cases. Hypoxia, fetal distress, maternal diabetes, and congenital syphilis also have been associated with adrenal hemorrhage. Adrenal hemorrhage can present as an abdominal mass.

59. **What are the manifestations of adrenal hemorrhage?**
    Even with bilateral adrenal hemorrhage, most infants are asymptomatic. On occasion, however, severe abnormalities of glucose, sodium, and potassium may be noted with signs of shock.

60. **Describe the evaluation of adrenal hemorrhage.**
    The evaluation should include a 60-minute adrenocorticotropic hormone stimulation test with measurement of baseline and 60-minute cortisols. The normal peak is greater than 20 μg/dL.

61. **A pregnant woman has a low urinary estriol level. At delivery, her male infant develops hyponatremia, hyperkalemia, and hypoglycemia. What diagnosis should you consider?**
    Congenital adrenal hypoplasia should be considered. A low maternal estriol level occurs because the fetus contributes to the precursors for placental formation of maternal estriols.

62. **How common is congenital adrenal hypoplasia?**
    Congenital adrenal hypoplasia is an X-linked disorder affecting 1 in 12,500 live births.

McCabe ERB. Adrenal hypoplasias and aplasias. In: Scriver CR, Beaudet AL, Valle D, Sly WS, Childs B, Kinzler KW, Vogelstein B, editors. The Metabolic and Molecular Bases of Inherited Diseases. 8th ed. Vol 3. New York: McGraw-Hill; 2001. p. 4263–74.

63. With what other disorders is congenital adrenal hypoplasia associated?

- Anencephaly
- Pituitary hypoplasia
- Gonadotropin deficiency

Bassett JH, O'Halloran DJ, Williams GR, et al. Novel DAX1 mutations in X-linked adrenal hypoplasia congenita and hypogonadotrophic hypogonadism. Clin Endocrinol (Oxf) 1999;50:69–75.

64. What is StAR protein?

StAR protein is necessary for proper reduction of aldosterone, cortisone, and sex hormones. Its absence leads to feminization of males as part of congenital lipoid adrenal hyperplasia. In a subset of patients with congenital lipoid adrenal hyperplasia, mutations in StAR protein result in severe impairment of steroid biosynthesis in the adrenal glands and gonads.

Jean A, Mansukhani M, Oberfield SE, et al. Prenatal diagnosis of congenital lipoid adrenal hyperplasia (CLAH) by estriol amniotic fluid analysis and molecular genetic testing. Prenat Diagn 2008;28:11–14.

65. What is the best time to obtain a cortisol level in premature neonates?

Collect the blood specimen at any time. Circadian rhythms do not affect the level of cortisol in very premature infants. Infants with extremely low birth weight may have quite low cortisol levels (9.2 ± 9.8 µg/dL) and lack the typical early-morning rise in cortisol. Whether such low corticosteroid levels in premature infants with very low birth weight indicate adrenal insufficiency is not fully known.

Metzger DL, Wright NM, Veldhuis JD, et al. Characterization of pulsatile secretion and clearance of plasma cortisol in premature and term neonates using deconvolution analysis. J Clin Endocrinol Metab 1993;77:458–63.

66. What is pseudohypoaldosteronism?

Pseudohypoaldosteronism is an inherited disease (autosomal recessive or dominant pattern) characterized by renal tubular unresponsiveness to the kaliuretic and sodium and chloride reabsorptive effects of aldosterone. In contrast to CAH or adrenal insufficiency, it is accompanied by excessive levels of renin and aldosterone. Unresponsiveness to aldosterone may be generalized, in which case sodium excretion is increased in sweat, saliva, stool, and urine, or limited to the renal tubule, in which case sodium excretion is increased in urine only.

67. How is pseudohypoaldosteronism treated?

Pseuduhypoaldosteronism is treated with massive salt supplementation and potassium-lowering agents such as Kayexalate (sodium polystyrene sulfonate).

✔ KEY POINTS: ADRENAL DISORDERS

1. CAH caused by 21-hydroxylase deficiency is the most common cause of ambiguous genitalia in a 46,XX newborn.

2. Even with bilateral adrenal hemorrhage, adrenal function is usually preserved.

3. Newborn infants lack established circadian rhythms for cortisol secretion.

PITUITARY DISORDERS

68. When does growth hormone first appear in fetal plasma?

Growth hormone first appears at 10 weeks' gestation. Levels increase in midgestation and decrease toward term.

69. Does placental growth hormone contribute to fetal levels?

No. Placental growth hormone is secreted only into the maternal circulation.

70. **When does the hypothalamic–pituitary–gonadal axis develop in the fetus?**
    Gonadotropin-releasing hormone is detectable in the hypothalamus at 8 weeks' gestation. Luteinizing hormone and follicle-stimulating hormone are present in the pituitary gland by 11 to 12 weeks' gestation and at term are found in low levels in cord blood. The fetal testis responds to human chorionic gonadotropin (hCG), but the fetal ovary does not respond because it lacks hCG receptors.

71. **What manifestations of adrenocorticotropic hormone insufficiency are seen in neonates?**
    - Hypoglycemia
    - Hyponatremia (without hyperkalemia)
    - Direct hyperbilirubinemia

72. **What are the symptoms of growth hormone deficiency in neonates?**
    The most common presenting symptom is hypoglycemia. Micropenis is also common in male neonates. Growth hormone deficiency may result in an exaggerated jaundice (direct and indirect hyperbilirubinemia). Because growth hormone is not necessary for intrauterine linear growth, intrauterine growth restriction is not a feature of growth hormone deficiency.

Palma Sisto PA. Endocrine disorders in the neonate. Pediatr Clin North Am 2004;1:1141–68.

✓ KEY POINTS: PITUITARY DISORDERS

1. Hypoglycemia and micropenis are commonly presenting symptoms and signs of neonatal hypopituitarism.

2. Midline facial defects are associated with pituitary hormone deficiencies.

3. Placental growth hormone is secreted only into the maternal circulation.

---

73. **What are the typical findings in neonates with hypogonadotropic hypogonadism (HHG)?**
    In male neonates HHG is associated with micropenis (stretched penile length <2.5 cm). Undescended testes also may be present. In female neonates there are no clinical findings of HHG.

74. **What major malformations may be associated with disorders of the hypothalamic–pituitary axis in neonates?**
    Cleft lip and palate, optic nerve atrophy, septo-optic dysplasia, and holoprosencephaly have been noted.

Traggiai C, Stanhope R. Endocrinopathies associated with midline cerebral and cranial malformations. J Pediatr 2002;140:252–55.

DISORDERS OF SEXUAL DEVELOPMENT

75. **What is the initial gene thought to be responsible for differentiation of the bipotential gonad into the testis?**
    Sex-determining region of Y-chromosome (SRY) is thought to be the first in a cascade of transcription factors that initiate the process of testicular development. SRY is located on the short arm of the Y chromosome, and the gonad loses bipotentiality at approximately 6 to 8 weeks' gestation. In the absence of SRY expression, the bipotential gonad will develop into an ovary.

76. **What two hormones, produced by the testes in utero, result in a phenotypic male?**
    Testosterone is produced by Leydig cells within the fetal testes by 6 weeks of gestation. In addition, the testes produce the peptide hormone, müllerian inhibitory substance (MIS), which eliminates all

müllerian structures in the male. An isolated deficiency in MIS produces a normal external male phenotype, but the internal phenotype is characterized by a fallopian tube running parallel to the vas deferens.

77. **What causes the XX male sex-reversal syndrome?**
There are a number of cases of 46,XX sex reversal in the literature. Only a minority of these cases have been shown to have been caused by translocation of SRY. At least one case of SOX9 duplication (a transcription factor downstream of SRY) has been reported. The majority of cases are unexplained at this time.

Ergun-Longmire B, Vinci G, Alonso L, et al. Clinical, hormonal and cytogenetic evaluation of 46,XX males and review of the literature. J Pediatr Endocrinol Metab 2005;18(8):739–48.

78. **You are asked to assess a neonate with nonpalpable gonads and genital ambiguity (i.e., severe hypospadias and an intermediate-sized phallic structure). What is the most likely diagnosis? Why?**
The most likely diagnosis is CAH caused by steroid 21-hydroxylase deficiency because it is the most common disorder of sexual development in a newborn female and because no gonadal tissue is palpable. Other diagnoses, such as mixed gonadal dysgenesis or hermaphroditism, generally present with one palpable gonad.

79. **Which one serum test has the greatest chance of confirming the correct diagnosis?**
Several steps leading to cortisol synthesis may be affected and produce the virilized female phenotype. The most likely missing enzyme is steroid 21-hydroxylase, and the result is a major accumulation of its immediate precursor, 17-hydroxyprogesterone. A serum radioimmunoassay for 17-hydroxyprogesterone should be diagnostic in almost all cases.

80. **A neonate presents with severe penoscrotal hypospadias and a palpable gonad in the left hemiscrotum; the right hemiscrotum is empty. Amniocentesis shows a classic 46,XX karyotype, and ultrasound shows a cystic structure behind the bladder but no uterus. The genitogram shows a vagina with low insertion and a tiny atretic uterine cavity. What is the differential diagnosis?**
The two most likely diagnoses are mixed gonadal dysgenesis and true hermaphroditism. The combination of a descended gonad and virilization indicates the presence of some functional testicular tissue. An ovary usually does not descend into the scrotum, and an ovotestis does so only in rare cases. In mixed gonadal dysgenesis, one gonad is a streak found within the abdomen, and one testis descends into an inguinal or scrotal position. True hermaphroditism is characterized by a combination of both ovarian-follicular and testicular tissue, which may be combined within one testis (ovotestis). The rudimentary vagina and uterus reflect inadequate production of MIS despite the presence of some testicular tissue. Because the action of MIS is also paracrine, the vaginal and uterine structures are lateralized primarily to the side opposite the testis.

81. **A neonate presents with genital ambiguity, including significant clitoromegaly and a palpable gonad on the left side in a labioscrotal fold. The right gonad is palpable in the right inguinal canal. The infant's family recently migrated from the Dominican Republic. What is the most likely diagnosis?**
The most likely diagnosis is 5-alpha reductase deficiency, which was first characterized by its striking clinical presentation. Cases are clustered in the Dominican Republic, where the culture is extremely supportive.

82. **You are asked to evaluate a neonate in the delivery room. Amniocentesis during pregnancy revealed a 46,XY karyotype, but the infant has a perfectly normal female phenotypic appearance. What is the most likely diagnosis?**
Androgen insensitivity syndrome (AIS) is the most likely diagnosis. Patients with AIS have a normal XY karyotype. The testes are fully developed but never descend, and the external genitalia are those

of a normal female. Serum testosterone levels are markedly elevated, but no virilization takes place. Because of a mutation in the androgen receptor, androgen has no effect on its target tissues. AIS, in effect, is end-organ failure based on molecular mutation; it is a syndrome in the sense that several point mutations have been identified.

83. **What are the likely findings on pelvic examination?**
Absence of the uterus and upper two thirds of the vagina is the most likely finding. These structures originate from the müllerian ducts, which involute in response to secretion of MIS. The testes are normal and produce normal amounts of testosterone and MIS.

84. **A male neonate in the intensive care unit has a right hernia and a left undescended testis. When the bulging hernia enlarges, intervention is recommended. The surgeon reports that a fallopian tube has been found in the hernia sac. What is the diagnosis?**
The diagnosis is hernia uteri inguinalis.

✓ KEY POINTS: DISORDERS OF SEXUAL DEVELOPMENT

1. Informative findings in narrowing the differential diagnosis in an infant with ambiguous genitalia are the presence or absence of palpable gonads, the presence or absence of a uterus, or a combination thereof.

2. MIS levels may be useful in documenting the presence of testicular tissue (Sertoli cells).

3. Complete androgen insensitivity is rarely diagnosed in infancy but may present in the newborn period when a phenotypically normal female infant is born after a prenatal karyotype of 46,XY has been documented on amniocentesis.

85. **What causes hernia uteri inguinalis?**
Absence of MIS, which is produced by the testis and results in involution of müllerian ducts during the course of normal male sexual differentiation, causes hernia uteri inguinalis. A normal-appearing testis that produces testosterone may lack the capacity to synthesize or secrete MIS. The result is a normal external prominent utricle.

http://omim.org/entry/261550

HYPOGLYCEMIA

86. **How is neonatal hypoglycemia defined?**
In adults hypoglycemia is defined as a condition involving a plasma glucose level below 40 mg/dL. A plasma glucose concentration of 70 to 100 mg/dL is considered normal, and the therapeutic target range for adults with hypoglycemia is above 60 mg/dL. The definition in neonates is controversial. Some physicians accept significantly lower plasma glucose concentrations as normal for neonates. However, in the absence of scientific evidence that neonates tolerate lower concentrations than adults, many clinicians now believe that values below 50 mg/dL are abnormal. This definition is supported by Koh and colleagues, who demonstrated electrophysiologic changes in the brains of infants when glucose reaches 50 mg/dL.

Stanley CA. Hypoglycemia in the neonate. Pediatr Endocrinol Rev 2006;4(Suppl 1):76–81.

Cornblath M, Hawdon JM, Williams AF, et al. Controversies regarding definition of neonatal hypoglycemia: suggested operational thresholds. Pediatrics 2000;105:1141–5.

Koh TH, Aynsley-Green A, Tarbit M. et al. Neural dysfunction during hypoglycaemia. Arch Dis Child 1988;63:1353–8.

87. **Why is glucose important?**
Glucose is the primary fuel for the brain and accounts for over 90% of total body oxygen consumption early in fasting. Because of their larger brain-to-body size ratio, infants have greater glucose requirements than adults. Hepatic glucose production rates in infants are approximately 6 mg/kg/min (3 to 6 times greater than those of adults).

88. **What causes hypoglycemia in neonates?**
Hypoglycemia results from either abnormal control of fasting adaptations or failure of a particular fasting metabolic system. In the first 12 to 24 hours of life, normal newborns are at increased risk for hypoglycemia because gluconeogenesis and especially ketogenesis are incompletely developed. Hypoglycemia occurring or persisting after the first 24 hours of life is abnormal and implies failure of one of the fasting systems.

88a. **Which infant catgories are at high risk for hypoglycemia?**
- Late-preterm infants
- Infants of diabetic mothers and large-for-gestational age infants
- Small-for-getational age infants

89. **What physical features suggest the cause of hypoglycemia in neonates?**
- Macrosomia: Because insulin is a growth factor, hyperinsulinism leads to macrosomia. Infants of diabetic mothers and infants with severe forms of congenital hyperinsulinism typically are large for gestational age. In addition, neonates with Beckwith–Wiedemann syndrome are macrosomic and may have hyperinsulinism.
- Midline defects: Congenital pituitary deficiency may be associated with midline defects such as cleft lip, cleft palate, single central incisor, and microophthalmia.
- Micropenis: Congenital gonadotropin deficiency can cause micropenis.
- Hepatomegaly: Glycogen storage diseases (GSDs) and fatty acid oxidation disorders may be associated with hepatomegaly.

90. **Which hormonal abnormalities cause hypoglycemia in neonates?**
- Hyperinsulinism is the most common cause of recurrent hypoglycemia in neonates.
- Hypopituitarism is the combination of growth hormone, thyroid hormone, and cortisol deficiencies.

91. **How is hypoglycemia treated acutely?**
Hypoglycemia can be treated emergently with oral or nasogastric tube feeding of dextrose or formula. If symptoms are severe, 2 mL/kg of 10% dextrose can be administered intravenously. Blood glucose should be checked within 15 minutes of intervention and subsequently monitored to ensure adequate treatment (plasma glucose above 60 mg/dL) and to prevent hypoglycemic episodes. If necessary, continuous IV dextrose is initiated (6 to 12 mg/kg/min).

92. **Which defects in fasting metabolic systems cause hypoglycemia in neonates?**
- Defects of glycogenolysis (i.e., GSDs) are associated with hepatomegaly. Examples include deficiencies of debranching enzyme (GSD type 3), liver phosphorylase (GSD type 6), and phosphorylase kinase (GSD type 9).
- Defects of gluconeogenesis include deficiencies of glucose-6-phosphatase (i.e., GSD type 1) and fructose-1,6-diphosphatase. Defects of gluconeogenesis and glycogenolysis rarely present in early infancy because neonates are not exposed to fasting for more than 4 hours at a time.
- Fatty acid oxidation disorders include medium-chain acyl dehydrogenase deficiency. Unless a neonate is breastfeeding poorly or experiences an illness that limits oral intake, a fatty acid oxidation disorder is unlikely to present in infancy. This disorder, however, can cause serious problems during fasting later in life and should be tested for as part of neonatal screening.

93. **List and explain the hormonal controls necessary for fasting adaptation.**
    - Insulin inhibits fasting metabolic systems.
    - Epinephrine stimulates hepatic glycogenolysis, hepatic gluconeogenesis, and hepatic ketogenesis.
    - Glucagon stimulates hepatic glycogenolysis.
    - Cortisol stimulates hepatic gluconeogenesis.
    - Growth hormone stimulates lipolysis.

94. **What tests should be included in the "critical sample" during a hypoglycemic episode?**
    Once hypoglycemia is confirmed (i.e., glucose ≤50 mg/dL), blood should be analyzed for the following:
    - Insulin
    - Free fatty acids
    - Growth hormone
    - Lactate/pyruvate
    - Bicarbonate
    - Ammonia
    - Ketones
    - Cortisol

95. **What causes transient hyperinsulinism?**
    Transient hyperinsulinism occurs in infants of diabetic mothers whose upregulated insulin secretion in response to a hyperglycemic fetal environment persists in the immediate postnatal period. In perinatally stressed neonates (e.g., infants who are small for gestational age or who have birth asphyxia or toxemia), hyperinsulinism caused by dysregulated insulin secretion may persist for up to several months after birth.

96. **How is transient hyperinsulinism treated?**
    Initial management consists of IV dextrose and frequent or continuous feeds. In persistent cases diazoxide (5 to 15 mg/kg/day) may be effective in controlling insulin secretion.

97. **What causes congenital hyperinsulinism?**
    Genetic defects of insulin secretion include recessive mutations of the β-cell sulfonylurea receptor/potassium channel genes and dominant gain of functional mutations of glucokinase and glutamate dehydrogenase. Dominant functional mutations are milder and usually appear later in infancy.

98. **What is the treatment for congenital hyperinsulinism?**
    Congenital hyperinsulinism caused by severe sulfonylurea receptor/potassium channel mutation is often resistant to diazoxide. Octreotide (a somatostatin analog) tempers excessive insulin secretion but rarely prevents hypoglycemia completely or normalizes fasting tolerance. Continuous glucagon infusion can stabilize blood glucose until surgery is performed, but experience with long-term use is limited. If the combination of octreotide and frequent feeds fails, pancreatectomy is necessary. Surgery may be curative if a focal lesion is present and completely resected.

Glaser B, Thornton P, Otonkoski T, et al. Genetics of neonatal hyperinsulinism. Arch Dis Child Fetal Neonatal Ed 2000;82:79–86.

Stanley C. Advances in diagnosis and treatment of hyperinsulinism in infants and children. J Clin Endocrinol Metab 2002;87:4857–9.

99. **What is the cornerstone of treatment for defects of glycogenolysis and gluconeogenesis?**
    These defects necessitate frequent feedings.

✓ KEY POINTS: HYPOGLYCEMIA

1. A work-up for hypoglycemia should be considered in any newborn who is documented to have a blood sugar level persistently lower than 50 mg/dL.

2. The three common etiologies for hypoglycemia in a neonate are decreased production owing to an inborn error of metabolism, increased utilization, and altered hormonal regulation.

3. An infant with hypoglycemia should be carefully examined for hepatomegaly, macroglossia, macrosomia, and midline abnormalities (including clefting defects).

4. The etiology of hypoglycemia is most readily identified by measuring metabolites and hormones at the time of hypoglycemia and should include measures of glucose, free fatty acids, ketones, lactate, pyruvate, ammonia, insulin, cortisol, and growth hormone. Abnormalities in any of these studies may then necessitate definitive diagnostic studies.

5. Treatment of hypoglycemia depends on the etiology but may include avoidance of fasting, a diet altered to circumvent a metabolic block, insulin suppression with diazoxide or pancreatic resection, or replacement of growth hormone or cortisol deficiency.

6. Abnormalities of both the β-cell sulfonylurea receptor and the potassium channel have been documented to cause congenital hyperinsulinism.

100. How are fatty acid oxidation disorders treated?
These disorders are treated by instituting a high-carbohydrate diet (and for certain long-chain fatty acid oxidation disorders, metabolic diets high in medium-chain triglyceride) and by ensuring that fasting is limited to 12 hours. If an affected infant is feeding poorly or experiences vomiting, IV dextrose must be initiated emergently. The finding of euglycemia in the setting of a concurrent illness should not deter the clinician from initiating IV dextrose. By the time hypoglycemia is detected in fatty oxidation disorders, liver failure, cerebral edema, and cardiac toxicity are already present or developing. Intervention must be prompt; the mortality rate during the first episode is greater than 25%.

NEONATAL SCREENING

101. Routine neonatal screening commonly tests for which diseases?
Routine neonatal screening tests for the following:
- Hypothyroidism
- Phenylketonuria (PKU)
- Glucose-6-phosphate dehydrogenase (G6PD) deficiency
- Galactosemia
- Maple syrup urine disease (MSUD) (G6PD deficiency)
- Biotinidase deficiency
- Medium-chain acyl-coenzyme A (CoA) dehydrogenase
- Fatty acid oxidation disorders
- Homocystinuria
- Sickle cell disease
- CAH
- Cystic fibrosis
- Severe combined immunodeficiency
- Hearing loss
- Cyanotic congenital heart disease

The American College of Medical Genetics recommends that clinicians screen for 29 disorders during the neonatal period.

102. **Which of these groups of diseases is likely to be life-threatening in the neonatal period: (1) galactosemia, MSUD, and CAH; or (2) sickle cell disease, G6PD deficiency, and biotinidase deficiency?**
The answer is (1). Galactosemia can cause acute liver failure promptly after institution of milk feedings. It also predisposes neonates to *Escherichia coli* septicemia. MSUD causes lethal depression of the function of the central nervous system in the neonatal period. Salt-losing CAH, caused by 21-hydroxylase deficiency, can cause addisonian crisis with hypovolemic/hyponatremic shock, hypoglycemia, and (most dangerous of all) severe hyperkalemia

103. **In which of these groups of diseases is delayed or impaired development of the central nervous system expected if effective treatment is begun at 3 months of age and not shortly after birth: PKU, hypothyroidism, MSUD, galactosemia, or homocystinuria?**
Effective treatment of PKU, hypothyroidism, and MSUD must begin within the first few weeks of life to prevent significant problems in development. In infants with galactosemia, learning disabilities are quite prominent if treatment is not initiated early. Developmental disabilities are found in 50% of untreated homocystinuric patients, but the age at which treatment must begin is not known.

Walter JH, Jahnke N, Remmington T. Newborn screening for homocystinuria. Cochrane Database Syst Rev. 2011;10(8):CD008840.

104. **In which of these groups of diseases may physical signs be present at or shortly after birth: (1) sickle cell disease, G6PD deficiency, and homocystinuria; (2) galactosemia and CAH; or (3) galactosemia, CAH, and PKU?**
The answer is (2). Some infants affected by galactosemia have cataracts shortly after birth. The female infant with CAH caused by 21-hydroxylase deficiency often has ambiguous genitalia (i.e., enlarged clitoris, labial fusion) at birth.

105. **What are the benefits of detecting sickle cell disease by neonatal screening?**
Sickle cell disease presents at various ages and in various ways, but the major threat to life for small infants is bacterial sepsis, with *Streptococcus pneumoniae* high on the list of causative organisms. Preclinical detection of sickle cell disease allows prophylaxis against pneumococcal infection.

Ellison AM, Ota KV, McGowan KL, et al. Pneumococcal bacteremia in a vaccinated pediatric sickle cell disease population. Pediatr Infect Dis J 2012;31:534–6.

106. **A 5-day-old breastfed infant has a strongly positive test result for urinary-reducing substance but a negative test result for urinary glucose. What action should be taken?**
In breastfed infants the dietary carbohydrate is lactose, which is hydrolyzed during absorption to glucose and galactose, both reducing sugars. Therefore a non–glucose-reducing substance in the urine is almost certainly galactose, and its presence strongly suggests the diagnosis of galactosemia. Intake of lactose should be stopped immediately and not re-instituted until galactosemia has been ruled out by assay for red blood cell galactose-1-phosphate uridylyltransferase. Because galactosemia can be rapidly lethal, do not delay this decision until the result of the screening test is known.

107. **How is newborn screening for cystic fibrosis performed?**
It most states it is a two-tiered test in which immunoreactive trypsinogen is first measured. Babies with the highest immunoreactive trypsinogen levels are then genetically tested for the most common mutations in cystic fibrosis transmembrane conductance regulator, including the most common delta F508 mutation.

Wagener JS, Zemanick ET, Sontag MK. Newborn screening for cystic fibrosis. Curr Opin Pediatr 2012;24:329–35.

108. How is genetic testing used in newborn screening?

To increase the specificity of newborn screening for diseases with a common genetic etiology, a two-tiered test is developed to screen for the disorder based on a metabolite or protein in the blood. The subset of newborns with the highest levels can then go on to genetic testing for the most common mutations to confirm the diagnosis genetically. This strategy has been commonly used for cystic fibrosis and medium-chain acyl-CoA dehydrogenase for which there are common mutations in the population.

✓ KEY POINTS: NEONATAL SCREENING

1. New technologic advances in tandem mass spectrometry have revolutionized newborn screening and allow for detection of dozens of inborn errors of metabolism from blood spots.

2. Specimens should be collected after 24 hours of life and, with the exception of sickle cell disease and G6PD deficiency, should not be affected by transfusions.

3. DNA diagnostic tests are also being added to newborn screening regimens to increase the specificity of testing and reduce the number of false-positive results.

4. The majority of positive results from newborn screening are false-positive results, and repeat or additional diagnostic testing is required to distinguish true positive results from false-positive results.

5. Treatment should be initiated as soon as the diagnosis is made; for some conditions, such as congenital hypothyroidism, PKU, and MSUD, permanent neurologic damage can result if treatment is delayed.

109. What new diagnostic method is being used in newborn screening to increase testing sensitivity and specificity, decrease cost, and increase the number of inborn errors of metabolism that can be effectively screened?

Tandem mass spectrometry (MS-MS) can be performed on dried blood spots and can measure hundreds of metabolites to facilitate screening of dozens of inborn errors of metabolism while more precisely quantitating the levels of the metabolites to improve screening sensitivity and specificity.

Chace DH, Spitzer AR. Altered metabolism and newborn screening: lessons learned from the bench to the bedside. Curr Pharm Biotechnol 2011;12:965–75.

110. What is the rationale for adding screening for Krabbe disease to one state's newborn screening panel?

Neonatal diagnosis before the onset of symptoms would allow for use of bone marrow transplantation as treatment at an age when it is most likely to be effective and allow for more normal brain development. Treatment initiation after the onset of symptoms often leaves children in a state of severe intellectual disability.

Perlman SJ, Mar S. Leukodystrophies. Adv Exp Med Biol 2012;724:154–71.

111. How is newborn screening for severe combined immunodeficiency (SCID) performed?

The newborn screening test for SCID based on measurement of T-cell receptor excision circles (TRECs) by real-time qPCR using DNA extracted from newborn screening of dried blood spots. RECs are by-products generated during T-cell maturation and are consistently absent or present in low numbers in newborns with SCID. Identification of infants with SCID allows for prevention of life threatening infections and early bone marrow transplantation.

INBORN ERRORS OF METABOLISM

112. What clinical signs suggest metabolic disease in neonates?
The following clinical signs suggest metabolic disease:
- Lethargy and coma
- Recurrent vomiting
- Jaundice
- Dysmorphism
- Ocular abnormalities, including cataracts
- Marked hypotonia
- Seizures
- Unusual odors
- Visceromegaly
- Abnormalities of skin or hair
- Unstable body temperature
- Bleeding
- Tachypnea unrelated to pulmonary disease

Note: The signs of metabolic disease are nonspecific. More common diseases, such as sepsis, must be considered in the differential diagnosis.

113. If a neonate misses one or two feedings, is large ketonuria likely to develop?
No. Large ketones usually are not detectable in the urine of normal newborn infants with fasting, including those with fasting-induced hypoglycemia. Conversely, ketonuria often is present in neonates with defects in gluconeogenesis and amino acid or organic acid metabolism. The rate of use of ketones as a fuel is greater in infants compared with children. Experimental data suggest that some inborn errors of metabolism may be associated with a secondary defect in ketone body use. Severe acidemia also may perturb the use of ketones.

114. Which metabolic disorders are associated with a distinctive odor?
The following metabolic disorders are associated with distinctive odors:
- PKU
- Multiple CoA carboxylase deficiency
- MSUD
- Beta-methylcrotonyl-CoA carboxylase deficiency
- Isovaleric acidemia
- Type II glutaric aciduria
- Type I tyrosinemia

115. Which metabolic disorders are commonly associated with acidosis?
The following metabolic disorders are associated with acidosis:
- Methylmalonic acidemia
- Holocarboxylase synthetase deficiency
- Propionic acidemia
- Fructose 1,6-diphosphatase deficiency
- Isovaleric acidemia
- Succinyl CoA acetoacetate CoA transferase deficiency
- MSUD
- Primary lactic acidosis due to mitochondrial disorders
- Ketothiolase deficiency, pyruvate dehydrogenase complex deficiency, citric acid cycle deficiencies, and respiratory chain deficiencies
- Type II glutaric aciduria

116. **What are the first items the neonatal transport team must address in an infant with a suspected inborn error of metabolism?**
The neonatal transport team should first address the following:
- ABCs: airway, breathing, circulation
- Hypoglycemia, metabolic acidosis

117. **What complications may the transport team encounter in infants with an inborn error?**
The transport team may encounter the following:
- Coma
- Seizures
- Cerebral edema
- Intracranial hemorrhage
- *E. coli* sepsis in infants with galactosemia
- Bleeding

118. **What congenital abnormalities are more common in infants born to women with PKU?**
Microencephaly (mental retardation) and congenital heart defects, which are thought to result from high levels of phenylalanine, are more commonly found in these infants.

119. **Which inborn errors of metabolism are commonly associated with neonatal seizures?**
The following inborn errors are common with neonatal seizures:
- Nonketotic hyperglycemia
- Pyridoxine-responsive seizure disorders
- Peroxisomal disorders (e.g., neonatal adrenoleukodystrophy)
- Sulfite oxidase deficiency
- Glucose transporter (e.g., GLUT 1) deficiency with hypoglycorrhachia
- Disorders of ammonia metabolism (e.g., ornithine transcarbamylase deficiency)
- Disorders causing hypoglycemia (e.g., fatty acid oxidation disorders, GSDs, hyperinsulinemia)

120. **What is the treatment for glucose transporter 1 deficiency syndrome?**
Treatment involves institution of a ketogenic diet, which shifts the brain's metabolism to the utilization of ketone bodies rather than carbohydrates.

Pong AW, Geary BR, Engelstad KM, et al. Glucose transporter type I deficiency syndrome: epilepsy phenotypes and outcomes. Epilepsia 2012;53:1503–10.

121. **What common metabolic diseases can cause Fanconi syndrome?**
The following are possible causes of Fanconi syndrome:
- Hereditary tyrosinemia
- Galactosemia
- Hereditary fructose intolerance
- Cytochrome C oxidase deficiency
- Pyroglutamic aciduria
- GSD type I

122. **What should the initial diagnostic assessment of an infant with suspected metabolic disease include?**
Diagnositic assessment should include the following:
- Serum electrolytes
- Blood amino acid quantitation

- Blood pH and partial pressure of carbon dioxide
- Liver function tests
- Ophthalmologic examination
- Blood lactate and pyruvate
- Urine Clinitest reaction (while the infant is ingesting a lactose-containing formula)
- Urine organic acid quantitation
- Blood ammonia (urine orotic acid, if elevated)

✓ KEY POINTS: INBORN ERRORS OF METABOLISM

1. Common presentations for inborn errors of metabolism include lethargy and coma, dysmorphism, recurrent vomiting, ocular abnormalities, tachypnea unrelated to pulmonary disease, visceromegaly, unusual odors, marked hypotonia, skin or hair abnormalities, seizures, unstable body temperature, bleeding, and jaundice.

2. Common strategies for treating inborn errors of metabolism include avoidance of fasting; dietary manipulation to avoid substrates that cannot be metabolized; medications to clear toxic by-product; supplementation with high doses of cofactors and vitamins used by the deficient enzyme; and, when appropriate, enzyme replacement therapy or organ transplants (e.g., liver or bone marrow transplant).

3. Infants with inborn errors of metabolism may not be symptomatic until metabolically stressed by an intercurrent illness or fasting.

4. Fetal development for inborn errors of metabolism may be normal if the metabolites are able to cross the placenta and may be metabolized by the mother for the fetus.

5. Sudden infant death syndrome can be caused by inborn errors of metabolism, and a family history of a death in infancy of unknown etiology should prompt screening for inborn errors of metabolism.

123. **What level of hyperammonemia should cause concern?**
Ammonia can be difficult to measure accurately because it must be run immediately by the laboratory. An ammonia level greater than 100 mmol/L is cause for concern and should be repeated. An ammonia level greater than 300 mmol/L is an emergency and may necessitate preparing for hemodialysis if it is confirmed.

124. **How should a neonate with a suspected urea cycle disorder be treated?**
Secure the airway; if necessary, intubate preemptively. Make sure that the infant receives nothing by mouth, and maintain on IV glucose only. Give IV arginine. Hemodialyze if ammonia levels are above 300 mmol/L and increasing. Administer sodium phenylbutyrate (trade name Buphenyl) and sodium benzoate as ammonia scavenger.

Bireley WR, Van Hove JL, Gallagher RC, et al. Urea cycle disorders: brain MRI and neurological outcome. Pediatr Radiol 2012;42:455–62.

125. **How should a newborn with hepatorenal tyrosinemia be treated?**
Treatment includes a diet low in phenylalanine, methionine and tyrosine. The drug 2-(2-nitro-4-trifluoromethylbenzoyl)-1,3-cyclohexanedione (NTBC) has been successful in the management of tyrosinemia. NTBC works by inhibiting the proximal tyrosine metabolic pathway. Babies should be monitored for coagulopathies resulting from problems with liver synthetic function.

126. **How can the five major kinds of metabolic diseases be distinguished?**
See Table 8-4.

TABLE 8-4. SUMMARY OF MAJOR FINDINGS IN THE FIVE MAJOR KINDS OF METABOLIC DISEASE

From Spitzer A. Intensive care of the neonate. St Louis: Mosby; 2005. p 1209.

FINDING	ORGANIC ACIDURIAS	PRIMARY LACTIC ACIDOSES	UREA CYCLE DEFECTS	CLASSIC GALACTOSEMIA	NONKETOTIC HYPERGLYCEMIA	FATTY ACID OXIDATION DEFECTS
Metabolic acidosis	Frequent	Frequent	No	No	No	Variable
Ketoaciduria	Frequent	Variable	No	No	No	No
Urine organic acids	Abnormal	Increased lactate	Normal	Nondiagnostic	Normal	Increased dicarboxylics
Lactic acidosis	No	Frequent	No	No	No	Not initially
Hyperammonemia	Usually <500 µmol/L	Usually <500 µmol/L	Usually >500 µmol/L	No	No	Possible
Blood aminogram	Nondiagnostic	Increased alanine	Very abnormal	Nondiagnostic	Marked glycine	Nondiagnostic
CSF aminogram	Nondiagnostic	Increased alanine	Very abnormal	Nondiagnostic	Marked glycine	Nondiagnostic
Urine orotic acid	Usually normal	Normal	Very high	Normal	Normal	Normal
Neutropenia	Frequent	Variable	Unusual	No	No	No
Thrombocytopenia	Frequent	Variable	Unusual	No	No	No
Urine Clinitest	Negative	Negative	Negative	Positive	Negative	Negative
Hepatic failure	No	Uncommon	No	Frequent	No	Frequent
Cataracts	No	No	No	Frequent	No	No
Cardiac disease	No	Variable	No	No	No	Frequent
Rhabdomyolysis	No	Variable	No	No	No	Frequent
Congenital malformation	Not usually	Variable	No	No	No	Variable

CSF, Cerebrospinal fluid.

127. **If an inborn error of metabolism is strongly suspected, what should the baby be fed?**
Nothing. The baby should not receive anything by mouth but should instead be given IV fluids containing only dextrose and electrolytes with enough dextrose to keep the baby anabolic.

128. **If an inborn error of metabolism is suspected, when is the best time to obtain samples for diagnostic testing?**
At the time the baby is most severely clinically affected, the diagnostic yield is highest.

129. **What is the treatment for children with PKU?**
Standard treatment is a phenylalanine-restricted formula providing just enough phenylalanine for normal growth and development. Tetrahydrobiopterin, the cofactor for phenylalanine hydroxylase, is now also approved by the Food and Drug Administration as an adjuvant to diet modification in some patients. Not all patients respond to tetrahydrobiopterin.

130. **What general treatment strategies can be used for inborn errors of metabolism?**
The following strategies can be used:
- Avoiding nonmetabolizable substrate (e.g., avoiding lactose in galactosemia and fructose in hereditary fructose intolerance)
- Supplementation with essential metabolites that are not synthesized (e.g., arginine in argininosuccinic aciduria and biotin in biotinidase deficiency)
- Supplementation with vitamins or cofactors (e.g., carnitine and riboflavin in fatty acid oxidation disorders)
- Inhibition of toxic by-product accumulation (e.g., NTBC in type I tyrosinemia)
- Enzyme replacement (e.g., Gaucher disease)
- Liver transplant (e.g., urea cycle defects)

CHAPTER 9

FLUID, ELECTROLYTE, ACID–BASE, AND RENAL-DEVELOPMENTAL PHYSIOLOGY AND DISORDERS

John M. Lorenz, MD, and Patricia L. Weng, MD

1. **How does the principal function of the kidney differ in fetal and neonatal life?**
   During fetal life the placenta is responsible for fetal water and electrolyte homeostasis. The principal function of the fetal kidney is the continuous excretion of water and electrolytes into the amniotic cavity, which is essential for maintenance of amniotic fluid volume. Normal amniotic fluid volume is essential for normal lung development. After birth the kidneys assume responsibility for maintenance of appropriate total body water and electrolyte homeostasis (Fig. 9-1).

2. **What is the urine flow rate in the fetus?**
   Urine is made by the fetus in increasing amounts as gestation advances. In fact, fetal urine output is quite high—in the range of 25% of body weight per day, approximately 750 to 1000 mL per day near term. Fetal urine, along with pulmonary secretions, is an important contributor to amniotic fluid. The process is dynamic, with amniotic fluid being produced continuously, then swallowed and reabsorbed

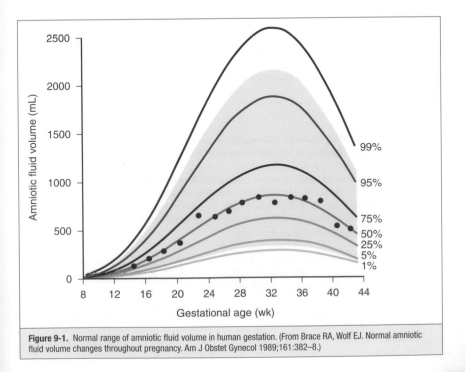

Figure 9-1. Normal range of amniotic fluid volume in human gestation. (From Brace RA, Wolf EJ. Normal amniotic fluid volume changes throughout pregnancy. Am J Obstet Gynecol 1989;161:382–8.)

from the gastrointestinal tract (Fig. 9-2). Fetal oliguria may produce oligohydramnios. Obstruction in the gastrointestinal tract or neurologic impairment of swallowing may result in polyhydramnios.

3. **When does nephrogenesis begin, and when is it complete?**
The first definitive nephrons form at 8 weeks of gestation. Renal function adequate to sustain extrauterine life develops by approximately 23 weeks of gestation. Nephrogenesis is complete at 36 weeks.

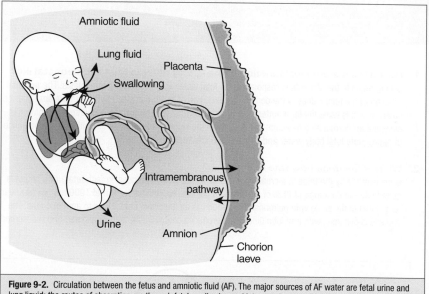

Figure 9-2. Circulation between the fetus and amniotic fluid (AF). The major sources of AF water are fetal urine and lung liquid; the routes of absorption are through fetal swallowing and intramembranous flow. (From Beall MH, van den Wijingarrd JPHM, van Germert M, et al. Placenta and fetal water flux. In: Oh W, Guignard J-P, Baumgart S, editors: Nephrology and fluid/electrolyte physiology: neonatology questions and controversies. 2nd ed. Philadelphia: Saunders; 2012. p 6.)

4. **When are the fetal kidneys detectable by ultrasound?**
By 22 weeks' gestation 95% of fetal kidneys are detectable.

5. **What proportion of cardiac output does the fetal kidney receive?**
Fetal renal blood flow (RBF) increases steadily from approximately 4% at 17 to 18 weeks of gestation to 6% at term. Adult kidneys receive between 20% and 25% of cardiac output. The low RBF in the fetus is due to high renovascular resistance caused by increased activity of the renin-angiotensis-aldosterone and sympathetic nervous systems.

6. **How does RBF change after birth? When does RBF reach adult levels?**
RBF increases sharply after birth at term to between 8% and 10% of cardiac output. Adult levels of RBF are not achieved until approximately 2 years of age.

7. **How does glomerular filtration rate (GFR) change in fetal life and after birth?**
Fetal GFR slowly increases during fetal life until approximately 36 weeks, when nephrogenesis is complete. Thereafter little increase occurs until birth, at which time there is a dramatic increase in GFR. The increase in GFR with birth is less dramatic in preterm infants (Fig. 9-3).

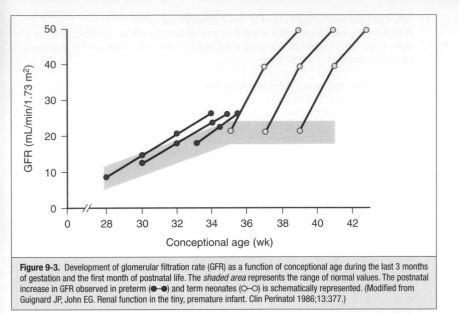

Figure 9-3. Development of glomerular filtration rate (GFR) as a function of conceptional age during the last 3 months of gestation and the first month of postnatal life. The *shaded area* represents the range of normal values. The postnatal increase in GFR observed in preterm (●–●) and term neonates (○–○) is schematically represented. (Modified from Guignard JP, John EG. Renal function in the tiny, premature infant. Clin Perinatol 1986;13:377.)

8. **What are the factors that cause the postnatal increase in GFR?**
   - Increase in net filtration pressure, which is the difference between hydrostatic pressure and oncotic pressure across glomerular capillaries
   - Increase in the ultrafiltration coefficient, which is a function of total glomerular capillary surface area and capillary permeability per unit of surface area

9. **What are normal values for GFR in a newborn infant?**
   See Table 9-1.

10. **What are normal values for serum creatinine concentration ([Cr]) in a newborn infant?**
    The answer to this question is complicated. In fact, it is the change in serum [Cr]—not a single value—after birth that is relevant. At birth serum [Cr] is largely a function of *maternal* serum [Cr]. The subsequent change varies with gestational age. In infants younger than 30 weeks' gestation, serum [Cr] either does not change or it increases 30% to 40% before declining to the birth level during the first 5 to 8 days of age, then subsequently declines before reaching a steady state by 7 to 10 weeks of age. The duration of the plateau is inversely related to gestational age; the rate of decline is directly related to gestational age. In infants at 30 weeks' gestation or older, serum [Cr] declines from birth to reach a steady value at 3 to 6 weeks of age. The rate of decline is directly related to gestational age.

TABLE 9-1. GLOMERULAR FILTRATION RATE ([mL/min/1.73 m²])			
	POSTNATAL AGE		
GESTATIONAL AGE	**1 WEEK**	**2-8 WEEKS**	**>8 WEEKS**
25-28 weeks	11.0 ± 5.4	15.5 ± 6.2	47.4 ± 21.5
29-34 weeks	15.3 ± 5.6	28.7 ± 13.9	51.4 ± 20.7
38-42 weeks	40.6 ± 14.8	65.8 ± 24.8	95.7 ± 21.7

11. **What determines urine output in the postnatal period?**

The volume of urine in the postnatal period is determined by water and sodium intake, GFR, the ability to maintain a concentration gradient in the renal medullary interstitium, and the presence or absence of antidiuretic hormone (ADH).

12. **What are the important differences in the regulation of sodium ion (Na^+) and potassium ion (K^+) balance?**

■ The vast majority of total body Na^+ is extracellular, whereas the vast majority of total body K^+ is intracellular.

■ Serum $[Na^+]$ is solely a function of total body water and sodium balance. Serum $[K^+]$ is a function of internal (the distribution of K^+ across cell membranes) and total body (or external) potassium balance. Urinary Na^+ excretion is a function of the amount of Na^+ filtered (which depends on the GFR and serum $[Na^+]$) and the amount of Na^+ which is reabsorbed along the renal tubules. The amount of K^+ filtered has little effect on urinary potassium because 5% to 10% of the filtered K^+ is delivered to the distal nephron regardless of serum $[K^+]$ or total body potassium balance. Urinary K^+ excretion, then, is a function of the amount of potassium secreted or reabsorbed in the distal nephron.

13. **What factors influence internal K^+ balance?**

Potassium uptake by cells is stimulated by the following:

■ High $[K^+]$
■ Beta$_2$-adrenergic agonists
■ Insulin
■ Respiratory and metabolic alkalosis

Potassium movement from the intracellular to extracellular space is stimulated by the following:

■ Low $[K^+]$
■ Alpha-adrenergic agonists
■ Beta$_2$-adrenergic antagonist
■ Respiratory acidosis (metabolic acidosis to a much lesser extent)
■ Ischemia
■ Cell damage
■ Hyperosmolality

14. **How does the capacity of preterm infants to conserve sodium differ from that of term infants?**

Term infants conserve sodium effectively after the first few hours of life (after contraction of the extracellular fluid space). Preterm infants conserve sodium less effectively for the following reasons:

■ Their proximal tubular capacity for sodium reabsorption is limited.
■ Their distal tubular response to aldosterone is diminished (Fig. 9-4).

15. **If preterm infants have a limited capacity to conserve sodium, is their ability to excrete a sodium load enhanced?**

No. Their ability to excrete a sodium load is limited by their low GFR.

16. **How does the concentrating capacity of the preterm and term infant compare to that of the adult?**

Concentrating ability is limited in infants for several reasons. Protein intake by the infant is used to make new cells during this period of rapid growth, and relatively little nitrogen is diverted to urea. Urea is an important component of the tonicity of the medullary interstitium and the osmolality of urine. Additional factors include (1) the relatively short loops of Henle in the neonatal nephrons that limit the surface area available for equilibration with the interstitium and (2) a high level of prostaglandins that can increase medullary blood flow and "wash out" the medullary concentration gradient. The maximum urine concentration in the preterm infant is approximately 600 mOsm/L, in the full term infant is 800 mOsm/L, and in the adult is 1500 mOsm/L.

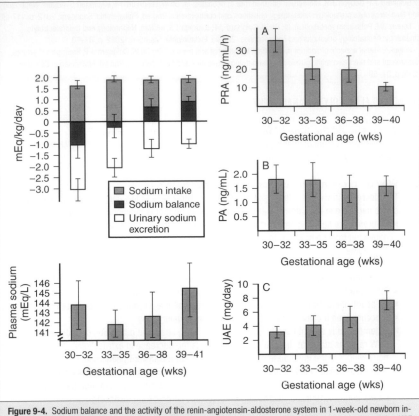

Figure 9-4. Sodium balance and the activity of the renin-angiotensin-aldosterone system in 1-week-old newborn infants with gestational ages of 30 to 41 weeks. *PA,* Plasma aldosterone concentration; *PRA,* plasma renin activity; *UAE,* urinary aldosterone excretion. (From Sulyok E, Németh M, Tényi J, et al. Relationship between maturity, electrolyte balance and the function of the renin-angiotension-aldosterone system in newborn infants. Biol Neonate 1979;35:60–5.)

17. **Preterm infants have a limited capacity to excrete a free water load. Is this because they cannot dilute their urine as much as full-term infants?**
    Not primarily. Preterm infants are capable of diluting their urine to 75 mOmol/L, compared with that of full-term infants and adults of 50 mOsm/L. The capacity of the newborn to excrete a free water load is limited by their lower GFR.

18. **Why do preterm infants have difficulty excreting a potassium load?**
    Data in animals suggest that potassium secretion by the immature distal nephron is limited by the following:
    - A relative paucity of K^+ channels in the apical membrane of principal cells in the distal nephron
    - Lower flow delivery to the distal tubule as the result of lower GFR
    - Lower sensitivity to aldosterone

Beall MH, van den Wijngaard J, van Germet M, et al. Water flux and amniotic fluid volume: understanding fetal water flow. In: Oh W, Guignard J-P, Baumgart S, editors. Nephrology and fluid/electrolyte physiology: neonatology questions and controversies. 2nd ed. Philadelphia: Saunders; 2012. p. 3–18.

Gallini F, Maggio L, Romagnoli C, et al. Progression of renal function in preterm neonates with gestational age < or = 32 weeks. Pediatr Nephrol 2000;15:119–124.

Gasser B, Mauss Y, Ghnassia JP, et al. A quantitative study of normal nephrogenesis in the human fetus: its implications in the natural history of kidney changes due to low obstructive uropathies. Fetal Diagn Ther 1993;8:371–84.

Guignard J-P, Gouyon J-B. Glomerular filtration rate in neonates. In: Oh W, Guignard J-P, Baumgart S, editors. Nephrology and fluid/electrolyte physiology: neonatology questions and controversies. 2nd ed. Philadelphia: Saunders; 2012. p. 117–35.

Lorenz JM. Potassium metabolism. In: Oh W, Guignard J-P, Baumgart S, editors. Nephrology and fluid/electrolyte physiology: neonatology questions and controversies. 2nd ed. Philadelphia: Saunders; 2012. p. 61–73.

Sulyok E. Renal aspects of sodium metabolism in the fetus and neonate. In: Oh W, Guignard J-P, Baumgart S, editors. Nephrology and fluid/electrolyte physiology: neonatology questions and controversies. 2nd ed. Philadelphia: Saunders; 2012, p. 31–59.

FLUID AND ELECTROLYTE MANAGEMENT

19. **When should the time of first voiding be considered delayed?**
Ninety-seven percent of infants pass urine in the first 24 hours of life and 100% by 48 hours. During the first 2 days of life, infants urinate two to six times per day (Table 9-2).

20. **Why do preterm infants lose weight after birth?**
This decrease in weight is the result of catabolism secondary to low caloric intake and a physiologic decrease in the extracellular water (ECW) volume that is independent of caloric intake. Most premature babies manifest a natriuretic diuresis in the first few days of life, which results in negative net total body water and sodium balance and, therefore, a decrease in extracellular fluid (ECF) volume.

21. **Why is the reduction in ECW volume in preterm infants considered physiologic?**
    - The diuresis occurs in spite of large variation in water and sodium intake.
    - Relatively large differences in water and sodium intake are required to moderate this reduction.
    - It occurs even if caloric intake mitigates postnatal weight loss.
    - When the body weight initially lost postnatally is regained, the proportion of body weight that is ECW remains stable at the new lower level. Thus the decrease in extracellular volume relative to body weight in the immediate postnatal period is not a transient phenomenon.
    - Water and sodium intakes high enough to prevent or markedly attenuate this decrease in extracellular volume have been associated with increased morbidity in premature newborns (e.g., patent ductus arteriosus, necrotizing enterocolitis, chronic lung disease).

22. **Which should be used, birth weight or daily weight, to calculate water and sodium requirements during the first week of life?**
The clinician should use what the attending physician requests. After the first day of life, however, it is important to understand that it is the absolute fluid and electrolyte intake (milliliters or millimoles per day) relative to that in the previous 8 to 24 hours that is relevant. In other words, should

TABLE 9-2. TIME OF FIRST VOID IN 500 INFANTS*

Adapted from Clark DA. Time of first void and first stool in 500 newborns. Pediatrics 1977;60:457.

	TERM INFANTS CUMULATIVE		PRETERM INFANTS CUMULATIVE		POSTTERM INFANTS CUMULATIVE	
	#	%	#	%	#	%
In delivery room	51	12.9	17	21.2	3	12
1-8 hr	151	51.1	50	83.7	4	38
9-16 hr	158	91.1	12	98.7	14	84
17-24 hr	35	100	1	100	4	100

*In 395 term infants, 80 preterm infants, and 25 postterm infants.

the absolute fluid or electrolyte intake be more or less than it was previously? The answer depends on what fluid and electrolyte balances resulted from the previous intakes and on what water and electrolyte losses are anticipated. There is no magic amount of water per kg/day that is appropriate for all infants, even infants at the same weight, gestational age, postnatal age, and in the same environment. If the infant loses more water (and therefore weight) than you judge to be appropriate and you anticipate that water losses will remain approximately the same, the absolute amount of water (milliliters per day) given should be increased. However, if the current weight is used to calculate fluid requirements, the absolute amount of water administered may be only slightly more or even less than the amount given the day before. For example, an 860-g infant loses 110 g (approximately 13% of birth weight) in the first day of life after receiving 100 mL/kg/day (86 mL/day). You decide this rate of weight loss is too great and increase water intake by 20% to 120 mL/kg/day. Based on the current weight of 750 gm, however, this is only 90 mL/day, which is barely more than that given the previous day. If water losses remain the same, weight loss will be only slightly less over the next 24 hours despite an increase in water intake per kilogram current body weight.

23. **What are the main variables to consider when estimating insensible water loss (IWL)?**
The most important determinants of IWL are gestational age, postnatal age, antenatal steroids, and environment. IWL decreases with increasing gestational and postnatal age (Fig. 9-5), exposure to antenatal steroids, and increasing ambient humidity.

24. **Why is accurate estimation of IWL so important in estimating fluid administration rate in preterms?**
   - It is the major route of water loss in very preterm infants.
   - It is not under feedback control—there is nothing the infant can do to reduce the rate of IWL if water intake to too low.

25. **What concentration of dextrose is needed for infants dependent on intravenous intake?**
The concentration of dextrose in the intravenous solution is an irrelevant number. The relevant variable is the dextrose administration rate. Neonates normally produce 4 to 8 mg/kg/min of glucose endogenously. Administration at this rate usually maintains serum glucose concentration in the normal range and conserves glycogen stores. Once the rate of water administration is determined, a dextrose concentration is selected that provides somewhere between 4 and 8 mg/kg/min. In some infants higher glucose infusion rates may be necessary, occasionally exceeding even 12 to 14 mg/kg/min in some circumstances to maintain appropriate blood glucose levels.

26. **Once the fluid administration rate is determined, how can the dextrose concentration necessary to provide a target dextrose administration rate be calculated?**

$$\text{Dextrose concentration }(\%) = \text{target dextrose administration rate (mg/kg/min)}$$
$$\div \text{ infusion rate (mL/kg/day)} \times 170$$

27. **Is there a simple way to calculate the dextrose administration rate that will be provided with a given dextrose concentration and administration rate of the intravenous fluid?**
Yes.

$$\text{Dextrose administration rate (mg/kg/min)} = \text{dextrose concentration }(\%)$$
$$\times \text{ infusion rate (mL/kg/day)} \times 0.006$$

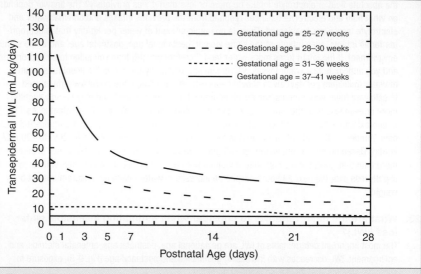

Figure 9-5. Transdermal loss as a function of gestational and postnatal age in naked, appropriate-for-gestational-age infants in a neutral thermal environment in incubators with 50% ambient humidity. (From Hammarlund K, Sedin G, Strömberg B. Transepidermal water loss in newborn infants. Part VIII: relation to gestational and post-natal age in appropriate and small-for-gestational-age infants. Acta Pediatr Scand 1983;72:721–8.)

28. **The specimen used for bedside glucose measurement by point of care (POC) analyzers is whole blood. Is it necessary to "correct" the glucose concentration determined with point of care analyzers to reflect the plasma concentration?**

    No. Although plasma blood glucose concentrations are approximately 10% to 18% higher than whole blood concentrations (because the water content of plasma is higher than that of blood cells), most POC analyzers are calibrated to plasma and therefore provide plasma glucose concentrations. However, POC analyzers have limited accuracy, with a tendency to read falsely lower than the actual plasma glucose concentration. Variation from the actual plasma glucose concentration may be as much as 10 to 20 mg/dL, with the greatest variation at low glucose concentrations. Because of limitations with rapid POC testing methods, any abnormal plasma glucose concentration must be confirmed by laboratory testing.

29. **How much sodium (Na⁺) should be given on the first day of life?**

    In the absence of unusual Na^+ losses (e.g., loss of gastrointestinal or cerebrospinal fluid), no Na^+ should be given. Under these conditions the kidney is the principal route of Na^+ loss. During the first day of life, urine Na^+ excretion is low (0.5 to 2 mEq/kg/day). With the onset of the postnatal diuresis (when the rate of net water loss often exceeds net Na^+ loss), the serum sodium $[Na^+]$ level often rises. Therefore it is usually best to withhold Na^+ initially, especially in extremely premature infants, in whom IWL is quite high and quite variable, therefore placing these infants at particular risk for developing significant hypernatremia in the first few days of life.

30. **When should maintenance potassium be started in an extremely premature infant?**

    The main route of potassium loss is in the urine. Urine potassium losses are low initially because GFR and urine output are relatively low after birth. Moreover, serum potassium concentration $([K^+])$ may rise in extremely premature infants even in the absence of exogenous potassium. Therefore potassium should be withheld until it can be ascertained that renal function is normal and, in extremely premature babies, the serum $[K^+]$ is normal and not increasing.

31. **Baby R is a 22-hour-old, 25-weeks'-gestation male infant in a humidified incubator. He has received 150 mL/kg/day of fluid during the first day of life. Serum sodium concentration ([Na]) is 128 mmol/L. Should sodium intake be increased?**

Not necessarily. Serum [Na] is the concentration, not the amount, of sodium in the ECF space. If it is abnormally low, the amount of sodium in the ECF space is "insufficient" for the amount of water in the ECF space. Thus serum [Na] may be low because there is too little extracellular sodium, too much ECW, or both. The most common cause of hyponatremia in neonates in the first 1 or 2 days of life is excessive fluid administration. In such situations free water intake should be restricted.

✓ KEY POINTS: FLUIDS AND ELECTROLYTES

1. Like the lung, the premature renal function is immature; there is a diminished capacity to excrete a free water load, to maintain plasma electrolyte homeostasis, to acidify the urine, and to concentrate the urine.

2. All premature neonates lose weight after birth. This results from a physiologic postnatal decrease in ECW volume. However, when more than 10% to 15% of body weight is lost in the first week of life, the possible pathophysiologic process should be considered and investigated.

3. Sodium and potassium should not usually be given on the first day of life, but glucose is necessary. Preterm infants may also require calcium.

Agren J, Sjors G, Sedin G. Transepidermal water loss in infants born at 24 and 25 weeks of gestation. Acta Paediatr 1998;87:1185–90.

American Academy of Pediatrics. Clinical report—postnatal glucose homeostasis in late-preterm and term infants. Pediatr 2011;127:575–79.

Bauer K, Boverman G, Roithmaier A, et al. Body composition, nutrition, and fluid balance during the first two weeks of life in preterm neonates weighing less than 1500 grams. J Pediatr 1991;118:615–20.

Bauer K, Versmold H. Postnatal weight loss in preterm neonates < 1599 g is due to isotonic dehydration of the extracellular volume. Acta Paediatr Scand Suppl 1989;360:37–42.

Bell EF, Acarregui MJ. Restricted versus liberal water intake for preventing morbidity and mortality in preterm infants. Cochrane Database Syst Rev 2008;1:CD000503.

Bell EF, Warburton D, Stonestreet BS, et al. Effect of fluid administration on the development of symptomatic patent ductus arteriosus and congestive heart failure in premature infants. N Engl J Med 1980;302:598–604.

Bell EF, Warburton D, Stonestreet BS, et al. High-volume intake predisposes premature infants to necrotizing enterocolitis [letter]. Lancet 1979;2:90.

Clark DA. Time of first void and first stool in 500 newborns. Pediatrics 1977;60:457–59.

Costarino AT, Gruskay JA, Corcoran L, et al. Sodium restriction versus daily maintenance replacement in very low birth weight premature neonates: a randomized, blind therapeutic trial. J Pediatr 1992;120:99–106.

Dimitriou G, Kavvadia V, Marcou M, et al. Antenatal steroids and fluid balance in very low birthweight infants. Arch Dis Child 2005;90:F509–F513.

Guignard J-P, Drukker A. Why do newborns have elevated plasma creatinine? Pediatr 1999;103:e49. www.pediatrics.org/cgi/content/full/103/4/e49.

Hammarlund K, Nilsson GE, Öberg PA, et al. Transepidermal water loss in the newborn I. Relation to ambient humidity and site of measurement and estimation of total transepidermal water loss. Acta Paediatr Scand 1977;66:553–62.

Hammarlund K, Sedin G, Strömberg B. Transepidermal water loss in newborn infants VIII. Relation to gestational age and post-natal age in appropriate and small for gestational age infants. Acta Paediatr Scand 1983;72:7.

Hartnoll G, Bétrémieux P, Modi N. Randomized controlled trial of postnatal sodium supplementation on body composition in 25 to 30 week gestation age infants. Arch Dis Child 2000;82:F24–F28.

Hawdon JM, Ward Platt MP, Aynsley-Green A. Prevention and management of neonatal hypoglycemia. Arch Dis Child 1994;70:F54–F65.

Heimler R, Doumas BT, Jendrzejcak BM, et al. Relationship between nutrition, weight change, and fluid compartments in preterm infants during the first week of life. J Pediatr 1993;122:110–14.

Kavvadia V, Greenough A, Dimitriou G, Forsling ML. Randomized trial of two levels of fluid input in the perinatal period—effect on fluid balance, electrolyte and metabolic disturbances in ventilated VLBW infants. Acta Paediatrica 2000;89:237–41.

Kelly LK, Seri I. Renal developmental physiology: relevance to clinical care. Neoreviews 2008;9:e150–e161.

Lorenz JM. Fluid and electrolyte therapy in the very low birth weight neonate. NeoReviews. 2008;9:e102–e108.

Lorenz JM, Kleinman LI, Ahmed G, et al. Phases of fluid and electrolyte homeostasis in the extremely low birth weight infant. Pediatr 1995;96:484–89.

Lorenz JM, Kleinman LI, Kotagal UR, et al. Water balance in very low birth weight infants: relationship to water and sodium intake and effect on outcome. J Pediatr 1982;101:423–32.

Omar SA, DeCristofaro JD, Agarwal BI, et al. Effect of prenatal steroids on water and sodium homeostasis in extremely low birth weight infants. Pediatr 1999;104:482–8.

Shaffer SG, Bradt SK, Hall RT. Postnatal changes in total body water and extracellular volume in preterm infants with respiratory distress syndrome. J Pediatr 1986;109:509–14.

Singhi S, Sood VI, Bhakoo NK, et al. Composition of postnatal weight loss and subsequent weight gain in preterm infants. Indian J Med Res 1995;101:157–62.

Stonestreet BS, Bell EF, Warburton D, et al. Renal response in low-birth-weight neonates: results of prolonged intake of two different amounts of fluid and sodium. Am J Dis Child 1983;137:215–19.

Shaffer SG, Bradt SK, Meade VM, et al. Extracellular fluid volume changes in very low birth weight infants during the first 2 postnatal months. J Pediatr 1987;111:124–8.

Shaffer SG, Meade VM. Sodium balance and extracellular volume regulation in very low birth weight infants. J Pediatr 1989;115:285–90.

Tammela OKT, Koivisto ME. Fluid restriction for preventing bronchopulmonary dysplasia? Reduced fluid intake during the first weeks of life improves the outcome of low-birth-weight infants. Acta Paediatrica 1992;81:207–12.

Van der Wagen A, Okken A, Zweens J, et al. Composition of postnatal weight loss and subsequent weight gain in small for dates newborn infants. Acta Paediatr Scand 1985;74:57–61.

Verma RP, Shibil S, Fang H, et al. Clinical determinants and utility of early postnatal maximum weight loss in fluid management of extremely low birth weight infants. Early Hum Dev 2009;85:59–64.

NONOLIGURIC HYPERKALEMIA IN PREMATURE INFANTS

32. **What is the definition of hyperkalemia in the newborn?**
    Hyperkalemia is defined as a serum potassium concentration that is equal to or greater than 6.7 mEq/L from a nonhemolyzed whole blood sample.

33. **What are the two ways that hyperkalemia develops in premature infants?**
    Hyperkalemia is caused by perturbations in internal or external K+ balance:
    - Internal K+ balance: shift of potassium from the intracellular to extracellular space
    and/or
    - Positive external K+ balance caused by either impaired renal potassium excretion or (less commonly) excessive intake. Increased K+ intake of a magnitude sufficiently severe to cause hyperkalemia is usually the result of a dosing error.

34. **What is nonoliguric hyperkalemia?**
    Nonoliguric hyperkalemia is a rise in the serum potassium concentration equal to or greater than 6.7 mEq/L in the absence of a falling or low urine output.

35. **What is the pathophysiology of nonoliguric hyperkalemia?**
    Nonoliguric hyperkalemia may develop in the first 24 to 36 hours of life even in the absence of potassium intake. In fact, most infants who develop nonoliguric hyperkalemia are in negative potassium balance. Therefore nonoliguric hyperkalemia is caused by a shift of potassium from the intracellular fluid to the extracellular space. Although the mechanisms responsible for this shift are unknown, infants with nonoliguric hyperkalemia are believed to have lower levels of Na+/K+ ATPase. It is noteworthy that serum [K+] increases after birth in nearly all extremely preterm infants, even those who do not develop hyperkalemia. The etiology of this shift is unknown, but it is only clinically significant in very preterm infants.

36. **What is the incidence of nonoliguric hyperkalemia in premature infants?**
    When originally reported in the literature in the early 1980s, the prevalence of nonoliguric hyperkalemia ranged from 25% to 50% of infants below 1000 g birth weight or younger than 28 weeks' gestational age. However, it is much less common now, even in infants younger than 25 weeks' gestational

age. This is probably the result of the increased prevalence of antenatal steroid therapy and more aggressive nutrition, which have been shown to reduce the risk of nonoliguric hyperkalemia.

37. **What are the consequences of hyperkalemia in a premature infant?**
Hyperkalemia increases the ratio of extracellular $[K^+]$ to intracellular $[K^+]$, depolarizing cells with excitable membranes, most importantly myocardial cells. This may causes bradyarythmias. These are uncommon with serum $[K^+]$s lower than 7 to 8 mmol/L. If serum $[K^+]$ continues to rise, asystole may occur. However, asystole is uncommon with serum $[K^+]$s lower than 8 to 9 mmol/L.

38. **What are the indications for treatment of nonoliguric hyperkalemia?**
There is no consensus regarding this issue. Treatment may be considered if serum $[K^+]$ is equal to or greater than 7 meq/L or there are electrocardiographic changes resulting from hyperkalemia. It is important to know that nonoliguric hyperkalemia normally resolves without treatment with the onset of physiologic natriuretic diuresis.

39. **How is nonoliguric hyperkalemia managed?**
Nonoliguric hyperkalemia is managed in the following ways:
- By antagonizing the arrythmagenic effect of hyperkalemia
  - 0.5 to 1 mEq/kg elemental calcium (1 to 2 mL/kg of 10% calcium gluconate solution) by slow intravenous push
  - Correct acidosis
- By stimulating cellular uptake of potassium
  - Correct respiratory and metabolic acidosis
  - Nebulized albuterol therapy—rapid effect; effectiveness documented in extremely premature infants with nonoliguric hyperkalemia in one randomized controlled trial; experience insufficient to confirm safety
  - Exogenous insulin—effective but takes time to initiate, and titration of insulin and glucose to avoid hypoglycemia is difficult
- By increasing renal potassium secretion
  - Furosemide does increase potassium excretion but is unproven in the management of hyperkalemia
- Peritoneal dialysis is rarely required except with hyperkalemia caused by renal failure.

40. **Is the use of a cation exchange resin (e.g., Kayexalate) an effective and safe way to treat hyperkalemia?**
Use of this method to treat hyperkalemia is no longer considered safe and effective.
Insulin therapy has been shown as more effective in lowering serum $[K^+]$ in extremely premature infants with nonoliguric hyperkalemia in a randomized controlled trial. Moreover, cation exchange resins have been associated with intestinal injury.

✓ KEY POINTS: HYPERKALEMIA

1. Nonoliguric hyperkalemia (potassium >6.7 mEq/L in plasma from a nonhemolyzed whole blood specimen) still occurs in extremely premature infants, but the current prevalence is less than originally reported (15% to 50%). This probably results from the increased prevalence of antenatal steroid exposure. Therefore the clinician should be particularly vigilant in checking for nonoliguric hyperkalemia in extremely preterm infants whose mothers have not received antenatal steroids before their birth.

2. Other causes of hyperkalemia of which to be cognizant are oliguric acute renal failure and drugs that inhibit K excretion (e.g., spironolactone and enalapril).

3. Hyperkalemia may be a life-threatening emergency. In this circumstance inhalation treatment with albuterol is most rapidly effective.

Fukuda Y, Kojima T, Ono A, et al. Factors causing hyperkalemia in premature infants. Am J Perinatol 1989;6:76–9.

Hu PS, Su BH and Peng CT, et al. Glucose and insulin infusion versus kayexalate for early treatment of non-oliguric hyperkalemia in very-low-birth-weight infants. Acta Paediatr Taiwan 1999;40:314.

Lorenz JM, Kleinman LI, Markarian K. Potassium metabolism in extremely low birth weight infants in the first week of life. J Pediatr 1997;131:81.

Malone TA. Glucose and insulin versus cation-exchange resin for the treatment of hyperkalemia in very low birth weight infants. J Pediatr 1991;118:121–3.

O'Hare FM, Molloy EJ. What is the best treatment for hyperkalemia in a preterm infant? Arch Dis Child 2008;93;174–6.

Omar SA, DeCristofaro JD, Agarwal BI, et al. Effect of prenatal steroids on potassium balance in extremely low birth weight neonates. Pediatr 2000;106:561–7.

Sato K, Kondo T, Iwao H, et al. Internal potassium shift in premature infants: cause of nonoliguric hyperkalemia. J Pediatr 1995;126:109–13.

Singh DS, Sadiq HF, Noguchi A, et al. Efficacy of albuterol inhalation in treatment of hyperkalemia in premature infants. J Pediatr 2002;141:16–20.

Yaseen H, Khalaf M, Dana A, et al. Salbutamol versus cation-exchange resin (Kayexalate) for the treatment of nonoliguric hyperkalemia in preterm infants. Am J Perinatol 2008;25:193–8.

ACID–BASE BALANCE

41. How are acid–base measurements made in blood gas analyzers?

Hydrogen ion concentration ($[H^+]$) is measured potentiometrically using a complicated system that employs two electrodes (usually Ag/AgCl) designed such that the potential between them is sensitive to the $[H^+]$ in the intervening medium. $[H^+]$ is expressed as pH, which equals the negative logarithm of $[H^+]$ ($-log[H^+]$). Because pH is defined as the negative log $[H^+]$, pH decreases as $[H^+]$ increases and increases when $[H^+]$ decreases.

Note: Unfortunately, as a result of expressing pH as $-log[H^+]$, the proportional change in $[H^+]$ is masked. To understand logarithm, think of "power." Thus $10^3 = 1000$ and log (1000) = 3. When the pH changes by 0.3 units (e.g., from 7.4 to 7.1), the hydrogen ion concentration nearly doubles from 40 to 79 nanoMol/L.

The partial pressure of oxygen is measured amperometrically by the Clark electrode. The reduction reaction of interest is: $4e^- + O_2 + 2H_2O = 4OH^-$. Current flows in linear proportion to the activity of dissolved oxygen.

The partial pressure of carbon dioxide (CO_2) is measured using an electrode with a semiperme-able membrane that allows only CO_2 to diffuse into the electrode compartment, where it is converted to carbonic acid. The hydrogen ions produced by this reaction are then measured as previously described. The semipermeable membrane ensures that this measurement is completely independent of blood pH.

Plasma bicarbonate concentration $[HCO_3^-]$ is not measured; it is calculated from the Henderson–Hasselbalch equation:

$$pH = pKa \times log \frac{[HCO_3^-]}{[H_2CO_3]}$$

The concentration of carbonic acid ($[H_2CO_3]$) is not measured, but it is proportional to the dissolved carbon dioxide (CO_2), with which it is in equilibrium. Dissolved carbon dioxide equals the product of the solubility coefficient of carbon dioxide in plasma at 37° C (0.031) and the partial pressure of carbon dioxide (pCO_2), which is measured. Therefore the $[HCO_3^-]$ can be calculated from the measured pH and measured pCO_2 as follows:

$$pH = pK' \times log \frac{[HCO_3^-]}{0.31 \times pCO_2}$$

The equation uses pK' (the apparent pK), to account for the equilibrium between dissolved CO_2 and HCO_3^-. The pK' for H_2CO_3 dissociation in adult human plasma is 6.1.

42. **What is base excess? How is it measured?**

The blood buffer bases of human adults are plasma HCO_3^-, plasma proteins, HCO_3^- in red blood cells, and hemoglobin (Hgb). The effect of these buffers is to establish and stabilize a pH of blood at approximately 7.4.

When *measured*, buffer base is the number of millimoles of strong base or strong acid needed to titrate 1 L of blood (Hgb = 15 g/dL) to pH = 7.4 at 37° C while pCO_2 is held at 40 mmHg (at which point the addition of base or acid has restored the total blood buffers to normal values). Base excess (BE) *in the blood* (actual BE) is the difference between what actually is measured in the test sample and the sum of these values.

In clinical practice it is the BE *in the extended extracellular space* (red blood cells + plasma + interstitial fluid [ISF]) that is of interest. The concentration of buffer base in the ISF is lower than whole blood, primarily because ISF contains no Hgb. Therefore the algorithm used in blood gas autoanalyzers to calculate ECF BE uses a model of the blood volume diluted with ISF. There are minor variations in the algorithm used to calculate ECF BE, but the most common one is as follows:

$$BE = 16.2 \times (pH - 7.40) - 25 + [HCO_3^-]$$

The normal total of extracellular buffers for infants is 3 to 4 mEq/L lower, so infants normally have a base deficit in this range.

43. **Serum HCO_3^- and BE are both measures of metabolic acid–base status. Which is better?**

This has been subject of some debate for some time. However, BE is easier to interpret than serum $[HCO_3^-]$ because it is less dependent on pCO_2. When an increase in $[H^+]$ is not due to an increase in respiratory acid (i.e., carbonic acid produced from the combination of CO_2 and H_2O), the added H^+ is bound by the buffer anions and base excess falls in direct proportion to the added H^+. However, when an increase in $[H^+]$ is due to an increase in CO_2, serum $[HCO_3^-]$ increases (because it is in equilibrium with CO_2) and the other buffer anions decrease in direct proportion; thus BE remains unchanged. Therefore at a pH of 7.4, what serum $[HCO_3^-]$ is *normal* depends on the measured pCO_2 (Table 9-3).

44. **Why is serum $[HCO_3^-]$ lower (and BE mildly negative) in newborns compared with that of the adult under baseline conditions? What serum $[HCO_3^-]$ is considered normal?**

The serum $[HCO_3^-]$ in preterm infants is normally 17 ± 1.2 mEq/L, with two standard deviations encompassing values as low as 14.5 mEq/L. During the first week of life, term infants have a serum

TABLE 9-3.   RELATION OF pCO_2 AND SERUM $[HCO_3^-]$ IN ADULTS WHEN pH IS 7.40 IN THE ADULT AND THERE IS NO CHANGE IN TOTAL BUFFER BASE

pCO_2 (mmHg)	PLASMA $[HCO_3^-]$ (mmol/L)
20	12
25	15
30	18
35	22
40	24
50	30
60	36

$[HCO_3^-]$ of 20 ± 2.8 mEq/L. During the first year of life, the serum $[HCO_3^-]$ is still only approximately 22 ± 1.9 mEq/L, compared with 23 ± 1 mEq/L and 26 ± 1 mEq/L in older children and adults.

These differences in normal serum bicarbonate levels with maturation result from the increased capacity of the mature kidney to conserve bicarbonate and to excrete $[H^+]$. These factors also impair the capacity of the newborn to excrete acid loads. This is the result of immaturity of carbonic anhydrase in the renal tubules and the intercalated cells of the collecting duct.

45. **Do infants excrete more or less titratable acid and ammonia per kilogram of body weight compared with older children?**
   Titratable acid is a term to describe acids such as phosphoric acid and sulfuric acid, which are involved in acid excretion. It excludes ammonium (NH_4^+) as a source of acid and is part of the calculation for net acid excretion. The titratable acid excretion rate in term infants younger than 1 month old is about one half of adult values, and the ammonium excretion rate about two thirds that of older children and adults. Preterm infants have even lower rates. After 1 month of age the net acid excretion rate in term infants is similar to that in older children and adults when expressed per 1.73 m^2. Preterm infants also increase their rates of titratable acid and ammonium excretion with maturation, but these rates still remain lower than in term infants, even up to the age of 4 months. After 1 month of age the amount of ammonia excreted also depends on diet (ammonia production is increased in infants fed cow's milk compared with that of infants fed breast milk).

46. **How low can a premature infant reduce the urine pH?**
   During the first 3 weeks of life a premature infant can reduce the urine pH only to 6 ± 0.1. After 1 month, the urine pH can be reduced to 5.2 ± 0.4.

47. **How can the oxygen saturation value reported with the blood gas be used clinically?**
   It is not useful. The oxygen saturation reported with the blood gas is calculated from the measured pO_2 using an algorithm based on the adult oxygen–Hbg desaturation curve.

48. **In acid–base disorders in human biology, in which body compartment are measurements made? What is the significance of this?**
   Acid–base measurements are made in the blood, but they are the same in the ISF space. Because $[HCO_3^-]$ is calculated from pH and pCO_2, it represents the plasma concentration of $[HCO_3^-]$. As calculated by blood gas autoanalyzers, the reported BE reflects the difference between the normal and actual buffer base concentrations. However, intracellular acid–base status cannot be measured in clinical practice. Because CO_2 diffuses across cell membranes much more rapidly than HCO_3^-, it is possible for rapid changes in pCO_2 to change the acid–base profile of the two compartments in different directions and at different rates. When attempting to treat acid-base disorders, the clinician must consider the possible consequences, such as worsening intracellular acidosis in the face of alkalinization of the ECF with infusions of bicarbonate.

49. **What is the difference between acidemia (or alkalemia) and acidosis (or alkalosis)?**
   Strictly speaking, acid*emia* and alkal*emia* refer to the actual pH of the blood relative to a pH of 7.4. A lower pH indicates acidemia; a higher pH indicates alkalemia. Acid*osis* and alkal*osis* refer to the respiratory and metabolic components of acid–base status compared with normal:
   - A pCO_2 greater than 40 indicates respiratory acidosis; a pCO_2 less than 40 indicates respiratory alkalosis.
   - A BE less than 0 mmol/L indicates metabolic acidosis; a BE greater than 0 mmol/L indicates metabolic alkalosis

50. **What are the principal mechanisms whereby infants compensate for abnormal acid–base abnormalities?**
   - Metabolic alkalosis compensation: hypoventilation
   - Metabolic acidosis compensation: hyperventilation

- Respiratory acidosis compensation: increased renal absorption of bicarbonate
- Respiratory alkalosis compensation: diminished renal absorption of bicarbonate

51. What is the importance of the volume of distribution in correcting acid–base derangements?

After a known amount of solute is introduced into a solution, the concentration is measured, and the apparent volume in which the solute is distributed is calculated. This volume is called the volume of distribution, and it is used to estimate how much solute is needed to change the measured concentration of that solute. For simple single compartments and inert solutes, the calculation measures the true volume. For multicompartment systems and unstable solutes, the solute may be distributed unevenly (i.e., either concentrated in or excluded from various compartments), metabolized, or otherwise eliminated. In these systems the calculated volume is different from the true volume in which the solute is distributed. Because of its interaction with a number of buffer systems, both intracellular and extracellular, and its elimination as CO_2 through the lungs, the volume of distribution of bicarbonate is larger than the ECF space. For metabolic acidosis in neonates the dosage should be based on the following formula if blood gases and pH measurements are available: HCO_3^- (mEq) = 0.3 × weight (kg) × base deficit (mEq/L). The usual dosage is 1 to 2 mEq/kg/dose.

52. What is the anion gap?

The anion gap is the difference in the serum between the concentrations of cations and anions. It its calculated as follows:

$$Anion\ gap = \{[Na^+] + [K^+]\} - \{[Cl^-] - [HCO_3^-]\}$$

The [K+] may be excluded from the calculation because wide variation in serum potassium is lethal. With [K+] in the equation the normal anion gap is approximately 12, and without [K+] in the equation it is approximately 8.

If there is an increase in unmeasured cations, the anion gap will be increased. If there is an increase in unmeasured anions, the anion gap will be decreased.

53. Is the anion gap useful in the differential diagnosis of acid–base disturbances?

Theoretically, it should be. Distinguishing between metabolic acidosis caused by bicarbonate loss and metabolic acidosis caused by increases in organic acid (an unmeasured cation) is a common and important problem. The anion gap will be normal when acidosis is caused by bicarbonate loss (because it is associated with increased renal tubular reabsorption of Cl^- and therefore increases in serum [Cl^-] without change in unmeasured anions. On the other hand, when metabolic acidosis results from an increase in organic acid (e.g., lactic acid), the sum of unmeasured cations will be higher. Unfortunately, there is so much overlap between a normal anion gap (no change in unmeasured cations or anions) and abnormal anion gaps resulting from a change in unmeasured cations or anions that the anion gap is clinically useful only in cases of extreme changes in unmeasured cations and anions. Because the serum lactic acid concentration can be readily measured clinically and because it is by far the organic acid most likely to be increased, the anion gap has fallen into disuse. It can be helpful, though, with marked elevation in organic acids whose measurements are less readily available.

54. What do we know about the efficacy of the therapeutic use of sodium bicarbonate to correct acidemia in pediatric patients?

As a general rule, replacement of bicarbonate when body losses of bicarbonate are excessive (e.g., through the stool or urine) is appropriate. On the other hand, there is minimal evidence documenting the value of sodium bicarbonate infusions to correct acidemia resulting from many, if not most, other causes (e.g. lactic acidosis). In fact, data in animals, children, and adults suggest that correction of lactic acidosis with sodium bicarbonate infusions may be detrimental. Although it is relatively easy to make the pH of the ECF change in the desired direction, it is much more difficult to know in what direction the associated change in intracellular pH will be, which is the relevant issue for cell function. Moreover, if the cause of the acidemia is ongoing, the improvement in pH will be temporary; the primary cause of the acidemia must be corrected. Therefore sodium bicarbonate treatment should be used cautiously, if at all.

✓ KEY POINTS: ACID–BASE BALANCE

1. A primary acid–base disturbance is always defined by the pH. A pH less than 7.3 indicates a primary acidemia, whereas a pH greater than 7.5 indicates a primary alkalemia.

2. The clinician must then turn to the pCO_2, [HCO_3^-], or base excess, and the underlying clinical situation to define the the the primary disturbance.

3. Sodium bicarbonate should be used sparingly to treat acidemia. The clinician should never administer bicarbonate until the ability to excrete carbon dioxide is ensured; otherwise, the clinical acid–base disturbance may be worsened.

Ammari AN, Schulze KF. Uses and abuses of sodium bicarbonate in the neonatal intensive care unit. Curr Opin Pediatr 2002;14:151–6.

Aschner J, Poland RL. Sodium bicarbonate: basically useless therapy. Pediatr 2008;122(4):831–5.

Berg CS, Barnette AR, Myers BJ, et al. Sodium bicarbonate administration and outcome in preterm infants. J Pediatr 2010;157:684–7.

Higgins C. An introduction to acid-base balance in health and disease. June 2004. Available at www.http://acutecaretesting.org/en/articles/an-introduction-to-acidbase-balance-in-health-and-disease. Accessed August 4, 2012.

Higgins C. Lactate and lactic acid. Oct 2007. Available at http://acutecaretesting.org/en/articles/lactate-and-lactic-acido sisosis. Accessed Aug 4, 2012.

Kecskes ZB, Davies MW. Rapid correction of early metabolic acidaemia in comparison with placebo, no intervention or slow correction in LBW infants. Cochrane Database Sys Rev. 2009;CD002976.

Kofstad J. All about base excess—to BE or not to BE. July 2003. www.http://acutecaretesting.org/en/articles/all-about-base-excess--to-be-or-not-to-be. Accessed August 4, 2012.

Lorenz JM, Kleinman LI, Markarian K, et al. Serum anion gap in the differential diagnosis of metabolic acidosis in critically ill newborns. J Pediatr 1999;135:751–5.

Seri I. Acid-base homeostasis in the fetus and newborn. In: Oh W, Guignard J-P, Baumgart S, editors. Nephrology and fluid/electrolyte physiology: neonatology questions and controversies. 2nd ed. Philadelphia: Saunders; 2012. p. 105–12.

DIURETICS

55. **Diuretics therapy may be complicated by hyponatremia. How should hyponatremia be managed in this situation?**

Hyponatremia is the result of too little sodium *relative* to water in the ECW compartment; therefore it may be caused by a deficit of sodium or an excess of water in the ECW compartment. The primary action of loop diuretics is to inhibit chloride (and thereby sodium) reabsorption in the loop of Henle. Therefore hyponatremia with loop diuretics could be caused by a sodium deficit resulting from excessive diuretic therapy or from excessive administration of free water. The former is managed by decreasing the frequency of loop diuretic administration, the latter by decreasing free water intake.

56. **What damage can chronic administrative loop diuretics inflict on the kidneys, urinary tract, or both?**

Loop diuretics induce hypercalciuria by inhibiting renal tubular calcium reabsorption. Therefore chronic administration of these agents can cause nephrocalcinosis, calcium nephrolithiasis, or both.

57. **What is the best way to treat the hypokalemic, hypochloremic metabolic alkalosis that occurs in newborns who receive chronic diuretic therapy?**

Diuretics cause metabolic alkalosis by increasing potassium secretion. This results from the increased delivery of water and sodium to the distal tubule and is treated with potassium chloride (KCl) supplementation. Diuretic therapy also induces a reduction in effective intraarterial volume and thereby activates the renin-angiotensin-aldosterone system, which stimulates secretion of potassium in the distal tubule. Blocking the effect of aldosterone on the distal tubule therefore counteracts the metabolic consequences of pharmacologic diuresis. Accordingly, adding spironolactone, a competitive inhibitor of aldosterone, to the diuretic regimen may prevent or improve derangements in serum bicarbonate and potassium concentrations. Caution should be used in adding spironolactone to the diuretic regimen *and* supplementing with KCl.

✓ KEY POINTS: DIURETICS

1. Infants receiving loop diuretics may require increased potassium and chloride intake to prevent potassium depletion and metabolic alkalosis.

2. Loop diuretics tend to be more effective in neonates but cause calciuresis, which can result in osteopenia, nephrocalcinosis, renal stone formation, or a combination of these.

3. Routine use of diuretic therapy has not been shown to significantly alter the course of bronchopulmonary dysplasia, although it may provide some immediate assistance in improving ventilation. The benefits should be carefully weighed against the risks of metabolic, bone, and renal complications.

Guignard J-P, Gouyon J-B. Use of diuretics in the newborn. In: Oh W, Guignard J-P, Baumgart S, editors. Nephrology and fluid/electrolyte physiology: neonatology questions and controversies. 2nd ed. Philadelphia: Saunders; 2012. p. 233–50.

DIFFERENTIAL DIAGNOSIS AND EVALUATION OF OLIGURIA

58. **The nurse reports that a 3-day-old infant is oliguric. You wonder, "How does she know the infant is oliguric?" What qualifies as oliguria?**

Your question is not so naïve, given the wide range of urine volumes from the most dilute to the most concentrated. The nurse likely responds on the basis of physical evidence; for example, he or she may say that the infant had only three wet diapers over the past 24 hours. If the baby is in an intensive care unit and the urine volume is being quantified, urine flow rate can be calculated. Within the first 24 hours after delivery the volume may be as low as 0.5 to 0.7 mL/kg/h, but beyond this period it is usually greater than 1 mL/kg/h. Oliguria is defined as a urine output persistently below 1 mL/kg/h.

59. **If an infant is found to be oliguric, what are the possible causes? How should it be evaluated and treated?**

In considering what the causes of oliguria are, you need to remember the determinants of urine flow rate (see Question 6). The *primary* causes of oliguria are as follows:

- *Dehydration.* Dehydration is defined as an inappropriately negative decrease in total body water, sodium, or both caused by insufficient water and sodium intake. If urine can be obtained for analysis, urine [Na$^+$] will be low and urine osmolality will be high with dehydration. Treatment depends on the cause but always includes replenishment of total body water and sodium.
- *Acute renal failure (ARF).* Renal failure by definition is a decrease in GFR below normal for gestational and postnatal age. Evaluation of serum [Cr] is required to judge whether GFR is reduced. However, a single value, especially in the first days of life when serum [Cr] is largely a function of maternal serum [Cr], will not be sufficient. The pattern of change over time, taking into account gestational and postnatal age, is more relevant. Treatment of ARF depends on the underlying etiology, but the principles of management are shown in Table 9-4.
  - *Syndrome of inappropriate antidiuretic hormone secretion (SIADH).* SIADH is the secretion of antidiuretic hormone by the hypothalamus in the absence of volume or osmolar stimuli. Treatment is restriction of free water.

It is important to note that all the aforementioned causes may occur without associated oliguria, but urine output should be relatively low. There is an extensive differential diagnosis for each of these primary causes, and the clinical context is important in narrowing the differential diagnosis.

TABLE 9–4. PRINCIPLES OF MANAGEMENT FOR ACUTE RENAL FAILURE

From Ringer SA. Acute renal failure in the newborn. Neoreviews 2010;11:e243.

Monitor weight.

Monitor urine output and fluid balance.

Monitor serum electrolytes, blood urea nitrogen, and creatinine.

Remove potassium from intravenous fluids until renal output is adequate.

Adjust doses of drugs excreted by the kidney.

Provide adequate nutrition.
 Adjust protein intake based on blood urea nitrogen to avoid overload.
 Add calories as carbohydrate and fat.

Correct acidosis with supplemental acetate, citrate, or bicarbonate.

Attempt a trial of furosemide to promote and maintain urine output.

Support blood pressure with dopamine.

Attempt dialysis, if necessary.

---

60. **An oliguric term infant had a serum creatinine of 0.7 mg/dL at birth and 1 mg/dL at 48 hours of life. How do you interpret these levels?**
 This would be consistent with ARF because serum [Cr] should fall after birth in a term newborn.

61. **In the face of an abnormal change in serum [Cr], how may the urine sodium concentration be helpful in evaluating oliguria?**
 Urinary indices to separate prerenal ARF from intrarenal ARF are not as useful in neonates as in older children and adults. However, the best index is the fractional excretion of sodium (FENa), which is calculated as follows:

$$FENa\,(\%) = \frac{urine\,[Na^+] \times serum\,\,[Na^+]}{urine\,[Cr] \times serum\,\,[Cr]} \times 100$$

 In prerenal failure in which renal tubular function is normal, FENa is 2.5% to 3%. A FENa above 2.5% to 3% indicates intrarenal ARF with associated renal tubular injury. Because of overlap between the two groups, specificity is limited. Note that during postnatal natriuretic diuresis or extracellular volume (ECV) expansion, FENa will be high; in this case, however, urine output should also be high. However, in the polyuric phase of ARF, urine output and FENa are abnormally high. The former and the latter can be differentiated by urine osmolality. With ECV expansion the urine is hypoosmolar; in the polyuric phase of ARF the urine is isoosmolar (Table 9-5).

62. **A 2-day-old baby is requiring significant ventilator support. His condition is complicated by bilateral pneumothoraces, and he has been anuric since birth. In reviewing his chart, you note that his mother had oligohydramnios. The baby is defined as "funny looking" in the admission note. Can you formulate an armchair differential diagnosis before going to see the baby?**
 The most likely diagnosis is oligohydramnios sequence.

63. **How should this infant be evaluated?**
 The most helpful initial test would be abdominal sonography concentrating on the kidneys, ureters, and bladder.

TABLE 9-5. URINE INDICES IN PRERENAL AND INTRINSIC RENAL FAILURE			
Data from Ringer SA. Acute renal failure in the newborn. Neoreviews 2010;11:e243			
	URINE OSMOLALITY (MOSM/L)	URINE SODIUM (MMOL/L)	FRACTIONAL EXCRETION OF SODIUM (%)
Prerenal failure (newborn/preterm Infant)	>350	<20 to 30	<2.5
Renal tubular injury (acute tubular necrosis)	<350	>30 to 40	>2.0

Andreoli SP. Kidney injury in the neonate. In: Oh W, Guignard J-P, Baumgart S, editors. Nephrology and fluid/electrolyte physiology: neonatology questions and controversies. 2nd ed. Philadelphia: Saunders; 2012. p. 285–303.

Ellis EN, Arnold WC. Use of urinary indexes in renal failure in the newborn. Am J Dis Child 1982;136:615–7.

Miall LS, Henderson MJ, Turner AJ, et al. Plasma creatinine rises dramatically in the first 48 hours of life in preterm infants. Pediatr 1999;104:e76. Available at www.pediatrics.org.cgi.content/full/104/6/e76. Accessed July 28, 2012.

Mathew OP, Jones AS, James E, et al. Neonatal renal failure: usefulness of diagnostic indices. Pediatrics 1980;65:57–60.

Pitkin RM, Reynolds A. Creatinine exchange between mother, fetus, and amniotic fluid. Am J Physiol 1975;228:231–7.

Rudd PT, Hughes EA, Placzek MM, et al. Reference ranges for plasma creatinine during the first month of life. Arch Dis Child 1983;58:212–5.

DIFFERENTIAL DIAGNOSIS AND EVALUATION OF POLYURIA

64. **What rate of urine flow constitutes polyuria?**
A urine flow rate greater than 4 to 5 mL/kg/h qualifies as polyuria.

65. **What are the primary causes of polyuria?**
Polyuria can be physiologic in response to excessive water and sodium intake or ECV expansion.
Pathologic causes of polyuria include the following:
- Impaired reabsorption of Na^+ by the kidney. This is often the result of renal tubular injury or disease.
- Osmotic diuresis. This is caused by the filtration of either a substance that is not reabsorbed by the renal tubules or a substance whose filtration rate greatly exceeds the capacity of the renal tubules to reabsorb it (e.g., glucose with marked hyperglycemia). In this case the offending substance impairs reabsorption of water and sodium, primarily in the proximal tubule. Because of the increased delivery of water and Na^+ to the distal tubule, K^+ secretion will also be stimulated, resulting in an inappropriate increase in urinary potassium excretion (or kaliuresis) and potassium depletion.
- Diabetes insipidus (DI). This results from the inability to concentrate the urine because of deficient production of antidiuretic hormone by the hypothalamus (central DI) or lack of responsiveness of the cortical collecting tubule to antidiuretic hormone.

66. **A newborn male infant is found to have renal failure caused by obstructive uropathy as the result of posterior urethral valves. A catheter is inserted into the bladder through the urethra. There is a large diuresis. The ARF gradually subsides with normalization of the serum creatinine level. Months later, the**

mother complains that her infant requires many more changes of diapers than did her other children. What is the likely explanation?

Severe obstruction of the urinary tract during nephrogenesis may lead to renal maldevelopment and can result in renal dysplasia. An early sign of dysplasia is a renal concentrating defect that manifests as polyuria and polydipsia. Some affected children maintain a normal GFR throughout their lives, but others have a slowly progressive decline in renal function, resulting in end-stage renal disease, often during the teenage years.

67. **An infant born prematurely to a mother who had polyhydramnios required mechanical ventilation for 1 week. At 6 days of life he had a rising serum creatinine level, hypotension with cool extremities, hyponatremia, and mild hypokalemia. Despite the appearance of ARF and hypovolemia, the infant had a large urine output with a high urinary concentration of sodium.**

The neonatal form of Bartter syndrome, also known as hyperprostaglandin E syndrome, may present this way. In such cases the mother has polyhydramnios caused by increased fetal urine excretion; affected infants are often born prematurely. Postnatally, polyuria and renal sodium wasting continue, resulting in hypovolemia and prerenal ARF. Infants with Bartter syndrome also have hypercalciuria and increased excretion of prostaglandin E_2. Additional findings may include hypokalemia and an elevated serum bicarbonate level, but this is not as common in infants as it is in older children with Bartter syndrome.

The defect appears to be in the ascending limb of the loop of Henle involving the NaCl, KCl cotransporter, or the potassium channel. There are two genetic forms of neonatal Bartter syndrome, one involving the gene that codes for the cotransporter (locus SLC12A1 on chromosome bands 15q–21) and one that results from mutation in the ROMK gene (locus KCNJ1 on chromosome bands 11q24–25), which controls the potassium channel.

67a. **How are infants with Bartter syndrome treated?**

Treatment with a prostaglandin synthetase inhibitor (e.g., indomethacin, ibuprofen) reverses many of the abnormalities. Salt-losing adrenal insufficiency must be excluded, but it is usually associated with hyperkalemia and acidosis.

Simon DB, Lifton RP. The molecular basis of inherited hypokalemic alkalosis: Bartter's and Gitelman's syndrome. Am J Physiol 1996;271:F961–F966.

 KEY POINTS: OLIGURIA AND POLYURIA

1. Oliguria is common in neonates during the first day of life because glomerular filtration is reduced. Nearly all babies will void, however, by 24 hours of life.

2. The creatinine measurement on the first day of life reflects the mother's creatinine level, whereas the change in creatinine over time, which varies with gestational age, is the best measure of the glomerular filtration rate in the newborn.

3. Normal urine output should exceed about 1 mL/kg/day in the neonatal period. Below that level can be considered oliguria after the first day of life. Polyuria can be considered when urine output exceeds 4 to 5 mL/kg/day.

RENAL TUBULAR ACIDOSIS

68. **What are the different types of renal tubular acidosis (RTA)?**
   - Type I (distal) : decreased distal H^+ secretion
   - Type II (proximal): decreased proximal tubular bicarbonate reabsorption
   - Type III: combination of types 1 and 2 (now rarely diagnosed as a separate entity)
   - Type IV: secondary to a lack of or insensitivity to aldosterone

All four types are associated with a hyperchloremic, normal anion gap acidosis.

69. What are the signs and symptoms of RTA?

RTA usually presents with nonspecific symptoms such as failure to thrive, lethargy, vomiting, and tachypnea. The hallmark of this syndrome is the presence of a normal anion gap hyperchloremic metabolic acidosis.

70. How does RTA usually present in the neonate?

In type I (distal) RTA the neonate presents with hypocitraturia, hypercalciuria, nephrocalcinosis, and failure to thrive with growth retardation. There are both dominant and recessive forms of distal RTA. The dominant form usually presents at an older age. The recessive form of distal RTA that presents in the neonatal period is associated with early onset bilateral sensorineural hearing loss. These patients often have vomiting and dehydration and can present with rickets.

Type II (proximal) RTA can present in infancy with ocular abnormalities such as band keratopathy, cataracts, and glaucoma. In addition to presenting with metabolic acidosis, these patients have growth restriction, defective dental enamel, developmental delay, and calcium deposits in the basal ganglia.

Type III RTA (combined proximal and distal) presents in infancy with osteopetrosis. These patients often have early nephrocalcinosis with blindness and deafness.

71. What are the usual causes of type IV RTA in neonates?

- Obstructive uropathy
- Adrenal insufficiency
- 21-Hydroxylase deficiency (congenital adrenal hyperplasia [CAH])
- Type I pseudohypoaldosteronism

Roth KS, Chan JC. Renal tubular acidosis: a new look at an old problem. Clin Pediatr 2001;40:533–43.

OBSTRUCTIVE UROPATHY

72. What is postnatal imaging likely to find on a newborn with antenatal hydronephrosis?

The most common finding is resolution of hydronephrosis (48%). Another 15% will show a nonobstructed, enlarged pelvis. The remaining will show the following:

- Ureteropelvic junction obstruction (11%)
- Vesicoureteral reflux (9%)
- Megaureter (4%)
- Multicystic dysplastic kidney (2%)
- Ureterocele (2%)
- Renal cyst (2%)
- Posterior urethral valves (1%)

Less common causes of hydronephrosis include ectopic ureter, prune-belly syndrome, urethral atresis, retrocaval ureter, ureteral stricture, hydrocolpos, pelvic tumor, and cloacal anomaly.

73. What is the natural history of fetal hydronephrosis?

In fetal hydronephrosis 50% of cases improve, 40% remain stable, and 10% progress.

74. What criteria justify prenatal intervention for fetal hydronephrosis? What are the goals of therapy?

Criteria for prenatal intervention are as follows:

- Significant diminution of amniotic fluid volume (bilateral hydronephrosis)
- No associated life-threatening conditions (55% of cases with bilateral hydronephrosis and oligohydramnios will be associated with other anomalies)
- Renal dysfunction reversible to some degree

- No ultrasonographic evidence of irreversible renal dysplasia
- Hypotonic urine

Prenatal intervention is generally limited to males with posterior urethral valves. The goals of intervention are to restore sufficient amniotic fluid volume to allow normal pulmonary development and maximize ultimate renal function.

75. **How should an infant with an abnormal genitourinary prenatal ultrasound be evaluated? When should the studies be done?**

Renal and bladder ultrasound is the first imaging needed in a neonate with an abnormal prenatal ultrasound. A normal 48-hour postnatal ultrasound is probably sufficient to exclude clinically significant disease, although some physicians will obtain an ultrasound later.

If unilateral hydronephrosis is present, a voiding cystourethrogram (to exclude vesicoureteral reflux) and serial ultrasounds are recommended. If there is progression of hydronephrosis, then a nuclear medicine scan (MAG-3 or DMSA) is indicated to assess kidney function. If there is bilateral hydronephrosis on the postnatal ultrasound, the neonate should have a vesicoureterogram (VCUG) within the first week of life.

76. **What is ureteropelvic junction obstruction? How is it diagnosed and managed?**

Ureteropelvic junction obstruction is the most common cause of hydronephrosis in children. Diagnosis requires the presence of hydronephrosis (ultrasound with dilated renal pelvis in the absence of a dilated ureter). Pyeloplasty, excision of the stenotic segment, is usually necessary in neonates with an abdominal mass, bilateral hydronephrosis, or a solitary kidney.

77. **What is a ureterocele? How does it cause obstruction?**

A ureterocele is a cystic dilation of the distal end of the ureter. It is obstructive because it may extend through the bladder neck (ectopic), but it may remain entirely within the bladder (intravesical). This condition affects girls more often than boys and is usually associated with the upper pole of a completely duplicated collecting system. Ultrasound commonly shows hydronephrosis in the upper pole, a dilated ureter, and a ureterocele in the bladder.

Chevalier RL. Perinatal obstructive nephropathy. Sem Perinatol 2004;28:124–31.

Chevalier RL. Obstructive uropathy: assessment of renal function in the fetus. In: Oh W, de Bruyn R, Marks SD, editors. Postnatal investigation of fetal renal disease. Sem Fetal Neonat Med 2008;13:133–41.

Guignard J-P, Baumgart S, editors. Nephrology and fluid/electrolyte physiology: neonatology questions and controversies. 2nd ed. Philadelphia: Saunders; 2012. p. 335–60.

EK S, Lidefeldt K-J, Varricio L. Fetal hydronephrosis: prevalence, natural history, and postnatal consequences in an unselected population. Acta Obstet et Gynecol Scand 2007;86:1463–6.

Estrada CR. Prenatal hydronephrosis: early evaluation. Curr Opin Urol 2008;18:401–3.

Sidhu G, Beyene J, Rosenblum ND. Outcome of isolated antenatal hydronephrosis: a systematic review and meta-analysis. 2006;21:218–24.

Yiee J, Wilcox D. Management of fetal hydronephrosis. Pediatr Nephrol 2008;23:347–53.

Lee RS, Cebdron M, Kinnamon DD, et al. Antenatal hydronephrosis as a predictor of postnatal outcome: a meta-analysis. Pediatr 2006;118:586–93.

POSTERIOR URETHRAL VALVES

78. **What is posterior urethral valves (PUV)?**

PUV is usually caused by an obstructing membrane extending from the verumontanum at the base of the prostatic urethra to the more distal anterior portion of the membranous urethra. This membrane contains only a small opening through which urine can pass; as the urine flows, the membrane billows out in a windsock fashion as a one-way flap valve, causing obstruction. The degree of obstruction varies depending on the size of the opening of the membrane.

79. Which conditions can be confused with PUV on fetal ultrasound?
- Prune-belly syndrome
- Severe bilateral vesicoureteral reflux with distended bladder

80. What is the most common presentation for an infant with PUV?
The most common presentation of PUV is poor urinary stream during the postnatal period. The ante-natal ultrasound often demonstrates bilateral hydroureteronephrosis, a dilated, thick-walled bladder with poor emptying, and occasionally oligohydramnios. A more severe clinical presentation of PUV in the postnatal period is with respiratory distress secondary to pulmonary hypoplasia, renal insuf-ficiency, urosepsis, and heart failure. Depending on the degree of obstruction, PUV may also present after the neonatal period with an abdominal mass, which indicates a distended bladder, ureter, or renal pelvis.

81. What are the short- and long-term consequences of PUV?
- Glomerular and renal tubular dysfunction causing renal insufficiency, poor urinary concentrating ability, and polyuria
- Urinary tract dilation, including hydroureteronephrosis and bladder dilation, and secondary to obstruction, polyuria, bladder dysfunction, and vesicoureteral reflux
- Vesicoureteral reflux, which is found in one third to one half of boys with valves
- Bladder dysfunction, including a wide spectrum ranging from bladder atony (poor contractil-ity), to bladder instability (hyperactive bladder with frequent bladder contractions), to poor bladder compliance caused by thickening of the bladder wall, to inability to store normal urine volumes

82. Does intervention after fetal diagnosis ultimately improve renal function?
Fetal intervention, including vesicoamniotic shunt placement, is performed when progressive oligo-hydramnios is noted on serial fetal ultrasounds to improve amniotic fluid levels. Oligohydramnios is detrimental to pulmonary development and may cause pulmonary hypoplasia. Correcting oligohy-dramnios is thought to allow better expansion of the chest wall and lung development, lessening the chance of pulmonary hypoplasia. Survival without intervention is 0% with a urinalysis consistent with a poor prognosis and 40% with a good prognosis. Prenatal intervention increases the chance of survival to 38% with a poor prognosis and 69% with a good prognosis.

83. Which conditions are associated with improved prognosis?
Conditions that allow decompression of the urinary tract (i.e., "pop-off" mechanism) have a better prognosis. Such conditions include bladder diverticular formation, urinary ascites, and unilateral vesiculoureteral reflux dysplasia (VURD) syndrome. Urinary ascites is caused by transudation of urine across a renal calyceal fornix into the peritoneal cavity; this transudation relieves the obstruction. VURD syndrome occurs when one kidney refluxes with subsequent renal dysplasia on that side, offer-ing protection for the contralateral kidney.

Gatti JM, Kirsch AJ. Posterior urethral valves: pre- and postnatal management. Curr Urol Report. 2001;2:138–45.
  Jee LD, Rickwood AM, Turnock RR. Posterior urethral valves: does prenatal diagnosis influence prognosis? Br J Urol 1993;72:830–3.

✓ KEY POINTS: OBSTRUCTIVE UROPATHY

1. Some fetuses appear to have obstructive uropathy on ultrasound that often resolves before birth.

2. Male patients with obstructive uropathy should be considered to have PUV until proved otherwise.

3. Prompt treatment of PUV does not always ensure normal renal function subsequently.

HEMATURIA

84. Is hematuria ever a normal finding in the newborn infant?
No. Hematuria is never physiologic, but it can be a common finding in sick premature infants.

85. How is hematuria typically defined?
Hematuria is defined as more than five red blood cells per high power field.

86. What are the causes of hematuria in the newborn infant?
- Perinatal asphyxia
- Renovascular accident (renal vein or renal artery thrombosis)
- Neoplasia
- Obstructive uropathy
- Coagulopathies
- Urinary tract infection
- Trauma (usually suprapubic aspiration)
- Congenital malformation of the kidney or urinary tract (or both), including polycystic disease

87. How should infants with hematuria be evaluated?
- Exclude other causes of red urine, such as urates, porphyrins, bile pigments, myoglobin, and hemoglobin.
- Obtain a microscopic evaluation on a fresh specimen (when examination is delayed, red blood cells can hemolyze).
- Decide whether the blood comes from upper or lower tracts (the presence of dysmorphic red cells or casts indicates parenchymal renal disease).
- Exclude extraurinary sources of blood, such as vaginal, rectal, or perineal sources.
- Obtain a urine culture if infection is suspected.
- Perform a renal ultrasound study if hematuria is persistent.
- Exclude a coagulopathy.
- Determine blood urea nitrogen and creatinine levels.

Emanuel B, Aronson N. Neonatal hematuria. Am J Dis Child 1974;128:204–6.

CONGENITAL NEPHROTIC SYNDROME

88. What is the definition of congenital nephrotic syndrome?
The term *congenital nephrotic syndrome* is used to describe a patient who develops the nephrotic syndrome during the first 3 months of life. Nephrotic syndrome is a constellation of abnormalities that includes (1) nephrotic-range proteinuria, defined as a urinary protein excretion greater than 100 mg/m^2 body surface area/24 h, calculated from a timed urine collection, or a ratio of urine protein concentration (mg/dL)/urine creatinine concentration (mg/dL) greater than 2, calculated from a single-spot urine sample; (2) nephrotic-range hypoalbuminemia with serum albumin concentrations less than 2.5 g/dL; (3) hyperlipemia, determined from the results of measurements of serum cholesterol or triglyceride concentrations (or both); and (4) peripheral edema that may be present in many patients.

89. Newborns may have proteinuria that occurs without complete nephrotic syndrome. How does the clinician interpret isolated proteinuria?
Abnormal proteinuria is defined as urine protein excretion greater than 100 mg/m^2 body surface area/24 h, calculated from a timed urine collection, or a ratio of urine protein (mg/dL)/urine creatinine (mg/dL) greater than 0.5, calculated from a single-spot urine specimen. Preterm infants are more likely to exhibit proteinuria than term infants. Abnormal proteinuria can occur in newborns as a result of various pathologic processes, including chronic volume depletion, congestive heart failure,

and interstitial nephritis caused by antibiotic administration. However, nephrotic-range proteinuria, as defined previously, suggests significant damage to glomerular epithelial cells caused by some pathologic process. Therefore discovery of nephrotic-range proteinuria, even in the absence of the full nephrotic syndrome, should prompt an evaluation.

90. **What is the most common cause of nephrotic syndrome in the first 3 months of life?**
The most common cause of nephrotic syndrome in the first 3 months of life is congenital nephrotic syndrome of the Finnish type, an autosomal recessive disease that is most common among Finns, although cases have been reported from all over the world. A less common cause of congenital nephrotic syndrome is diffuse mesangial sclerosis (DMS). DMS seems to have a genetic basis, but the exact mode of inheritance is unknown. Patients with DMS tend to develop nephrotic syndrome between 3 months and 2 years of age. Other renal lesions that can cause neonatal nephrotic syndrome may be associated with malformations that are not inherited in a known mendelian fashion. An example is Denys–Drash syndrome, a combination of ambiguous or female external genitalia with gonadal dysgenesis, a 46,XY genotype, and a predilection for the development of nephroblastoma.
Congenital infections may also cause nephrotic syndrome in a neonate. Congenital syphilis is the most common infectious association, but hepatitis B, C, human immunodeficiency virus (HIV), and cytomegalovirus (CMV) infections are also associated with congenital nephrotic syndrome. Many patients with congenital nephrotic syndrome resulting from a congenital infection demonstrate depressed serum concentrations of one or more components of the complement system.

91. **What prenatal or perinatal abnormalities should alert the perinatologist to the possibility that a newborn may have or develop congenital nephrotic syndrome?**
Infants with congenital nephrotic syndrome of the Finnish type (CNF gene map locus 19q13.1) generally have a large placenta (mean placental/fetal weight, 0.4) and are born preterm and small for gestational age. Prenatal evaluation of the mother of a patient with congenital nephrosis, Finnish variant (CNF), commonly demonstrates elevated concentrations of alpha-fetoprotein in both the amniotic fluid and the mother's blood. These abnormalities are not observed in mother–infant pairs afflicted with other forms of congenital nephrotic syndrome.

92. **Which evaluation is appropriate for a newborn with the nephrotic syndrome?**
The evaluation should be, as usual, driven by the differential diagnosis. Although the most likely underlying diagnosis is congenital primary glomerular disease, causes of secondary nephrotic syndrome should be pursued. A careful physical examination and renal/pelvic imaging (ultrasonogram) are helpful to identify any abnormalities of the external genitalia, the internal reproductive organs, or the kidneys (such as a Wilms tumor) that may suggest Denys–Drash syndrome or other malformation syndromes associated with congenital nephrotic syndrome. A family history of consanguinity, fetal or neonatal demise, or renal failure may be useful in suggesting a genetic cause for the nephrotic syndrome. Blood should be drawn to measure the levels of serum complement and complement components and to uncover evidence of prenatal infection with syphilis, hepatitis B or C, HIV, CMV, *Toxoplasma gondii*, or malaria. If the imaging and serologic evaluations reveal nothing, a renal biopsy should be performed to help make a diagnosis and guide future management.

93. **What is the prognosis for children who develop nephrotic syndrome in the newborn period?**
As a group, patients who develop nephrotic syndrome in the newborn period have a guarded prognosis. With the initiation of renal replacement therapy (usually peritoneal dialysis) in these neonates, the long-term survival rates have increased dramatically in the past few decades. Possible causes of increased morbidity and mortality in this population include the development of bacterial infections,

developmental delay, growth failure, thrombotic events, acute or chronic renal failure, complications of renal transplantation, and Wilms tumor among patients with Denys–Drash syndrome.

Penaflor G. Congenital nephrotic syndrome. Pediatr Rev 2001;22:32.

NEPHROCALCINOSIS

94. **How is the diagnosis of nephrocalcinosis usually made in an infant?**
Nephrocalcinosis is usually suggested by the findings on a renal ultrasound of a hyperechoic renal medulla, commonly in a very-low-birth-weight infant. Nephrocalcinosis results from microscopic calcification in the medullary portion of the kidney but often is accompanied by hyperechoic foci in the calyces, which represent renal calculi as well. Nephrocalcinosis can present with hematuria or urinary tract infection, but it is usually an incidental finding.

95. **A 6-week-old premature infant of 28 weeks' gestation with bronchopulmonary dysplasia is found to have nephrocalcinosis. The infant has been treated for several weeks with furosemide. Is chronic treatment with furosemide the most likely diagnosis in this case?**
Yes. The association of long-term furosemide therapy and nephrocalcinosis has been well recognized since the original description by Hufnagle et al. in 1982. There are, however, other diagnostic considerations for infants with nephrocalcinosis, which are outlined in Table 9-6.

96. **Hypercalciuria is an important diagnostic consideration in an infant with nephrocalcinosis. What is the normal range for calcium excretion in infants?**
The value for hypercalciuria, if defined as calcium excretion of greater than the 95th percentile for an age-matched cohort, is different in infants than it is in older children. In infants younger than 7 months old the 95th percentile for urinary calcium/creatinine (mg/mg) was reported by Sargent et al. to be 0.86, and in children 7 to 18 months old the value was 0.60. In another study very-low-birth-weight infants with nephrocalcinosis had a mean urinary calcium/creatinine of 0.49 compared with 0.11 in control subjects.

97. **What is the suggested therapy for an infant with nephrocalcinosis?**
Treatment of the primary cause can be important in cases not caused by long-term furosemide therapy. In infants being given furosemide, substitution of a thiazide diuretic for furosemide can decrease the calcium excretion and result in shrinkage of calculi and improvement of the medullary nephrocalcinosis. The long-term prognosis has been correlated with the course of the urinary calcium excretion.

TABLE 9-6.   DIFFERENTIAL DIAGNOSIS OF NEPHROCALCINOSIS IN INFANTS

Adapted from Karlowicz MG, Adelman RD. Renal calcification in the first year of life. Pediatr Clin North Am 1995;42:1397–1413.

NORMOCALCEMIC HYPERCALCIURIA	HYPERCALCEMIC HYPERCALCIURIA	NORMOCALCIURIC NEPHROCALCINOSIS
Furosemide therapy	Hyperparathyroidism	Primary hyperoxaluria
Bartter syndrome	Hypophosphatasia	Enteric hyperoxaluria
Distal renal tubular acidosis	Williams syndrome	Renal candidiasis
Hyperprostaglandin E	Idiopathic infantile	Long-term hypercalcemia
Subcutaneous fat necrosis	Acetazolamide therapy	
	Dystrophic calcifications	

98. **What is the prognosis in infants with nephrocalcinosis?**

Long-term studies of premature infants with nephrocalcinosis have suggested that 30% to 50% of the children continue to have evidence of renal calcification up to 5 years after diagnosis. There is some evidence of a slightly decreased GFR in patients with nephrocalcinosis, but these findings may be the result of prematurity and not specific for the history of nephrocalcinosis.

Hufnagle KG, Khan SN, Penn D, et al. Renal calcifications: a complication of long-term furosemide therapy in preterm infants. Pediatrics 1982;70:360–3.

Karlowicz MG, Adelman RD. Renal calcification in the first year of life. Pediatr Clin North Am 1995;42:1397–1413.

Porter E, McKie A, Beattie TJ, et al. Neonatal nephrocalcinosis: long term follow up. Arch Dis Child Fetal Neonatal Ed 2006;91;333–6

Sargent JD, Stukel TA, Kresel J, et al. Normal values for random urinary calcium to creatinine ratios in infancy. J Pediatr 1993;123:393–7.

HYPERTENSION

99. **What are the environmental and technical factors that can affect blood pressure measurements in the newborn?**

Various factors can alter the relationship between blood pressure as recorded on the NICU flow sheet and the patient's true average baseline blood pressure. For example, blood pressure readings are affected by the patient's position (pressures measured when the patient is supine are slightly higher than those obtained when the patient is prone), by recent medical manipulations, and by recent feedings. Cuff inflation, by itself, can stimulate the startle response, which can cause a transient increase in blood pressure. In addition, body geography has an impact on blood pressure measurements: Pressures measured in the legs are normally somewhat higher than those measured in the arms.

100. **What is the definition of neonatal hypertension?**

This question is often difficult to answer. Data regarding the normal ranges of systolic and diastolic blood pressures for term newborns and premature infants at various gestational ages have been published. Studies have shown that blood pressure in the neonatal period increases with gestational age, birth weight, and postmenstrual age.

A single random recording of elevated blood pressure may not be clinically significant because it may not exemplify the patient's average blood pressure. A more representative blood pressure measurement is recorded when the infant has not been fed or manipulated for 90 minutes before the evaluation; further refinement is achieved when several blood pressure measurements are made over a period of 5 to 10 minutes.

The diagnosis of hypertension should be made only if the systolic and diastolic blood pressures are above the 95th percentile on at least three separate blood pressure measurements recorded at 2-minute intervals during a time when the infant is quiet and otherwise undisturbed (Table 9-7).

101. **What is the most common cause of hypertension among patients in the NICU?**

The majority of hypertension in the NICU is renovascular in etiology. Umbilical artery catheter (UAC)–associated thrombosis can release thrombotic emboli to the aorta, the renal arteries, or both and thus induce the release of renin leading to hypertension. Thrombus formation at the time of UAC line placement is most likely secondary to disruption of the vascular endothelium of the umbilical artery.

102. **What are some other common causes of neonatal hypertension?**

Extremely-low-birth-weight infants with bronchopulmonary dysplasia appear to develop hypertension in the absence of clear evidence of renal artery occlusion at a rate higher than that seen with renal thrombosis. The etiology in many of these cases cannot be determined, although it is postulated that hypoxemia might be involved. Over 50% of these infants with bronchopulmonary dysplasia develop elevated blood pressures after discharge from the NICU. Extremely-low-birth-weight infants who have been hospitalized for a prolonged period should therefore have routine blood pressure

TABLE 9-7. NEONATAL AND INFANT BP NORMATIVE DATA AFTER 2 WEEKS' CHRONOLOGICAL AGE BASED ON POSTMENSTRUAL AGE (GESTATIONAL AGE + CHRONOLOGICAL AGE)

Data From Dionne JM, Arbitol CL, Flynn JT. Hypertension in infancy: Diagnosis, management and outcome. Pediatr Nephrol 2012;27:17–32.

POSTMENSTRUAL AGE	50TH PERCENTILE	95TH PERCENTILE	99TH PERCENTILE
44 weeks			
SBP	88	105	110
MAP	63	80	85
DBP	50	68	73
42 weeks			
SBP	85	98	102
MAP	62	76	81
DBP	50	65	70
40 weeks			
SBP	80	95	100
MAP	60	75	80
DBP	50	65	70
38 weeks			
SBP	77	92	97
MAP	59	74	79
DBP	50	65	70
36 weeks			
SBP	72	87	92
MAP	57	72	77
DBP	50	65	70
34 weeks			
SBP	70	85	90
MAP	50	65	70
DBP	40	55	60
32 weeks			
SBP	68	83	88
MAP	49	64	69
DBP	40	55	60
30 weeks			
SBP	65	80	85
MAP	48	63	68
DBP	40	55	60

TABLE 9-7. NEONATAL AND INFANT BP NORMATIVE DATA AFTER 2 WEEKS' CHRONOLOGICAL AGE BASED ON POSTMENSTRUAL AGE (GESTATIONAL AGE + CHRONOLOGICAL AGE)—cont'd

POSTMENSTRUAL AGE	50TH PERCENTILE	95TH PERCENTILE	99TH PERCENTILE
28 weeks			
SBP	60	75	80
MAP	45	58	63
DBP	38	50	54
26 weeks			
SBP	55	72	77
MAP	38	57	63
DBP	30	50	56

BP, blood pressure; SBP, systolic blood pressure; MAP, mean arterial blood pressure; DBP, diastolic blood pressure.

TABLE 9-8. DIFFERENTIAL DIAGNOSIS OF NEONATAL HYPERTENSION

AORTIC OBSTRUCTION

Coarctation of the aorta
Aortic arch interruption
Descending aorta thrombosis

RENAL AND RENOVASCULAR PROBLEMS

Renal artery thrombosis or embolus
Renal artery stenosis
Renal vein thrombosis (late)
Cystic renal disease
Obstructive uropathy

PHARMACOLOGIC ADVERSE EFFECTS

Catecholamines
Cocaine
Dexamethasone
Theophylline

OTHER CAUSES

Exogenous fluid administration
Environmental cold or noise stress
Seizures
Chronic lung disease

measurements made during their well-baby visits throughout the first year of life. Blood pressure measurement is often neglected by pediatricians because of the difficulty in obtaining an accurate determination in these tiny babies. Other causes of neonatal hypertension are listed in Table 9-8.

103. **What is the blood pressure profile of a patient whose hypertension is caused by a complication related to a UAC?**
Most patients who develop hypertension as a result of complications from a UAC are normotensive until the UAC is pulled. When the UAC is removed, hypertension often develops abruptly. The onset

of hypertension in this situation coincides with the embolization of renal vessels by clots that are sheared from the tip of the catheter during its withdrawal. Hypertension associated with UAC thrombosis usually resolves by 2 years of age.

104. What is the treatment of choice for newborns with hypertension related to a complication from the UAC?

UAC-related hypertension is generated by high circulating concentrations of angiotensin II. Angiotensin II production can be blocked by use of drugs that inhibit angiotensin-converting enzyme (ACE) inhibitors. Captopril is usually the ACE inhibitor of choice, with a starting dose of 0.01 to 0.5 mg/kg/dose given three times a day. The daily dose may be increased to a maximum of 6 mg/kg/day, if needed. Other ACE inhibitors such as enalapril or lisinopril may be used with equally beneficial effects, but dosing of these drugs for very small patients may be problematic for pharmacists. The use of ACE inhibitors is somewhat controversial because they may cause an exaggerated fall in blood pressure in the preterm infant. In addition, ACE inhibitors may hinder the final stages of renal maturation. For both those reasons, some clinicians do not use an ACE inhibitor until the infant has reached 44 weeks' postmenstrual age. For other causes of hypertension, calcium channel blockers are recommended. Table 9-9 summarizes the dosing for the commonly used antihypertensive agents.

105. What role do endocrine hormones play in neonatal hypertension?

Most cases of hypertension in newborns are caused by excessive circulating concentrations of hormones that cause hypertension as a result of their ability to increase peripheral vascular resistance and/or their ability to cause salt and water retention.

Renin produced by the kidney in response to either UAC-related renal artery thrombosis or to congenital renal artery stenosis generates angiotensin I. Angiotensin I is converted to angiotensin II by the action of ACE that is present in the kidney, lung, placenta, brain, and other organs. Angiotensin II has multiple effects when it circulates in the blood, including increased peripheral vascular resistance, augmented production and release of aldosterone by the adrenal glands, and stimulation of thirst and salt craving. All of these angiotensin II actions can increase blood pressure.

Rare endocrine disorders such as virilizing adrenal hyperplasia caused by 11β-hydroxylase deficiency and primary hyperaldosteronism may cause neonatal hypertension owing to overproduction of mineralocorticoid (desoxycorticosterone in the case of 11β-hydroxylase deficiency; aldosterone in patients with hyperaldosteronism). The overproduction of mineralocorticoid in these diseases causes hypertension by way of inappropriate renal salt and water retention. There may also be a mineralocorticoid-mediated hypokalemic metabolic alkalosis.

Prenatal or postnatal exposure to exogenous steroids (e.g., betamethasone, prednisone, or methylprednisolone) can likewise cause hypertension in newborns.

106. What abnormality of the physical examination of a hypertensive infant suggests that coarctation of the aorta may be the cause of the elevated blood pressure?

Despite the conventional wisdom that coarctation of the aorta is associated with a cardiac murmur and absent femoral pulses, many newborns with aortic coarctation do not fit the mold. In hypertensive infants measurement of blood pressure in both upper and lower extremities is crucial. Coarctation of the aorta should be suspected if the systolic pressure in the leg is more than 10 mmHg lower than the systolic pressure in the arms. It is also important to note that hypertension may persist in these infants even after the coarctation has been surgically repaired.

Flynn JT. Neonatal hypertension: diagnosis and management. In: Oh W, Guignard J-P, Baumgart S, editors. Nephrology and fluid/electrolyte physiology: neonatology questions and controversies. 2nd ed. Philadelphia: Saunders; 2012. p. 251–65.

Nawankwo MU, Lorenz JM, Gardiner JC. A standard protocol for blood pressure measurement in the newborn. Pediatrics 1997;99:E10.

Tan KL. Blood pressure in very low birth weight infants in the first 70 days of life. J Pediatr 1988;112:266–70.

TABLE 9–9. DOSING OF SELECTED ANTIHYPERTENSIVE AGENTS IN NEONATES

Data from Dione JM, Flynn JT. Hypertension in the neonate. Neoreviews 2012;13:e401.

CLASS	DRUG	ROUTE	DOSE	INTERVAL
ACEI*	Captopril	Oral	<3 mo: 0.01-0.5 mg/kg/dose Max 2 mg/kg/day	tid
			>3 mo: 0.15-3.0 mg/kg/dose Max 6 mg/kg/day	tid
	Enalapril	Oral	0.08-0.6 mg/kg/day	bid
	Lisinopril	Oral	0.07-0.6 mg/kg/day	qd
Alpha- and beta-antagonists	Labetalol	Oral	0.5-1 mg/kg/dose up to 10 mg/kg/day	bid-tid
		IV	0.20-1 mg/kg/dose (bolus)	q4-6 h
		IV	0.25-3 Mg/kg/h	Infusion
	Carvedilol	Oral	0.1 mg/kg/dose to 0.5 mg/kg/dose	bid
Beta-antagonists	Esmolol	IV	100-500 µg/kg/min	Infusion
	Propranolol	Oral	0.5-1 mg/kg/dose Max 8-10 mg/kg/day	tid
Calcium channel blockers	Amlodipine	Oral	0.05-0.3 mg/kg/dose up to 0.6 mg/kg/day	qd
	Isradipine	Oral	0.05-0.15 mg/kg/dose up to 0.8 mg/kg/day	qid
	Nicardipine	IV	0.5-4 µg/kg/min	Infusion
Central alpha-agonist	Clonidine	Oral	5-10 µg/kg/day up to 25 µg/kg/day	tid
Diuretics	Chlorothiazide	Oral	5-15 mg/kg/dose	bid
	Hydrochlorothiazide	Oral	1-3 mg/kg/dose	qd-bid
	Spironolactone	Oral	0.5-1.5 mg/kg/dose	bid
Vasodilators	Hydralazine	Oral	0.25-1.0 mg/kg/dose Up to 7.5 mg/kg/day	tid-qid
		IV	0.15-0.6 mg/kg/dose	q4h
	Minoxidil	Oral	0.1-0.2 mg/kg/dose	bid-tid
	Sodium Nitroprusside	IV	0.5-10 µg/kg/min	Infusion

*Avoid use in preterm infants until 44 weeks' postmenstrual age

✓ KEY POINTS: HYPERTENSION

1. Neonatal hypertension during or after NICU hospitalization is not rare and should be monitored in all patients.

2. Hypertension related to umbilical catheterization usually occurs during treatment or immediately after removal of the catheter.

3. Hypertension unrelated to catheters typically appears later during NICU hospitalization in an extremely-low-birth-weight infant with chronic lung disease.

4. Coarctation of the aorta should be considered in any neonate with hypertension.

RENAL VEIN THROMBOSIS

107. What are some maternal and infant factors that increase the risk of renal vein thrombosis (RVT) in the newborn infant?

Maternal factors known to increase the risk of RVT in the newborn include diabetes mellitus, elevated levels of immunoglobulin G anticardiolipin antibody, and activated protein C resistance. In addition, infants born to mothers who have required anticoagulation during pregnancy for thrombotic disorders should be treated with special caution.

Infants with inherited thrombophilic disorders, such as a deficiency of protein S, protein C, or anti-thrombin III, have an increased risk of RVT. Newborns who are otherwise healthy may develop RVT if they have experienced perinatal asphyxia, an episode of sepsis, or hyperosmolarity and dehydration caused by, for example, administration of intravenous radiocontrast or fluid losses as a result of vomiting or diarrhea.

108. What signs and symptoms suggest the occurrence of RVT in a newborn?

Clinicians should suspect the diagnosis of RVT if a newborn develops hematuria (often gross hematuria) in association with a swollen kidney, palpable as a flank mass, and abrupt or progressive elevation of the plasma creatinine concentration. Suspicion of RVT is especially warranted if these abnormalities are accompanied by thrombocytopenia. RVT may not, however, always induce dramatic clinical or laboratory changes. For example, a newborn with RVT may produce urine that is clear yellow; microscopic hematuria with or without proteinuria may be the only urinary abnormality. Even when the RVT does not cause major changes in the urinalysis, however, there is usually a measurable deterioration of renal function, thrombocytopenia, and perhaps a transient elevation of blood pressure.

109. Which imaging studies are helpful, and which may be harmful, in the diagnosis of RVT?

Renal ultrasonography is a useful tool. It is noninvasive and usually identifies areas of the kidney that are affected by RVT. The renal parenchyma that experiences obstruction to venous drainage appears swollen and hyperechoic.

Renal scans using intravenous injections of technetium diethylenetriaminepentaacetic acid (DTPA) or technetium dimercaptosuccinic acid demonstrate perfusion defects in the areas that are drained by the thrombosed renal vessels. These scans, however, do not provide anatomic detail, nor are they able to differentiate between arterial and venous renovascular disease. Furthermore, the utility of renal scans is limited by the fact that they generally require the sick infant to be transported from the neonatal unit to the nuclear medicine department.

Because RVT may be caused by serum hyperosmolarity, intravenous administration of hypertonic radiocontrast agents may be ill-advised. Therefore the clinician should not order studies that may require administration of intravenous contrast agents (e.g., intravenous pyelography, computed tomography).

110. **Which fluid and electrolyte abnormalities may occur in an infant with RVT?**
Infants with RVT commonly experience a period of renal insufficiency that results in the following fluid and electrolyte abnormalities:
- Oliguria, fluid retention, and hyponatremia
- Metabolic acidosis
- Hyperphosphatemia and hypocalcemia

111. **Is there a role for thrombectomy or nephrectomy in infants with RVT?**
Neither thrombectomy nor nephrectomy has a role. Thrombectomy is unlikely to provide benefit because most cases of RVT begin in the peripheral renal venous circulation; therefore removal of a clot present in the main renal vein is not likely to restore venous drainage to the bulk of the affected renal parenchyma. Some experts advocate attempting thrombectomy when bilateral RVT also involves the inferior vena cava; however, there is little evidence to support the notion that the procedure, even in the direst circumstances, improves either long-term patient survival or ultimate renal function.

Because many, if not most, kidneys with RVT ultimately recover some function as a result of recanalization of thrombosed vessels, nephrectomy of the affected kidney in the acute or subacute phase of RVT should be discouraged. Evidence that nephrectomy improves patient survival is unsubstantiated, and this procedure certainly leads to a decrease in functional nephron mass.

112. **Is thrombolytic (e.g., urokinase, tissue plasminogen activator) or anticoagulant therapy useful in neonates with RVT?**
The usefulness of thrombolytic or anticoagulant therapy must be qualified by such terms as *maybe* or *sometimes*. Infusion of thrombocytic agents, either locally or systemically, has been used with some success in patients with RVT or renal arterial thrombosis. The risk of hemorrhagic complications, however, is significant. Because thrombolysis and venous recanalization occur as part of the normal resolution of RVT, it is not clear that pharmacologic thrombolytic therapy carries a favorable risk-to-benefit ratio.

Anticoagulant intervention that aims to prevent extension of RVT into previously uninvolved venous structures may be appropriate for some patients, particularly those who have congenital thrombophilic disorders. The prothrombotic factors that lead to RVT formation and propagation in most newborns can be eliminated without anticoagulant therapy (e.g., hyperosmolarity, dehydration). However, anticoagulants may protect infants with intrinsic abnormalities of the coagulation cascade from experiencing secondary thrombotic events.

Rosendaal FR. Thrombosis in the young: epidemiology and risk factors. A focus on venous thrombosis. Thromb Haemost 1977;78:1–6.

PRUNE–BELLY SYNDROME

113. **What is prune-belly syndrome?**
Prune-belly syndrome is a rare congenital anomaly that consists of genital (usually undescended testes) and urinary tract abnormalities with absent or decreased abdominal wall musculature (Fig. 9-6). Prune-belly syndrome is caused by urethral outlet obstruction early in development.

114. **What are the most common urinary tract anomalies that occur in patients with prune-belly syndrome?**
From bottom to top, the most common urinary tract anomalies are as follows:
- The bladder neck is patulous.
- The bladder is capacious. The bladder wall may be thickened, but the internal contour of the bladder is smooth, without trabeculations or diverticuli. Often the bladder communicates with a patent urachus.

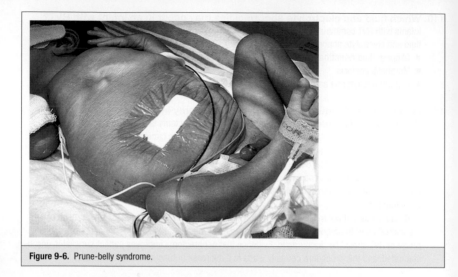

Figure 9-6. Prune-belly syndrome.

- Ureteral abnormalities commonly consist of irregular dilations and narrowings, usually most dramatic in the lower ureteral segments.
- The kidneys are often small, with or without dilation of the collecting system.

It is important to note that the anatomic abnormalities of the urinary tract in patients with prune-belly syndrome may be caused by primary, intrinsic, and diffuse defects of embryologic development of the structures involved, which are different from the discrete lesions of obstruction or reflux that may occur in the urinary tract of otherwise normal newborns. However, the abnormalities may appear similar to those that occur in prune-belly syndrome. For example, the large, thick-walled bladder of patients with prune-belly syndrome may occur in the absence of bladder outlet obstruction, although the bladder may bear a resemblance to that of a patient with PUV. Similarly, although ureteral dilation in otherwise normal infants is commonly associated with vesicoureteral reflux or obstruction, a similar ureteral lesion in a patient with prune-belly syndrome may occur in the absence of reflux or obstruction.

115. **What other anomalies occur outside the genitourinary system in infants with prune-belly syndrome? What are their causes?**

Patients with prune-belly syndrome often have additional problems, including pulmonary hypoplasia and Potter facies (flattening of the nose, redundant skin, receding chin, ocular hypertelorism, and low-set ears); hip dislocation or subluxation; talipes equinovarus; congenital cardiac disease, especially atrial septal defect, ventricular septal defect, and tetralogy of Fallot; and gastrointestinal anomalies.

The urologic/renal dysfunction in patients with prune-belly syndrome is almost certainly responsible for some of the nonurologic complications. For example, oligohydramnios, a common complication of prune-belly syndrome pregnancies, accounts for the pulmonary hypoplasia, the hip dislocation or subluxation, and the talipes equinovarus that may be seen in these newborns. It has been suggested that the underlying defect in prune-belly syndrome is abnormal mesoderm development.

116. **Which diagnostic studies assist the neonatologist in evaluating a child with prune-belly syndrome?**

The initial work-up should include (1) abdominal and pelvic ultrasonography to provide a basic road map of the genitourinary anomalies and (2) voiding cystourethrography to diagnose vesicoureteral reflux and reflux into a patent urachus. Either of these two diagnoses mandates initiation of antibiotic prophylaxis. If the infant is stable enough to be transported, other imaging studies significantly enhance understanding of the genitourinary pathology. Computerized axial tomograms of the abdomen, performed before and after intravenous administration of radiocontrast material, will usually reveal more anatomic detail than ultrasound; in addition, they provide a qualitative assessment of comparative renal function (i.e., right versus left kidney). A renal scan using DTPA or MAG3 will localize any points of obstruction between the kidneys and the bladder and provides a quantitative estimate of the comparative function of the two kidneys.

Because an infant with prune-belly syndrome may also harbor gastrointestinal and cardiac anomalies, an upper gastrointestinal tract series with small bowel follow-through, a barium enema, an electrocardiogram, and an echocardiogram are also needed as part of the initial work-up.

117. What is the role for surgical intervention in patients with prune-belly syndrome?

Every newborn with prune-belly syndrome should be evaluated by a pediatric urologist. However, intervention during the newborn period should be limited to the least invasive procedures available and should be used only when necessary to relieve high-grade obstruction in the urinary tract. More extensive genitourinary reconstructive procedures should be postponed to a later date and, in fact, may not be necessary at all. There is considerable controversy about whether surgical intervention is appropriate in boys with prune-belly syndrome when their genitourinary anomalies are not associated with obstruction or vesicoureteral reflux.

At some point the surgeon must deal with the intraabdominal cryptorchidism. Orchidectomy, as a means to prevent testicular neoplasia, is an option because the reproductive potential of boys with prune-belly syndrome is probably low. An alternate approach is to relocate the abdominal testes into the scrotum by one of a variety of complex surgeries. In any case these surgical interventions can wait until the infant is several months old.

Surgical plication of the lax abdominal musculature is important for the psychological well-being of patients with prune-belly syndrome, but this cosmetic reconstruction should probably not be performed in a newborn.

Hassett S, Smith GH, Holland AJ. Prune belly syndrome. Pediatr Surg Int 2012;28:219–28.

Lesavoy MA, Chang EI, Suliman A, et al. Long-term follow-up of total abdominal wall reconstruction for prune belly syndrome. Plast Reconstr Surg 2012;129:104e.

Routh JC, Huang L, Retik AB, et al. Contemporary epidemiology and characterization of newborn male with Prune Belly Syndrome. Urology 2010;76:44–8.

CYSTIC KIDNEY DISEASE

118. What is the definition of multicystic renal disease?

A multicystic kidney is the result of abnormal metanephric differentiation. There is no continuity between glomeruli and calyces, and the kidney does not function. The contralateral kidney may be normal, absent, hydronephrotic, ectopic, or dysplastic.

119. What is the definition of renal cystic dysplasia?

Renal cystic dysplasia may be unilateral or bilateral. The kidneys are usually cystic and exhibit disorganized architecture. They often contain ectopic tissue (e.g., cartilage, muscle) and do not function normally.

120. What is the definition of polycystic renal disease?

In polycystic renal disease there are many cysts in both kidneys, no dysplasia, and continuity between glomeruli and calyces. The kidneys are often large.

121. Describe the management of autosomal recessive polycystic kidney disease in a neonate.

- Treat the hypertension (usually requires multiple antihypertensive agents, one of which should be an ACE inhibitor).
- Ventilate; drain pneumothoraces.

- Perform uninephrectomy or bilateral nephrectomy if there is massive nephromegaly that interferes with feeding or ventilation.
- Order peritoneal dialysis in cases of chronic renal failure.

122. **What are some complications that can occur in infants with autosomal recessive polycystic disease?**

- Hypertension
- Bleeding from gastroesophageal varices
- Hypersplenism with combinations of anemia, leukopenia, and thrombocytopenia
- Urinary tract infections in 30%
- Growth restriction in 25%
- Rare cases of cholangiocarcinoma

123. **Can autosomal dominant polycystic kidney disease occur in the neonate?**
Yes. Affected neonates have extremely large cystic kidneys and respiratory distress, and they usually manifest significant renal failure immediately after birth.

124. **What are the indications for liver and renal biopsies in neonates with polycystic kidneys?**
There are no indications for biopsies in these patients. Careful evaluation with ultrasonography is sufficient for diagnostic and treatment purposes.

125. **In which conditions is congenital hepatic fibrosis associated with renal disorders?**

- Congenital hepatic fibrosis and polycystic kidneys (autosomal recessive and dominant)
- Hereditary tubulointerstitial nephritis
- Juvenile nephronophthisis
- Bardet–Biedl syndrome
- Jeune syndrome (asphyxiating thoracic chondrodystrophy)
- Congenital hepatic fibrosis and hereditary renal dysplasia
- Meckel syndrome
- Chondrodysplasia syndromes
- Renal-hepatic-pancreatic cystic dysplasia (Ivemark syndrome)
- Zellweger syndrome

Avni FE, Hall M. Renal cystic diseases in children: new concepts. Pediatr Radiol 2010;40:939–46.
Fick GM, Gabow PA. Hereditary and acquired cystic disease of the kidney. Kidney Int 1994;46:961–4.
Kaplan BS, Fay J, Shah V, et al. TM autosomal recessive polycystic kidney disease. Pediatr Nephrol 3:1989;43–9.
Ogborn MR. Polycystic kidney disease—a truly pediatric problem. Pediatr Nephrol 1994;8:762–7.
Roy S, Dillon MJ, Trompeter RS, et al. Autosomal recessive polycystic kidney disease: Long-term outcome of neonatal survivors. Pediatr Nephrol 1997;11:302–6.

EXSTROPHY OF THE BLADDER

126. **What are the correct terms for the developmental defect shown in Figure 9-7?**
The correct terms for the developmental defect shown in Figure 9-7 are *bladder exstrophy* and *epispadias*.

127. **When does this developmental defect occur?**
Bladder closure takes place between the sixth and eighth weeks of fetal life.

128. **When should the exstrophy–epispadias complex be repaired?**
Bladder exstrophy should be closed in the first 48 hours of life to ensure the best possible technical results for achieving long-term continence.

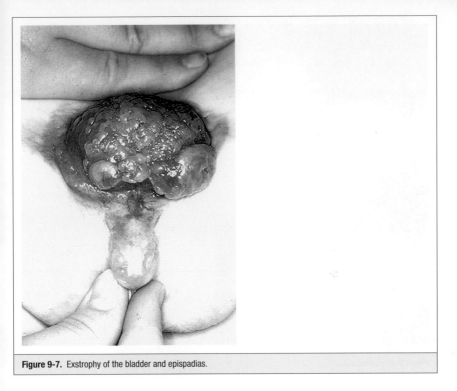

Figure 9-7. Exstrophy of the bladder and epispadias.

129. **Should the clinician be concerned with upper urinary tract anomalies in children with bladder exstrophy?**
The upper urinary tract is almost always normal in these children. Evaluation of these children should include assessment of the hips, however, because some of them will have hip dysplasia.

130. **What is the risk of recurrence in subsequent pregnancies?**
The risk is no greater than that for the general population, which is 1:50,000 live births.

131. **Why is exstrophy–epispadias complex decreasing in incidence?**
The reasons are not entirely clear; however, it appears that the widespread use of prenatal ultrasonography and elective termination have had a significant impact on the incidence of bladder exstrophy worldwide.

Phillips TM. Spectrum of cloacal exstrophy. Semin Pediatr Surg 2011;20:113–8.
  Woo LL, Thomas JC, Brock JW. Cloacal exstrophy: a comprehensive review of an uncommon problem. J Pediatr Urol 2010;6:102–11.

HYPOSPADIAS

132. **What is the developmental defect shown in Figure 9-8?**
The developmental defect shown in Figure 9-8 is called hypospadias.

133. **Does the child shown in Figure 9-8 need immediate surgical attention?**
No. Surgical correction is best done somewhere between 6 and 12 months of life, assuming there are no additional medical issues.

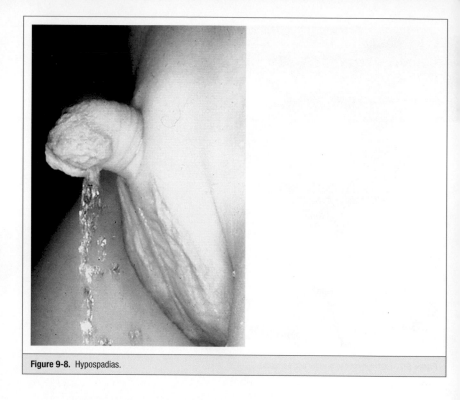

Figure 9-8. Hypospadias.

134. When during development did this lesion occur?

Penile development takes place between 12 and 15 weeks of gestation.

135. Hypospadias in association with bilateral nonpalpable gonads demands what kind of evaluation?

Chromosomal evaluation is mandatory in infants with hypospadias and nonpalpable gonads. The clinician must rule out virilizing congenital adrenal hyperplasia to prevent errors in gender assignment and avoid the risk of a salt-losing crisis in the infant.

136. How common are other genitourinary abnormalities in infants with distal hypospadias?

Rare. There is no greater incidence of other genital urinary anomalies in infants with distal hypospadias than in other infants.

137. What is happening to the incidence of hypospadias?

The incidence of hypospadias is increasing nationwide. The reason is not entirely clear, but it may have to do with increased use of *in vitro* fertilization or exposure to environmental estrogens and antiandrogens.

Erickson JD. Epidemiology of hypospadias. Adv Exper Med Biol 2004;545:25–9.

Kalfa N, Philibert P, Sultan C. Is hypospadias a genetic, endocrine or environmental disease, or still an unexplained malformation? Int J Androl 2008; 32:187–97.

Silver RI. Endocrine abnormalities in boys with hypospadias. Adv Exper Med Biol. 2004;545:45–72.

Snodgrass WT. Consultation with the specialist: hypospadias [Review]. Pediatr Rev 2004;25:63–7.

CHAPTER 10

GASTROENTEROLOGY AND NUTRITION

Sarah A. Taylor, MD, and Joel E. Lavine, MD, PhD

DEVELOPMENT OF THE GASTROINTESTINAL SYSTEM

1. **How does the primitive gut develop in the fetus, and what are its three divisions?**

   Folding occurs along the embryo in a cephalocaudal progression that leads to the incorporation of some of the endodermal-lined yolk sac into the embryo, which in turn results in the creation of the primitive gut. The primitive gut is composed of the foregut, midgut, and hindgut. The foregut is most cephalic and will become the esophagus and stomach. The midgut becomes the small intestines, and the hindgut becomes the colon (Fig. 10-1).

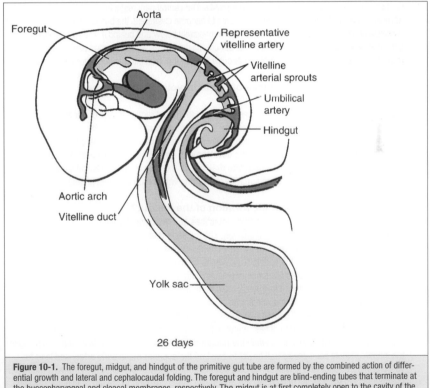

Figure 10-1. The foregut, midgut, and hindgut of the primitive gut tube are formed by the combined action of differential growth and lateral and cephalocaudal folding. The foregut and hindgut are blind-ending tubes that terminate at the buccopharyngeal and cloacal membranes, respectively. The midgut is at first completely open to the cavity of the yolk sac. (From Larsen WJ, Sherman LS, Potter SS, Scott WJ, editors. Human embryology. 3rd ed. New York: Churchill Livingstone; 2001. p. 237.)

2. **When does the lung bud separate from the esophagus?**

At approximately 4 weeks of gestation, the lung buds appear on the ventral surface of the foregut. This outpocketing from the esophagus will eventually separate completely, forming separate walls known as the esophagotracheal septum. This separation is critical, and any remnant in connection leads to esophageal atresia, a tracheoesophageal fistula, or both. The most common type of developmental abnormality that can occur as a result of this splitting is proximal esophageal atresia with a distal esophagotracheal fistula, which accounts for about 85% of all esophageal atresias.

3. **When does the liver develop?**

The liver forms at about the third week of gestation as an outgrowth, known as the hepatic diverticulum or liver bud, of the endodermal epithelium of the foregut. This connection grows and narrows to form the bile duct to connect the developing liver to the foregut. A small ventral outgrowth forms that will develop into the gallbladder and connecting cystic duct. The intrauterine failure to develop a complete biliary tree can lead to extrahepatic biliary atresia of embryonic or fetal form, which occurs in 10% to 35% of all cases.

Petersen C. Biliary atresia: the animal models. Semin Pediatr Surg 2012;21(3):185–91.

4. **How does the pancreas develop?**

The pancreas develops in two separate locations as a bud from the endodermal-lined foregut. The dorsal pancreas develops from a bud on the dorsal surface opposite the developing biliary tree. The dorsal pancreatic bud is located within the dorsal mesentery and grows with a central dorsal pancreatic duct draining to the foregut through the minor papilla. The ventral pancreatic bud develops close to the developing bile duct. When the duodenum rotates to become C-shaped, the bud is rotated onto the dorsal surface along the dorsal pancreas in a position immediately below and behind it. The two developing pancreas parts grow together, and the dorsal pancreatic duct fuses with the ventral pancreas to form the main pancreatic duct (of Wirsung) draining through the major papilla into the duodenum (Fig. 10-2).

5. **What is the clinical significance of the embryologic development of the pancreas?**

If the connection from the dorsal pancreas continues to drain directly into the duodenum by way of this secondary drainage system (the accessory pancreatic duct of Santorini), the condition is known as pancreas divisum. This connection drains through the minor papilla at a separate location and is the most common anomaly of pancreatic development. Any variation in this process can lead to completely separated drainage to a duplicate drainage of the pancreas. The clinical significance of this condition is the higher risk of pancreatitis in patients with pancreatic duct anomalies.

6. **What is the significance of the rotation of the midgut?**

During the sixth week of gestation the small intestines and the colon herniate into the umbilical cord as a result of the rapid growth of the liver. The intestine then rotates around a central axis formed by the superior mesenteric artery. This counterclockwise rotation is completed, and the intestine migrates back into the abdominal cavity to be fixed in position. This rotation results in the colon being located anterior to the small intestines, with the cecum being located in the right lower quadrant. An interruption during this physiologic herniation and rotation will result in abnormalities. When the gut fails to return to the abdominal cavity, an omphalocele is formed. This abnormality occurs in approximately 2.5 in 10,000 births. There is a high rate of associated developmental defects, such as cardiac abnormalities, spinal defects, and chromosomal abnormalities. Malrotation is another abnormality that occurs when the midgut fails to rotate completely. Malrotation can cause the inappropriately positioned small bowel to twist on the superior mesenteric artery and lead to vascular insufficiency and volvulus. The gold standard for diagnosis of malrotation remains the upper gastrointestinal tract series that shows the duodenal C-loop crossing to the left of midline at a level equal to or greater than the pylorus.

Martin V, Shaw-Smith C. Review of genetic factors in intestinal malrotation. Pediatr Surg Int 2010;26(8):769–81.

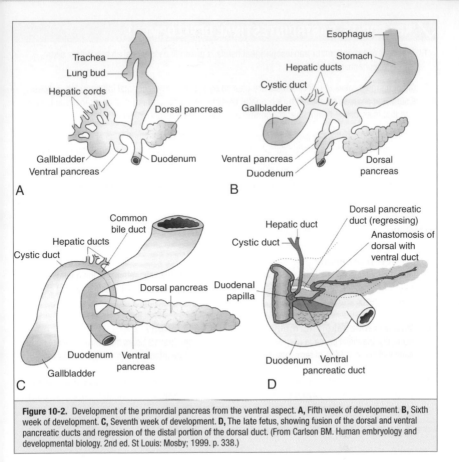

Figure 10-2. Development of the primordial pancreas from the ventral aspect. **A,** Fifth week of development. **B,** Sixth week of development. **C,** Seventh week of development. **D,** The late fetus, showing fusion of the dorsal and ventral pancreatic ducts and regression of the distal portion of the dorsal duct. (From Carlson BM. Human embryology and developmental biology. 2nd ed. St Louis: Mosby; 1999. p. 338.)

7. **How does the hindgut develop?**

The hindgut forms the most distal part of the primitive gut. It develops into the distal third of the transverse colon and the upper part of the rectal canal. Initially the urogenital system and the hindgut join together in the cloaca. The two systems separate from each other, and the rectal canal fuses with the surface to form an open pathway that will form the anus and rectum. Any abnormalities with this development can result in a continued connection, or urorectal fistula, between the urologic and gastrointestinal tracts. When the anorectal canal fails to fuse with the surface, a rectoanal atresia occurs with resulting imperforate anus. Imperforate anus occurs in 1 in 50,000 live births and has a high incidence of other associated birth defects.

Juang D, Snyder CL. Neonatal bowel obstruction. Surg Clin North Am 2012;92(3):685–711.

8. **What is the enteric nervous system (ENS)?**

The ENS is the nervous system that regulates intestinal smooth muscle to control gastrointestinal motility. The ENS is composed of a complex network of ganglia that function independently from the central nervous system. Although independent, the ENS can be influenced by vagal and pelvic nerves of the parasympathetic nervous system and spinal nerves. Within the ENS the interstitial cells of Cajal are the pacemaker cells and are responsible for the coordinated smooth muscle contractions within the gut.

✓ KEY POINTS: GASTROINTESTINAL DEVELOPMENT

1. The most common form of transesophageal fistula is proximal esophageal atresia with a distal tracheoesophageal fistula.

2. Although most cases of biliary atresia are caused by a destructive, perinatal inflammatory process, a subset appears to be caused by a prenatal developmental abnormality of the extrahepatic biliary tree that is associated with other congenital anomalies, such as polysplenia.

3. Rotational abnormalities of pancreas development can be observed either as an annular pancreas presenting with obstruction or as ductal abnormalities presenting with pancreatitis later in childhood.

4. Delayed passage of meconium should raise consideration of both anatomic abnormalities (e.g., variants of imperforate anus) and motility disorders (e.g., Hirschsprung disease).

MECONIUM

9. **What is meconium?**
   Meconium is the material and secretions created by or swallowed by the fetus in the gastrointestinal tract while *in utero*. It contains ingested amniotic fluid, lanugo, intestinal cells, bile salts and pigments, and pancreatic enzymes.

10. **When is meconium normally passed in a term infant?**
    Normally, the initial passage of meconium occurs within the first 12 hours after birth. Meconium passage will occur in 99% of term infants and 95% of premature infants within 48 hours of birth.

11. **What is the significance of the lack of passage of meconium at the normal time?**
    When meconium is not passed by 48 hours of life, the possibility of an anatomic or neuromuscular abnormality must be considered, such as Hirschsprung disease.

Kenny SE, Tam PK, Garcia-Barcelo M. Hirschsprung's disease. Semin Pediatr Surg 2010;19(3):194–200.

FETAL GROWTH AND ASSESSMENT

12. **Why is it important to routinely monitor fetal growth during pregnancy?**
    Intrauterine growth is one of the most important signs of fetal well-being and one of the most reliable indicators of the pathologic conditions that affect the mother and fetus during pregnancy. Early identification of alterations in fetal growth can allow for early intervention to prevent long-term complications for the fetus and newborn infant.

13. **What do the terms low birth weight (LBW), very low birth weight (VLBW), and extremely low birth weight (ELBW) indicate?**
    - LBW: less than 2500 g
    - VLBW: less than 1500 g
    - ELBW: less than 1000 g

    This classification is clinically relevant because neonatal morbidity and mortality are strongly correlated with the infant's gestational age and birth weight.

14. **What are the most common causes of intrauterine growth restriction (IUGR)?**
    Intrinsic (fetal causes):
    - Constitutional
    - Genetic

- Toxic
- Infectious
- Teratogenic
- Behavioral
- Intrauterine constraint

Extrinsic (maternal/placental) causes:

- Maternal age younger than 16 years or older than 35 years
- Maternal illness
- Placental dysfunction
- Multiple gestation
- Demographic

15. What causes neonates to be large for gestational age?

Infants with birth weight above the 90th percentile on the intrauterine growth chart are classified as large for gestational age. Maternal diabetes is the most common cause of fetal growth acceleration owing to the induction of fetal hyperinsulinism during gestation. Other causes include fetal hydrops (edema), Beckwith–Wiedemann syndrome, transposition of the great vessels, and maternal obesity.

16. Why is it clinically useful to classify small-for-gestational-age infants as symmetric or asymmetric?

Infants who are symmetrically growth retarded have proportionally reduced size in weight, length, and head circumference. This type of growth retardation starts early in pregnancy, and it is often secondary to congenital infection, chromosomal abnormalities, and dysmorphic syndromes. Most babies with IUGR, however, are asymmetrically growth retarded, with the most severe growth reduction in weight, less severe length reduction, and relative head sparing. Asymmetric IUGR is caused by extrinsic factors that occur late in gestation, such as pregnancy-induced hypertension. Distinguishing between symmetric and asymmetric IUGR is important because infants with asymmetric IUGR have a better long-term growth and developmental outcome.

MEDICAL PROBLEMS OF THE GROWTH-RESTRICTED INFANT

17. What are the long-term risks of IUGR?

- Development: Because this group is heterogeneous, the outcome depends on perinatal events, the etiology of growth retardation, and the postnatal socioeconomic environment. In general, the asymmetric growth-retarded baby does not show significant differences in intelligence or neurologic sequelae but does demonstrate differences in school performance related to abnormalities in behavior and learning.
- Health effects: An increased risk of hypertension is found in adolescents and young adults. Growth-retarded infants with a low ponderal index (measurement of leanness calculated by body mass divided by height cubed) are at increased risk for syndrome X (non–insulin-dependent diabetes mellitus, hypertension, and hyperlipidemia) and death resulting from cardiovascular disease by the age of 65 years (Barker hypothesis).
- Growth: Fetuses that experienced growth failure after 26 weeks' gestation (asymmetric growth retardation) exhibit a period of catch-up growth during the first 6 months of life. However, their ultimate stature is frequently less than an appropriate-for-gestational-age (AGA) baby.

CALORIC REQUIREMENTS

18. What is the significance of energy balance?

Energy, being neither created nor destroyed, conforms to classic balance relationships. Energy balance is a state of equilibrium when energy intake equals expenditure plus losses. If energy intake exceeds expenditure plus losses, the infant is in positive balance, and excess calories are stored. If energy intake is less than expenditure plus losses, the infant is in negative balance, and calories are mobilized from existing body stores. Maintenance, or basal, energy requirements are the energy needs required to cover basal metabolic rate or resting energy expenditure; total energy expenditure in infants is the sum of the energy required for basal metabolic rate, activity, thermoregulation, diet-induced thermogenesis, and growth. The energy balance equation may be stated as follows:

$$\text{Gross energy intake} = \text{energy excreted} + \text{energy expended} + \text{energy stored or}$$
$$\text{Metabolizable energy} = \text{energy expended} + \text{energy stored}$$

19. **What are the caloric requirements for LBW infants?**
    LBW infants require at least 120 cal/kg/day, partitioned to approximately 75 cal/kg/day for resting expenditure and the remainder for specific dynamic action (10 cal/kg/day), replacement of inevitable stool losses (10 cal/kg/day), and growth (25 cal/kg/day) (Table 10-1).

20. **What is the respiratory quotient (RQ), and what is its significance?**
    The RQ is the ratio of the volume of carbon dioxide (CO_2) produced to the volume of oxygen (O_2) consumed per unit of time (V_{CO_2}/V_{O_2}). This ratio varies with the type of nutrient oxidized. In addition, the energy produced varies with the type of substrate burned. Thus various substrates have different RQs, and varying proportions of different nutrients result in different energy production per liter of O_2 consumption or CO_2 production. The RQs and caloric equivalents of O_2 and CO_2 for carbohydrate, fat, and protein are shown in Table 10-2.

21. **What is the energy cost of growth?**
    The energy cost of growth includes the energy used for synthesis of new tissues (e.g., absorption, metabolism, and assimilation of fat and protein) and the energy stored in these new tissues. The energy cost of growth varies with the type of tissue added during growth. The precise caloric requirements for growth are unknown. A wide range of values for energy cost of growth in neonates has been

TABLE 10-1. CALORIC REQUIREMENTS OF LOW-BIRTH-WEIGHT INFANTS

	REQUIREMENTS (kcal/kg/day)
Resting*	50 to 75
Specific dynamic action	5% to 8% of total intake
Stool losses	10% of total intake
Growth	25 to 45
Total†	85 to 142

*Estimate includes caloric expenditure for maintenance of basal metabolism plus activity and response to cold stress.
†Includes sum of resting and growth requirements for specific dynamic action and replacement of stool losses plus an increment of 15% to 18%.

TABLE 10-2. RESPIRATORY QUOTIENTS AND CALORIC EQUIVALENTS

	RESPIRATORY QUOTIENT	ENERGY PRODUCED/L OF O_2 (kcal)	ENERGY PRODUCED/L OF CO_2
Carbohydrate	1	5	5
Fat	0.71	4.7	6.6
Protein	0.80	4.5	5.6

determined (1.2 to 6 kcal/g of weight gain). Separate evaluations of energy expenditure requirement for fat and protein deposition in premature newborns estimate that 1 g of protein deposition requires 7.8 kcal, and 1 g of fat requires 1.6 kcal.

CARBOHYDRATE REQUIREMENTS

22. **How can carbohydrate requirements be estimated in newborn infants?**
    Strict carbohydrate requirements are difficult to estimate because glucose, a preferred metabolic fuel for many organs (including the brain), is synthesized endogenously from other compounds. Several methods have been used to assess carbohydrate requirements in neonates:
    - Breast milk intake of lactose (assuming breast milk provides optimal intakes of all nutrients)
    - Constant infusion of labeled glucose to determine the rates of glucose production and oxidation (as a reflection of overall carbohydrate metabolism)
    - Altering the amount of the carbohydrate intake in the diet and determining its effect on energy metabolism and nitrogen retention

23. **The rate of endogenous glucose production in neonates has been estimated to range from 4 to 6 mg/kg/min. Do these values represent the ideal carbohydrate intake in neonates?**
    No. The rates of endogenous glucose production should be regarded as only the minimal carbohydrate requirement because of the methods and conditions in which these measurements were performed. These studies were done in neonates under basal or resting metabolic conditions and during fasting periods. In addition, these studies did not take into account the energy cost of physical activity, growth, and thermal effect of feeding. Higher values ranging from 5.8 to 6.8 mg/kg/min have been used as guidelines for the initiation of glucose infusion in neonates receiving parenteral nutrition with the ability to increase toward 13 mg/kg/min, depending on the infant.

24. **What problems can be associated with excessive carbohydrate intake?**
    Excessive intake of carbohydrate in infant feedings may lead to delayed gastric emptying, emesis, diarrhea, and abdominal distention caused by excessive gas formation as colonic bacteria digest the extra carbohydrates. The excessive administration of intravenous glucose, at rates exceeding 13.8 mg/kg/min, may be associated with metabolic complications such as hyperglycemia, glycosuria, and osmotic diuresis. In addition, the excessive glucose metabolized is stored mainly as fat. Early overfeeding may be an important factor in later childhood and adult obesity, though more recent work suggests that genetic factors may be as important.

Zhao J, Grant SF. Genetics of childhood obesity. J Obes 2011;2011:845148.

25. **Why do infant formulas contain comparable amounts of lactose and glucose polymers?**
    - Premature infants have a limited ability to digest lactose because intestinal lactase does not reach maximal activity until near term.
    - Glucose polymers are well digested and absorbed by premature infants.
    - The use of glucose polymers allows the osmolarity of the formula to remain low, even at high caloric density of 24 kcal/30 mL (<300 mOsm/L), thereby providing premature infants with adequate caloric intake and preventing such consequences as osmotic diarrhea.

26. **What is the metabolic fate of the lactose malabsorbed by the small intestine?**
    The malabsorbed lactose is fermented in the colon, forming various gases such as CO_2, methane, and hydrogen and short-chain fatty acids such as acetate, propionate, and butyrate. These short-chain fatty acids are absorbed in the colon, reducing energy losses in the stools and maintaining the nutrition and function of the colon. Despite these putative benefits of lactose fermentation, metabolic

concerns that result from the reduced digestion and absorption of lactose in the small intestine include the following:

- Decreased insulin secretion and a reduced effect on protein synthesis
- Lower adenosine triphosphate formation when lactose is fermented to acetate instead of following the glucose metabolic pathways
- Possible increased risk of necrotizing enterocolitis

PROTEIN REQUIREMENTS

27. What are the essential amino acids?

The amino acids that cannot be synthesized in the body are regarded as essential amino acids:

- Leucine
- Threonine
- Phenylalanine
- Isoleucine
- Methionine
- Tryptophan
- Valine
- Lysine
- Histidine

28. Which of the amino acids are considered conditionally essential for the preterm infant?

Cysteine, tyrosine, and taurine are essential because of immaturity of the enzymes (decreased activity) involved in their synthesis.

29. What is the whey-to-casein ratio of cow's milk and human milk protein?

The whey-to-casein ratio of cow's milk protein is 18:82 and that of human milk protein is 60:40. In total, most formulas contain up to 1.5 times more protein than human milk in order to approximate the protein quality of human milk.

Martinez JA, Ballew MP. Infant formulas. Pediatr Rev 2011;32:179–89.

30. How does the whey-to-casein ratio change during lactation?

The ratio of whey to casein is about 90:10 at the beginning of lactation and rapidly decreases to 60:40 (or even 50:50) in mature milk.

31. What is the predominant whey protein in human milk and cow's milk?

The predominant whey protein in cow's milk is beta-lactoglobulin, and the predominant whey protein in human milk is alpha-lactalbumin.

32. What are the non-nutritive roles of protein in human milk?

- Whey proteins are known to be involved in the immune response (immunoglobulins), lactose synthesis (alpha-lactalbumin), and other host defenses (lactoferrin).
- Casein phosphopeptides are believed to enhance the absorption of minerals.
- Casein fragments are thought to increase intestinal motility.
- Glycoproteins may promote the growth of certain beneficial bacteria.

33. Name the methods used for determining protein requirements.

- Factorial method (based on reference data of infant body composition)
- Balance method (protein intake = protein retention − inevitable protein losses)
- Indices of protein nutritional status (e.g., plasma albumin and transthyretin concentrations; protein intake required to maintain these indices within an acceptable range)

- Stable isotope tracer techniques (insight into the way metabolism changes with clinical state or nutritional status and thus an assessment of protein requirement)

34. **What is a lactobezoar?**
Lactobezoars are intragastric masses composed of partially digested milk curd (i.e., casein, fat, and calcium). Rarely seen now, lactobezoars were reported in LBW infants (<2000 g) fed casein-predominant formulas because casein can form large curds when exposed to gastric acid that are difficult for the LBW infant to digest. Whey protein, however, is less likely to precipitate and is emptied more rapidly from the stomach.

35. **What is the protein requirement of term and preterm infants?**
The recommended protein intake for term infants is approximately 2 to 2.5 g/kg/day; for preterm infants it is 3 to 4 g/kg/day.

36. **What factors may affect protein use in the neonate?**
- Energy intake
- Quality of protein intake
- Intake of other nutrients
- Infections and stress

37. **What is the protein content of currently available formulas?**
Term formulas:
- Milk-based formulas (e.g., Similac Advance, Enfamil LIPIL, Good Start Supreme): 2.1 to 2.8 g/100 kcal or about 1.5 to 1.8 g/100 mL
- Soy-based formulas (e.g., Similac Isomil Advance, Enfamil Prosobee LIPIL, Good Start Supreme Soy): 2.3 to 2.5 g/100 kcal or about 1.4 to 1.6 g/100 mL
  Preterm formulas (e.g., Similac Special Care, Enfamil Premature LIPIL):
- 2.5 to 2.9 g/100 cal, 1.6 to 2 g/100 mL
  Follow-up formulas for LBW weight infants (e.g., Similac NeoSure Advance, EnfaCare LIPIL):
- 2.6 to 2.8 g/100 kcal, 1.6 to 1.8 g/ 100 mL

38. **What is the rate of protein loss in premature infants who receive only 10% dextrose and water in the immediate newborn period?**
ELBW infants (<1000 g) who receive only glucose lose approximately 1.2 g/kg/day. More mature infants lose protein at a slower rate (0.9 g/kg/day at 28 weeks and 0.7 g/kg/day at 31 weeks). Any protein deficits that are accrued must be replaced.

39. **How can the protein losses be minimized?**
Early provision of protein (1 to 1.5 g/kg/day) along with minimal calories (30 cal/kg/day) can minimize the protein losses in ELBW infants. Even with good early protein administration, however, rates of intrauterine growth are virtually never achieved and some degree of extrauterine growth failure is the norm.

40. **How do protein requirements differ when protein is delivered parenterally versus enterally?**
Protein requirements are higher parenterally because preterm infants retain only 50% of amino acids administered intravenously but 70% to 75% of formula or human milk protein.

41. **What is the ideal calorie-to-protein ratio to ensure complete assimilation of protein?**
- Enteral feedings: approximately 30 cal/g of protein
- Parenteral feedings: 20 to 30 cal/g of protein (based on limited data)

LIPID REQUIREMENTS

42. What are the beneficial effects of lipid emulsions in a premature infant?
- Provision of calories (in a calorically dense form)
- Prevention of essential fatty acid deficiency

43. What is the percentage of calories provided by fat in human milk?
The percentage of fat calories in human milk is between 40% and 55%.

44. What is the source of fat in breast milk?
Most of the fat in breast milk is formed from circulating lipids derived from the mother's diet. A small amount of fat is synthesized by the breast itself, with that percentage increasing in women receiving a low-fat, high-carbohydrate diet.

45. What structural features of fatty acids improve enteral absorption?
- Shorter-chain-length to medium-chain triglycerides are absorbed more efficiently than long-chain triglycerides.
- Fatty acids with double bonds are absorbed more efficiently.

46. What are the energy contents of long-and medium-chain triglycerides?
- Long-chain triglycerides: 9 cal/g
- Medium-chain triglycerides: approximately 7.5 cal/g

47. What is the energy cost of synthesizing fat from carbohydrate?
Synthesis of fat from glucose requires about 25% of the glucose energy invested in synthesis. In comparison, synthesis of fat from fat requires only 1% to 4% of the energy invested.

48. What fatty acids are essential for fetuses and premature infants?
All humans have a requirement for linoleic and linolenic acid. These are 18-carbon, omega-6 and omega-3 fatty acids, respectively. Linoleic and linolenic acid serve as precursors for long-chain polyunsaturated fatty acids (LCPUFAs) such as arachidonic (a 20-carbon omega-6 fatty acid), eicosapentaenoic (a 20-carbon omega-3 fatty acid), and docosahexaenoic acid (a 22-carbon omega-3 fatty acid). LCPUFAs are essential components of membranes and are particularly important in membrane-rich tissues such as the brain and retina, thereby affecting visual and neurodevelopmental outcomes in children. In addition, eicosapentaenoic and arachidonic acids are precursors for prostaglandins, leukotrienes, and other lipid mediators. The fetus receives essential fatty acids (including LCPUFAs) transplacentally, and breastfed babies receive them in breast milk. Vegetable oil–based formulas do not contain LCPUFAs, and the ability of preterm infants to synthesize LCPUFAs from linoleic and linolenic acid may be limited.

49. What are the current recommendations for LCPUFA supplementation?
Currently all formulas contain the addition of LCPUFAs, particularly docohexaenoic acid (range of 0.15% to 0.32% total fatty acids) and arachidonic acid (range of 0.4% to 0.64% total fatty acids), because studies have consistently found significant benefit with such supplementation.

50. What are the side effects of LCPUFA depletion?
- Omega-6 LCPUFA: reduced growth
- Omega-3 LCPUFA: alterations in electroretinogram responses, reduced visual acuity, and possible cognitive abnormalities

51. What is the advantage of supplying calories as lipid rather than carbohydrate in infants with chronic lung disease?
The RQ of lipids is lower than that of carbohydrate. Therefore the use of lipid infusions should theoretically decrease CO_2 production in infants with bronchopulmonary dysplasia, one of the cardinal problems of infants with chronic lung disease in the neonatal period.

52. **What is the advantage of using a 20% lipid emulsion versus a 10% lipid emulsion in newborn infants?**
Twenty-percent lipid emulsions are cleared from the circulation more rapidly than 10% emulsions. Ten-percent lipid emulsions contain proportionately more emulsifier (egg yolk phospholipid). In 10% emulsions the phospholipid-to-triglyceride ratio is 0.12, and in 20% emulsions the ratio is 0.06. The excess phospholipid forms bilayer vesicles that extract free cholesterol from peripheral cell membranes to form lipoprotein X. Lipoprotein X is cleared very slowly from the circulation (half-life, 2 days).

53. **What is the maximum acceptable triglyceride level in infants receiving lipid emulsions, and how often should they be checked?**
The maximum level is 150 mg/dL. Routine monitoring of serum triglycerides is necessary as they are being advanced.

TOTAL PARENTERAL NUTRITION: MONITORING AND COMPLICATIONS

54. **What is the usual distribution of nutrients in total parenteral nutrition (TPN) solutions used for neonates?**
TPN is written with a calorie distribution of 8% to 10% from amino acids, 30% to 40% from lipid emulsions, and 50% to 60% from dextrose.

55. **What are the metabolic advantages of using different regimens containing high carbohydrate (67%) and low fat (5%) or low carbohydrate (34%) and high fat (58%)?**
There are none. The administration of TPN solutions containing a moderate carbohydrate (60%) to fat (32%) ratio has been shown to result in a higher nitrogen retention rate than that of the unbalanced regimens.

Nose O, Tipton JR, Ament ME, et al. Effect of energy source on changes in energy expenditure, respiratory quotient and nitrogen balance during total parenteral nutrition in children. Pediatr Res 1987;21:538–41.

56. **Hyperglycemia is a common complication observed in ELBW infants receiving parenteral nutrition. Should insulin infusions be provided routinely to these infants?**
In most infants hyperglycemia is a transient problem and resolves when the rate of glucose or lipid administration is reduced. Insulin infusions have been used for infants weighing less than 1000 g who develop hyperglycemia (serum glucose level in excess of 150 mg/dL) and glycosuria during the course of parenteral nutrition, providing low glucose infusion rates (<12 mg/kg/min). In these infants insulin infusions at rates of 0.04 to 0.1 U/kg/h have been shown to improve glucose tolerance and promote weight gain, compared with infants in a control group.

Sinclair JC, Bottino M, Cowett RM. Interventions for prevention of neonatal hyperglycemia in very low birth weight infants. Cochrane Database Syst Rev. 2011 Oct 5;10:CD007615.
    Bottino M, Cowett RM, Sinclair JC. Interventions for treatment of neonatal hyperglycemia in very low birth weight infants. Cochrane Database Syst Rev. 2011 Oct 5;10:CD007453 [Review].

57. **The clearance of intravenous fat emulsions in neonates is improved by all the following measures except for which of the following? (A) Increasing the period of infusion from 8 to 24 hours; (B) adding a low dose of heparin to the TPN solutions (1 U/mL); (C) exposing the fat emulsions to ambient light or to phototherapy lights; (D) using 20% instead of 10% lipid emulsions.**
The answer is (C). Exposure of lipid emulsions to ambient or phototherapy lights increases the formation of triglyceride hydroperoxide radicals but does not enhance lipid clearance. Lipid clearance in neonates is improved by prolonging the infusion period; by adding heparin to TPN solutions (which

releases lipoprotein lipase from capillary endothelial cells); and by using 20% lipid emulsions, which contain a lower phospholipid content than 10% lipid emulsions.

58. **Why do premature infants who receive prolonged courses of parenteral nutrition develop osteopenia resulting in pathologic bone fractures?**

The development of osteopenia during the course of TPN in premature infants is believed to result from the inability to provide the calcium and phosphorus required for proper bone mineralization. The solubility of calcium and phosphorus in TPN solutions can be improved by providing a high amino acid intake and by the supplementation of cysteine hydrochloride. These measures allow for a greater, though still inadequate, intake of calcium and phosphorus. The administration of calciuric diuretics such as furosemide, the use of postnatal steroids, and the development of cholestatic liver disease further aggravate calcium homeostasis in these patients. The intravenous administration of vitamin D does not prevent the occurrence of TPN-induced osteopenia.

59. **Which of the trace elements in TPN solutions can be potentially toxic for patients with cholestatic liver disease?**

Copper and manganese are potentially toxic for these patients. Both of these trace elements are metabolized in the liver and primarily excreted in bile. Therefore the chronic administration of trace elements in patients with cholestasis may result in toxic states. Manganese and copper supplements should be withheld from TPN solutions when hepatic cholestasis is present. Monitoring of serum levels of copper and manganese is indicated in patients with cholestasis who require a prolonged course of TPN.

60. **What is the most common complication of TPN administered by peripheral vein catheters?**

The most common complication is the accidental infiltration of TPN solution into the subcutaneous fat tissue that results in skin necrosis. This complication can be minimized by lowering the osmolality of TPN solution through the administration of dextrose concentrations that do not exceed 10% and by the concomitant administration of lipid emulsions.

61. **What is the most common cause of bacterial infection in neonates receiving TPN by central vein catheter?**

Staphylococcus epidermidis remains the most common cause of bacterial sepsis during the course of TPN. Other organisms include *Staphylococcus aureus, Escherichia coli, Pseudomonas* species, *Klebsiella* species, and *Candida albicans.* TPN-related infections are more common in the smallest and sickest infants who receive prolonged courses of TPN through a central catheter. The rate of these infections can be reduced by aseptic preparation of TPN solutions and by avoiding the use of the TPN catheter for blood transfusions, administration of medications, and blood sampling. Most important, TPN should be discontinued (and central lines removed) when "full" enteral volume feedings have been achieved (approximately 100 mL/kg/day).

In recent years many NICUs have demonstrated that the rates of catheter-related infections can be substantially reduced through careful aseptic technique and thoughtful, conscientious management of indwelling lines. A number of NICUs have been able to go beyond 1 year without a single catheter-related infection. It is evident that this complication is far more preventable than was once thought possible.

ENTERAL NUTRITION

62. **What is the carbohydrate source in human milk and in term and preterm formulas?**

Lactose is the major source of carbohydrate in human milk and in formulas for term infants. The preterm formulas contain a mixture of lactose and glucose polymers to compensate for the developmental lag and lower concentration of lactase in the intestinal mucosa. Lactose, however, remains important both in calcium absorption and as a prebiotic. Glycosidase enzymes involved in the digestion of glucose polymers are active in preterm infants.

63. **Why is the fat absorption of preterm infants lower than that of term infants?**
The lower fat absorption reported in preterm infants is attributed to their relative deficiency of pancreatic lipase and bile salts.

64. **Why is the fat of human milk well absorbed by preterm infants?**
The human milk triglyceride molecule has palmitic acid in the beta position and is more easily absorbed compared with triglyceride molecules of cow's milk, vegetable fats, and animal fats that have palmitic acid in the alpha position. The presence of human milk lipase also improves fat absorption.

65. **When should soy protein–based formulas be used for feeding infants?**
Soy formulas are recommended for the following:
   ▪ Infants with congenital lactase deficiency and galactosemia (soy formulas are lactose free)
   ▪ Infants with an immunoglobulin E–mediated allergy to cow's milk protein (8% to 14% of these infants will also react to soy)
   ▪ Infants of parents requesting a vegetarian-based diet

66. **What essential amino acid is added to soy-based infant formulas?**
Because soy protein has low concentrations of methionine, this amino acid is added to all soy-based formulas.

67. **When can preterm infants successfully use the nipple to feed?**
The success of feeding a preterm infant by nipple depends on the ability of the infant to coordinate sucking and swallowing, which develops at approximately 33 to 34 weeks of gestational age.

68. **Why may transpyloric feedings result in fat malabsorption?**
Transpyloric feedings may result in fat malabsorption as a result of bypassing the lipolytic effect of gastric lipase.

69. **Why are early minimal enteral feedings recommended for preterm infants receiving parenteral nutrition?**
Gastrointestinal hormones such as gastrin, enteroglucagon, and pancreatic polypeptide may have a trophic effect on the gut. Postnatal surges of these hormones occur in preterm infants receiving minimal enteral feedings. Minimal enteral feeding has also been reported to produce more mature small intestinal motor activity patterns in preterm infants. Thus early minimal enteral feedings given along with parenteral nutrition may improve subsequent enteral feeding tolerance and may shorten the time to achieve full enteral intake. Furthermore, enteral feedings stimulate the enterohepatic circulation and are known to lessen parenteral nutrition–associated liver disease. The most recent Cochrane Review, however, suggests that the evidence for this effect is unclear, at best.

Bombell S, McGuire W. Early trophic feeding for very low birth weight infants. Cochrane Database Syst Rev 2009;3:CD000504.

70. **What are the reported advantages of feeding human milk to preterm infants over the commercially available infant formulas?**
   ▪ A lower incidence of necrotizing enterocolitis in preterm infants fed human milk
   ▪ Faster gastric emptying in preterm infants fed human milk compared with those fed bovine milk–derived formulas
   ▪ Improved long-term cognitive development, which has been correlated with human milk feedings in preterm infants

71. **Does human milk completely meet the nutritional requirements of VLBW preterm infants (birth weight below 1500 g)?**
Growth rates of preterm infants fed banked human milk or their own mother's milk are lower than those of infants fed preterm formulas. In addition, the calcium and phosphorus content of human milk is insufficient to fully support adequate skeletal mineralization. Supplementation of human milk with available human milk fortifiers that provide protein, calcium, phosphorus, sodium, zinc, and up to 23 vitamins helps overcome these nutritional inadequacies. Newly designed preparations of pooled human breast milk (Prolacta) do contain adequate calories and minerals for growth.

BREASTFEEDING

72. **What are the determinants of milk volume (milk production)?**
Initially, hormonal factors (prolactin and oxytocin) affect the synthesis and secretion of milk. Once mother's milk "comes in," tight junctions close, and lactation shifts from endocrine control to autocrine control, or control driven by milk removal. The frequency of breastfeeding then becomes the most important factor affecting the continuation of adequate milk production. The term infant should receive between 8 and 12 feedings per day in the first week and more than 5 daily thereafter. To minimize the volume of residual milk, mothers should alternate the breast they start with at the next feeding. When breastfeeding is first initiated, mothers should switch the infant from one side to the other approximately every 5 to 10 minutes. Maternal diet and fluid intake rarely affect milk volume; however, in the setting of severe malnutrition there may be diminished milk production.

73. **How can milk production be increased?**
There are no magic potions or medications that increase milk production, though increasing maternal fluid intake may be of modest help. The administration of metoclopramide will occasionally increase serum prolactin and increase milk production. Unfortunately, this medication has side effects, including sedation and extrapyramidal neurologic signs. Oxytocin will not increase milk production, but it may help milk ejection (once milk already has been synthesized). Herbal remedies have been advocated, but no data are available that determine their efficacy or associated risks. Fatigue and stress also affect milk production adversely. A small percentage of women (2% to 5%) have lactation insufficiency and cannot produce adequate quantities of milk.

74. **What are the contraindications for breastfeeding?**
   - Galactosemia
   - Use of controlled substances such as cocaine, narcotics, and stimulants.
   - Miliary tuberculosis: Breastfeeding should not take place until adequate therapy has been received for approximately 2 weeks.
   - Human immunodeficiency virus (HIV): This contraindication has far-reaching global concerns. In the United States women who test positive for HIV should not breastfeed. The risk-to-benefit ratio must be determined for particular populations outside the United States. Efforts are under way to determine the risk-to-benefit ratio and cost-to-benefit ratio for the use of antiretroviral therapy along with breastfeeding or the use of infant formula in high-risk populations.

   Only a few medications are incompatible with breastfeeding, although most medications do enter breast milk in low concentrations. The following are some of the contraindicated drugs:
   - Bromocriptine (suppresses lactation)
   - Amiodarone
   - Ergotamine
   - Thiouracils
   - Chemotherapeutic agents
   - Metronidazole
   - Radiopharmaceuticals
   - Klonapin

- Phenindione
- Salts containing bromide and gold
- Amantadine

75. **Does energy expenditure differ between breastfed and formula-fed infants?**

In studies of AGA gavage-fed infants, there was significantly lower energy expenditure in the infants fed human milk compared with those fed formula.

Lubetzky R, Vaisman N, Mimouni F, et al. Energy expenditure in human milk– versus formula-fed preterm infants. J Pediatr 2003;143:750–3.

76. **A mother has breastfed her 5-week-old infant exclusively. She now calls with the concern that she has recently noticed a burning pain in her nipple during breastfeeding. You examine the mother and note some erythema of her areola. You diagnose a fissure and advise her to use dry heat and a few drops of milk on her areola after breastfeeding. She calls back in a few days to report that the pain is increasing. What other diagnosis should you consider?**

This is not an uncommon presentation for a Candida infection of the nipple. You should examine the infant for evidence of perioral thrush. If thrush is evident, the baby should be treated with an oral medication and the mother with an antifungal.

77. **A mother calls you and explains that she is worried because her 4-day-old baby is not receiving enough breast milk. How do you assess whether a newborn is receiving sufficient amounts of breast milk during the first week after birth?**

Understand why the mother is concerned. Some of the following factors should influence your decision either to see the mother and baby or to reassure the mother over the phone: frequency of feeding (8 to 12 times in 24 hours, no interval longer than 4 hours), urine output (light yellow–stained diapers), and stool output (no more meconium stools after day 3). Some practitioners use the following rough guide for urine and stool output in the first week: minimum of one urine output in the first 24 hours, two to three in the next 24 hours, about four to six on day 3, and six to eight on day 5; stools should be one per day on days 1 and 2, two per day on day 3, and four or more afterward, although this can vary substantially among infants. The mother should sense that her milk has "come in" between the second and fourth days postpartum. The baby should have established feeding activities, such as lip smacking and rooting. You should hear swallows, and the baby should be satisfied after a feeding. Feeding activities, however, vary widely. Some adequately hydrated infants are sleepy and need coaching with feedings. If a mother experiences leaking from one breast while the child is nursing at the other, her milk supply is usually quite adequate. Weighing an infant before and after feeding can provide an accurate assessment of milk intake. The technique requires an electronic scale and strict attention to details such as not unwrapping the infant or changing diapers before the reweighing is done.

78. **You see a 5-day-old male infant in the office for a routine check after early hospital discharge. The mother reports no particular problems; he is much easier to manage than she thought a newborn would be. She is breastfeeding every 3 hours but lets him sleep at night (last night he slept for 6 hours). About once a day she notes that he has dark yellow urine in his diaper. He had a dark-green, tarry stool yesterday. The mother thinks her milk has "come in," but she acknowledges no signs of engorgement. You examine the infant and note jaundice to the level of the umbilicus and dry skin but moist mucous membranes. He is responsive and alert. You examine the mother and note that her breasts are moderately engorged. The infant's body weight is 11 ounces below his birth weight of 7 pounds, 8 ounces. You check his serum bilirubin**

concentration, which is 11 mg/dL. There is no blood group incompatibility. How would you manage this case, and what would you advise the mother?

You should observe a breastfeeding to ensure that the baby has a good latch-on to the breast and is able to suck and swallow. You advise the mother to breastfeed every 2 hours. You do not advise water supplements because the baby needs calories. His bilirubin level should decline with this strategy. If the mother had not been making milk, you might suggest that she mechanically express her milk after every feeding to increase stimulation. You must schedule a return visit in 24 hours to reassess the Infant.

79. **What is the most variable nutrient in human milk?**
Fat is the most variable content of all nutrients in human milk. The fat content rises slightly during lactation, increases from the beginning (foremilk) to the end (hindmilk) of the feeding, varies among women (probably a direct effect of body fat stores), and varies over the course of the day. If the mother does not completely empty her breast after feeding, the baby will not receive all the calories (fat). Mothers using mechanical methods to express their milk may not completely empty the breast.

80. **Breastfeeding a premature infant can be a challenge. How do you advance from tube-feeding to breastfeeding in a premature infant?**
Note the sucking and swallowing ability of the infant. Parental skills, infant feeding cues, and timing of feedings should also be considered. Begin one breastfeeding in place of a tube feeding or in addition to the tube feeding. If the latch-on is good and clinical signs of sucking, swallowing, and some drooling of milk are noted, then continue the process each day. Withdrawing milk from an indwelling feeding tube to assess milk intake from breastfeeding will not yield accurate results because gastric emptying from the stomach occurs rapidly after a human milk feeding. Furthermore, clinical signs of feeding activity and maternal assessment of breast emptying are inexact measures of milk intake and may not reflect small amounts consumed. Weighing the infant before and after breastfeeding is the most accurate way to assess milk intake.

Funkquist EL, Tuvemo T, Jonsson B, et al. Influence of test weighing before/after nursing on breastfeeding in preterm infants. Adv Neonatal Care 2010;10(1):33–9.

81. **Do mothers benefit from breastfeeding?**
Postpartum weight loss and uterine involution may be more rapid with breastfeeding. The postpartum amenorrhea during lactation is an acknowledged method of child spacing, especially for 4 to 6 months. This technique is most reliable if breastfeeding is practiced around the clock. Several reports now suggest that women who breastfed their infants had a decreased incidence of premenopausal breast cancer and ovarian cancer. Women who breastfed their infants also may have a decreased incidence of osteoporosis.

Labbok MH: Health sequelae of breastfeeding for the mother. Clin Perinatol 1999;26:491–503.

VITAMINS AND TRACE NUTRIENTS

82. **A 2-month-old preterm infant (with an estimated gestational age of 26 weeks) develops osteopenia of prematurity and fractures of both humeri. The infant is receiving 400 units of vitamin D daily. Should the dose of vitamin D be increased?**
No. Contrary to an earlier theory, osteopenia of prematurity results primarily from inadequate intake of mineral substrate (calcium and phosphorus) and not vitamin D. High doses of vitamin D do not appear to aid in the prevention or treatment of osteopenia of prematurity. Infants born prematurely are at risk for developing osteopenia because of limited accretion of bone mass *in utero* (fetal accretion rates for calcium and phosphorous range from 92 to 119 mg/kg/day and 59 to 74 mg/kg/day, respectively). Preterm infants often cannot receive the ideal amount of calcium by way of parenteral

nutrition and thus do not receive the daily goal of calcium until full enteral feedings are established. Diuretics, steroids, and physical inactivity have a negative effect on bone mineralization. To mimic fetal accretion, an enteral intake of 120 to 230 mg/kg/day of calcium and 60 to 140 mg/kg/day of phosphorus is recommended for preterm infants. This amount is provided by 150 cc/kg/day of premature infant formula or fortified breast milk.

83. **A 6-week-old infant is recovering from necrotizing enterocolitis that necessitated resection of two thirds of the jejunum and placement of an ileostomy. When enteral feedings are restarted, the drainage from the ileostomy becomes excessive. The infant is growing poorly (despite an adequate caloric intake) and develops vesiculobullous and eczematous lesions around the eyes, mouth, and genitals. What mineral deficiency should be considered?**
Infants with abnormal gastrointestinal losses (persistent diarrhea, excessive ileostomy drainage) may be at risk for zinc deficiency because fecal loss is the major excretory route. Signs of zinc deficiency include poor wound healing, poor linear growth, decreased appetite, hair loss, depressed immune function, and skin lesions that commonly mimic a diaper rash but are also perioral in location.

84. **What are the causes of zinc deficiency in LBW infants?**
   - Poor zinc stores
   - Increased requirement for growth
   - Prolonged intravenous nutrition containing inadequate zinc
   - Abnormally low zinc content of mother's milk
   - Supplements of iron or copper that compete with zinc for absorption

Adapted from Atkinson SA, Zlotkin S. Recognizing deficiencies and excesses of zinc, copper, and other trace elements. In: Tsang RC, Zlotkin SH, Nichols BL, Hansen JW, editors. Nutrition during infancy. 2nd ed. Cincinnati: Digital Educational Publishing; 1997.
   Shah MD, Shah SR. Nutrient deficiencies in the premature infant. Pediatr Clin North Am 2009;56(5):1069–83.

85. **The requirements for what nutrient are increased under phototherapy?**
Riboflavin is a photosensitive vitamin, and requirements may be increased in infants receiving phototherapy.

86. **Is fluoride an essential nutrient for a newborn infant?**
Although fluoride has been considered "beneficial for humans," whether it is essential remains unknown. Fluoride supplementation is not recommended from birth because of questions concerning whether the benefit of fluoride warrants the risk of dental fluorosis. Commercial infant formulas do not contain fluoride.

✓ KEY POINTS: GROWTH AND NUTRITION

1. The parents of IUGR infants should be aware that significant catch-up growth will occur in the first year of life but that ultimate stature may be less than that of an AGA infant.

2. Lactose malabsorption is extremely uncommon in infants unless they have had a significant insult to the intestinal mucosa (e.g., infection, short gut syndrome) or have the very rare disorder of congenital lactase deficiency.

3. The infant with an ostomy should be carefully monitored for excessive sodium losses and zinc deficiency, both of which can impair growth.

4. A critical nutritional goal for the infant with short gut syndrome is to advance enteral feeds as clinically tolerated to enable intestinal adaptation and ultimate discontinuation of TPN.

TABLE 10-3. WATER-SOLUBLE VITAMINS IN MATURE HUMAN MILK

Adapted from Schanler RJ. Who needs water soluble vitamins? In: Tsang RC, Zlotkin SH, Nichols BL, Hansen JW, editors. Nutrition during infancy. 2nd ed. Cincinnati: Digital Educational Publishing; 1997.

	HUMAN MILK (RANGE)	AAP, CON* (UNITS/100 kcal)
Thiamin (μg)	31 (21-26)	40
Riboflavin (μg)	56 (42-85)	60
Niacin (mg)	0.29 (0.27-0.34)	0.25 (0.8)
Vitamin B_6 (μg)	20 (15-30)	35
Pantothenic acid (mg)	0.6 (0.3-1.0)	0.3
Biotin (μg)	0.7 (0.6-1.1)	1.5
Folate (μg)	7 (6-12)	4
Vitamin B_{12} (μg)	0.10 (0.07-0.16)	0.15
Vitamin C (mg)	8 (5-13)	8

*Committee on Nutrition of the American Academy of Pediatrics.

87. **What is the scientific rationale for administering vitamin A to prevent bronchopulmonary dysplasia?**
    - Lung differentiation is regulated in part by vitamin A.
    - Vitamin A deficiency causes replacement of mucus-secreting epithelium by stratified squamous keratinizing epithelium in the trachea and bronchi.
    - Bronchopulmonary dysplasia has been associated with vitamin A deficiency in VLBW preterm infants.
    - Premature birth deprives the newborn infant of the supply of retinol (vitamin A).
    - The histopathology of bronchopulmonary dysplasia includes findings commonly seen with vitamin A deficiency (e.g., loss of ciliated cells and keratinizing metaplasia).

88. **What are the concentrations of water-soluble vitamins in mature human milk, and how do they compare with the recommended dietary allowances for healthy term infants?**
    See Table 10-3.

IRON REQUIREMENTS

89. **How long can iron stores meet the needs of term, LBW, and preterm infants before supplementation is necessary?**
    The quantity of iron stored is proportional to the birth weight of the infant. On average, the iron stores in a term infant can meet the infant's iron requirement until 4 to 6 months of age and that of LBW and preterm infants until 2 to 3 months of age. Transfused infants, however, likely have greater iron stores.

90. **What are the daily dietary iron requirements for term, LBW, and preterm infants?**
    The estimated daily requirement is 1 mg/kg/day for term infants and 2 to 4 mg/kg/day for LBW and preterm infants.

91. **Do breastfed infants require iron supplementation?**
    Although the bioavailability of iron in breast milk is high (because of the presence of lactoferrin, which enhances iron absorption), the content is relatively low. Additional sources of iron are recommended for breastfed infants after 4 to 6 months of age.

92. **What is the iron content of hemoglobin?**
Each gram of hemoglobin contains 3.4 mg of iron.

93. **Where is iron absorbed, and what factors can influence iron absorption?**
Dietary iron is absorbed in the duodenum and the proximal jejunum. Absorption is influenced by the body's demand and also by the dietary source. The majority of the dietary iron (in plant foods and fortified food products) is nonheme iron. Ascorbic acid enhances the absorption of nonheme iron, whereas calcium, phytates, manganese, and polyphenols decrease it.

94. **Do premature infants need more or less iron than term infants?**
Overall, premature infants need more iron than term infants during their first postnatal year. The reason for this increased need stems from two factors. First, iron is accreted primarily during the last trimester. The fetus maintains a fairly steady level (75 mg of elemental iron per kilogram of body weight) during this period. At 24 weeks' gestation the fetus has 37.5 mg of total body iron, whereas at term the newborn has 225 mg. Therefore premature birth results in significantly reduced total body iron. Second, premature infants exhibit a more rapid rate of growth per kilogram of body weight than the term infant. Iron intake must increase to support the increase in hemoglobin mass. Whereas the term newborn needs approximately 1 mg/kg of iron per day, the preterm infant needs between 2 and 4 mg/kg/day. The more premature the infant, the greater the need.

95. **What groups of term neonates are at increased risk of low iron stores at birth?**
Growth-retarded infants and infants of diabetic mothers are at risk for reduced iron stores. Approximately 50% of IUGR infants and 65% of infants of diabetics have cord serum ferritin concentrations below the fifth percentile (60 ng/L). In growth-restricted infants the etiology is probably related to impaired placental transport of nutrients. The pathophysiology of low iron stores in infants of diabetic mothers is more complex. Chronic maternal hyperglycemia results in chronic fetal hyperglycemia and hyperinsulinemia, both of which increase the oxygen consumption of the fetus by approximately 30%. Chronic fetal hypoxia leads to increased erythropoietin secretion and secondary polycythemia, which in turn requires increased iron delivery. Each extra gram of hemoglobin synthesized by the fetus requires an additional 3.49 mg of elemental iron delivered by the placenta. The human placenta is not capable of upregulating placental transport to that extent, leaving the fetus of a diabetic mother dependent on its accreted iron stores to support its expanding fetal blood volume. The result is that iron is redistributed away from storage and nonstorage tissues and into the red cell mass. It does not appear that either group needs additional dietary iron postnatally, supporting the principle that the neonatal intestine avidly absorbs iron.

Verner AM, Manderson J, Lappin TR, et al. Influence of maternal diabetes mellitus on fetal iron status. Arch Dis Child Fetal Neonatal Ed. 2007;92(5):F399–401.

Siddappa AM, Rao R, Long JD, et al. The assessment of newborn iron stores at birth: a review of the literature and standards for ferritin concentrations. Neonatology. 2007;92(2):73–82.

96. **What is the effect of recombinant human erythropoietin (rhEPO) on the iron needs of the premature infant?**
Erythropoietin increases the need for iron by up to threefold to 6 mg/kg/day. A recent study suggested that once weekly dosing at 1200 units/Kg/dose was adequate to maintain hematocrit levels in premature neonates. Studies of erythropoietin given to sheep with varying degrees of iron sufficiency demonstrated that the degree of hemoglobin response is directly related to the iron sufficiency of the animal. In addition, some recent evidence suggests that EPO may have neuroprotective effects, including reduction of risk of retinopathy of prematurity.

Ohls RK, Roohi M, Peceny HM, et al. A randomized, masked study of weekly erythropoietin dosing in preterm infants. J Pediatr 2012;160(5):790–5.

Romagnoli C, Tesfagabir MG, Giannantonio C, et al. Erythropoietin and retinopathy of prematurity. Early Hum Dev 2011;87(Suppl 1):S39–42.

97. True or false: premature infants are iron overloaded at hospital discharge.
This is a trick question. In fact, preterm infants could be iron deficient, iron neutral, or iron overloaded. Preterm AGA infants start with approximately 75 mg of iron per kilogram of body weight. This amount of iron is considered sufficient for the neonatal period, and iron supplementation probably should not begin until the preterm infant is at least 2 weeks of age. Preterm infants are born with very immature antioxidant systems, and there is a concern that large doses of iron could overwhelm the system and lead to disease related to oxidant stress (e.g., retinopathy of prematurity, bronchopulmonary dysplasia). On the other hand, the rapid growth rate of preterm infants results in a rapid expansion of the blood volume, and iron is required to support this growth. Those who are born at low gestational ages, who have a benign neonatal course, and who are fed a low-iron diet (e.g., breast milk without iron supplementation) are at high risk of using up all the available stores soon after discharge. These infants should have their iron and hemoglobin status checked earlier than the usual 9 months of age recommended for term infants. In contrast, a sick preterm infant who requires multiple transfusions to maintain cardiovascular stability may be at high risk for iron overload. Preterm infants can have ferritin concentrations of 500 ng/dL at discharge, suggesting significant iron loading of the liver.

98. Does placental iron transport depend on maternal iron status, fetal iron status, or both?
Both. Early studies clearly establish a relationship between maternal iron stores, as indexed by the mother's ferritin concentration and the infant's cord serum ferritin concentration. This relationship appears to be particularly strong when the mother is suffering from profound iron deficiency. However, lesser degrees of iron deficiency do not seem to influence fetal iron status. In fact, the fetus manages to maintain iron sufficiency in the face of maternal iron deficiency. Conversely, certain fetuses can become iron deficient in spite of maternal iron sufficiency. This occurs when placental iron transport is disturbed by uteroplacental vascular insufficiency (resulting in IUGR) and when fetal iron demand exceeds placental iron transport ability. The latter occurs in pregnancies complicated by diabetes mellitus and chronic fetal hypoxia with augmented secondary fetal erythropoiesis.

99. How can the fetus increase placental transport of iron?
In pregnancies complicated by fetal iron deficiency, as indexed by a low cord serum ferritin concentration or decreased placental iron content, the expression of iron transport proteins such as the transferrin receptor is increased on the apical (maternal-facing) membrane of the syncytiotrophoblast. Studies have shown that this upregulation is most likely in response to the iron status of the syncytiotrophoblast. This upregulation is achieved by intracellular iron regulatory proteins that bind transferrin receptor mRNA, stabilizing it to produce more copies of the receptor and leading to greater iron transport. Thus the fetus appears to regulate its own iron accretion. A similar system has been described for the transport of certain amino acids by the placenta.

Georgieff MK, Berry SA, Wobken JA, et al. Increased placental iron regulatory protein-1 expression in diabetic pregnancies complicated by fetal iron deficiency. Placenta 1999;20:87–93.
    Petry CD, Wobken JD, McKay H, et al. Placental transferrin receptor in diabetic pregnancies with increased fetal iron demand. Am J Physiol 1994;267:E507–E514.

GASTROESOPHAGEAL REFLUX

100. How common is gastroesophageal reflux (GER)?
Gastroesophageal reflux is seen in up to 50% of infants with recurrent emesis.

101. What is the course of GER in a healthy infant?
During infancy GER is very common because of the immaturity of the lower esophageal sphincter. Recurrent vomiting is the most common manifestation of reflux in this age group and is usually effortless. It is clinically evident in 50% of infants in the first 3 months of life. Only 5% to 10% of

children have reflux at the age of 1 year. There is gradual resolution of vomiting by the age of 1 to 2 years. If regurgitation has not resolved by 24 months of age, further evaluation is recommended.

102. What does the term "happy spitter" signify?
These infants have uncomplicated GER. They have no concerning signs or symptoms and have effortless, painless vomiting. Weight gain is normal, and the children develop normally. Reassurance, education, and anticipatory guidance are generally the only interventions required.

103. What are the red flags of GER disease (GERD) in infants?
- Bilious or forceful vomiting
- Hematemesis
- Failure to thrive

Any of these findings should suggest severe GERD, or an alternative diagnosis to GERD should be sought.

104. What is the differential diagnosis for GERD in infants and children?
A key point is differentiating GERD from the causes of recurrent or persistent vomiting:
- Gastrointestinal obstruction
- Pyloric stenosis
- Malrotation with intermittent volvulus (Fig. 10-3)
- Intermittent intussusception
- Intestinal duplication
- Hirschsprung disease
- Antroduodenal web
- Incarcerated hernia
- Gastrointestinal disorders
- Gastroparesis
- Gastroenteritis
- Eosinophilic esophagitis or gastroenteritis
- Food allergy or intolerance
- Achalasia
- Peptic ulcer disease
- Neurologic problems: Increased intracranial pressure

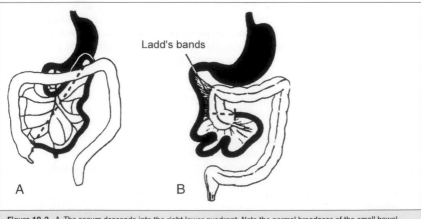

Figure 10-3. **A,** The cecum descends into the right lower quadrant. Note the normal broadness of the small bowel mesentery *(dashed line).* **B,** In malrotation the duodenal loop lacks 90 degrees of its normal 270-degree rotation such that the duodenojejunal flexure does not cross midline, and the cecocolic loop lacks 180 degrees of its normal rotation.

- Infectious disorders
- Sepsis
- Meningitis
- Urinary tract infection
- Hepatitis
- Pneumonia
- Metabolic/endocrine disorders
- Galactosemia
- Urea cycle defects
- Hereditary fructose intolerance
- Amino and organic acidemias
- Congenital adrenal hyperplasia
- Maple syrup urine disease
- Renal disorders
- Obstructive uropathy
- Renal insufficiency
- Environmental causes
- Ingestion of or exposure to toxins
- Munchausen syndrome by proxy
- Cardiac disorder: congestive heart failure

105. What diagnostic tests are available to evaluate GER?
See Table 10-4.

106. What are nonmedical treatment options for GER?
- Smaller-volume feeds given more frequently
- Thickened formula
- Avoidance of seated or supine positions after feeding
- Elevation of the head of the crib
- Elimination of second-hand smoke (which causes relaxation of the lower esophageal sphincter)
- Trial of cow's milk protein–free formula

Infants with GER may be placed in an upright position for at least 30 minutes after meals, and the head of the crib may be elevated to 30 to 45 degrees. Placing the child in a car seat in the home is not recommended. Thickening of the formula with rice cereal or commercial thickening agents may help decrease the amount of regurgitation and lessen irritability. The recommended starting amount is 1 teaspoon per ounce of formula; this may be increased to 1 tablespoon per ounce as needed. Modification of the feeding schedule to offer smaller feeds at more frequent intervals can help decrease gastric distention and regurgitation of less frequent larger feeds.

107. What are the medical treatments for GER?
Pharmacologic:
- Antacids
- Prokinetic agents (e.g., metoclopramide, bethanechol, erythromycin)
- H_2-receptor antagonists (e.g., ranitidine, cimetidine, famotidine, nizatidine)
- Proton-pump inhibitors (e.g., omeprazole, lansoprazole, esomeprazole, pantoprazole, rabeprazole)
- Surface agents (sucralfate gel)
Surgical:
- Transpyloric feeding tubes
- Fundoplication
- Pyloroplasty

TABLE 10-4.	DIAGNOSTIC TESTS FOR THE EVALUATION OF GASTROESOPHAGEAL REFLUX	
TEST	**ADVANTAGES**	**DISADVANTAGES**
Upper gastrointestinal tract series (UGIS)	Evaluates for structural abdnormalities	Short duration (<1 h) that may miss a reflux episode Manipulation during study can produce a reflux event in an otherwise healthy infant Low sensitivity and specificity for GER
Gastroesophageal scintigraphy	Evaluates for gastric emptying time, reflux, and aspiration in lungs Longer study period than UGIS (1 to 2 h) to better assess frequency and degree of aspiration	Study limited to time period of feeding bolus May underestimate frequency of daily events if volume or composition of feed is altered for the study Lacks standardized technique and age-specific normative data.
24-hour pH probe monitoring	Evaluates pH changes over extended period of time, ideally 24 h, to better assess frequency of reflux Can correlate with symptom scales No activity restriction during testing	Must be on bolus feeds and off acid suppression medications for 72 h for an accurate study Invasive Does not evaluate for alkaline reflux
Impedance probe	Evaluates for pH changes as well as impedance Extended study, ideally 24 h, as with pH probe Can detect non–acid reflux episodes Can correlate with symptom scales No activity restriction during testing	Must be on bolus feeds and off acid suppression medications for 72 h for an accurate study. Invasive
Esophago-gastroduodenoscopy	Evaluates gross and histologic mucosal changes of the esophagus, stomach, and duodenum	Most invasive test; often requires anesthesia
GER, Gastroesophageal reflux.		

EOSINOPHILIC GASTROINTESTINAL DISORDERS

108. What are eosinophilic enteropathies?

Eosinophilic enteropathies are eosinophilic inflammatory conditions that can be present throughout the entire gastrointestinal tract. The inflammatory process is characterized by the selective infiltration of large numbers of eosinophils into the bowel mucosa, smooth muscle, or both. The initial trigger for this process is unknown, but antigens in food are believed to contribute to ongoing disease.

109. What is the differential diagnosis for eosinophils in the gastrointestinal lining in newborns?

The differential diagnosis includes idiopathic eosinophilic gastroenteritis, formula protein intolerance, GERD, and normal variation.

110. How does this process present in neonates?

This disease process can present as failure to thrive, diarrhea, malabsorption, regurgitation and irritability (identical to GER), and colitis. In neonates the protein found in cow's milk or soy protein may be the offending antigen for the inflammatory process. When this occurs, the process is called dietary protein–induced colitis, milk protein colitis, enteritis, and so forth. A common presentation is an infant who has a history of irritability, diarrhea with mucus and blood, poor weight gain or failure to thrive, and some degree of anemia. It is the most common cause of bloody stools in the first year of life. The second common presentation in neonates is that of reflux that does not respond to therapeutic management. In this clinical picture the neonate has symptoms of GER and irritability that do not improve as expected despite appropriate medical and nonmedical therapeutic interventions.

111. What is the prognosis of eosinophilic colitis in the neonate?

Eosinophilic colitis in infants has a very good prognosis. The vast majority of patients are able to tolerate milk protein by the age of 1 to 3 years. Some studies associate eosinophilic colitis with the later development of inflammatory bowel disease, but this association is under debate.

112. What treatment options are available?

Multiple medications have been tried and used depending on the location of the involved portion of the gastrointestinal tract. These medications, which mostly work by attempting to modify the immune response, include systemic steroids, protein pump inhibitors, histamine receptor-2 blockers, topical steroids, antacids, cromolyn, leukotriene antagonists, sucralfate, and prokinetics if there is secondary dysmotility. Elimination from the diet of the offending milk or soy protein allergen is accomplished in neonates by changing to a protein-hydrolyzed or amino acid formula or, on occasion, by eliminating dairy from the maternal diet for breastfed infants.

✓ KEY POINTS: INFLAMMATORY GASTROINTESTINAL DISORDERS

1. Features of gastroesophageal reflux and allergic esophagitis may be clinically similar; the latter should be considered when standard antireflux therapy is ineffective.

2. Allergic colitis is a relatively common cause of rectal bleeding and bloody stools in the otherwise healthy-appearing infant.

3. The presence of *Clostridium difficile* toxin in stools is a common finding in healthy infants.

4. Hirschsprung disease can be associated with an inflammatory enterocolitis that can be quite severe and life-threatening.

MALABSORPTION

113. What is an easy method of differentiating between osmotic and secretory diarrhea?

Patients with secretory diarrhea continue to have diarrhea even after they are not fed enterally. The laboratory method of differentiating between osmotic and secretory diarrhea is the measurement of the osmotic gap in the stool, which is achieved by measuring the stool osmolarity, sodium (Na), and potassium (K) concentrations in a random stool sample. Normal fecal osmolality is 290 mOsm/kg water, and the normal osmotic gap is less than 40 mEq/L.

$$\text{Osmotic gap} = \text{fecal osmolality} - 2 \times ([\text{Na}]\ [\text{K}])$$

Osmotic gap and sodium and potassium concentrations are expressed as mEq/L and fecal osmolality as mOsm/kg H_2O.

114. What are the most common causes of lactose malabsorption?

Almost any process damaging the mucosa of the small intestine can result in malabsorption of lactose owing to secondary lactase deficiency. The most common cause of secondary lactase deficiency is mucosal damage resulting from infection (e.g., postviral damage). Lactase enzyme has the lowest activity of any brush border disaccharidases and is localized at the tip of the villus, thus making it most vulnerable to brush border injury at the time of infection. It is the first enzyme to be affected and the last one to recover after mucosal damage.

115. What are the stool characteristics of carbohydrate malabsorption? Why does diarrhea occur?

Stools in carbohydrate malabsorption are acidic, with a pH of less than 5.5 (owing to fermentation), and are positive for reducing substances (sugar). Reducing substances will be negative in the stool in the face of carbohydrate malabsorption if the sugar is not a reducing sugar (e.g., sucrose). In that situation the stool sample should be hydrolyzed with 0.1 N hydrogen chloride and boiled briefly to break up the sucrose before being tested to yield a positive result for reducing substances.

The malabsorbed carbohydrate induces an osmotic fluid shift in the small intestine, resulting in an increase in fluid delivery to the colon. There the carbohydrate is fermented by colonic bacterial flora to organic acids such as lactic acid, yielding an increase in the osmolality beyond the colon's salvage capacity, thereby leading to diarrhea. Colonic bacteria ferment the carbohydrate in a process known as colonic scavenging. The main by-products of fermentation are short-chain fatty acids, which can be used as a source of energy by the epithelial cells of the colon.

116. Is a 72-hour fecal fat collection useful for detecting fat malabsorption in the neonate?

The 72-hour fecal fat collection is useful only if patients are receiving a diet containing long-chain triglycerides as the only source of fat in the diet. The standard method used for quantitation of fat does not detect medium-chain triglycerides. A 72-hour dietary record must be obtained simultaneously so that the coefficient of fat absorption can be obtained.

117. What is the coefficient of fat absorption in infants younger than 6 months of age?

The coefficient is 85%.

118. How common is primary lactase deficiency in neonates?

Contrary to common belief, primary or congenital lactase deficiency is a very rare disease, with only a few dozen cases reported in the literature. The disease is manifested by severe diarrhea while the infant is receiving a lactose-containing formula or breastfeeding, and it starts within the first few hours or days of life. The diarrhea resolves after the infant is switched to a lactose-free formula.

119. What is microvillus inclusion disease?

This very rare congenital disease is often quoted as a cause of severe neonatal diarrhea. The major manifestation is severe secretory diarrhea unresponsive to the withdrawal of oral diet. Diagnosis is based on a small bowel biopsy in which shortened enterocyte microvilli with microvillus inclusions are seen on electron microscopy. The etiology is unknown, and prognosis is poor. Patients often become dependent on TPN and have a shortened life expectancy.

Other uncommon causes of congenital diarrhea include autoimmune enteropathy, enterocolitis associated with Hirschsprung disease, primary lactase deficiency, congenital chloride diarrhea, congenital sodium diarrhea, primary bile acid malabsorption, and enterokinase deficiency.

120. What is the cause of diarrhea in a neonate fed exclusively Pedialyte?

If other causes of diarrhea, such as that resulting from an infectious source, are excluded, congenital glucose-galactose malabsorption is high on the differential diagnosis because the carbohydrate in Pedialyte is dextrose (a form of glucose monohydrate). Glucose or galactose malabsorption is an autosomal recessive disease caused by a missense mutation in the *SGLT1* gene resulting in a complete loss of the Na-dependent glucose transporter, which mediates glucose absorption in the brush border of the intestine. The treatment is elimination of glucose and galactose from the diet with resolution of the diarrhea.

121. **Is there a test to assess the absorptive integrity of the small intestine?**

The delta-xylose absorption test is a useful tool frequently used for the evaluation of small intestine integrity and to screen for carbohydrate malabsorption. Delta-xylose is a five-carbon sugar handled similarly to natural six-carbon sugars by way of high-efficiency proximal small bowel uptake. It is not metabolized and is rapidly excreted in the urine. Thus it is ideally suited to test the most basic of carbohydrate pathways. The test is performed in a fasting patient who is given 14.5 g/m^2 of delta-xylose orally as a 10-g% solution. A serum level of the delta-xylose is measured 1 hour later. Small intestinal biopsies can be used to confirm anatomic disruption of the mucosal surface or reduced disaccharidase levels to complement the functional absorptive results obtained from a delta-xylose test.

122. **A 21-year-old pregnant woman was diagnosed with polyhydramnios. A prenatal ultrasound study demonstrated distended loops of small intestine. The baby was delivered at 33 weeks' gestation by cesarean section, and at the time of delivery the amniotic fluid was noted to contain yellow-green stool. On day 2 of life the infant developed a hypochloremic metabolic alkalosis and loose stools. A stool sample contained high concentrations of chloride. What is the most likely diagnosis in this case?**

The following features of this case suggest a diagnosis of congenital chloride diarrhea:
- High concentrations of fecal chloride (exceeding the sum of sodium and potassium)
- Polyhydramnios
- Distended loops of bowel on a prenatal ultrasound
- Prematurity

This is an autosomal recessive disease caused by a defect in the chloride-bicarbonate exchange transport system in the ileum and colon resulting in lifelong secretory diarrhea. The diagnosis is made by the high concentration of fecal chloride. Treatment consists of fluid and electrolyte replacement—initially intravenously and then orally. If the condition is diagnosed and treated early, the prognosis is excellent.

123. **What are the anatomic causes of gastric outlet obstruction in neonates and infants?**
- Hypertrophic pyloric stenosis
- Antral and pyloric membranes or webs
- Eosinophilic gastroenteritis
- Aberrant pancreatic tissue
- Duplication of antrum or duodenum
- Pyloric channel ulcer
- Pyloric atresia

124. **What type of surgery is typically performed in complicated cases of meconium ileus?**

In 1957 Bishop and Koop described the technique of resection of the dilated ileal segment and proximal end-to-distal side ileal anastomosis with distal ostomy, also known as the Bishop–Koop ileostomy. This procedure minimizes contamination, allows for anastomosis between appropriately sized bowel segments, provides access to the distal bowel for decompression and irrigation, and allows for bedside closure of the stoma once the obstruction has resolved. Various irrigating solutions have been used, including normal saline, Gastrografin, hydrogen peroxide, and 2% to 4% solutions of N-acetylcysteine. Figures 10-4 and 10-5 illustrate the typical findings of meconium ileus with obstruction and the Bishop–Koop ileostomy technique.

125. **What is the operative approach if the patient has meconium ileus with suspected intestinal perforation?**

If the infant has had a perforation with peritonitis, the clinician must determine the degree of peritonitis. If perforation occurs just before delivery, meconium ascites without calcification is usually present, whereas if it occurs several weeks or months before delivery, calcification and dense adhesions

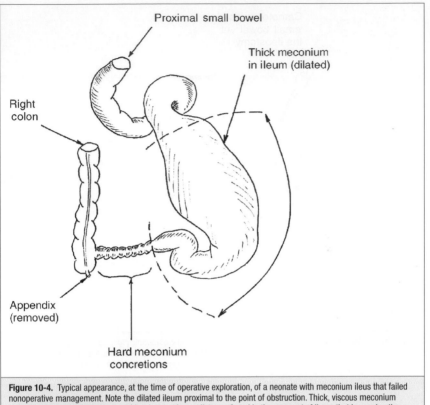

Proximal small bowel

Thick meconium
in ileum (dilated)

Right
colon

Appendix
(removed)

Hard meconium
concretions

Figure 10-4. Typical appearance, at the time of operative exploration, of a neonate with meconium ileus that failed nonoperative management. Note the dilated ileum proximal to the point of obstruction. Thick, viscous meconium is found in the dilated segment, and hard meconium pellets are found in the segment of ileum that is causing the complete mechanical obstruction. For this degree of disease the massively dilated bowel must be resected.

will develop. Occasionally, a fibrous wall forms around the meconium, leading to a pseudocyst, often referred to as giant cystic meconium peritonitis. Operative repair of the obstruction can be difficult because the adhesions are usually quite vascular, carrying a high risk of intraoperative mortality. The goal is relief of the obstruction and, if possible, restoration of bowel continuity or creation of a temporary Bishop–Koop ileostomy. Ostomy closure is usually safe 6 to 8 weeks later. TPN may be necessary if inadequate bowel length is available for feeding.

✓ KEY POINTS: INHERITED DISORDERS OF ABSORPTION AND MOTILITY

1. An infant who continues to produce significant amounts of stool in the absence of oral intake should be evaluated for an inherited or acquired disease of secretory diarrhea.

2. Congenital disorders of carbohydrate malabsorption that cause significant diarrhea in the infant are extremely rare.

3. The diagnosis of cystic fibrosis should be considered in any infant with meconium ileus.

4. An abnormal stooling pattern in an infant with Down syndrome should raise the possibility of Hirschsprung disease.

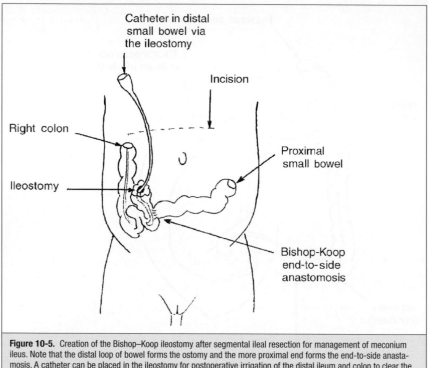

Figure 10-5. Creation of the Bishop–Koop ileostomy after segmental ileal resection for management of meconium ileus. Note that the distal loop of bowel forms the ostomy and the more proximal end forms the end-to-side anastomosis. A catheter can be placed in the ileostomy for postoperative irrigation of the distal ileum and colon to clear the remaining bowel of partially obstructing thick meconium.

126. **In newborns what are the three most common gastrointestinal manifestations of cystic fibrosis?**
   - Meconium ileus is the earliest clinical manifestation of cystic fibrosis. Between 10% and 20% of patients with cystic fibrosis develop intestinal obstruction *in utero* during the last trimester of development. Abdominal distention is marked, with no passage of meconium. The obstruction is secondary to a mass of extremely thick, tenacious meconium, which adheres to the wall of the distal small bowel and impacts the lumen.
   - The most common complication is volvulus of meconium-laden loops, frequently associated with ischemia, necrosis, perforation, and peritonitis. Twisted devitalized loops may become adherent, lose their continuity with the intestinal lumen, and form a gelatinous pseudocyst.
   - Spillage of meconium into the peritoneal cavity after antenatal intestinal perforation results in the development of meconium peritonitis. Meconium peritonitis may be seen before birth on ultrasound, and if it occurred early in utero, it can present as calcifications of the abdomen during the newborn period.

SHORT GUT SYNDROME

127. **What is short gut syndrome?**
   The healthy newborn intestine is approximately 200 to 300 cm in length. Traditionally, the definition of short gut was less then 75 cm of total small bowel, thus an approximate loss of about half of the small bowel. Short gut syndrome is presently defined on the basis of the constellation of symptoms,

signs, and metabolic and nutritional alterations associated with a physiologically significant loss of gut. The overall prognosis would depend on what specific sections were lost and the overall remaining bowel function, including the following:

- Amount of remaining small intestine
- Whether it is proximal (jejunal) or distal (ileal)
- Whether the ileocecal valve is resected
- Whether the colon is resected
- Degree of intestinal adaptation
- Presence of residual bowel disease

128. What are the mechanisms responsible for diarrhea in short gut syndrome?

- Decreased absorptive surface area
- Rapid transit time
- Bacterial overgrowth
- Hypersecretion and impaired regulation of gut motility
- Decreased absorption of bile salts, particularly with the loss of the terminal ileum: The unabsorbed bile salts are deconjugated by anaerobic bacteria, causing inhibition and even net secretion of water and electrolytes.
- Steatorrhea: secondary to decreased availability of bile salts necessary for fat absorption
- Loss of the ileocecal valve: This permits reflux of colonic bacteria into the small intestine, thereby contributing to bacterial overgrowth.
- Colonic resection: The colon is where most fluid reabsorption occurs.

129. What problems may be associated with enteral feeding in patients with short gut syndrome?

Enteral feeds should be initiated early and aggressively advanced as tolerated to promote intestinal adaptation and help diminish the complications associated with TPN. Formula is given through a feeding tube at a continuous rate initially to maximize absorption during advancement. No conclusive data prove that one type of formula or breast milk is ideal, and many different regimens have been used successfully. The major limiting factor in the formulas is the amount of carbohydrate, because unabsorbed sugars increase the osmotic load in the colon and cause an osmotic diarrhea that can lead to significant water loss and acidosis. The excessive malabsorption is accompanied by an increase in stool volume (stool outputs greater then 40 to 50 mL/kg/day), positive reducing substances, and a stool pH below 5.5.

130. What are the long-term complications of short gut syndrome?

- TPN-related liver disease
- Nutrient deficiencies
- Failure to thrive
- Small bowel bacterial overgrowth
- Catheter-related sepsis
- Motility disturbances
- Gastric acid hypersecretion
- Delta-lactic acidosis
- Renal stones and gallstones

IMPERFORATE ANUS

131. How is imperforate anus diagnosed?

Imperforate anus is often diagnosed in the nursery as the nursing staff attempts to obtain a rectal temperature from the neonate or during the newborn examination. Rectal atresia might be missed during the examination because the anal opening can appear normal. However, failure to pass meconium and increasing abdominal distention should warrant further evaluation.

132. How frequently is imperforate anus associated with other abnormalities?
Associated spinal and genitourinary anomalies are rather common, occurring in 20% to 50% of patients with imperforate anus. Imperforate anus may be seen as part of the vertebral defects, imperforate anus, tracheoesophageal fistula, and radial and renal dysplasia (VATER) or vertebral abnormalities, anal atresia, cardiac abnormalities, tracheoesophageal fistula and/or esophageal atresia, renal agenesis and dysplasia, and limb defects (VACTERL) association. The evaluation of an infant with imperforate anus includes looking for other associated anomalies.

133. What tests determine initial management of an infant with imperforate anus?
The initial testing should include a complete physical examination and a urine analysis. If the baby has a flat bottom without a well-developed gluteal fold or has meconium in the urine, a colostomy is indicated. Conversely, in the setting of a bucket-handle deformity or meconium staining in the perineal midline, a minimal anorectoplasty is indicated without colostomy. In girls a colostomy is warranted barring demonstration of a perineal fistula. These decisions are all made after 16 to 24 hours to permit increased luminal pressures to force meconium through a fistula so that it is noted on examination. In all cases an abdominal ultrasound should be obtained to rule out other anomalies.
- Colostomy not required: Perineal (cutaneous) fistula.
- Colostomy required: Rectourethral fistula (bulbar or prostatic), rectovesical fistula, imperforate anus without fistula, rectal atresia

HIRSCHSPRUNG DISEASE

134. When and by whom was Hirschsprung disease first classically described?
The classical description of Hirschsprung disease is attributed to Harald Hirschsprung, a pathologist, who described this condition in two children in 1888. This abnormality occurs in 1 in 5000 live births. Male children are four times more likely to be affected than female children.

135. Why does Hirschsprung disease occur?
The parasympathetic fibers that innervate the colonic bowel wall (to form the myenteric [Auerbach] and the submucosal [Meissner] nervous plexi) are derived from neural crest cells in the neural folds. During embryologic development the cells migrate along the bowel in a cranial to caudal migration, providing innervation. Hirschsprung disease results when the progression of such migration stops prematurely. Without this parasympathetic innervation, the intestine cannot relax when nitric oxide is released from the postganglionic nerve fibers. Approximately 80% of the time, the progression stops in the rectum, and only 20% of cases involve the total bowel or small bowel. Short-segment Hirschsprung disease does not extend beyond the rectosigmoid region, whereas long-segment Hirschsprung disease extends more proximally.

136. How is Hirschsprung disease diagnosed?
The diagnosis of Hirschsprung disease can be made with a barium enema, rectal suction or surgical full-thickness biopsy, or anorectal manometry. The initial test of choice is the unprepared barium enema. The test looks for the classic finding of a transition zone where the distal noninnervated section of bowel is smaller than the more proximal dilated bowel. The transition zone will occur in the location where the neurons stopped normal progression. The diagnosis by pathologic examination uses rectal biopsies to look for evidence of nerve cells directly. The biopsy will show absence of ganglion cells or presence of nerve cell hypertrophy or increased acetylcholinesterase with special staining. Anorectal manometry can be used to demonstrate the absence of the normal rectoanal inhibitory reflex that is present in the internal anal sphincter when innervated by the parasympathetic plexi.

137. Is there a genetic component to the disease?
Approximately 10% of children have a family history, especially with longer-segment Hirschsprung disease. A higher incidence occurs in children with Down syndrome and other genetic abnormalities.

Recent studies indicate the presence of mutations in the RET proto-oncogene in 17% to 38% of children with short-segment disease and in 70% to 80% of those with long-segment disease. Additional genes linked to the RET activation pathway and other mechanisms have now been identified.

Carter TC, Kay DM, Browne ML, et al. Hirschsprung's disease and variants in genes that regulate enteric neural crest cell proliferation, migration and differentiation. J Hum Genet 2012;57(8):485–93.

138. What are the complications after surgical repair of Hirschsprung disease?

- Obstruction
- Mechanical obstruction
- Incomplete resection of aganglionic bowel segments
- Motility disorder
- Functional megacolon
- Internal sphincter achalasia
- Enterocolitis
- Incontinence

GASTROINTESTINAL HEMORRHAGE

139. How does one determine whether swallowed maternal blood is the cause for gastrointestinal bleeding in the neonate?

This determination is made using the Apt–Downey test. For this test 1 part stool is mixed with 5 parts water and centrifuged for 2 minutes to separate out fecal material. The supernatant is removed, and 1 mL of 0.25 N (1%) sodium hydroxide is mixed with the 5 mL of supernatant. After 2 minutes there is a color change; if the hemoglobin is fetal, the color stays pink; if it is from the mother, it turns yellow-brown.

140. What are the sources of neonatal gastrointestinal bleeding?

See Table 10-5.

141. What are some of the risk factors and clinical features that help distinguish necrotizing enterocolitis (NEC) from other causes of gastrointestinal bleeding in the neonate?

NEC tends to be more common in premature infants and often occurs in those who have experienced some type of perinatal stress, such as hypoxia, need for mechanical ventilation, or sepsis. The

TABLE 10-5. SOURCES OF NEONATAL GASTROINTESTINAL BLEEDING	
HEMATEMESIS/MELENA	**HEMATOCHEZIA**
Swallowed maternal blood	Swallowed maternal blood
Gastritis or stress ulcers	Dietary protein intolerance
Duplication cyst	Duplication cyst
Coagulopathy: Vitamin K deficiency or DIC	Coagulopathy: Vitamin K deficiency or DIC
Maternal NSAID use	Maternal NSAID use
Maternal idiopathic thrombocytopenic purpura	Maternal idiopathic thrombocytopenic purpura
Vascular malformation	Colitis: infectious, NEC, Hirschsprung disease with enterocolitis
Hemophilia	Hemophilia
Esophagitis	Rectal fissure, tear, or hemorrhoids
DIC, Disseminated intravascular coagulopathy; NEC, necrotizing enterocolitis; NSAID, nonsteroidal antiinflammatory drug.	

addition of gross or occult blood in stools, feeding intolerance, abdominal distention or discoloration, bilious emesis, and lethargy should all lead to the consideration of NEC in the differential diagnosis.

142. What is the first step in the management of an acutely ill infant with significant gastrointestinal bleeding?

The key initial step is to obtain stable intravenous access for patient resuscitation. Particularly with hematemesis, the rapidity and severity of gastrointestinal bleeding can be significant, and the need for urgent intravenous access should not be underestimated. Once the ABCs of resuscitation have taken place, it is appropriate to focus on diagnosis and etiology.

NECROTIZING ENTEROCOLITIS

143. What is NEC?

NEC is a disease of unknown origin that primarily affects premature infants (80% of cases), typically after the onset of enteral alimentation during convalescence from the common cardiopulmonary disorders associated with prematurity. Manifestations cover a broad spectrum, from mild abdominal distention with hematochezia to a fulminant septic shock–like picture with transmural necrosis of the entire gastrointestinal tract (NEC totalis).

144. Which infants are at risk for developing NEC?

NEC typically occurs in infants with a corrected gestational age of 30 to 32 weeks and at a time when most premature infants are progressing on enteral feedings. Onset of NEC is unusual on the first day of life and highly uncommon among infants who have not received enteral feeds. NEC can occur sporadically, but often cases are clustered in place and time, which suggests an infectious etiology, although no consistent agent has been isolated from reported epidemics.

Many associated risk factors have been suggested but have not been shown to be directly associated with the pathogenesis of NEC. When investigated in carefully controlled studies, risk factors such as perinatal asphyxia, respiratory distress syndrome, umbilical catheters, patent ductus arteriosus, hypotension, and anemia have not been demonstrated to be more common among patients who developed NEC than among unaffected age-matched control subjects. The most dominant known risk factor for NEC is the degree of immaturity.

145. How are breast milk–fed infants thought to be protected from NEC?

Breast milk may reduce the risk of NEC. Breast milk offers many nutritive advantages in addition to protective immunologic substances. Milk macrophages and phagocytes, immunoglobulins A and G, and immunocompetent T and B lymphocytes may offer a protective advantage to the mucosa. These components potentiate the effect of the complement components C3 and C4, lysozyme, lactoferrin, and secretory immunoglobulin A. Furthermore, breast milk contains hormones (e.g., thyroid, thyroid-stimulating hormone, prolactin, steroid), enzymes (e.g., amylase, lipase), and growth factors (endothelial growth factor). Breast milk also favors the growth of *Lactobacillus bifidus* and promotes the development of a healthy gut microbiome.

Gephart SM, McGrath JM, Effken JA, et al. Necrotizing enterocolitis risk: state of the science. Adv Neonatal Care 2012;12(2):77–87.

146. What feeding risk factors have been associated with the development of NEC?

The absence of NEC *in utero* suggests an absolute requirement for gut colonization in its pathogenesis. Host luminal pH, proteases, oxygen tension, temperature, and osmolarity of enteral feedings have been implicated in the pathogenesis of NEC. The volume of milk fed to infants may also predispose them to NEC. Excessively rapid increments of milk feeding may overcome the infant's intestinal absorptive capability (especially in the presence of altered motility), resulting in malabsorption.

Large-volume milk feedings that are increased too rapidly during the feeding schedule may place undue stress on a previously injured or immature intestine. Two studies have shown that volume increments in excess of 20 to 25 mL/kg/day have been associated with NEC, whereas another two studies have shown the safety of 30 to 35 mL/kg/day increments. The evidence therefore is unclear as to the role of rapid feeding advancement in the development of NEC. Volume increments probably should not be more than 20 to 35 mL/kg/day and should be advanced on the basis of the clinical examination, physiologic stability, and feeding tolerance.

Morgan J, Young L, McGuire W. Slow advancement of enteral feed volumes to prevent necrotising enterocolitis in very low birth weight infants. Cochrane Database Syst Rev 2011 Mar 16;3:CD001241.

147. Are probiotics useful in the prevention of NEC?

Recent prospective randomized trials have looked at the effects of probiotics and their ability to prevent NEC. Studies have shown that the use of probiotics decreases the incidence of NEC but not the mortality rates among those patients that do develop NEC. However, a higher incidence of sepsis was reported in those infants receiving probiotics. Thus probiotics can be considered but should be used with caution, based on current data. To date, no large-scale trial of probiotics has been successfully carried out, and there are currently many different bacterial components in available probiotics. No probiotic is currently approved by the Food and Drug Administration for neonatal use.

Neu J, Walker WA. Necrotizing entercolitis. N Engl J Med 2011;364:255–64.

148. What is the gas in pneumatosis intestinalis?

Malabsorbed carbohydrates are fermented by colonic bacteria and cause increased intestinal gas production, resulting in abdominal distention. This gas, which is 30% to 40% hydrogen gas, dissects into the submucosa and subserosa, producing pneumatosis intestinalis. High intraluminal pressure resulting from gaseous distention may reduce mucosal blood flow, producing secondary intestinal ischemia.

149. What infective agents are associated with NEC?

In many cases of NEC, no infective agent is identifiable. Bacteria identified by positive blood cultures are seen in only 20% to 30% of patients with NEC. *S. epidermidis* is the most common organism, followed by gram-negative bacilli such as *E. coli* and *Klebsiella* species. Epidemics have been associated with a single pathogen such as *E. coli*, *Klebsiella* species, *Salmonella* species, *S. epidermidis*, *Clostridium butyricum*, *Coronavirus* species, *Rotavirus* species, and enteroviruses. NEC has also been associated with fungal sepsis. NEC may also result from an enterotoxin-mediated illness, such as toxins from *Clostridium* species or *S. epidermidis*. It is important to emphasize that, unlike in adults, *Clostridium difficile* and associated toxins are found in the intestinal tracts of many neonates who are entirely asymptomatic. The asymptomatic carrier state in some infants may be due to differences in intestinal immaturity, local differences in the intestinal milieu, absence of toxin-related receptors, or other protective factors.

150. What are the criteria for considering the diagnosis of NEC?

NEC is a common cause of systemic inflammatory response syndrome in neonates. Based on systemic signs, intestinal signs, and radiologic signs, staging of NEC is performed as shown in Table 10-6.

151. A 1000-g infant, born at 28 weeks' gestation, had an initial course characterized by respiratory distress syndrome and suspected sepsis. He was initially treated with surfactant and mechanical ventilation. The antibiotics were stopped after 3 days because the blood culture results were negative. On day 5 he was placed on nasal continuous positive airway pressure until day 18. He began enteral gavage feeds on day 5, at 20-cc/kg/day increments, and finally achieved "full feeds" (150 cc/kg/day) by day 20. He then developed an increased frequency of apnea and bradycardia associated with temperature instability. The gavage feeds were held because of

TABLE 10-6. STAGING OF NECROTIZING ENTEROCOLITIS

STAGE	SYSTEMIC SIGNS	INTESTINAL SIGNS	RADIOGRAPHIC SIGNS	TREATMENT
IA (suspected NEC)	Temperature instability, apnea bradycardia, lethargy	Increased gastric residuals, mild abdominal distention, emesis, guaiac-positive stools	Normal or mild intestinal dilation, mild ileus	NPO with antibiotics × 3 days
IB	Same as IA	Bright red blood per rectum	Same as IA	Same as IA
IIA (definite, mild NEC)	Same as IA	Same as IA/IB plus decreased or absent bowel sounds ± abdominal tenderness	Intestinal dilation with pneumatosis intestinalis	NPO with antibiotics × 7 to 10 days
IIB (definite, moderate NEC)	Same as IIA plus mild metabolic acidosis and thrombocytopenia	Same as IIA plus definite abdominal tenderness, absent bowel sounds, possible abdominal cellulitis or right lower quadrant mass	Same as IIA with definite ascites and possible portal vein gas	NPO with antibiotics × 14 days
IIIA (advanced, severe NEC)	Same as IIB plus hypotension, bradycardia, severe apnea, combined respiratory and metabolic acidosis, DIC, neutropenia, anuria	Same as IIB plus peritonitis; abdominal tenderness, distention, and erythema	Same as IIB	NPO with antibiotics × 14 days, fluid resuscitation, possible pressors or mechanical ventilation, paracentesis
IIIB (advanced, severe NEC with perforated bowel)	Same as IIIA	Sudden, severely increased abdominal distention with bowel perforation	Same as IIIA with pneumoperitoneum	Same as IIIA plus surgery

DIC, Disseminated intravascular coagulopathy; NEC, necrotizing enterocolitis; NPO, nothing by mouth.

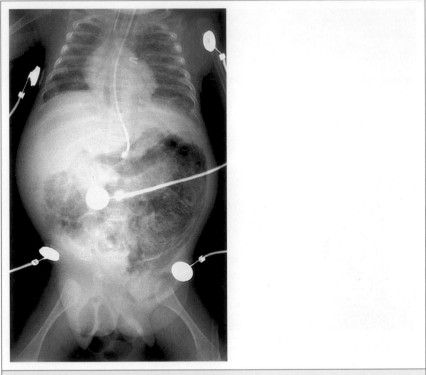

Figure 10-6. Abdominal radiograph 1 day after treatment for necrotizing enterocolitis stage IB. (Courtesy Dr. Jack Sty, Department of Pediatric Radiology, Children's Hospital of Wisconsin, Medical College of Wisconsin, Milwaukee, Wisconsin.)

increasing gastric residuals, presence of blood in stools, and abdominal distention. What should be done next?

This infant falls into stage IB because of the temperature instability, apnea and bradycardia, increased gastric residuals, presence of blood in stools, and abdominal distention. An abdominal x-ray is recommended to view the bowel gas pattern. Dilated bowel loops are expected. Management includes the following: (1) consultation with a pediatric surgeon, (2) withdrawing all enteral feeds, (3) gastric decompression by placing an orogastric tube to low wall suction, and (4) beginning antibiotics after appropriate cultures are collected. Meanwhile, TPN is necessary for nutritional support. It is important to carefully follow up with this infant to monitor for progression to NEC and exclude other diagnostic possibilities that may mimic NEC at this age.

152. **One day after beginning appropriate management, the same infant (see Question 151) develops persistent abdominal distention, right lower quadrant tenderness, and diminished bowel sounds. The abdominal radiographs are shown in Figures 10-6 and 10-7. How do you interpret these signs? What should be done next?**

At this stage the infant is showing definite signs of NEC (stage II), as demonstrated by the failure to recover from stage IB and worsening intestinal signs, such as diminished bowel sounds, guarding, and abdominal distention and tenderness. These clinical findings may herald the beginning of dilated viscus, submucosal or subserosal dissection of air, and peritonitis. Such an infant should be regarded

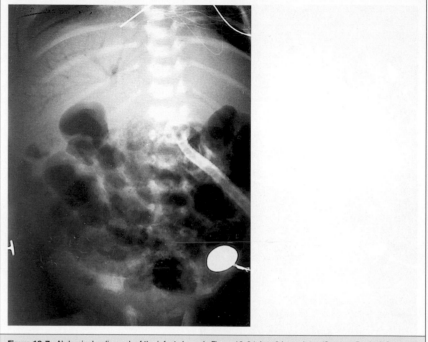

Figure 10-7. Abdominal radiograph of the infant shown in Figure 10-6 taken 8 hours later. (Courtesy Dr. Jack Sty, Department of Pediatric Radiology, Children's Hospital of Wisconsin, Medical College of Wisconsin, Milwaukee, Wisconsin.)

as having NEC and is moderately ill. The radiograph in Figure 10-6 shows grossly dilated bowel loops and submucosal and subserosal pneumatosis intestinalis. Management based on this radiograph includes careful monitoring for worsening of clinical status (e.g., metabolic acidosis and thrombocytopenia) and a course of antibiotics for a minimum of 7 to 10 days. However, the second radiograph in Figure 10-7 shows worsening disease, as manifested by portal vein gas (within the liver). At this stage it is imperative to anticipate the possibility of intestinal perforation. Management should now include correction of hypovolemia and metabolic acidosis using colloids and sodium bicarbonate, respectively. If NEC does not progress further, 2 weeks of appropriate antibiotics would suffice, with hopes to avoid surgical intervention.

153. **The infant's condition suddenly deteriorates 24 hours later. He develops generalized abdominal tenderness and periumbilical erythema. An arterial blood gas determination shows a pH of 7.10, PCO_2 of 80 mmHg, PO_2 of 32 mmHg, HCO_3^- of 12 mEq/L, and a base deficit of 16. The blood count is remarkable for a platelet count of 22,000/µL. The abdominal radiography is shown in Figure 10-8. How do you interpret these signs? What should be the approach to the management of this infant?**
The infant at this stage has advanced NEC and is severely ill. This condition is characterized by worsening hypotension, a combined respiratory and metabolic acidosis, thrombocytopenia, and anuria. Thrombocytopenia usually represents a consumptive thrombocytopenia with or without intestinal perforation. The sudden deterioration is ominous for a bowel perforation, and progressive abdominal distention with erythema signifies worsening peritonitis and pneumoperitoneum. The lateral decubitus abdominal radiograph is remarkable for worsening pneumatosis and free air (see Figure 10-8).

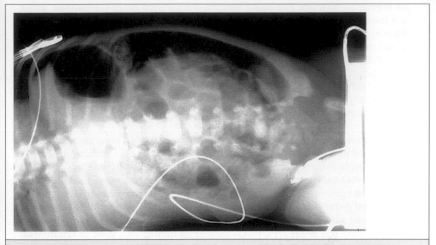

Figure 10-8. Abdominal radiograph of advanced necrotizing enterocolitis. (Courtesy Dr. Jack Sty, Department of Pediatric Radiology, Children's Hospital of Wisconsin, Medical College of Wisconsin, Milwaukee, Wisconsin.)

This infant needs vigorous fluid resuscitation with colloids (i.e., fresh frozen plasma, albumin) and cellular products (i.e., packed red cells, platelets). Inotropic support using dopamine and epinephrine drips may be needed. Surgical exploration is indicated in this setting to facilitate abdominal decompression and salvage the viable bowel. If it is difficult to ventilate the infant at this stage, an abdominal paracentesis may be helpful.

154. When is surgery indicated for an infant with NEC? What are the complications of performing surgery on an infant with advanced NEC with bowel perforation?

Absolute indications for surgery include pneumoperitoneum and intestinal gangrene (as demonstrated by positive results of abdominal paracentesis testing). Relative indications include progressive clinical deterioration (metabolic acidosis, ventilatory failure, oliguria, thrombocytopenia), fixed abdominal mass, abdominal wall erythema, portal vein gas, and persistently dilated bowel loop.

The postoperative complications occurring immediately after surgery are usually related to the stoma (retraction, prolapse, or peristomal hernia) or wound (infection, dehiscence, enterocutaneous fistula). Rarely, intraabdominal abscesses, recurrence of NEC, and bowel obstruction can develop. Chronic complications result from the dysfunctional ostomies, strictures, or short gut syndrome depending on the amount of remaining healthy bowel.

In some extremely sick ELBW infants, the placement of an intraperitoneal drain may be an option as opposed to a laparotomy, which may be excessively stressful for the deteriorating infant. In the presence of obvious perforation, this approach is an extremely difficult one, but it may allow time for another therapy to exert an effect before the child is taken to the operating room.

155. A 30-week-gestation male infant had been diagnosed with stage IIA NEC and was appropriately managed medically for 10 days. He subsequently tolerated feeds poorly. The stooling pattern was reported as normal (small green stools). Different formulas and prokinetics were tried without any positive result. An abdominal x-ray revealed what was reported as a "gassy abdomen." Treatment with antibiotics was begun again, and feedings were held for 3 days. A sepsis work-up yielded negative results at 3 days. Feedings were then resumed with

an elemental formula. The same feeding-intolerance pattern prevailed. What are the diagnostic considerations in this infant?

Recovery after NEC occurs by second intention, with areas of patchy necrosis often healing by fibrosis and stricture formation. The repair process also involves the peritoneum, resulting in adhesions. Both of these processes can result in signs of functional or mechanical obstruction. An upper gastrointestinal contrast radiograph may show a prolonged transit time and gross dilation of jejunum consistent with more distal stricture formation. A lower gastrointestinal contrast x-ray may be necessary to identify strictures in the large bowel. At laparotomy this infant was found to have multiple strictures, which were resected and ultimately resulted in a short bowel syndrome.

156. **A 3500-g term female infant born after an uncomplicated pregnancy was discharged home from the newborn nursery after a normal transition. She was fed exclusively with breast milk. On her seventh day of life she presented acutely with bilious emesis. The clinical examination was remarkable for a pulse rate of 180 bpm, respiratory rate of 70/min, mean blood pressure of 30 mmHg, abdominal distention, and marked tenderness with diminished bowel sounds. She passed a dark, bloody stool. Laboratory study results were notable for an arterial blood gas of pH 7.15, PCO_2 level of 30 mmHg, PO_2 level of 120 mmHg, and HCO_3^- level of 10 mEq/L. The complete blood count was remarkable for a hematocrit level of 24 and platelet count of 400,000/µL. What is the approach to management in this infant? How would you establish a diagnosis in this infant?**

The infant's examination is consistent with an acute abdomen. She also has signs of hypovolemia and shock. She needs immediate fluid resuscitation and correction of metabolic acidosis. Because sepsis is common in the neonatal period, antibiotics are indicated after blood cultures are obtained. A nasogastric tube should be placed and the stomach decompressed. An abdominal x-ray reveals gassy distended bowel loops with air-fluid levels. An upper gastrointestinal contrast radiograph is shown in Figure 10-9. The contrast fails to flow distally, suggesting intestinal obstruction. Furthermore, the pig-tail appearance of the contrast is classic for a diagnosis of volvulus, and surgical exploration should be considered.

157. **How do you differentiate NEC from volvulus? In what conditions is pneumatosis intestinalis seen?**

Table 10-7 summarizes the features that differentiate NEC from volvulus. Apart from NEC, pneumatosis intestinalis is also seen in midgut volvulus, acute or chronic diarrhea, postoperative gastrointestinal surgery, Hirschsprung disease, short gut syndrome, mesenteric thrombosis, postcardiac catheterization, structural disease of the hindgut (colonic atresias and stricture, imperforate anus), and intestinal malignancies.

NEONATAL HEPATITIS

158. **What are the common causes of neonatal liver failure, and what are the diagnostic tests for each?**

See Table 10-8.

159. **What are the components of neonatal biliary disease?**

Any disease process in the neonate with altered bile acid transport or biliary structure is a biliary disease. The clues to its presence include cholestasis (elevated serum bile acids), conjugated hyperbilirubinemia, and altered serum levels of enzymes resulting from biliary inflammation or obstruction (e.g., gamma-glutamyl transferase [GGT] and alkaline phosphatase).

160. **What is cholestatic jaundice?**

Conjugated bilirubin greater than 2 mg/dL or exceeding 15% of the total bilirubin is referred to as direct hyperbilirubinemia and is a clinical indicator of cholestatic jaundice. Unlike indirect

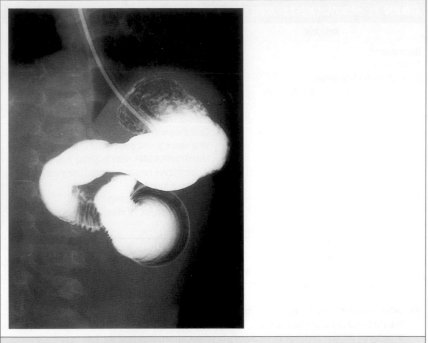

Figure 10-9. Upper gastrointestinal contrast radiograph. (Courtesy Dr. Jack Sty, Department of Pediatric Radiology, Children's Hospital of Wisconsin, Medical College of Wisconsin, Milwaukee, Wisconsin.)

TABLE 10-7. NECROTIZING ENTEROCOLITIS DIFFERENTIATED FROM VOLVULUS

Modified from Kliegman R. Necrotizing enterocolitis: differential diagnosis and management. In: Polin RA, Yoder MC, Burg FD, editors. Workbook in practical neonatology. 2nd ed. Philadelphia: Saunders; 1993. p. 449–70.

CHARACTERISTICS	NEC	VOLVULUS
Preterm	90%	30%
Onset by 2 weeks	90%	60%
Male:female ratio	1:1	2:1
Associated anomalies	Rare	25% to 40%
Bilious emesis	Unusual	75%
Grossly bloody stools	Common	Less common
Pneumatosis intestinalis	90%	2%
Marked proximal obstruction	Rare	Common
Thrombocytopenia without DIC	Common	Rare

DIC, Disseminated intravascular coagulopathy; NEC, necrotizing enterocolitis.

TABLE 10-8. NEONATAL CAUSES OF ACUTE LIVER FAILURE AND DIAGNOSTIC TESTS	
DISEASE	**DIAGNOSTIC FINDINGS**
Galactosemia	Red cell galactose-1-phosphate uridyl transferase
Tyrosinemia	Urine succinyl acetone
Neonatal hemochromatosis	Elevated ferritin, extrahepatic iron deposition
Hemophagocytic lymphohistiocytosis and congenital leukemia	Bone marrow findings
Sepsis, shock	Positive blood cultures
Giant cell hepatitis with hemolytic anemia	Coombs-positive hemolytic anemia
HHV-6, Hepatitis b, adenovirus, parvovirus	Viral serology and polymerase chain reaction
Mitochondrial hepatopathy	Mitochondrial DNA, muscle and/or liver biopsy for quantitative respiratory chain enzymes
Vascular malformations and congenital heart disease	Echocardiography
Maternal overdose	History, toxicology screen
Hypocortisolism	Cortisol levels, ACTH stimulation test

ACTH, Adrenocorticotropic hormone; HHV-6, human herpesvirus 6.

hyperbiloirubinemia, cholestatic jaundice is always physiologically abnormal and warrants a medical evaluation. Note that biliary disease can present with or without cholestatic jaundice.

161. **What are the causes of direct hyperbilirubinemia?**
The mechanisms include the following:
- Impaired bilirubin metabolism secondary to parenchymal disease of the liver
- Inherited disorders of bilirubin excretion
- Mechanical obstruction to biliary flow, either intrahepatic or extrahepatic
- Excessive bilirubin loads, such as may occur in massive hemolysis

162. **When should an infant's fractionated bilirubin be obtained?**
Evaluation of jaundice persisting beyond the normal physiologic period (2 weeks) in newborns must always include a fractionation of bilirubin.

163. **How should the evaluation of cholestatic jaundice in infants be approached?**
Neonatal cholestasis can be a manifestation of (1) extrahepatic biliary disease, (2) intrahepatic biliary disease, or (3) hepatocellular disease. All can present with similar symptoms. Therefore differentiation based on history and physical examination alone is usually not diagnostic.
The clinician should initiate further evaluation to promptly identify clinical conditions amenable to therapy (Table 10-9), particularly those in which any delay in treatment could be tragic (e.g., sepsis; urinary tract infection; hypothyroidism; biliary atresia; and congenital metabolic disorders requiring special diets such as galactosemia, hereditary fructose intolerance, and tyrosinemia).

164. **What tests should be obtained during the initial evaluation of neonatal cholestasis?**
See Table 10-10.

165. **When should the infant be referred to a gastroenterologist?**
As soon as cholestatic jaundice is diagnosed and sepsis ruled out, a gastroenterologist should be consulted. The tests mentioned in the previous question can be scheduled, but the clinician should not wait for the results before making the referral. In most cases a liver biopsy is needed to help make the final diagnosis. The hepatologist will also conduct a broad laboratory evaluation to make a diagnosis and initiate therapy. In addition to medical therapy, preventive therapy can be provided

TABLE 10-9. TREATABLE CAUSES OF NEONATAL CHOLESTASIS

Adapted from Dhawah A, Mieli-Vergani G. Acute liver failure in neonates. Early Hum Dev 2005;81:1005–10.

INFECTIOUS	SURGICAL	METABOLIC	OTHER
Urinary tract infection	Biliary atresia	Galactosemia	Hypothyroidism,
Sepsis	Choledochal cyst	Hereditary fructose	panhypopituitarism
TORCH* infections	Cholelithiasis	intolerance	Bile acid synthetic
Neonatal hepatitis	Biliary strictures	Tyrosinemia	anomalies
	Bile duct perforation	Iron storage disorders	Histiocytosis X
	Congenital duct		Mass (neoplasia)
	anomalies		Alpha 1 antitrypsin
	Intestinal obstruction		deficiency

*TORCH is an acronym for *To*xoplasmosis, *O*ther infections, *R*ubella, *C*ytomegalovirus, and *H*erpes simplex virus 2.

TABLE 10-10. TESTS FOR THE INITIAL EVALUATION OF NEONATAL CHOLESTASIS

	INDICATION
Blood	
Fractionated bilirubin	Detect cholestatic jaundice
Complete blood count	Rule out sepsis
Blood cultures if clinically indicated	Rule out sepsis
Hepatic function panel	Detect hepatobiliary disease
Thyroid-stimulating hormone and free T$_4$	Rule out hypothyroidism
Coagulation studies	Assess liver synthetic function
Urine	
Urinalysis and culture	Detect urinary tract infection, sepsis
Reducing sugars	Detect galactosemia
Protein	Support galactosemia, hereditary fructose intolerance, or tyrosinemia
Imaging Studies	
Abdominal ultrasound	Detect choledochal cyst, stones, mass, or biliary stricture
Diisopropyl immodiacetic acid (DISIDA) scan	Differentiate between biliary atresia (non-excreting) and neonatal hepatitis (delayed uptake with excretion)

through genetic counseling. Time is of the essence to identify treatable causes of cholestasis and intervene early in such cases as biliary atresia for better outcomes.

166. What is spontaneous bile duct perforation?

Spontaneous perforation of the bile ducts is a rare occurrence but has been documented in infants between 4 and 12 weeks of age. The cause is currently unknown. It most often occurs at the point at which the cystic duct is joined to the common bile duct. Infants can present with lethargy, nonbilious vomiting, acholic stools, mild jaundice, dark urine, abdominal distention, and a mildly elevated conjugated hyperbilirubinemia. Definitive diagnosis can be made with a hepatoiminodiacetic acid scan or abdominal paracentesis.

TABLE 10-11.   CHARACTERISTIC FEATURES IN PROGRESSIVE FAMILIAL INTRAHEPATIC CHOLESTASIS

Adapted from Hori T, Nguyen JH, Uemoto S. Progressive familial intrahepatic cholestasis. Hepatobiliary Pancreat Dis Int 2010;9(6): 570–8.

	PFIC1	*PFIC2*	*PFIC3*
Functional deficiency	*FIC1* gene	*BSEP* gene	*MDR3* gene
Age of onset	Neonates	Neonates	1 month to 20 years
Cholestasis	Chronic	Chronic	Chronic
Ductular proliferation	Absent	Absent	Absent
Progression to cirrhosis	Yes	Yes	Yes
Portal fibrosis	Present	Pronounced	Rare
Giant cell transformation	Present	Pronounced	Rare
Pruritis	Severe	Severe	Moderate
Serum GGT levels	Normal	Normal	High
Serum cholesterol levels	Normal	Normal	Normal

GGT, Gamma-glutamyl transferase.

167. **How do the bile salt transporter defects present?**
This group of conditions is collectively known as progressive familial intrahepatic cholestasis. They typically present as neonatal cholestasis but individually have distinct clinical, laboratory, and histologic features that differentiate them (Table 10-11).

BILE DUCT AND BILIARY ATRESIA

168. **A 6-week-old healthy term breast-fed infant was noted to be jaundiced at the routine well-baby visit. She was growing well. Examination of the abdomen revealed a palpable liver (1 cm below right costal margin) and spleen (2 cm below left costal margin). Her history revealed that she had pigmented stools since birth. Total and direct bilirubin levels were 6.9 and 4.3 mg/dL, respectively. Other findings include alanine aminotransferase (ALT), 138 U/L; aspartate aminotransferase (AST), 120 U/L; alkaline phosphatase (ALK), 205 U/L; GGT, 420 U/L; albumin, 3 g/dL; and prothrombin time (PT) 13.9 sec. Calcium, phosphate, and magnesium levels were normal; complete blood count, urinalysis, and culture had normal results. What do the laboratory results suggest, and which further tests need to be performed?**
Apart from ruling out sepsis and urinary tract infection, the preceding tests are nondiagnostic. The liver enzymes, albumin level, and PT are useful for following the degree of hepatic injury and course of hepatic function. The following are some of the other tests that should be performed:

■ Ultrasound: This is a quick, noninvasive test useful for detecting causes of extrahepatic cholestasis (e.g., choledochal cysts, biliary stones, tumors). Finding a gallbladder on ultrasound does not rule out biliary atresia, although the absence of a gallbladder would rasie the suspicion of biliary atresia.

■ Radionuclide scans (diisopropyl iminodiacetic acid [DISIDA]): Good hepatic uptake of radionuclide with absence of excretion into the gut lumen suggests an obstructive process such as biliary atresia. Delayed excretion may also occur in hepatitis. If the hepatocytes are damaged to a degree that they cannot take up the tracer, there would also be no secretion on the scan, further complicating the test results.

169. **In the infant described in the preceding question, the ultrasound revealed hepatosplenomegaly, and no gallbladder was seen. The DISIDA scan showed normal uptake but no excretion at 24 hours. A liver biopsy specimen was**

TABLE 10-12.	CAUSES OF PEDIATRIC ELEVATIONS OF GAMMA-GLUTAMYL TRANSFERASE
DISEASE	**VARIATION OF GGT**
Extrahepatic biliary atresia	Increased up to 10 times upper limit
Alagille syndrome	Increased 3 to 20 times upper limit
Sclerosing cholangitis	Increased 50 to 100 times upper limit
PFIC types I and II	Normal or decreased
PFIC type III	Increased
Bile acid disorders	Normal

GGT, Gamma-glutamyl transferase; PFIC, progressive familial cholestasis.

obtained, which showed intrahepatic cholestasis with proliferation of the bile ducts. Is the evaluation now complete for making a definitive diagnosis?
The evaluation is very suggestive of biliary atresia; however, the gold standard diagnostic test is an intraoperative cholangiogram. Other causes of neonatal cholestasis such as Alagille syndrome may clinically mimic biliary atresia and may be differentiated only by intraoperative cholangiogram.

170. **What are the causes of extrahepatic neonatal cholestasis?**
In general, these lesions lead to the extrahepatic obstruction of bile flow from the liver to the duodenum. These processes lead to bile buildup in the duct, causing inflammation and damage to the liver. The result is elevations of GGT and ALK consistent with biliary duct damage and varying degrees of elevation of liver enzymes and direct hyperbilirubinemia. Examples of extrahepatic bile duct disorders include the following:
- Biliary atresia
- Choledochal cyst and choledochocele
- Biliary hyperplasia
- Bile duct perforation
- Neonatal sclerosing cholangitis

171. **What are the causes of pediatric elevations of GGT?**
See Table 10-12.

172. **Why is it critical to make an early diagnosis of biliary atresia?**
The effectiveness of surgical therapy (Kasai procedure) for biliary atresia depends on the patient's age at surgery. Best outcomes are achieved when intervention occurs before 8 to 10 weeks of age. Biliary atresia is the leading indication for liver transplantation in children.

173. **A 10-week-old, former 34-week premature, breastfed boy was referred for evaluation of jaundice and elevated liver enzymes. His test results indicated a conjugated bilirubin, 3.8 mg/dL; ALK 650 U/L; AST, 120 U/L; ALT, 138 U/L; and GGT, 1200 U/L. During the newborn period he had mild respiratory distress syndrome, was treated for sepsis, and received TPN for 7 days. He was discharged home on breast-milk feeds at the age of 3 weeks. How should the evaluation proceed?**
The laboratory results show a disproportionately elevated serum GGT and ALK as well as a high conjugated bilirubin level, all of which suggest biliary disease. However, because the clinical manifestations of neonatal cholestasis are independent of the etiology, the initial basic evaluation should be broad, as previously described in Table 10-10.

174. **A careful physical examination revealed that the patient in Question 173 had a prominent forehead, small chin, and a systolic heart murmur consistent with peripheral pulmonary stenosis. The ultrasound yielded normal results. The**

DISIDA scan showed excretion at 24 hours. Is this sufficient for making the diagnosis of Alagille syndrome?

A liver biopsy is necessary to confirm the diagnosis and differentiate this syndrome from biliary atresia. Alagille syndrome is also referred to as syndromic bile duct paucity. During infancy the histologic studies may show bile duct proliferation. However, in later childhood and adulthood the liver histology commonly shows bile duct paucity. The genetic defect has been identified as jagged 1 *(JAG1)* located on chromosome 20p12. Inheritance occurs in an autosomal dominant pattern. Alagille syndrome is the most common form of familial intrahepatic cholestasis and consists of five characteristics:

- Chronic cholestasis: associated with hypercholesterolemia and paucity of intralobular bile ducts
- Congenital heart disease: most commonly peripheral pulmonic stenosis
- Bone defects: commonly butterfly vertebrae
- Eye findings: posterior embryotoxon
- Typical facies: frontal bossing, deep-set eyes, bulbous tip of nose, and pointed chin

Turnpenny PD, Ellard S. Alagille syndrome: pathogenesis, diagnosis and management. Eur J Hum Genet 2012;20(3):251–7.

✓ KEY POINTS: LIVER DISEASE

1. Direct hyperbilirubinemia is always abnormal.

2. The key to the evaluation of an infant with cholestatic jaundice requires early assessment for treatable causes and surgical intervention if biliary atresia is confirmed.

3. Significant hypoglycemia or coagulopathy in an infant with cholestatic jaundice may be an important sign of significant hepatocellular disease.

4. Do not forget silent urinary tract infection as an important, treatable cause of cholestatic jaundice in the infant.

---

175. **What clinical conditions are associated with cholelithiasis?**
- Hemolytic disease
- TPN
- Diuretic use
- Short gut syndrome
- Small bowel bacterial overgrowth
- Sepsis

176. **What are common mistakes in the evaluation of an infant with neonatal cholestasis?**
- Attributing all jaundice beyond the physiologic period in healthy infants to breast milk
- Not obtaining a fractionated bilirubin
- Not performing the basic evaluation in an expedited fashion
- Relying only on the clinical history and physical examination to make a diagnosis
- Delaying referral to a specialist

177. **What is extrahepatic biliary atresia?**
Extrahepatic biliary atresia is the term given to idiopathic progressive obliteration or discontinuity of the extrahepatic biliary tree in infancy. The process is a progressive destruction of the biliary tree. Two forms are recognized, depending on when the obliteration occurs.
The embryonic/fetal type of biliary atresia occurs in 10% to 35% of cases:
- Direct hyperbilirubinemia present at birth without any true jaundice-free period after physiologic jaundice
- More often associated with congenital malformations
- Bile duct remnants often not seen at time of surgery

The perinatal type of biliary atresia occurs in 65% to 90% of cases:
- Direct hyperbilirubinemia occurs at 4 to 8 weeks of age.
- There is a jaundice-free period after physiologic jaundice.
- Bile duct remnants are often seen at the time of surgery.

Hinds R, Davenport M, Mieli-Vergani G, et al. Antenatal presentation of biliary atresia. J Pediatr 2004;144:43–6.

178. What are the demographics of extrahepatic biliary atresia?

Extrahepatic biliary atresia occurs in 1 in 10,000 to 15,000 live births, with females affected 1.4 times more frequently than males. Approximately 10% to 20% of infants with biliary atresia will have associated anomalies (syndromic biliary atresia), including splenic abnormalities (polysplenia or asplenia), malrotation, and situs inversus.

179. What are the typical presenting clinical features of an infant with extrahepatic biliary atresia?

The usual presentation is that of an otherwise healthy infant who develops jaundice between 4 and 8 weeks of age. If an infant appears ill (e.g., vomiting, acidosis, failure to thrive), metabolic (nonobstructive) causes of jaundice should be considered promptly.

180. What are the typical radiographic findings in extrahepatic biliary atresia?

- Ultrasound: Hepatic parenchyma is often normal, and the gallbladder and common bile duct are generally not visualized. It is important to note that the gallbladder may not be visualized in healthy infants because of contraction; failure to visualize the gallbladder should not be considered evidence of biliary atresia. The main purpose of ultrasound in this setting is to rule out an obstructing choledochal cyst.
- DISIDA scan: There should be uptake of the radiotracer by the hepatic parenchyma, although uptake may be delayed secondary to associated hepatocyte injury. In biliary atresia absolutely no contrast will reach the bowel after 12 to 24 hours but instead will ultimately appear in the kidneys and urinary bladder as it is cleared through the urinary tract.

181. What are the typical histopathologic findings in extrahepatic biliary atresia?

Liver biopsy is the final step in preoperative diagnosis of biliary atresia. The biopsy will demonstrate proliferation of bile ducts and bile plugs in response to extrahepatic obstruction. The main purpose of the biopsy is to differentiate between obstructive and nonobstructive causes of cholestasis. A variable amount of fibrosis is also present, the degree of which depends on the age of the infant and the rapidity of disease progression.

182. How do the radiologic and histopathologic findings in biliary atresia compare with those of neonatal hepatitis?

See Table 10-13.

183. What is the natural history of untreated biliary atresia?

- Untreated biliary atresia is uniformly fatal within 2 years, with a median survival of 8 months. Untreated biliary atresia leads to biliary cirrhosis, portal hypertension, esophageal varices, failure to thrive, and liver failure with subsequent death from any of a number of complications.

184. What is appropriate surgical and medical therapy for biliary atresia, and how does therapy affect survival?

- Surgical: If the liver biopsy suggests biliary atresia, the infant undergoes exploratory laparotomy and an intraoperative cholangiogram. If biliary atresia is confirmed, an attempt to restore biliary drainage using the Kasai procedure (i.e., hepatic portoenterostomy) is made. During the Kasai procedure a loop of bowel is anastomosed directly to the hepatic capsule at the porta hepatis after resection of the fibrous biliary remnants. Bowel continuity is restored by formation of a Roux-en-Y intestinal anastomosis. The success of the procedure depends on the age of the infant at the time of the operation and the experience of the surgeon. Long-term survival rates may exceed 60% for infants younger

TABLE 10-13.   BILIARY ATRESIA VERSUS NEONATAL HEPATITIS

IMAGING STUDY	BILIARY ATRESIA	NEONATAL HEPATITIS	OTHER DISORDERS OF INTEREST
Ultrasound	Nonvisualization of gallbladder, common bile duct	Normal gallbladder and common bile duct; echogenic liver	Choledochal cyst would show dilation of bile ducts
DISIDA scan	Good or delayed uptake without excretion into the bowel	Delayed uptake of trace with some excretion into the bowel	Spontaneous rupture of biliary tree would show bile leak.
Liver biopsy	Proliferation of the bile ducts, bile plugs in the ducts, fibrosis of portal tracts or hepatocytes, cirrhosis	Inflammation of the hepatic parenchyma, cholestasis, possible giant cell transformation, hepatic acini (rosettes), variable inflammation	PFICs would show chronic cholestasis without ductular proliferation, cirrhosis, variable portal fibrosis and giant cell transformation

PFIC, Progressive Familial Intrahepatic Cholestasis

than 2 months of age at the time of portoenterostomy, compared with only 25% for those older than 2 months of age. The first sign of a successful portoenterostomy is the passage of green (bile-stained) stools rather than the acholic stools seen preoperatively. A retrospective study of 81 patients in the United States noted a success rate of approximately 38% with the Kasai procedure alone.

■ Medical: Any child with biliary atresia, regardless of the status of portoenterostomy, should be treated for chronic liver disease and its potential complications. Infants should receive fat-soluble vitamin supplementation (vitamins A, D, E, and K). Many infants require supplemental tube feedings, particularly if the portoenterostomy is unsuccessful. Good nutritional status will optimize the infant's survival if liver transplantation becomes necessary. Medical treatment with steroids after the Kasai procedure has been found to be beneficial in many studies and is implemented in practice at various institutions.

Wildhaber BE, Coran AG, Drongowski RA, et al. The Kasai portoenterostomy for biliary atresia: a review of a 27-year experience with 81 patients. J Pediatr Surg 2003;38:1480–5.

185. What are the potential complications of the Kasai portoenterostomy?
Specific complications include failure to achieve drainage, ascending cholangitis where drainage is achieved, and biliary cysts at the portoenterostomy site.

186. What are the therapeutic options for children who do not undergo portoenterostomy or in whom drainage is not achieved?
Liver transplantation is the only definitive therapy and has an approximately 80% expected 5-year survival rate.

187. Other than biliary atresia, what are the causes of obstructive jaundice in infancy?
Choledochal cysts and spontaneous perforation of the extrahepatic biliary tree are two causes of obstructive jaundice in infancy. Cholelithiasis is not a major cause of biliary obstruction in infancy, although gallstones may be seen as incidental findings on ultrasound of premature infants and occasionally even on prenatal ultrasound.

188. What are the demographics and presentation of choledochal cysts?
Choledochal cysts are much less common than biliary atresia, with estimates of incidence ranging from 1 in 13,000 to 1 in 2,000,000 live births. Girls are affected four times more frequently than boys. The classic triad of abdominal pain, mass, and jaundice occurs in fewer than 20% of cases. Choledochal cysts may present as jaundice, mass, vomiting, fever, and even pancreatitis. Fewer than half of choledochal cysts present in infancy.

TABLE 10-14. COMMON ABDOMINAL MASSES IN NEONATES

MASS LOCATION	EXAMPLES	CHARACTERISTICS
Lateral	Renal cysts, hydronephrosis	Smooth, moderate mobility, transilluminates
	Renal tumor	Smooth, minimally mobile, does not transilluminate
	Neuroblastoma	Irregular contour, minimally mobile, frequently crosses midline
Midabdominal	Mesenteric cyst	Smooth, mobile, transilluminates
	Gastrointestinal duplication cyst	Smooth, mobile, does not transilluminate, associated with obstruction
	Ovarian cyst	Smooth, mobile, transilluminates
Upper abdominal	Hepatic tumors	Hard, immobile, do not transilluminate
	Choledochal cyst	Smooth, immobile, does not transilluminate, associated with jaundice
Lower abdominal	Hydrometrocolpos	Smooth, immobile, does not transilluminate, associated with imperforate hymen
	Urachal cyst	Smooth, fixed to abdominal wall, extends to umbilicus
	Sacrococcygeal teratoma	Hard, fixed, does not transilluminate, associated with external sacral component

189. **What are the types of choledochal cysts?**
   - Type I: diffuse enlargement of the common bile duct (the majority fall in this category)
   - Type II: diverticular cyst from the common bile duct
   - Type III: choledochocele
   - Type IV: multiple cysts of the intrahepatic and extrahepatic biliary tree
   - Type V: caroli disease or cystic dilation of the intrahepatic biliary tree

ABDOMINAL MASSES

190. **What is the origin of most neonatal abdominal masses?**
   More than half of all abdominal masses in the neonate arise from the urinary tract.

191. **List the two most common causes of abdominal masses of urologic origin in the neonate.**
   - Hydronephrosis secondary to ureteropelvic junction obstruction
   - Multicystic kidney disease

192. **A pregnant woman has an antenatal ultrasound scan that reveals an intraabdominal mass in the fetus. Are any special arrangements necessary for the timing and mode of delivery?**
   No.

193. **How do the location and other physical examination characteristics of the common abdominal masses in newborn infants provide clues for their identification?**
   Physical examination may significantly narrow the diagnostic possibilities, even if it does not provide an absolute answer (Table 10-14). Of note:
   - Large masses may fill the entire abdomen, making it impossible to determine the site of origin on examination and therefore requiring further imaging studes.
   - Hard, nodular masses are usually malignant tumors.
   - A highly mobile mass is usually a mesenteric cyst, a duplication, or an ovarian cyst.

CHAPTER 11

GENETICS

Wendy K. Chung, MD, PhD

1. **What are the most common major congenital anomalies in the United States?**
   Anencephaly and spina bifida, occurring with a prevalence of about 0.5 to 2 of 1000 live births, and congenital heart disease, with a prevalence of approximately 1%, are the most common.

Hoffman JI, Kaplan S. The incidence of congenital heart disease. J Am Coll Cardiol 2002;39:1890–1900.

2. **Should an asymptomatic infant with a single umbilical artery have a screening ultrasound scan done for renal anomalies?**
   This point has been argued for years. A single umbilical artery is a rare phenomenon. In one study of nearly 35,000 infants, examination of the placenta showed that only 112 (0.32%) had a single umbilical artery. All 112 underwent renal ultrasonography, and 17% had abnormalities (45% of which persisted). A more recent study demonstrated that left umbilical arteries tend to be absent more often than right umbilical arteries when only a single artery is present. In addition, there was a high incidence of associated congenital malformations in nearly 25% of the infants diagnosed prenatally with a single umbilical artery. Because of the rarity of the condition and the increased association of abnormalities, patients with single umbilical arteries probably should receive a screening renal ultrasound.

Murphy-Kaulbeck L, Dodds L, Joseph KS, et al. Single umbilical artery risk factors and pregnancy outcomes. Obstet Gynecol 2010;116(4):843–50.

3. **Excluding chromosomal analysis, what laboratory test results suggest that a woman is carrying a fetus with trisomy 21 syndrome?**
   There is some variation in the sensitivity of the screening methods, depending on the tests used and the timing of the screening. Maternal serum alpha-fetoprotein (AFP), unconjugated estriol (uE3), and human chorionic gonadotropin (hCG) make up the "triple test" and the addition of inhibin A makes up the "quadruple screen." Maternal serum pregnancy–associated plasma protein (PAPP)-A and free beta-hCG are used at 11 to 13 weeks along with nuchal translucency followed by maternal serum AFP, hCG, uE3, and inhibin at 15 to 18 weeks of gestation to provide an integrated first- and second-trimester screen with a sensitivity of 91% and 4.5% false-positive results. Absent fetal nasal bone is another marker under investigation for Down syndrome screening.

   Recently a new test has been developed that analyzes circulating cell-free DNA extracted from a maternal blood sample. The test detects an increased representation of chromosome 21 material, which is associated with trisomy 21. The Down syndrome detection rate was 98.6% with a false-positive rate of 0.20% This test is not recommended for population-based screening but may be used for women who screen positive on serum screening before proceeding to an invasive diagnostic test.

Palomaki GE, Kloza EM, Lambert-Messerlian GM, et al. DNA sequencing of maternal plasma to detect Down syndrome: an international clinical validation. Genet Med 2011;13(11):913–20.

Cuckle HS, Malone FD, Wright D, et al. Contingent screening for Down syndrome—results from the FaSTER trial. Prenat Diagn 2008;28(2):89–94.

4. **Which other conditions may be detected by a raised amniotic fluid AFP level?**
   - Multiple gestation
   - Intrauterine fetal death
   - Omphalocele and gastroschisis
   - Bowel and esophageal atresias
   - Turner syndrome (cystic hygroma)
   - Meckel syndrome
   - Congenital nephrosis (Finnish type)
   - Sacrococcygeal teratoma
   - Bladder exstrophy
   - Focal dermal hypoplasia or aplasia cutis congenita

5. **A woman had a positive serum screen in the second trimester and normal fetal ultrasound results but declined amniocentesis. She delivers a healthy-appearing infant. What further studies are indicated given the triple screen?**
   None. A positive triple screen is a screening test, not a diagnostic test. If the infant looks healthy without features of Down syndrome or other anomalies, no further testing is necessary. Chromosome tests do not need to be performed on a normal-appearing infant just because the triple test result was abnormal.

6. **How would you evaluate a newborn with Down syndrome to ensure you are discharging a healthy infant? What serious abnormalities are likely?**
   - Order a chromosome study on peripheral blood (G-banding) to rule out translocation or mosaicism.
   - Perform a cardiac evaluation (40% of infants with Down syndrome have congenital heart disease, with the most common defect being an atrioventricular canal).
   - Ensure there is no bowel obstruction. Duodenal atresia, duodenal web, and Hirschsprung disease are more common in Down syndrome. Anal stenosis may mimic Hirschsprung disease.
   - Assess hearing.
   - Monitor feeding and sucking.
   - Perform a thyroid screen (included in all newborn screens automatically).
   - Refer for genetic counseling and early intervention.

✓ KEY POINTS: COMMON CAUSES OF BIRTH DEFECTS

1. Chromosomal disorders (aneuploidy, deletions, duplications)

2. Maternal diabetes

3. Insufficient maternal micronutrients (folic acid and neural tube defects)

4. Teratogenic exposures

5. Maternal infection

6. Inborn errors of metabolism

7. Monogenic disorders

8. Multifactorial (cleft lip and cleft palate)

9. Developmental deformation

10. Developmental disruption

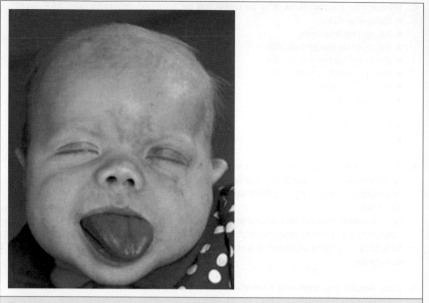

Figure 11-1. Beckwith–Wiedemann Syndrome. Macroglossia can be significant in babies with Beckwith–Wiedemann Syndrome

7. **A macrosomic infant is born with an omphalocele and large tongue. What would you anticipate monitoring closely in this baby, and why?**
   This baby may have Beckwith–Wiedemann syndrome and may be at risk for hypoglycemia. Other signs of Beckwith–Wiedemann syndrome include grooves or pits on the ear lobes, hemihypertrophy, and visceromegaly (Fig. 11-1). These children are at risk for Wilms tumor and hepatoblastoma and should be monitored with an abdominal ultrasound and AFP testing every 4 months for the first 6 years of life.

8. **Are there any known factors that increase the risk of having a child with Beckwith–Wiedemann syndrome?**
   Yes, *in vitro* fertilization is associated with an increased risk of Beckwith–Wiedemann syndrome and other rare imprinting disorders.

9. **What is the difference between an omphalocele and gastroschisis?**
   Omphalocele:
   - This midline anterior abdominal well defect is covered by a transparent sac consisting of amnion and peritoneum with Wharton jelly between them.
   - Intraabdominal viscera is herniated through the umbilical ring. The size varies with contents.
   - The umbilical cord inserts into the sac.
   - Other malformations are present in 67% of cases.
   - This defect can be associated with chromosome abnormalities, especially trisomy 13.
   Gastroschisis:
   - The umbilical cord is attached to the abdominal wall to the left of the defect. There is a normal umbilical cord insertion.
   - Herniated organs usually consist of thickened loops of small intestine with no membranous covering. The intestine floats freely in the amniotic fluid *in utero*.
   - In 15% of cases, gastroschisis is associated with other major malformations.
   - It is not commonly found in fetuses with chromosome abnormalities.

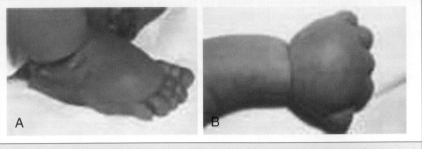

Figure 11-2. Lymphedema is often visible in the feet (**A**) and hands (**B**) at birth in girls with Turner syndrome.

10. **What are the most common syndromes associated with congenital diaphragmatic hernia?**
    Congenital diaphragmatic hernia is an associated inherited condition in the following syndromes:
    - Fryns syndrome
    - Donnai-Barrow syndrome
    - Cornelia de Lange syndrome
    - Beckwith–Wiedemann syndrome
    - Simpson–Golabi–Behmel syndrome
    - Denys–Drash syndrome
    - Pallister–Killian syndrome (mosaic tetrasomy 12p)
    - Perlman syndrome
    - Aneuploidy and chromosomal disorders, including numerous microdeletions and microduplication

11. **A female infant is born with the following features: puffiness of the dorsum of the hands and feet, excessive skin at the nape of the neck with a low posterior hairline, and a broad chest and widely spaced nipples. What is the differential diagnosis?**
    - Turner syndrome (Fig. 11-2)
    - Noonan syndrome

12. **How would you work up the baby in Question 11?**
    - Chromosome study on peripheral blood (G-banding)
    - Genetic testing for Noonan syndrome if chromosomes are normal
    - Cardiac evaluation, including echocardiogram
    - Renal ultrasound
    - Referral for genetic counseling and early intervention

✓ KEY POINTS: PRINCIPLES OF BIRTH DEFECTS

1. Single minor anomalies such as an isolated simian crease are common and not necessarily associated with an underlying genetic problem. However, as the number of minor anomalies increases, the likelihood of an underlying genetic diagnosis also increases.

2. Susceptibility for some birth defects such as cleft lip and palate are multifactorial and caused by a combination of genetic and environmental factors.

3. The findings of intrauterine growth restriction or birth defects (or both) should warrant investigation into genetic, infectious, and teratogenic etiologies.

4. The most common birth defect is a neural tube defect.

13. **How do you perform genetic testing for Noonan syndrome?**
Noonan syndrome overlaps with LEOPARD, cardiofaciocutaneous, and Costello syndromes. All are autosomal dominant disorders typically caused by gain-of-function mutations in genes encoding signaling molecules of the RAS/MAPK pathway *(PTPN11, RAF1, SOS1, KRAS, BRAF, MAP2K1, MAP2K2, HRAS, NRAS, CBL, SHOC2)*. Genetic testing can be performed on a blood sample and ideally should include testing for this panel of genes to maximize the sensitivity to make the diagnosis. Identification of a specific mutation will provide some prognostic information about risk of arrhythmias, cardiomyopathy, and learning or intellectual disabilities. Genetic testing will also provide the family with important information about the risk of recurrence within the family. Noonan syndrome is autosomal dominantly inherited, but for cases diagnosed prenatally or neonatally, many result from *de novo* mutations.

14. **Can Noonan syndrome be diagnosed prenatally, and if so, what are the most common prenatal features?**
Yes, the panel of 11 genes can be tested prenatally for Noonan syndrome using either a chorionic villus or amniocentesis sample. The most common ultrasound findings are increased nuchal translucency or cystic hygroma.

15. **How is fetal growth restriction defined?**
Fetal growth restriction is the failure of a fetus to achieve its growth potential. In practice, measures of size relative to the population mean for gestational age and sex are used. Fetal growth retardation is variably defined as an infant who is either below the 10th percentile or less than two standard deviations (SDs) below the population mean for that gestational age and sex.

16. **Intrauterine growth restriction (IUGR) has many causes. What approach would you use to evaluate a newborn with IUGR?**
   - Establish whether the growth restriction is proportionate or disproportionate.
   - Perform a detailed physical examination for anomalies or dysmorphic features.
   - If dysmorphic or multiple anomalies are present, chromosome studies are indicated.
   - Take a detailed pregnancy history to look for teratogenic exposures, smoking, infection history, or maternal illness (e.g., hypertension and preeclampsia).
   - Viral studies and antibody titers should be ordered as indicated.
   - Uncontrolled maternal phenylketonuria can be associated with IUGR and microcephaly.
   - An infant with disproportionate IUGR should be worked up for skeletal dysplasia or metabolic bone disease.
   - Proportionate IUGR may be associated with many dysmorphic syndromes that may be recognized by a geneticist.
   - Placental examination for size and infarction and placental genetic studies should be performed for confined placental mosaicism and uniparental disomy (UPD).

17. **What is confined placental mosaicism?**
The abnormal cell line in this condition is "confined" either to the cytotrophoblast or chorionic stroma cells of the placenta and is not present in the fetus itself. This situation may be discovered when an abnormal karyotype results from chorionic villous sampling (CVS) reflecting the placenta, but the fetus appears to be healthy and amniocentesis is normal. The diagnosis of confined placental mosaicism postnatally is usually made retrospectively by follow-up studies on the infant or fetus, placenta, and membranes. Confined placental mosaicism may be associated with growth impairment in chromosomally normal fetuses. It may increase the risk of a spontaneous abortion. Overall, there appears to be a low risk of adverse pregnancy outcome with confined placental mosaicism.

18. **What is uniparental disomy (UPD)?**
UPD occurs when both members of a chromosome pair are derived solely from one parent in a diploid offspring. Many cases of UPD are the result of resolved trisomies in which the embryo was initially trisomic but lost one of the extra chromosomes and ended up with two chromosomes from

the same parent. The disomy may be two copies of the same chromosome (i.e., isodisomy) or one copy of each of the given parent's chromosomes (i.e., heterodisomy).

19. **What conditions are associated with UPD?**
    - Maternal UPD 15 is associated with Prader–Willi syndrome, whereas paternal UPD 15 is associated with Angelman syndrome.
    - Paternal UPD 11 is associated with Beckwith–Wiedemann syndrome.
    - Maternal UPD 7 has been seen in some cases of Russell–Silver syndrome.
    - Paternal UPD 6 causes growth retardation (sometimes severe) and transient neonatal diabetes.
    - Maternal UPD 16 is associated with growth retardation and variable congenital anomalies but a generally good prognosis.

20. **What conditions are commonly diagnosed by fluorescent *in situ* hybridization (FISH)?**
    - DiGeorge syndrome
    - Williams syndrome
    - Prader–Willi syndrome
    - Angelman syndrome
    - Wilms tumor, aniridia, genitourinary anomalies, and retarded growth and development (i.e., WAGR syndrome)
    - Kallmann syndrome
    - Smith–Magenis syndrome
    - Miller–Dieker syndrome

21. **Can microdeletion syndromes such as DiGeorge syndrome be detected by a routine karyotype?**
    Whereas large deletions (greater than 5 megabases in size) are sometimes detectable on a karyotype, submicroscopic deletions cannot be visualized even on high-resolution chromosome banding. These deletions can be detected by FISH. In this technique a DNA probe specific for the chromosomal region of interest is hybridized to the chromosomes. A fluorescent signal is attached to the probe so that the number of copies of the DNA corresponding to the probe can be determined for each cell. Normally, two copies of each region, one on each chromosome, should be present. If a deletion has occurred, only one of the copies will be seen. FISH is not always reliable for detecting duplications, however. This technique has aided in the diagnosis of microdeletion syndromes that were once difficult to detect because of their small size.

22. **When is FISH most useful in clinical practice?**
    An example of the use of FISH is for rapid prenatal diagnosis of trisomies on amniotic fluid or chorionic villi, using interphase cells from cultured specimens and probes for the most common chromosomal abnormalities (13, 18, 21, X, and Y). Although interphase FISH for prenatal diagnosis has low false-positive and false-negative rates, it is considered investigational and is used only in conjunction with standard cytogenetic analysis. FISH is also useful in diagnosing the microdeletion genetic syndromes noted in Question 20.

✓ KEY POINTS: CHROMOSOMAL DEFECTS

1. The risk of aneuploidy increases with advanced maternal age; however, most aneuploid births are to mothers who are not of advanced maternal age. The majority of trisomies are a result of maternal meiotic errors; however, almost half of Klinefelter cases are caused by errors in paternal meiosis.

2. Screening for Down syndrome with a combination of noninvasive ultrasound markers of nuchal translucency and maternal serum markers allows for greater than 95% sensitivity in detecting Down syndrome.

Continued

✓ KEY POINTS: CHROMOSOMAL DEFECTS—cont'd

3. Microdeletions are too small to be resolved by a karyotype and require fluorescence *in situ* hybridization. The majority are *de novo* and not inherited. They are associated with a variety of clinical syndromes such as DiGeorge syndrome, Williams syndrome, Angelman syndrome, Miller–Dieker syndrome, Smith–Magenis syndrome, and Kallmann syndrome.

4. Balanced translocations have the total correct amount of DNA. If the balanced translocation is inherited, the phenotype in the child is predicted to be that of the balanced translocation carrier parent. If the translocation is *de novo*, there is an approximately 15% chance it will be associated with a phenotypic consequence such as a birth defect, cognitive impairment, or medical problem.

5. UPD means that for one set of chromosomes, both chromosomes were inherited from the same parent. If genes on that chromosome are imprinted, this can produce specific clinical symptoms, such as Prader–Willi syndrome. UPD cannot be detected by a standard karyotype but can be detected with other molecular genetic techniques.

23. **What is a chromosome microarray? To whom should this test be offered?**
This is analogous to series of thousands of FISH probe panels that cover all known microdeletion and microduplication syndromes and can detect deletions or duplications of at least 1 megabase on all the chromosomes to detect genomic imbalances. The resolution of the chromosome microarray varies by laboratory, and higher and lower density arrays are available depending on the needs of the clinical situation. All fetuses with major anomalies or IUGR should be offered this test. Patients with dysmorphic features, major congenital anomalies, developmental delay, intellectual disability, seizures, and failure to thrive should have this test.

24. **For a newborn baby with congenital heart disease and a diaphragmatic hernia, which test should you order first, a karyotype or a chromosome microarray?**
Chromosome microarray is now considered the first line test to evaluate chromosomes. The only anomalies missed by a chromosome microarray are balanced translocations and low levels of mosaicism, but the prevalence of these types of chromosomal disorders is low.

Miller DT, Adam MP, Aradhya S, et al. Consensus statement: chromosomal microarray is a first-tier clinical diagnostic test for individuals with developmental disabilities or congenital anomalies. Am J Hum Genet 2010;86(5):749–64.

25. **The geneticist cannot be reached, and you have to evaluate an intrauterine fetal demise. What do you do?**
   - Obtain the pregnancy history and a family history.
   - Take photographs and obtain an x-ray (i.e., babygram) of the fetus.
   - Do a detailed clinical exam of the fetus.
   - Perform a skin biopsy for fibroblasts to allow chromosome studies, genetic studies, and possible metabolic studies.
   - Examine the placenta and culture the placenta or fetal membranes if available.
   - If possible, obtain blood samples from the cord or perform a cardiac puncture for immunoglobulin M and cultures if you suspect a congenital infection.
   - Obtain autopsy permission (freeze liver, heart, and muscle from autopsy for additional metabolic studies, if indicated).

26. **What is anophthalmia?**
Anophthalmia is the medical term used to describe the absence of the globe and ocular tissue from the orbit. Anophthalmia and microphthalmia are often used interchangeably because, in most cases, the magnetic resonance imaging (MRI) or computed tomography (CT) scan shows some remnants of either the globe or surrounding tissue. Anophthalmia may be unilateral or bilateral and is often

associated with other anomalies. There are many causes of anophthalmia including single gene mutations, syndromes, chromosome abnormalities, and teratogenic exposures. Anophthalmia is rare, with an incidence of about 1 in 10,000.

27. **How would you evaluate a newborn with anophthalmia?**
    - Ophthalmology evaluation and referral to an oculoplastic surgeon and ocularist
    - CT scan or MRI of brain and globe to determine whether any ocular tissue is present and whether the optic nerve is present; brain anomalies may help point to a specific diagnosis
    - Genetic evaluation
    - Renal ultrasound
    - Chromosome study, G-banding
    - Referral to early intervention and nearest school for the blind

28. **What are the main advantages of CVS over amniocentesis?**
    CVS is the aspiration of chorionic villi through a transcervical catheter or transabdominal needle using ultrasound guidance. The main advantage of CVS is that it can be done between 10 and 12 weeks of gestation compared with the usual 16-week timing for amniocentesis. This permits the termination of pregnancy at a significantly earlier date in the event of major chromosomal or genetic anomalies. CVS does not permit analysis of the amniotic fluid AFP levels, so screening for neural tube defects must be performed with maternal serum AFP and ultrasound.

29. **What are the major characteristics of the three major chromosomal malformations: trisomy 21, trisomy 18, and trisomy 13?**
    See Table 11-1.

29. **What is the chance that a newborn with a simian crease has Down syndrome?**
    A single transverse palmar crease is present in 4% of normal newborns. Bilateral palmar creases are found in 1%. These features occur twice as commonly in males than in females. However, 50% to 55% of newborn infants with Down syndrome have a single transverse crease. Because Down syndrome occurs in 1 of every 800 live births, the chance that a newborn with a simian crease has Down syndrome is only 1 in 60.

30. **What is the expected intelligence and personality of a child with Down syndrome?**
    The IQ range is generally 35 to 65, with a mean reported IQ of 54. Occasionally the IQ may be higher. Intelligence deteriorates in adulthood, with clinical and pathologic findings consistent with advanced Alzheimer disease. Autopsy results from the brains of deceased adults with Down syndrome reveal both neurofibrillary tangles and senile plaques, as found in Alzheimer disease. By age 40 the mean IQ is 24. Children with Down syndrome are generally affectionate and docile. They tend toward mimicry and are noted usually to enjoy music, having a good sense of rhythm. However, 13% have serious emotional problems, and their coordination is usually poor.

31. **Why was the maternal age of 35 years at delivery chosen as the cutoff for recommending amniocentesis for chromosome analysis, and is this still relevant?**
    There is a well-known association between advanced maternal age and trisomies (including XXY; XXX; and trisomies 13, 18, and 21). Most cases of Down syndrome involve nondisjunction at meiosis I in the mother. This may be related to the lengthy stage of meiotic arrest between oocyte development in the fetus and ovulation, which may occur as many as 40 years later (Table 11-2). With the advent of multiple noninvasive methods to screen for aneuploidies, invasive testing is driven more by results on the screening tests rather than maternal age alone.

TABLE 11-1. COMMON AUTOSOMAL TRISOMIES

	TRISOMY 21	TRISOMY 18	TRISOMY 13
Eponym	Down syndrome	Edward syndrome	Patau syndrome
Live-born incidence	Hypotonia	Hypertonia	Hypotonia or hypertonia
Tone	1/800	1/8000	1/15,000
Cranium/brain	Mild microencephaly, flat occiput, three fontanels	Microcephaly, prominent occiput	Microcephaly, sloping forehead, occipital scalp defects holoprosencephaly
Eyes	Upslanting, epicanthal folds, speckled iris (Brushfield spots)	Small palpebral fissures, corneal opacity	Microphthalmia hypotelorism, iris coloboma, retinal dysplasia
Ears	Small, low-set, over-folded upper helix	Low-set, malformed	Low-set, malformed
Facial features	Protruding tongue; large cheeks; low, flat nasal bridge	Small mouth, micrognathia	Cleft lip and palate
Skeletal	Clinodactyly fifth digit, gap between toes 1 and 2, excessive nuchal skin, short stature	Clenched hand, absent fifth finger distal crease, hypoplastic nails, short stature, thin ribs	Postaxial polydactyly, hypoconvex fingernails, clenched hands
Cardiac defect	40%	60%	80%
Survival	Long-term	90% die in first year	80% die in first year
Other	Abnormal palate, single palmar crease (i.e., simian crease)	Rocker bottom feet, dermatoglyphic arch pattern	Polycystic kidneys

TABLE 11-2. ASSOCIATION BETWEEN MATERNAL AGE AND RISK OF TRISOMY 21 SYNDROME

MATERNAL AGE (YEARS)	APPROXIMATE RISK
30	1/1000
35	1/365
40	1/100
45	1/50

32. **What percentage of babies with Down syndrome are born to women over the age of 35?**

Only 34% of babies are born to mothers older than 35 years of age. Although their individual risk is higher, women in this age bracket account for only 5% of all pregnancies in the United States.

Olsen CL, Cross PK, Gensburg LJ, et al. The effects of prenatal diagnosis, population ageing, and changing fertility rates on the live birth prevalence of Down syndrome in New York State, 1983-1992. Prenat Diagn;16(11):991–1002.

33. **What percentage of cases of Down syndrome are caused by translocations?**
Of all cases of Down syndrome, 3.3% are caused by unbalanced Robertsonian translocations in which a third copy of chromosome 21 is present, attached to an acrocentric chromosome. The chance of translocation Down syndrome is two to three times greater in children of younger mothers (6% to 8% of mothers younger than 30). One of three infants with translocation Down syndrome will have a parent with a Robertsonian translocation. Two thirds of the time, translocation Down syndrome occurs as a *de novo* event in the infant.

34. **What is the overall recurrence risk of Down syndrome?**
The answer depends on the chromosome complement of the parents. In chromosomally normal women under the age of 40, the recurrence risk for Down syndrome after having had one fetus or baby with Down syndrome is 1% (assuming the father's chromosomes are also normal). When the mother is older than age 40, the risk of having a child with Down syndrome increases, primarily as a function of her age. If the mother carries a translocation, the recurrence risk is 10% to 15%. If the father carries a transloca-tion, the recurrence risk is 2% to 5%. One theory for this observed discrepancy between maternal and paternal rates of translocation Down syndrome is hindered motility of chromosomally abnormal sperm. If either parent is balanced and carries a 21;21 translocation, the recurrence risk for that parent is 100%.

35. **With what genetic abnormality is advanced paternal age associated?**
Advanced paternal age is associated with *de novo* point mutations in all genes.

✓ KEY POINTS: MONOGENIC CONDITIONS

1. Genetic susceptibility to some neurologic conditions that are dominantly inherited is due to expan-sion of triplet repeats. The likelihood of repeat expansions depends on the sex of the transmitting parent and is specific to each disease. For instance, triplet repeats in the gene for myotonic dystro-phy are more likely to expand when transmitted maternally, whereas the triplet repeats in the gene for Huntington disease are more likely to expand when transmitted paternally.

2. Most monogenic conditions affecting children are autosomal recessively inherited.

3. Genes encoding mitochondrial proteins can be found either in the mitochondrial genome and be maternally inherited or in the nuclear genome and autosomal recessively inherited.

4. Genetic mosaicism may be detectable by differences in skin pigmentation that appear as swirls.

5. Genetic testing is currently clinically available for more than 2500 disorders.

36. **What genetically inherited disease has the highest known mutation rate per gamete per generation?**
Neurofibromatosis. The estimated mutation rate for this disorder is 1×10^4 per haploid genome. The clinical features are café-au-lait spots and axillary freckling in childhood, followed by development of neurofibromas in later years. Learning disabilities are common in *NF1*.

37. **Which disorders with ethnic and racial predilections most commonly warrant maternal screening for carrier status?**
See Table 11-3.

38. **Why are mitochondrially encoded disorders transmitted from generation to generation by the mother and not the father?**
Mitochondrial DNA abnormalities (e.g., many cases of ragged red fiber myopathies) are passed on from the mother because mitochondria are present in the cytoplasm of the egg and not the sperm. Transmission to male or female offspring is equally likely; however, expression can be variable

TABLE 11-3.	SCREENING FOR GENETIC DISORDERS	
DISORDER	**ETHNIC GROUP**	**TEST**
Tay–Sachs disease	Ashkenazi Jewish, French Canadian	Hexosaminidase A enzymatic testing and genetic testing
Sickle cell disease	African, Black, Hispanic, Arab, Indian, Mediterranean	Hemoglobin electrophoresis
Alpha- and beta-thalassemia	Mediterranean, southern southeastern Asian, Chinese	MCV <80
Cystic fibrosis	All ethnicities; more common among Caucasians	Genetic testing for the common mutations

within a family because of heteroplasmy with normal and abnormal mitochondria in differing proportions in different family members.

DiMauro S, Schon EA. Mitochondrial respiratory-chain diseases. N Engl J Med 2003;348(26):2656–68.

39. **Are all mitochondrial diseases encoded by DNA in the mitochondria?**
No. Many of the proteins found in the mitochondria are encoded within the nucleus. Those encoded within the nuclear genome are most commonly autosomal recessively inherited. They are still referred to as mitochondrial or oxidative phosphorylation defects and tend to result in more similar manifestations among affected family members.

40. **Which syndromes are associated with advanced paternal age?**
Advanced paternal age is associated with new dominant mutations. The assumption is that the increased mutation rate is caused by accumulation of new mutations from many cell divisions in the spermatid as men age. The more cell divisions, the more likely that an error (mutation) will occur. The mutation rate in fathers older than 50 years is five times higher than the mutation rate in fathers younger than 20 years of age. New, common autosomal dominant mutations that are often the result of *de novo* mutations are achondroplasia, craniosynostosis, neurofibromatosis, and Marfan syndrome.

Goriely A, Wilkie AO. Paternal age effect mutations and selfish spermatogonial selection: causes and consequences for human disease. Am J Hum Genet 2012;90(2):175–200.

41. **What is the most common genetic disease that is lethal without intervention within the first year of life?**
The most common is spinal muscular atrophy, an autosomal recessively inherited disease of the anterior motor neuron associated with decreased reflexes and progressive neuromuscular degeneration.

42. **What is the H₃O of Prader–Willi syndrome?**
Hyperphagia, hypotonia, hypogonadism, and obesity. Up to 75% of patients have a paternal microdeletion on the long arm of chromosome 15. The gene or genes responsible for Prader–Willi syndrome are subject to parental imprinting. Imprinting is the process by which expression of a gene depends on whether it has been inherited from the mother or the father. The gene or genes associated with Prader–Willi syndrome are maternally imprinted or maternally silenced, meaning that loss of the paternal copy will result in the phenotype of Prader–Willi (Fig. 11-3) because only the father's copy is active. A closely related area of the long arm of chromosome 15 is maternally imprinted, and loss of the maternal copy leads to Angelman syndrome. Angelman syndrome is characterized by severe

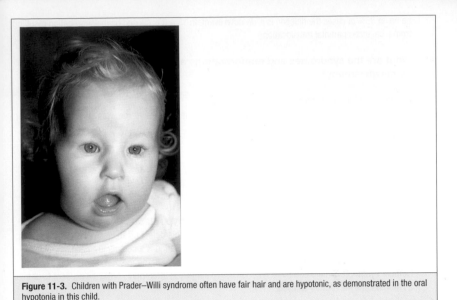

Figure 11-3. Children with Prader–Willi syndrome often have fair hair and are hypotonic, as demonstrated in the oral hypotonia in this child.

developmental delay; abnormal ataxic gait; seizures; inappropriate laughter; and jerking movements, especially of the arms.

Cassidy SB, Schwartz S, Miller JL, et al. Prader-Willi syndrome. Genet Med 2012;14(1):10–26.
Buiting K. Prader-Willi syndrome and Angelman syndrome. Am J Med Genet C Semin Med Genet 2010;154C(3):365–76.
Williams CA, Driscoll DJ, Dagli AI. Clinical and genetic aspects of Angelman syndrome. Genet Med 2010;12(7):385–95.

43. Name the two most common forms of dwarfism recognizable at birth.

Twenty-one different skeletal dysplasia syndromes were classified at the International Nomenclature of Constitutional Diseases of Bone meeting as recognizable at birth. The most common is thanatophoric dwarfism, a lethal chondrodysplasia characterized by flattened, U-shaped vertebral bodies, telephone receiver–shaped femurs, macrocephaly, and redundant skin folds causing a puglike appearance. Thanatophoric means death-loving, and this is a lethal disorder. The incidence is 1 in 6400 births.

Achondroplasia is the most common viable skeletal dysplasia, occurring 1 in 26,000 live births. Its features are short stature (mean adult height, 4 feet 2 inches), macrocephaly, depressed nasal bridge, lordosis, and a trident hand. Some patients develop hydrocephalus because of a small foramen magnum. Radiographic findings include narrowing of the interpedicular distance as one proceeds caudally. Both achondroplasia and thanatophoric dysplasia are due to mutations in fibroblast growth factor receptor 3. In achondroplasia the mutation is in the transmembrane domain, whereas the mutation in thanatophoric dysplasia is either in the intracellular domain (type 2) or in the extracellular domain (type 1).

Tavormina PL, Shiang R, Thompson LM, et al. Thanatophoric dysplasia (types 1 and 2) caused by mutations in fibroblast growth factor receptor 3. Nature Gen 1995;9:321–8.

44. What chromosomal abnormality is found in cri du chat syndrome and what are the clinical features?

Cri du chat syndrome is due to a deletion of material from the short arm of chromosome 5 (i.e., 5p-) that causes many problems, including growth retardation, microcephaly, and severe mental retardation. Patients have a characteristic catlike cry during infancy from which the syndrome derives its name. In 85% of cases the deletion is a *de novo* event. In 15% it is caused by malsegregation resulting from a balanced parental translocation.

45. **What are the syndromes and malformations associated with congenital limb hemihypertrophy?**
    - Russell–Silver syndrome
    - Conradi–Hünermann syndrome
    - CHILD syndrome (congenital hemidysplasia with icthyosiform erythroderma and limb defects)
    - Klippel–Trénaunay–Weber syndrome
    - Beckwith–Wiedemann syndrome
    - Neurofibromatosis

    One of every 32 patients with isolated hemihypertrophy is at risk for developing Wilms tumor or hepatoblastoma. For this reason renal and abdominal ultrasound and AFP should be followed every 4 months until 6 years of age as screening for patients with hemihypertrophy.

46. **Which genetic disorders are associated with hypoplastic left heart syndrome?**
    Most newborns with hypoplastic left heart syndrome have this defect as an isolated abnormality, but several syndromes with which this congenital heart malformation is a component have been identified: Down syndrome, Turner syndrome, Smith–Lemli–Opitz syndrome, trisomy 13, trisomy 18, and Ivemark syndrome. Before extensive reconstructive surgery is attempted, it may be prudent to obtain a chromosome microarray analysis.

✓ KEY POINTS: GENETIC CARE IN PREGNANCY

1. Standard genetic care in pregnancy should include evaluating the family history; screening for hemoglobinopathies; offering carrier testing for cystic fibrosis; and evaluating for aneuploidy, including noninvasive testing such as nuchal translucency and serum screening or invasive testing such as chorionic villus sampling or amniocentesis. Certain populations or individuals should be offered specific genetic testing for monogenic disorders depending on their personal or family history or their ethnicity.

2. When taking a family history, the clinician should gather information about the number and relationships of family members with birth defects, growth problems, mental retardation, serious medical problems (especially those at a young age), auditory or visual impairment, ethnicity, and consanguinity.

3. Prenatal genetic testing can be performed by chorionic villus sampling or amniocentesis. There is a chance that a genetic abnormality could be identified by chorionic villus sampling that is confined to the placenta (confined placental mosaicism) that will have little bearing on the fetus if the placenta develops normally.

4. Carrier screening for cystic fibrosis is currently offered to all couples contemplating pregnancy or currently pregnant, regardless of ethnicity.

5. The sensitivity of carrier screening for diseases such as cystic fibrosis depends critically on the ethnicity of the patient.

47. **In the evaluation of a stillborn infant, how does the general appearance of the fetus suggest a likely etiology?**
    A fresh embryo or fetus implies a rapid expulsion after intrauterine or intrapartum death. These fetuses are usually without major anomalies and have normal karyotypes. Common causes of death are placental abruption, cord accidents, and infection. A macerated fetus indicates prolonged retention and is more likely to be associated with structural malformations or chromosomal anomalies.

48. **In which fetal and infant deaths are autopsies strongly advised?**
    - Infants with external or suspected internal structural abnormalities
    - Infants with no obvious cause of death

- Macerated fetuses
- Infants with IUGR
- Infants with nonimmune hydrops
- Families with a previous unexplained loss

In addition to an autopsy, other studies that should be considered include chromosomal analysis; skeletal radiographs; placental and cord histologic studies; titers for congenital infection; and, if hydropic, evaluation for a hemoglobinopathy (e.g., alpha-thalassemia) or possible metabolic storage disease.

Bove KE. Practice guidelines for autopsy pathology: the perinatal and pediatric autopsy. Autopsy Committee of the College of American Pathologists. Arch Pathol Lab Med 1997;121(4):368–76.

49. How should women with recurrent pregnancy loss be evaluated?

Couples with recurrent pregnancy loss, defined as three or more losses, should be considered for the following evaluations:

- Cytogenic analysis of both parents to rule out mosaicism or a balanced translocation
- Hysterosalpingography to rule out malformations of the uterine cavity (e.g., congenital, diethylstilbestrol-induced, myomas, and intrauterine synechiae)
- Infectious work-up for *Mycoplasma* species, *Chlamydia* species, and other pathogens
- Immunologic evaluation for antiphospholipid antibody, anticardiolipin antibody, and antinuclear antibody (e.g., systemic lupus erythematosus)
- Hormonal-endometrial biopsy or progesterone level analysis to rule out a luteal phase defect
- Thyroid function tests
- Thrombophilia
- Evaluation of any suspected systemic illnesses

It is particularly important to initiate these studies before pursuit of any *in vitro* fertilization approach because the pregnancy may be adversely affected again with a number of these problems.

50. How are structural dysmorphisms categorized?

- Malformation: a problem of poor formation (likely genetically based) in which the abnormality is present at the onset of development (e.g., hypoplastic thumbs of Fanconi anemia)
- Disruption: an extrinsic destructive process interfering with previously normal development (e.g., amniotic banding causing limb abnormalities)
- Deformation: an extrinsic mechanical force causing abnormalities, which are usually asymmetric (e.g., breech position causing tibial bowing and positional club feet)
- Dysplasia: an abnormal cellular organization or function that generally affects only a single tissue type (e.g., cartilage abnormalities that result in achondroplasia)

51. What is the difference between a major and a minor malformation?

Major malformations are unusual morphologic features that cause significant cosmetic, medical, or developmental consequences for the patient. Minor anomalies are features that do not have associated medical problems. Approximately 14% of newborns will have a minor malformation, whereas only about 2% to 3% will have a major malformation.

52. What are the features of most common associations, CHARGE, VATER, and VACTERL?

- CHARGE: coloboma of the eye, heart defects, atresia of the choanae, retardation (mental and growth), genital anomalies (in males), ear anomalies. Some cases of CHARGE association are due to mutations in the gene chromodomain helicase DNA-binding protein 7 (CHD7).
- VATER: vertebral, anal, tracheoesophageal, renal or radial anomalies
- VACTERL: VATER anomalies plus cardiac and limb anomalies

53. What malformations and conditions are associated with oligohydramnios?

In early pregnancy (before 4 months), the majority of amniotic fluid is produced by transudation through the placental membranes and fetal skin. Later in pregnancy the bulk of amniotic fluid arises

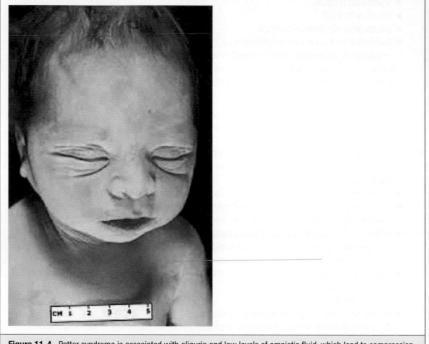

Figure 11-4. Potter syndrome is associated with oliguria and low levels of amniotic fluid, which lead to compression of the face during development and dysmorphic facial features that can include hypertelorism.

from fetal urination and fetal lung fluid production. At term the fetus swallows approximately 500 mL of amniotic fluid per day and urinates an equivalent amount. Fetal urine production increases rapidly from 3.5 mL/h at 25 weeks to 25 mL/h at term. Any malformation that leads to impaired urine production will cause oligohydramnios, including renal dysplasia, renal agenesis, and bladder outlet obstruction. When uteroplacental insufficiency occurs, the fetus is often faced with poor nutritive and volume support. The fetus becomes intravascularly depleted, leading to increased fluid conservation and decreased urine output, causing oligohydramnios. Oligohydramnios is often associated with IUGR.

54. What are the causes of polyhydramnios?

The etiology of polyhydramnios may be broken down into maternal causes (30%), fetal causes (30%), and idiopathic causes (40%). Maternal disorders, such as diabetes, erythroblastosis fetalis, and pre-eclampsia, are often associated with excessive amniotic fluid. Fetal disorders that commonly predispose to polyhydramnios are central nervous system (CNS) anomalies (e.g., anencephaly, hydrocephaly, neurologic disorders), gastrointestinal disorders (e.g., tracheoesophageal fistula, duodenal atresia), fetal circulatory disorders, and multiple gestation. The etiology for polyhydramnios in fetuses with CNS and upper gastrointestinal tract anomalies is presumed to be impaired fetal swallowing ability.

55. What causes Potter syndrome?

Potter syndrome has come to be synonymous with fetal malformations caused by extreme oligohydramnios. A lack of amniotic fluid leads to fetal compression; a squashed, flat face; clubbing of the feet; pulmonary hypoplasia; and, commonly, breech presentation (Fig. 11-4). Normal fetal lung development depends on *in utero* "breathing" and production of fetal lung fluid. In the absence of amniotic fluid, pulmonary hypoplasia occurs and is the cause of death for most fetuses with Potter syndrome. The underlying mechanism in Potter syndrome was initially reported to be renal agenesis or renal

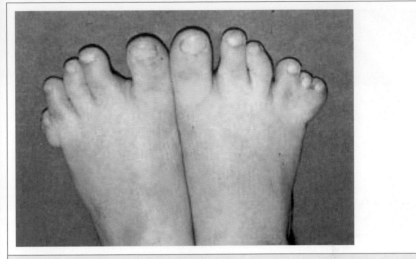

Figure 11-5. Syndactyly and postaxial polydactyly can be observed with genetic conditions such as Bardet–Biedl syndrome.

dysplasia. However, bladder outlet obstruction and prolonged premature rupture of the membranes may also cause this sequence. Some prefer that Potter syndrome be defined solely as renal agenesis.

Often, these children present in the neonatal period with severe respiratory distress beginning shortly after birth. Pneumothorax is common because high ventilatory pressures are often used in an attempt to initiate gas exchange. Survival rarely lasts longer than a few hours in the most severe cases.

56. **If an infant is born with Potter syndrome, why should the parents undergo a renal ultrasound?**
Renal agenesis is thought to be a sporadic or multifactorial condition, although autosomal dominant inheritance with variable expression (i.e., unilateral renal agenesis in a parent) has also been postulated. For this reason obtaining a renal ultrasound on parents of a child with renal agenesis is advised. If the parents have normal renal evaluations, the empirically determined recurrence risk is approximately 3%. If one of the parents has unilateral renal agenesis, the recurrence risk may be as high as 50% because of a presumed autosomal dominant gene.

57. **How do clinodactyly, syndactyly, and camptodactyly differ?**
 - Clinodactyly: Curvature of a toe or finger (usually the fifth) due to hypoplasia of the middle phalanx, which is the last fetal bone to develop in the hands and feet. Normal curvature can consist of up to 8 degrees of in-turning. Curvature beyond this is considered a minor anomaly.
 - Syndactyly: An incomplete separation of fingers (usually third and fourth) or toes (usually second or third) (Fig. 11-5).
 - Camptodactyly: Abnormal persistent flexion of fingers or toes.

58. **Are preauricular ear tags a significant finding?**
Preauricular pits and tags are minor anomalies that occur in about 0.3–1.0% of persons, with a wide variance in frequency among racial groups (Fig. 11-6). They are twice as common in females as in males and can be inherited as an autosomal dominant trait. They are believed to represent remnants of early embryonic bronchial cleft or arch structures. As isolated findings, they do not warrant additional evaluations.

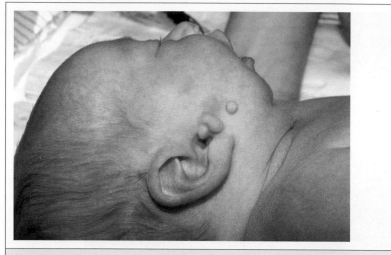

Figure 11-6. Preauricular tags can be observed with genetic conditions such as Goldenhar syndrome.

59. What is the proper way to test for low-set ears?

This designation is made when the upper portion of the ear (i.e., helix) meets the head at a level below a horizontal line drawn from the lateral aspect of the palpebral fissure. The best way to measure is to align a straight edge between the two inner canthi and determine whether the ears lie completely below this plane. Normally, approximately 10% of the ear is above this plane.

Feingold M, Bossert VM. Normal values for selected physical parameters: an aid to syndrome delineation. In: Bergsma D, editor. The National Foundation-March of Dimes Birth Defects Series 10:9. White Plains, NY: March of Dimes Birth Defects Foundation; 1974. p. 1–16.

60. Why do the sclerae of patients with osteogenesis imperfecta (OI) appear blue?

OI is a disease of bone, in which the affected neonate with osteogenesis imperfecta type II or III often manifests severe fractures prenatally, at birth, or shortly after birth. Although the disease has several levels of severity, in its most problematic forms growth is significantly impaired and life expectancy is very short. The primary component of sclera in humans is collagen. Given that abnormal collagen formation is the underlying defect in many of these disorders, it is not surprising that in OI types I, II, and III and many other connective tissue diseases the sclerae are abnormally thin and transparent. The bluish color of the sclera in patients with connective tissue (especially collagen) diseases is thought to be caused by visualization of the bluish uvea (the eye layer behind the retina) as seen through a more transparent sclera.

61. How should you genetically test for OI?

There is a genetic blood test for OI, and skin biopsies are no longer routinely required for testing. *COL1A1* and *COL1A2* are the two genes associated with OI types I, II, III, and IV. Mutation detection rates are approximately 100% for OI type I, 98% for OI type II, 60% to 70% for OI type III, and 70% to 80% for OI type IV.

62. What is the inheritance pattern of cleft lip and palate?

Most cases of cleft lip and palate are inherited in a polygenic or multifactorial pattern. The male-to-female ratio is 3:2, and the incidence in the general population is approximately 1 in 1000. The recurrence risk after one affected child is 3% to 4%; after two affected children, it rises to 8% to 9%.

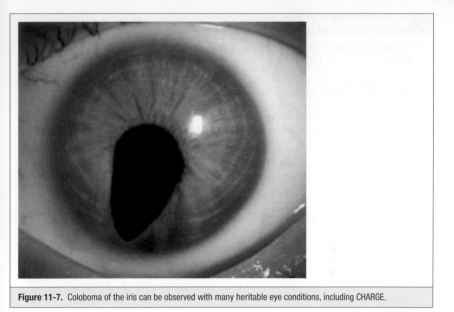

Figure 11-7. Coloboma of the iris can be observed with many heritable eye conditions, including CHARGE.

63. **How can hypertelorism be rapidly assessed?**
If an imaginary third eye would fit between the eyes, hypertelorism is possible. Precise measurement involves measuring the distance between the center of each eye's pupil. This is a difficult measurement in newborns and uncooperative patients because of eye movement. In practice the best way to determine hypotelorism or hypertelorism is to measure the inner and outer canthal distances, then plot these measurements on standardized tables of norms.

64. **Which syndromes are associated with colobomas of the iris?**
Colobomas of the iris result from abnormal ocular development and embryogenesis. They are frequently associated with chromosomal syndromes, most commonly trisomy 13, 4p-, 13q-, and triploidy. In addition, they may be commonly found in the CHARGE association, Goltz syndrome, and Axenfeld-Rieger syndrome (Fig. 11-7). Whenever iris colobomas are noted, chromosome microarray is recommended.

65. **How large is the posterior fontanel in a healthy term infant?**
In 97% of term infants, the posterior fontanel is normally the size of a fingertip or smaller. Large posterior fontanels can be seen in infants with congenital hypothyroidism, skeletal dysplasias, or increased intracranial pressure.

66. **On which side does a newborn "crown" usually sit?**
In the fetus hair follicles on the skin surface grow downward during weeks 10 through 16. During this time the brain and scalp expand outward in a domelike fashion, pulling the follicles in different directions, and at 18 weeks when the hair erupts, patterns are set. The "crown," or parietal hair whorl, is the focal point of this outgrowth. At birth it is usually a few centimeters anterior to the posterior fontanel. Approximately 55% of single parietal scalp whorls are left of midline (presumably secondary to the larger size of the left brain), 30% are right-sided, and 15% are midline. Bilateral hair whorls are present in 5% of normal persons. Abnormal positioning of the hair whorl (particularly a posterior location) can be seen in microcephaly.

✓ KEY POINTS: RISK OF RECURRENCE

1. The risk of having an affected child with an autosomal recessive condition if both parents are carriers is 25%.

2. The risk of having an affected child with an autosomal recessive condition after having three previously affected children (if both parents are carriers) is still 25%. Each pregnancy is an independent event.

3. The risk of having a child with Duchenne muscular dystrophy if the mother is a carrier is 25%. None of the girls will be affected for this X-linked disorder, but 50% of the boys will be affected.

4. A karyotype should be determined for every baby with Down syndrome to determine whether the condition was caused by an inherited translocation of chromosome 21, because this would significantly increase the risk of recurrence for the parents.

67. **How does mosaicism develop?**

Mosaicism is the possession of multiple genetically different cell lines in a single person. Most chromosomal mosaicism involves the sex chromosomes and occurs because of defects in mitosis in an early embryo. Normally, chromosomes duplicate and separate equally in mitotic division. Mosaicism can occur when the chromosomes fail to separate (mitotic nondisjunction) or fail to migrate (anaphase lag). In general, the greater the proportion of abnormal cell lines, the more abnormal the phenotype. The earlier in embryonic development an abnormal cell is established, the higher the percentage of abnormal cells in that person.

68. **What causes chimerism in infants?**

The term *chimera* is derived from the Greek mythologic monster that, according to Homer, had the head of a lion, body of a goat, and tail of a dragon. In cytogenetic parlance chimerism is the presence of two or more cell lines in a person that are derived from two separate zygotes. The most common cause of chimerism is the mixing of blood from unlike-sexed twins, resulting in a karyotype of 46,XX/46,XY. Chimerism can also result from the admixture of cells from a nonviable twin into a surviving fetus or, rarely, from incorporation of two zygotes into a single embryo.

69. **What is the risk of having a child with a recessive disorder when the parents are first or second cousins?**

First cousins may share mutations in one or more deleterious recessive genes. They have one eighth of their genes in common, and their progeny are homozygous at one sixteenth of their gene loci. Second cousins have only a one in 32 chance of having genes in common. The risk that consanguineous parents will produce a child with a severe or lethal abnormality is 6% for first-cousin marriages and 1% for second-cousin marriages. Expanded carrier screening panels are available containing several hundred mutations that may be useful for consanguineous couples before conception.

70. **How does a reciprocal translocation differ from a Robertsonian translocation?**

A chromosome translocation is a transfer of chromosomal material between two (or more) nonhomologous chromosomes. The exchange is usually reciprocal (the two segments trading places). The genetic content of the person is therefore complete but rearranged. A Robertsonian translocation represents a special variety of chromosome translocation in which the long arms of two acrocentric chromosomes (13, 14, 15, 21, or 22) fuse at their centromeres. The breaks may occur within, above, or below the centromeres. The short arms are usually lost, but this does not produce an abnormality because the genetic material on the short arms of acrocentric chromosomes occurs in multiple copies throughout the genome. A phenotypically normal person with a Robertsonian translocation has only 45 chromosomes inasmuch as the long arms of two acrocentric chromosomes are fused into one.

71. **How can an autosomal recessive disease occur when only one parent is a carrier?**

Uniparental disomy is an inheritance pattern in which a child receives two identical chromosomes from one parent and none from the other. The most likely explanation is an abnormality in meiosis whereby one gamete receives an extra copy of a homologous chromosome owing to an error in separation. This gamete with two copies from one parent then unites with the gamete of the other parent. If the second gamete lacks that particular chromosome (i.e., nullisomic gamete), a normal karyotype results. If the second gamete contains that particular chromosome, a trisomic zygote results. During embryonic development this trisomy may be lost, resulting in a normal karyotype. UPD has been reported in some patients with Prader–Willi, Angelman, and Beckwith–Wiedemann syndromes as well as cystic fibrosis.

72. **46,XY, t(4:8)(p21; q22)—what does it all mean?**
    - 46: normal number of chromosomes
    - XY: genetic male
    - t(4:8): The first set of parentheses refers to the chromosomes. The symbol in front indicates the change: *t* stands for reciprocal translocation, *del* for deletion, *dup* for duplication, and *inv* for inversion.
    - (p21; q22): The second set of parentheses refers to the bands on the chromosomes. The short arm symbol is p; the long arm symbol is q.

    In this case a genetic male with a normal number of chromosomes has a reciprocal translocation between the short arm of chromosome 4 at band 21 and the long arm of chromosome 8 at band 22.

73. **What are the features of the four most common sex chromosome abnormalities?**

See Table 11-4.

74. **Is it possible to get identical twins of different sexes?**

Rarely, yes. If anaphase lag (loss) of a Y chromosome occurs at the time of cell separation into twin embryos, a female fetus with karyotype 45,X (Turner syndrome) and a normal male fetus (46,XY) result.

75. **What are the possible placental appearances for monozygotic twins? For dizygotic twins?**

Monozygotic twins can be monochorionic monoamniotic, monochorionic diamniotic, or dichorionic diamniotic. Dizygotic twins will be dichorionic diamniotic.

76. **Of the four most common types of sex chromosomal abnormalities, which is identifiable at birth?**

Only infants with Turner syndrome have physical features easily identifiable at birth.

77. **Describe the similarities and differences between Turner syndrome and Noonan syndrome.**
    - Similarities include short stature, web neck, cardiac defects, low posterior hairline, broad chest, wide-spaced nipples, edema of the dorsum of the hands and feet, and cubitus valgus.
    - Differences are summarized in Table 11-5.

78. **What is the most common inherited form of mental retardation?**

Fragile X syndrome is most common.

79. **What is the nature of the mutation in fragile X syndrome?**

When the lymphocytes of an affected male are grown in a folate-deficient medium and the chromosomes examined, a substantial number of X chromosomes demonstrate a break near the distal end of the long arm. This site, the fragile X mental retardation 1 gene *(FMR1)*, was identified and

TABLE 11-4. CHARACTERISTICS OF SEX CHROMOSOME DISORDERS

	47,XXY (KLINEFELTER SYNDROME)	47,XYY	47,XXX	45,X (TURNER'S SYNDROME)
Frequency of live births	1/2000	1/2000	1/2000	1/5000
Maternal age association	Yes	No	Yes	No
Phenotype	Tall, eunuchoid habitus, underdeveloped secondary sex characteristics, gynecomastia	Tall, severe acne, indistinguishable from healthy male subjects	Tall, indistinguishable from healthy female subjects	Short stature, web neck, shield chest, pedal edema at birth, coarctation of aorta
IQ and behavior	80 to 100; behavioral problems	90 to 100; aggressive behavior Common	90 to 110; behavioral problems Common	Mildly deficient to normal IQ, spatial and perceptual problems Extremely rare
Fertility	Rarely fertile	Fertile	Fertile	Rarely fertile
Gonad	Hypoplastic testes, Leydig cell hyperplasia, Sertoli cell hypoplasia, seminiferous tubule dysgenesis, few spermatogenic precursors	Normal-size testes, normal testicular histology	Normal-size ovaries, normal ovarian histology	Streak ovaries with deficient follicles

TABLE 11-5. DIFFERENCES BETWEEN TURNER AND NOONAN SYNDROMES

TURNER SYNDROME	NOONAN SYNDROME
Females only	Both males and females
Chromosomal disorder (45,X)	Normal chromosomes (autosomal dominant) Near-normal IQ, mild to moderate intellectual disability
Coarctation the most common	Pulmonary stenosis the most common, cardiac defect
Amenorrhea and sterility	Normal menstrual cycle in females

sequenced in 1991. At the center of the gene is a repeating trinucleotide sequence (CGG) that in normal persons repeats between 6 and 45 times. However, in carriers the sequence expands to between 50 and 200 times (called a premutation), and in fully affected persons it expands to between 200 and 600 copies. These longer sequences cause malfunctioning of the gene. The repeat expansion is most sensitively and accurately determined by Southern blot analysis. Male as well as female subjects can be affected, although it is an X-linked disorder.

80. **What are some potential manifestations in women who are carriers of the Fragile X premutation?**
Premature ovarian failure is one potential manifestation.

81. **What are the most common genetic causes of aniridia?**
Isolated aniridia is most commonly caused by mutations in *PAX6* and is prognostically associated with a multitude of ophthalmologic abnormalities that significantly impair vision but do not result in involvement of other organ systems. A contiguous gene deletion of 11p13 can produce syndromic aniridia associated with WAGR syndrome (Wilms tumor, aniridia, genitourinary anomalies, and retarded growth and development). When initially diagnosing a neonate with aniridia, it may not be obvious at birth whether this will be isolated or syndromic, and genetic testing for these two disorders is useful to determine the prognosis and the potential for associated problems.

82. **What findings on ultrasound scan may suggest the diagnosis of aneuploidy?**
Short femurs, IUGR, congenital heart disease, pyelectasis, echogenic cardiac focus, echogenic bowel, choroid plexus cyst, and cystic hygroma are all associated with aneuploidy.

83. **What disorder should be considered in a neonate with a maternal history of acute fatty liver of pregnancy or Hemolysis, Elevated Liver enzymes, and Low Platelet count (HELLP) syndrome?**
Long-chain 3-hydroxyacyl-CoA dehydrogenase (LCHAD), a fatty acid oxidation disorder.

84. **What types of congenital heart disease are classically associated with DiGeorge syndrome?**
Conotruncal defects such as tetralogy of Fallot, interrupted aortic arch, truncus arteriosus, and ventricular septal defects are associated with DiGeorge syndrome.

85. **What other features are associated with DiGeorge syndrome?**
Cleft lip, cleft palate, hypothyroidism, hypocalcemia owing to hypoparathyroidism, immunodeficiency with thymus hypoplasia and altered T cell function, failure to thrive, and developmental delay are also associated with DiGeorge syndrome.

86. **What inborn errors of metabolism are associated with birth defects?**
Smith–Lemli–Opitz syndrome (congenital heart disease and genitourinary anomalies), peroxisomal disorders (congenital heart disease, epiphyseal stippling, renal cysts, CNS malformations), congenital disorders of glycosylation (CNS malformations, renal cysts, genitourinary anomalies), and fatty acid oxidation disorders (renal cysts; hypertrophic cardiomyopathy; CNS malformations, including cerebellar hypoplasia).

87. **What disorders are associated with triplet repeat expansions?**
Fragile X syndrome, myotonic dystrophy, Huntington disease, spinocerebellar ataxia, and spinal bulbar muscular atrophy (Kennedy disease).

88. **What genetic disorders should you suspect in the severely hypotonic neonate?**
Prader–Willi syndrome, congenital myopathy or muscular dystrophy, myotonic dystrophy, and inborn error of metabolism.

89. **If you suspect a baby has congenital myotonic dystrophy, which parent would you examine for symptoms, and what would you look for?**
You would examine the mother for evidence of a myopathic face, difficulty with speech or swallowing, myotonia and inability to release her grip, or cataracts. The AGC/CTG repeat size is unstable and much more likely to expand when transmitted through a female patient than through a male patient. As the repeat increases in size, the severity increases, and age of onset decreases.

90. **If there is a maternal history of long QT syndrome, what should be done for the neonate?**

If the long QT syndrome is genetically based, it is most likely to be autosomal dominantly inherited, putting the baby at 50% risk of long QT syndrome. The baby should be screened by electrocardiograph, and the QTc interval should be calculated. If it is prolonged more than 440 msec, the baby should be started on beta blockers. Additionally, genetic testing is now available for long QT syndrome, a genetically heterogeneous disorder caused by mutations in at least 12 currently known genes. Once a familial mutation is identified, the baby can be tested to determine whether he or she has inherited the mutation. Electrocardiographic screening is not perfectly sensitive, especially in children. Whenever possible, genetic screening of the at-risk child should always be performed to increase the sensitivity and specificity of screening. Additionally, medical management and risk of sudden cardiac death depends on which of the genes is affected and is definable only with genetic testing.

91. **What is a marker chromosome?**

A marker chromosome is a small piece of a chromosome seen on routine karyotype that is hard to define by conventional cytogenetics.

92. **What is the prognosis for a fetus with a marker chromosome?**

This depends on the genetic content of the marker chromosome. If it contains a significant number of genes, it is more likely to be associated with birth defects, growth problems, and intellectual disability.

93. **If a marker chromosome is identified prenatally, what additional studies should be performed?**

A chromosome microarray should be performed to define the source of the marker and characterize the gene content. If the genetic material is derived from chromosome 6, 7, 11, 15, or 16, uniparental disomy testing for that chromosome should be performed to rule out associated imprinting disorders observed with UPD of those chromosomes.

94. **What is the most common cause of nonsyndromic hearing loss?**

Mutations in the autosomal recessive genes *GJB2* and *GJB6* account for approximately 50% of cases of nonsyndromic hearing loss, and genetic testing for hearing loss should start with these genes. Genetic testing for a panel of genes associated with the most commons forms of syndromic and nonsyndromic hearing loss is also available and can be helpful to diagnose Pendred and Usher syndromes before other manifestations become apparent.

95. **A fetus is found to have a cardiac rhabdomyoma on prenatal ultrasound, and both parents are healthy. What is the most likely diagnosis, how would you confirm this, and how would you counsel the parents?**

The diagnosis is most likely tuberous sclerosis complex (TSC). Cardiac rhabdomyomas are present in 47% to 67% of individuals with TSC. These tumors regress with time and eventually disappear and are largest during the neonatal period. Surgical intervention immediately after birth is necessary only when cardiac outflow obstruction occurs.

TSC is autosomal dominantly inherited and caused by mutations in *TSC1* (31%) and *TSC2* (69%). Molecular genetic testing for both genes is available on a clinical basis both prenatally and postnatally.

TSC involves other organ systems, including abnormalities of the skin later in life (facial angiofibromas, shagreen patches, ungual fibromas); cortical tubers in the brain; seizures; intellectual disability or developmental delay; kidney problems (angiomyolipomas, cysts, renal cell carcinomas); and, rarely, lymphangioleiomyomatosis in the lungs.

Northrup H, Koenig MK. Tuberous Sclerosis Complex, <http://www.ncbi.nlm.nih.gov/books/NBK1220/>; 2011 [accessed 11.05.13]

96. **A fetus is found to have polycystic kidneys on prenatal ultrasound. What is the most likely diagnosis, what would you do to confirm the diagnosis, and how would you counsel the parents?**

The fetus most likely has polycystic kidney disease. If both parents have normal renal ultrasounds, this is most likely autosomal recessive polycystic kidney disease (ARPKD). The diagnosis can be confirmed with molecular genetic testing for *PKHD1*, the only gene known to be associated with ARPKD. In the prenatal and neonatal period there are enlarged echogenic kidneys. Approximately 45% of infants also have liver abnormalities. Pulmonary hypoplasia resulting from oligohydramnios is common. Approximately 30% of affected infants die in the neonatal period or within the first year of life, primarily as a result of respiratory insufficiency or superimposed pulmonary infections. More than 50% of affected children progress to end-stage renal disease, usually in the first decade of life.

CHAPTER 12

HEMATOLOGY AND TRANSFUSION MEDICINE

Robert D. Christensen, MD

NORMAL ERYTHROCYTE VALUES OF NEONATES

1. **A term newborn infant on the day of birth has a hemoglobin (Hgb) of 11.8 g/dL. Is that value low or is it within the expected (normal) reference range?**
   Expected values, also called "reference ranges," for Hgb and hematocrit on the day of birth are a function of gestational age, increasing gradually through the second and third trimesters. Studies with very large sample sizes of neonates on the day of birth reveal no differences in Hgb or hematocrit associated with the infants' sex. Reference ranges for blood Hgb concentrations are shown as Figure 12-1. The fifth percentile value (the lowest expected limit) at term is 14 g/dL. Thus the value of 11.8 g/dL in this patient is low.

Christensen RD, Henry E, Jopling J, et al. The CBC: reference ranges for neonates. Semin Perinatol 2009;33:3–11.

2. **A term newborn infant on the day of birth has an Hgb of 24 g/dL. Is that value high, or is it within the expected (normal) reference range?**
   The 95th percentile reference range at term is 22.5 g/dL (see Figure 12-1). The value of 24 g/dL in this patient is therefore high.

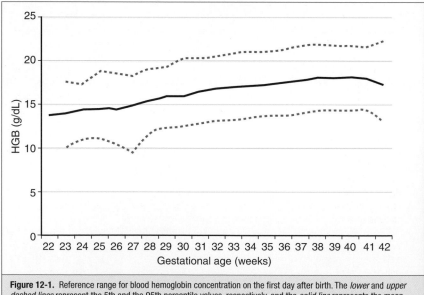

Figure 12-1. Reference range for blood hemoglobin concentration on the first day after birth. The *lower* and *upper* dashed lines represent the 5th and the 95th percentile values, respectively, and the *solid line* represents the mean value. (From Jopling et al. Pediatrics 2009;123(2):e333–337.)

3. **Are Hgb and hematocrit values of newborn infants higher when obtained from capillary blood than when obtained from venous or arterial blood?**
Yes. Values from capillary beds (heel stick) are generally about 15% higher and also more variable than venous or arterial values. This observation is due in part to the changing peripheral perfusion in the hours after birth. Poorly perfused heels seem to have capillary pooling or sludging of red blood cells (RBCs) that result in higher values. This phenomenon of higher Hgb level in capillary as opposed to central blood sources is not so significant in older children and adults. If the Hgb value of 24 g/dL in the patient in Question 2 was drawn from a heel stick, you would want to repeat it using a central vascular determination before you decide whether the neonate is truly polycythemic.

4. **Which one of the following RBC measurements in a fetus or newborn infant does *not* normally diminish gradually with maturation during the second and third trimesters of pregnancy?**
    - MCV (mean corpuscular volume) fL
    - MCH (mean corpuscular Hgb) pg
    - MCHC (mean corpuscular Hgb concentration) g/dL

The MCV and the MCH both diminish gradually through the second and third trimesters, as shown in Figure 12-2. The MCHC, however, does not change during this period but remains in the range of 31 to 34 g/dL. MCHC values greater than 36 g/dL should alert you to the possibility of hereditary sphero-cytosis or pyropoikilocytosis, two conditions that generally present with a low MCV and a high MCHC. They commonly also demonstrate hyperbilirubinemia and sometimes a diminishing Hgb concentra-tion. If the MCV is consistently greater than 36 g/dL you should assess the morphology of the RBCs, and you will need to ask whether other family members have abnormally shaped RBCs and have had anemia, neonatal jaundice, or early cholelethiasis (bilirubin stones).

5. **The complete blood count (CBC) of a term neonate is reported to show greater than 100 nucleated red blood cells (NRBCs) per 100 white blood cells (WBCs). Is this value high, or is it within the expected (normal) reference range?**
NRBCs can be reported as the number of NRBCs per 100 WBCs or as NRBCs per μL. The latter pro-vides a more accurate accounting because of changing WBC counts over the first several days. The former is more commonly used in clinical practice. Reference ranges for NRBCs per 100 WBCs are shown in Figure 12-3. For term infants on the day of birth, the 95th percentile (highest expected limit) is 15 per 100 WBCs. Therefore the value of 100 in this patient is abnormally high.

6. **A newborn infant at 28 weeks' gestation has no NRBCs per 100 WBCs. Is that value low, or is it within the expected (normal) reference range?**
A value of zero (0) NRBCs per 100 WBCs is always within the reference range, regardless of gesta-tional age. Thus the value of 0 in this patient is within the expected (normal) range.

7. **You are asked to evaluate the result of a Hgb electrophoresis from a state metabolic screen, drawn on a nontransfused, extremely-low-birth-weight (less than 1 kg) neonate. The report reads as follows: 85% Hgb F, 5% Hgb A, and 10% Hgb Barts. What is your interpretation?**
Hgb is a tetramer of globin chains, usually of two distinct types, bound to a heme moiety. Adult hemo-globin (Hgb A) consists of two alpha chains and two beta chains, whereas fetal hemoglobin (Hgb F) consists of two alpha chains and two gamma chains (Figure 12-4).

   Embryonic Hgbs are present in the first 8 weeks after conception and consist of Hgb Gower 1 (zeta 2, epsilon 2), Hgb Gower 2 (alpha 2, epsilon 2), and Hgb Portland (zeta 2, gamma 2). Hgb Barts con-sists of four gamma chains and occurs in the absence or deficiency of alpha chains. Thus 10% of the Hgb observed as Barts is abnormal and suggests a deficiency of at least one, and probably two, of the four alpha chain genes. Deletion of one alpha gene results in a phenotypically normal individual, and deletion of two can result in mild microcytic anemia with the presence of Barts Hgb during the fetal and early newborn period. Deletion of three genes gives rise to Hgb H disease; deletion of all

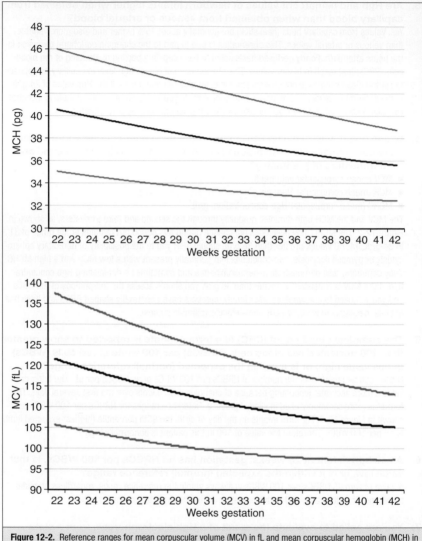

Figure 12-2. Reference ranges for mean corpuscular volume (MCV) in fL and mean corpuscular hemoglobin (MCH) in pg on the first day after birth. The *lower* and *upper lines* represent the 5th and the 95th percentile values, respectively, and the *center line* represents the mean value. (From Christensen, et al. J Perinatol 2008;28:24–28.)

four gives rise to a lethal syndrome of hydrops fetalis with all or most of the Hgb being Barts, and no Hgb A or F or alpha 2 (because there are no alpha chains).

Kemper AR, Knapp AA, Metterville DR, et al.Weighing the evidence for newborn screening for Hemoglobin H disease. J Pediatr 2011;158:780–3.

8. **How does Hgb F differ from Hgb A?**
   Hgb F binds oxygen more avidly. The oxyhemoglobin dissociation curve for Hgb F is shifted to the left of the adult curve. The higher affinity for oxygen facilitates transfer of oxygen from maternal

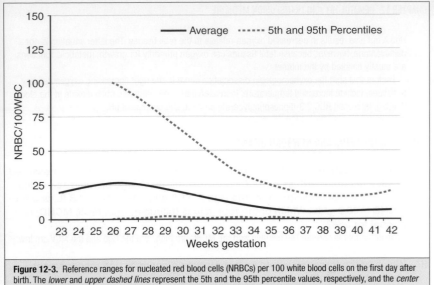

Figure 12-3. Reference ranges for nucleated red blood cells (NRBCs) per 100 white blood cells on the first day after birth. The *lower* and *upper dashed lines* represent the 5th and the 95th percentile values, respectively, and the *center line* represents the mean value. (From Christensen, et al. Neonatol 2011;99:289–294.)

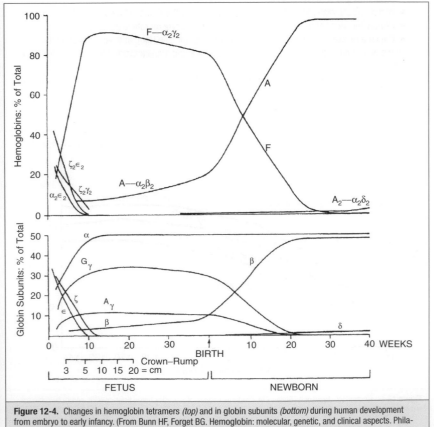

Figure 12-4. Changes in hemoglobin tetramers *(top)* and in globin subunits *(bottom)* during human development from embryo to early infancy. (From Bunn HF, Forget BG. Hemoglobin: molecular, genetic, and clinical aspects. Philadelphia: Saunders; 1986.)

Hgb A but also results in decreased oxygen release to the fetal tissues. The latter situation is not a disadvantage, however, because fetal tissues use oxygen primarily for growth; metabolic functions are mostly handled by the mother.

Factors that shift the oxyhemoglobin dissociation curve to the right (increasing oxygen delivery to tissues) include increased temperature, increased partial pressure of carbon dioxide in the blood ($PaCO_2$), increased RBC 2,3-diphosphoglycerate content, and decreased pH.

ANEMIA IN THE FETUS AND NEWBORN INFANT

9. **A term neonate has a total serum bilirubin (TSB) level of 18.8 mg/dL measured at 48 hours after birth as part of a pre–hospital-discharge bilirubin screening program. A CBC indicates that the Hgb is 11.2 g/dL, the MCV is 88 fL, and the MCHC is 38.2 g/dL. Which of the four values (bilirubin, Hgb, MCV, MCHC) is normal for age?**
   None of the four is normal. The bilirubin and the MCHC are high, and the Hgb and the MCV are low.

10. **Which of the following would be appropriate diagnostic and management steps at this point?**
    - Initiate intensive phototherapy.
    - Take a careful family history of neonatal jaundice and anemia, chronic jaundice and anemia, and gallstones (bilirubin cholelethiasis) at an early age.
    - Determine the maternal and neonatal blood type and the direct antiglobulin test (Coombs test).
    - Review the blood film, specifically looking for erythrocyte morphologic abnormalities.
    - Obtain a reticulocyte count, urine analysis (looking for free Hgb), and serum haptoglobin.

    All the preceding steps may be helpful in the diagnosis and management of this case. Consider the following:
    - Intensive phototherapy and careful follow-up of the TSB are needed because the TSB plots well into the "high risk" zone (Figure 12-5).

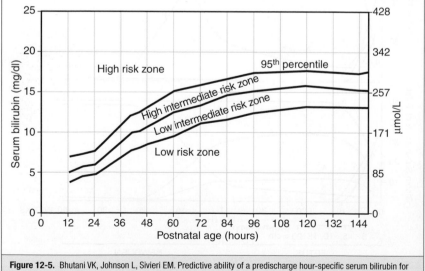

Figure 12-5. Bhutani VK, Johnson L, Sivieri EM. Predictive ability of a predischarge hour-specific serum bilirubin for subsequent significant hyperbilirubinemia in healthy term and near-term newborns. Pediatrics 1999;103:6-14.

- The family history might reveal that the father or mother has hereditary spherocytosis (HS). Approximately two thirds of cases of HS are inherited in an autosomal dominant fashion. HS in this neonate would be compatible with the laboratory findings given. Between 40% and 50% of neonates with HS have a mutation in *ANK1* (at 8p11.2) encoding the RBC cytoskeletal protein component ankyrin 1. Between 20% and 35% have a mutation in *SLC4A1* (at 17q21) encoding band 3, and 15% to 30% have a mutation in *SPTB* (at 14q23-24.1) encoding beta-spectrin.

- Alternatively, the family history might reveal that either father *or* mother has hereditary ellipto-cytosis (see the discussion later in this chapter explaining how this could explain this neonate's findings). On the other hand, the family history might be completely unrevealing because about one third of HS cases in neonates are either *de novo* mutations or autosomal recessive variet-ies. The latter includes mutations in *SPR1* (1q22-23) encoding alpha-spectrin and *EPB42* (at 15q15-21) encoding protein 4.2. The latter mutation is more likely among neonates of Japanese descent.

- Type and Coombs testing should be done when the TSB falls in the "high risk" zone. The MCHC can be high in ABO hemolytic disease associated with spherocytes, but it generally does not exceed 36.5 fL. The value greater than 38 in this case suggests that HS is more likely.

- It is appropriate to examine the blood film for the presence of spherocytes or other morphologic abnormalities. Although microspherocytes can be seen in ABO hemolytic disease (sometimes presenting a dilemma between HS and ABO hemolytic disease in neonates with Coombs-positive jaundice), the high MCHC in this case suggests that HS is more likely. Figure 12-6 shows an example of a blood smear of a neonate with HS.

- Hereditary elliptocytosis (HE) in a neonate does not generally result in significant hemolytic jaundice and anemia, and the RBC indices are not generally abnormal. However, a related condi-tion called pyropoikilocytosis does indeed present similarly to this case, including early jaundice, anemia, low MCV, and high MCHC. Pyropoikilocytosis generally occurs when a father or mother has HE, consisting of an alpha-spectrin deficiency, and the other spouse has an asymptomatic alpha-spectrin defect. As a result, the neonate has a genetic condition similar to autosomal recessive inheritance as a compound heterozygote. Figure 12-7 shows an example of a blood film of HE, and Figure 12-8 shows an example of neonatal pyropoikilocytosis.

Cohen RS, Wong RJ, Stevenson DK. Understanding neonatal jaundice: a perspective on causation. Pediatr Neonatol 2010;51:143–8.

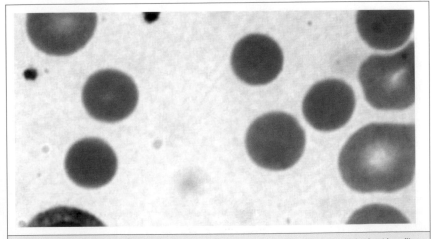

Figure 12-6. Photomicrograph of a Wright-stained blood film of a newborn infant with autosomal dominant hereditary spherocytosis. Note that many erythrocytes lack a zone of central pallor.

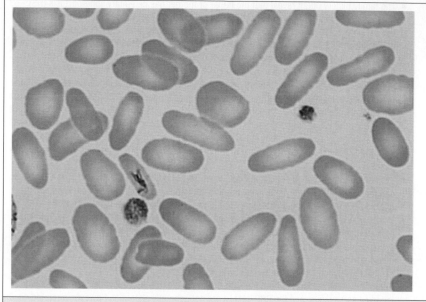

Figure 12-7. Photomicrograph of a Wright-stained blood film of a newborn infant with hereditary elliptocytosis. Note that most of the erythrocytes do have a zone of central pallor, but they vary in shape from round to oval to elliptical.

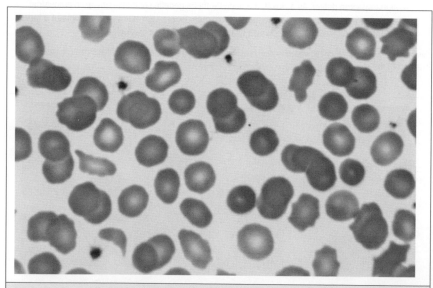

Figure 12-8. Photomicrograph of a Wright-stained blood film of a newborn infant with the diagnosis of pyropoikilocytosis. The mother had autosomal dominant hereditary elliptocytosis, and the father had a "silent" mutation in alpha-spectrin. Neither parent had problematic jaundice during the neonatal period or subsequently, but the baby required phototherapy for more than 1 week. Note that some of the erythrocytes appear normal, but many have abnormal shapes, varying from spherocytes to schistocytes to acanthocytes. This high degree of poikilocytosis was termed *pyropoikilocytosis* because the cells resemble those after thermal burns ("pyro").

11. Following a long labor of a term primipara, vacuum extraction is successfully accomplished. A capillary blood gas reading obtained within a few minutes of delivery was normal, including an Hgb count of 16 g/dL. Over the next hour the site of the vacuum attachment to the crown of the head becomes progressively larger and more fluctuant. A repeat Hgb count is still 16 g/dL. One clinician suggests that this finding might represent a subgaleal hemorrhage, but another states that the stable Hgb level is more likely to represent caput succedaneum. Which of the following would be appropriate diagnostic and management decisions?

- Order continuous heart rate and respiratory rate monitoring with frequent blood pressure measurements, looking for any signs of compensated hypovolemia.
- Obtain a CBC (at least a Hgb and hematocrit) now and again in about 2 hours.
- Obtain a blood type and cross match in case an early transfusion is needed.
- Wrap the head very tightly with an elastic bandage to prevent further head swelling.
- Consider imaging the head to determine whether the swelling is consistent with blood in the subgaleal space.

The initially stable Hgb level does not exclude the diagnosis of a subgaleal hemorrhage. Hemorrhage itself does not lower the Hgb and hematocrit. The fall occurs only when extravascular fluid moves into the vascular space as a physiologic response to hypovolemia.

Although much less common than a caput, a subgaleal hemorrhage can be life-threatening and therefore demands aggressive monitoring and support. Head wrapping has been attempted in the past as a potential method for tamponade, but in general this approach has not been successful because it tends to increase the intracranial pressure.

With signs of hypovolemia, transfusion support may be warranted. Coagulopathy can occur, generally secondary to shock and disseminated intravascular coagulopathy (DIC), and can worsen the hemorrhage. Portable cranial ultrasound will generally confirm the presence of a subgaleal hemorrhage. Computed tomography or magnetic resonance imaging will provide more accurate and detailed information, but these are usually not needed to make the diagnosis of a subgaleal hemorrhage.

12. All neonatal subgaleal hemorrhages follow vacuum extraction delivery (true or false).

False. Most neonatal subgaleal hemorrhages do indeed follow vacuum extraction, but some follow forceps delivery and some occur with nonoperative delivery. However, in a series from Intermountain Healthcare, we found that every neonate with a subgaleal hemorrhage that required one or more RBC transfusions was delivered by either vacuum or forceps extraction.

All neonates who had a "spontaneous" subgaleal hemorrhage (not delivered by vacuum or forceps extraction) lacked signs of shock, had no transfusions, and generally had a good outcome. Thus vacuum delivery is the most significant risk factor for developing a neonatal subgaleal hemorrhage.

Reid J. Neonatal subgaleal hemorrhage. Neonatal Netw 2007;26(4):219–27.

13. A subgaleal hemorrhage following vacuum extraction delivery is rare, occurring in fewer than 1 percent of all vacuum deliveries (true or false).

True. In a recent report from Taiwan, one in 218 vacuum deliveries developed a subgaleal hemorrhage. In a study from Intermountain Healthcare, a subgaleal hemorrhage was diagnosed in one in 598 vacuum deliveries. A subgaleal hemorrhage is therefore rare, even after a vacuum delivery, but because of the vigilance needed for proper diagnosis and management, the possibility of a subgaleal hemorrhage should be considered after any operative delivery in which scalp fluctuance is observed.

14. If a subgaleal hemorrhage is diagnosed, the expected mortality rate is about 25% (true or false).

False. Some publications describing cases from the 1980s and earlier did indeed report a mortality rate this high, but more recent series suggest the mortality rate is 5% to 10%. Regardless, this injury is devastating. Vigilance and aggressive management are likely responsible for the observed improvement in outcome.

15. **Hemolytic disease of the fetus and newborn (HDFN) can occur when a woman has immunoglobulin G antibodies directed against paternal RBC antigens inherited by the fetus. What is a typical clinical presentation for a case of HDFN?**

Neonatal hemolytic jaundice is typical, particularly manifesting in the following ways:

- Hyperbilirubinemia typically results in an elevated cord blood TSB; also, a TSB in the "high risk" zone within 24 or 48 hours of birth is possible.

- Reticulocytosis: After day of life one or two, the reticulocyte count generally falls to near zero percent. However, in most cases of HDFN the reticulocyte count remains elevated, sometimes higher than 10%.

- Hemolysis: Evidence includes a falling Hgb, free Hgb in the urine, and an absent serum haptoglobin concentration.

- Erythroblastosis: Most cases other than anti-D have a normal or only a slightly elevated NRBC count. Severe cases of HDFN can have marked anemia, erythroblastosis, and hydrops fetalis.

Wennberg RP, Ahlfors CE, Aravkin AY. Guidelines for neonatal hyperbilirubinemia: an evidence based quagmire. Curr Pharm Des 2009;15:2939–45.

16. **HDFN arising from maternal anti-Kell (Kell$_1$) antibody can present in a manner very different from the typical presentation described previously. What is that presentation, and why is that variety of HDFN different from the rest?**

HDFN resulting from maternal anti-Kell antibody presents with fetal or neonatal anemia but no reticulocytosis, no evidence of hemolysis, and no hyperbilirubinemia. These cases present with hyporegenerative anemia. The explanation is that the Kell antigen is expressed on erythroid progenitor cells, whereas most other blood group antigens are not expressed until the cells clonally mature. As a consequence of maternal anti-Kell antibody binding to fetal erythroid progenitors, fetal RBC production is reduced and hyporegenerative anemia results. The *KEL* gene (7q33) encodes a 93 kilodalton transmembrane zinc-dependent endopeptidase that is responsible for cleaving endothelin-3. The Kell protein has recently been designated CD238.

17. **In developed countries ABO incompatibility is now the leading cause of HDFN (true or false).**

True. Women lacking the A and the B erythrocyte antigens often have anti-A and anti-B antibodies even before pregnancy. In the case of women with blood type O, their anti-A and anti-B antibodies are sometimes of the immunoglobulin G type and therefore can cross the placenta and bind to fetal antigens. Unlike the situation observed with maternal anti-D, in neonates with ABO hemolytic disease the principal problem is usually jaundice. Anemia, erythroblastosis, and hydrops are all very rare. The ABO locus is on chromosome 9 and has three main allelic forms: A, B, and O. The A and B alleles encode glycosyltransferases. The O allele differs from the A allele by deletion of only one nucleotide—guanine at position 261. This deletion causes a frame shift and results in premature termination of translation of the mRNA.

Geaghan SM. Diagnostic laboratory technologies for the fetus and neonate with isoimmunization. Semin Perinatol 2011;35(3):148–54.

18. **What is the H antigen, and what does it have to do with the ABO blood type?**

The H antigen is the precursor to the ABO blood group antigens. The H locus is on chromosome 19 and encodes the H antigen, which is expressed on the RBC surface. The H antigen is then modified by the A or the B antigen to produce the final A, B, or O antigen. Very rarely an individual lacks the H antigen because of a mutation in the H gene. This results in type O blood, but because the precursor molecule (the H antigen) is also missing, even type O blood cannot be transfused because the individual recognizes the H antigen in the type O blood as foreign. This unusual O blood type is called Bombay blood group and occurs in approximately four per million people, except in parts of India where it may be as common as 1 in 10,000. Neonates who are type O on the basis of Bombay can hemolyze if transfused with type O blood.

19. **A mother about to deliver at 29 weeks' gestation requests that the obstetrician and the neonatal team do everything possible to avoid an RBC transfusion in the neonate. What options are available to help the family with this request?**
   - Delay clamping of the umbilical cord, or cord "stripping" or "milking." These maneuvers, roughly equivalent in terms of the volume of fetal blood transferred from the placenta to the fetus, can be expected to result in an Hgb concentration of about 2 g/dL. Ask the obstetrician to consider these approaches.
   - Draw all laboratory tests on NICU admission (e.g., blood culture, CBC, state metabolic screen) using fetal blood in the placenta after placental delivery, thereby removing no blood from the neonate initially.
   - Carefully consider the need for all blood tests you order during the first several days to weeks, with the understanding that many early RBC transfusions in very-low-birth-weight infants are generally needed on the basis of anemia that results from phlebotomy for laboratory testing.
   - Consider slightly lowering the Hgb value you consider as a "transfusion trigger." For instance, if your guidelines call for RBC transfusion at 10 g/dL or lower, consider lowering it to 9 g/dL or lower for this patient.
   - Consider administering the long-acting erythropoietin analog darbepoetin (Aranesp) once in the first few days and again 1 week later. Use 10 µg/kg as a unit dose.
   - Let the parents know that despite your best efforts to help them with their request, the baby's best interests might force you to administer an RBC transfusion if the baby would be critically compromised otherwise. Explain all the steps that you are taking to avoid transfusing the infant.

McPherson RJ, Juul SE. Erythropoietin for infants with hypoxic-ischemic encephalopathy. Curr Opin Pediatr 2010;22:139–45.

20. **A twin-twin transfusion is expected on the basis of discordant-sized monochorionic twins. Fetal ultrasonography indicates the likelihood of anemia in the smaller twin because of the middle cerebral artery blood flow. It appears that the larger twin has pleural fluid and ascites, although these are subtle findings. You are anticipating that the smaller twin will be anemic and the larger twin may be polycythemic, but what other hematologic differences do you anticipate?**
   The donor (anemic, smaller) twin is more likely to have a hyporegenerative neutropenia, similar to that seen in neonates born after pregnancy-induced hypertension. This situation is likely to present with no left shift (a normal immature-to-total neutrophil ratio) and a duration of only about 2 or 3 days. Similarly, the donor twin is more likely to have a moderately low platelet count with a normal mean platelet volume (MPV). The pathogenesis of these findings is not known with certainty but likely relates to the accelerated erythropoietic effort in the anemic twin, with a concomitant temporary reduction in platelet and neutrophil production. Also, the anemic twin will usually have a higher NRBC count, generally above the reference range for age (see Figure 12-3).

Mosquera C, Miller RS, Simpson LL. Twin-twin transfusion syndrome. Semin Perinatol 2012;36:182–9.

21. **RBC transfusion can be life-saving for neonates with acute hemorrhage or severe anemia. However, before ordering any RBC transfusion, the clinician must assess the potential risks and potential benefits. What are some of the risks associated with RBC transfusion in the NICU?**
   Typical transfusion reactions (i.e., those commonly reported for adult recipients) are only rarely observed in transfused neonates. These include febrile nonhemolytic reactions, urticarial (allergic)

reactions, hypothermia, circulatory overload, hypotensive reactions, citrate toxicity (e.g., peripheral paresthesia, tingling, buzzing, cramps, nausea, vomiting), and acute hemolysis resulting from undetected incompatibility. Transfusion-transmitted diseases include bacterial contamination, which is considerably more common than the hepatitis and other viruses transmitted in past decades, before development and implementation of modern hemovigilance techniques and procedures.

Adverse associations with transfusions that are unique to neonates include transfusion-associated necrotizing enterocolitis (generally very-low-birth-weight neonates 3 to 4 weeks old receiving a "late" transfusion) and severe intraventricular hemorrhage in extremely-low-birth-weight neonates after an "early" transfusion. Transfusion-related acute lung injury (TRALI) reactions involve acute onset of (or acute worsening of) respiratory distress after transfusion. All plasma-containing blood products have been implicated in TRALI reactions. TRALI is now among the three leading causes of transfusion-related fatalities, along with ABO incompatibility and bacterial contamination, but it is rarely reported (perhaps because it is rarely recognized) in neonatal transfusion recipients.

Strauss RG. How I transfuse red blood cells and platelets to infants with the anemia and thrombocytopenia of prematurity. Transfusion 2008;48:209–17.

Strauss RG. Anaemia of prematurity: pathophysiology and treatment. Blood Rev 2010;24:221–5.

22. **After a double-volume exchange transfusion for extreme hyperbilirubinemia in a term neonate, you obtain a CBC. The exchange was performed with packed RBC reconstituted with plasma to a hematocrit concentration of approximately 60%. Before the exchange transfusion a CBC revealed a hematocrit concentration of 30%, an Hgb of 10 g/dL, a platelet count of 230,000/μL, and an absolute neutrophil count of 2000/μL. What significant differences do you anticipate finding in the CBC after the exchange?**
   Several differences can be anticipated. Awareness of these differences prevents confusion when you compare the CBCs before and after the exchange.
   - The hematocrit and Hgb will be higher than before the exchange. If they are not higher, you might want to check the hematocrit and Hgb in the remaining unused reconstituted unit to ensure that the product you received approximated what you ordered.
   - The erythrocyte indices, particularly the MCV and MCH, will fall because adult donor erythrocytes have partly replaced erythrocytes of the neonate. The MCHC will likely be about the same because this measurement is generally in the same range in neonates and adults.
   - The platelet count will be considerably lower after the exchange because of the lack of platelets in the reconstituted donor unit. It is not uncommon to find a platelet count below 100,000/μL after an exchange transfusion. The count will not likely fall to a level requiring a platelet transfusion, however, unless you must repeat the double-volume exchange transfusion within a few hours. Indeed, if a repeat exchange transfusion is needed soon after the first, be aware that the platelet count after the second exchange might fall to exceedingly low levels. Because there is no large marrow ready reserve of platelets, the platelet count will not rebound rapidly (within hours) of the exchange.
   - The neutrophil count, already on the low side (2000/μL) before the exchange will be lower still afterward. Similar to the anticipated fall in platelet count, the reconstituted donor unit will lack neutrophils, and the count will fall. It would be expected that the post–exchange transfusion neutrophil count would be below 1000/μL in this patient.

POLYCYTHEMIA: DIAGNOSIS AND MANAGEMENT

23. **Are the terms *polycythemia* and *hyperviscosity* synonymous?**
   Technically, these two words describe different aspects of illness, but in neonates the two tend to occur together. In older children and adults marked increases in blood concentrations of leukocytes and serum proteins can result in hyperviscous blood, even with a normal hematocrit level, and they can therefore have hyperviscosity without polycythemia. Neonates with leukocyte concentrations up

to and over 100,000/μL, however, have been reported to have normal blood viscosity measurements. In neonates hyperviscosity is nearly always secondary to polycythemia, and polycythemia (particularly a "central" hematocrit exceeding 70%) essentially always indicates hyperviscosity.

deAlarcón PA, Werner EJ, Christensen RD, editors. Neonatal hematology. Cambridge: Cambridge University Press; 2012.

24. **Is a reduction transfusion needed for neonates with polycythemia?**
A hematocrit (or blood Hgb concentration) exceeding the 95th percentile limit (see Fig. 12-1) on the first day of life is, by definition, abnormal. However, not all neonates with a hematocrit above the 95th percentile need a reduction transfusion. If they did, 5% of all neonates would be subjected to a reduction transfusion. A general recommendation is that if the central (noncapillary) value exceeds 70% *and* the neonate has physiologic disturbances consistent with hyperviscosity, a reduction transfusion is warranted. Those disturbances include tachypnea, tachycardia, plethora, hypoglycemia, and tremulousness. An additional general recommendation is that if the central hematocrit exceeds 75%, a reduction transfusion may be warranted even if the neonate is asymptomatic. Ideally, avoiding the signs associated with hyperviscosity by reducing the hematocrit before intravascular problems result is preferable.

25. **What method is recommended for reduction transfusion?**
An isovolemic reduction is better tolerated than simply withdrawing blood. In hyperviscocity syndrome withdrawal of blood alone may produce increased intravascular sludging and increase the risk of symptoms. To accomplish this process, the clinician can simultaneously administer sterile saline while removing an equal volume of blood. This exchange can be done using two separate sites (pushing through one intravenous line and pulling through the other) or through one site, such as an umbilical venous catheter, pushing and then pulling in increments not exceeding 5 mL/kg body weight in each cycle. The procedure should be set up in a sterile manner, using continuous heart rate, respiratory rate, and pulse oximetry monitoring. In general, the total volume of saline infused will equal exactly the total volume of blood removed. This volume can be calculated as follows.

Multiply the estimated blood volume (about 80 to 90 mL/kg body weight) by the observed hematocrit minus the desired hematocrit (aim for 60%) divided by the observed hematocrit. In general, you will be performing a reduction on a term neonate (3 kg) with a hematocrit of 75%, so the equation will be calculated as follows:

80 mL/kg × 3 kg = The estimated blood volume is 240 mL.
The percentage reduction you want to achieve is (75% to 60%) ÷ 75% or 20% of the blood volume. 20% of 240 mL is 48 mL. Therefore 48 mL of saline is to be infused and 48 mL of blood is to be withdrawn to drop the hematocrit from 75% to 60% in an isovolemic reduction.

This type of reduction transfusion has been documented to reverse the clinical symptoms of neonatal hyperviscosity, but it is not clear whether any long-term improvements occur as a result.

NORMAL PLATELET VALUES OF MOTHERS AND NEONATES

26. **You are informed that an apparently healthy term neonate was delivered to a woman with "mild" thrombocytopenia, and you wonder whether it would be of value to obtain a platelet count on the neonate. The mother's platelet count on her first prenatal visit (at 10 weeks) was 205,000/μL, but it was 132,000/μL at delivery; her MPV was 9.2 fL at 10 weeks and again at delivery. Her pregnancy, labor, and delivery were completely normal. Is her platelet count low, or is it within the expected (normal) reference range? Is it good practice to check a platelet count on her normal-appearing neonate on the basis of her count of 132,000/μL?**
Reference ranges for platelet counts during pregnancy are shown in Figure 12-9. The 5th percentile value (the lowest expected limit) at term is 100,000/μL; thus a value of 135,000/μL is within the

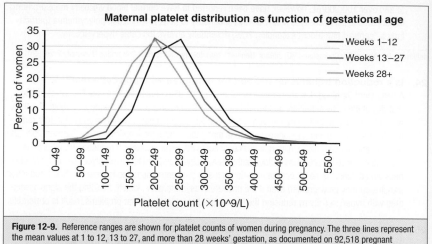

Figure 12-9. Reference ranges are shown for platelet counts of women during pregnancy. The three lines represent the mean values at 1 to 12, 13 to 27, and more than 28 weeks' gestation, as documented on 92,518 pregnant women. (From Jensen, et al. Am J Perinatol 2010;28:597–604.)

normal range. As the figure shows, the reference range diminishes steadily throughout gestation, generally falling by an increment of about 50,000/μL from early pregnancy to term. This fall is at least partly caused by the normal hemodilution of pregnancy. In contrast, no change in MPV normally occurs during pregnancy. Neonates born to women who have platelet counts in the range of 100,000 to 150,000/μL do not have an increased risk of neonatal thrombocytopenia. Therefore if the neonate appears healthy, it is not necessary to obtain a platelet count on the basis of the mother's count of 135,000/μL.

Wiedmeier SE, Henry E, Sola-Visner MC, et al. Platelet reference ranges for neonates, defined using data from over 47,000 patients in a multihospital healthcare system. J Perinatol 2009;29:130–6.

27. **A neonate delivered at 30 weeks' gestation is admitted to the NICU. Aside from mild respiratory distress, the patient seems stable. A CBC on NICU admission reveals a platelet count of 129,000/μL with an MPV of 8.8 fL. Is this platelet count low, or is it within the expected (normal) reference range?**
Reference ranges for platelet counts on the day of birth, according to gestational age, are shown in Figure 12-10. The 5th percentile (lower) expected range at 30 weeks' gestation is about 110,000/μL, and thus the observed count of 129,000/μL is normal.

28. **Approximately 3 weeks later, the same neonate discussed in Question 27 is doing well and growing appropriately, but a CBC shows that the platelet count is now 595,000/μL. Is that value high, or is it within the expected (normal) reference range?**
Reference ranges for platelet counts during the first 90 days after birth are shown in Figure 12-11. The 95th percentile (upper limit) value at 3 weeks is about 650,000/μL, and the value of 595,000/μL is therefore within the expected reference range. The reference range for platelets increases after birth, reaching a first peak at 14 to 20 days. This change is most likely due to the physiologic thrombopoietin surge that occurs at birth. This surge—and the subsequent increase in platelet count—occurs after either vaginal or cesarean delivery and in preterm as well as term neonates. A comparable increase in MPV also occurs during the first 2 to 3 weeks, consistent with increased platelet production. The cause of the second peak in platelet count at 40 to 50 days (see Figure 12-11) is not known.

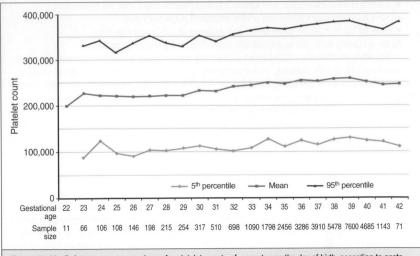

Figure 12-10. Reference ranges are shown for platelet counts of neonates on the day of birth, according to gestational age. The *lower* and *upper lines* represent the 5th and the 95th percentile values, respectively, and the *center line* represents the mean value. (From Wiedmeier, et al. J Perinatol 2009;29:130–136.)

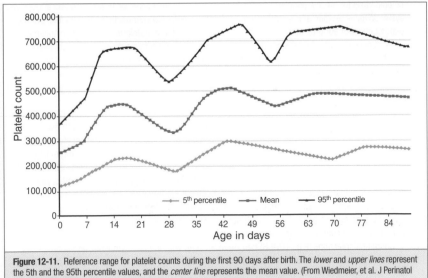

Figure 12-11. Reference range for platelet counts during the first 90 days after birth. The *lower* and *upper lines* represent the 5th and the 95th percentile values, and the *center line* represents the mean value. (From Wiedmeier, et al. J Perinatol 2009;29:130–136.)

THROMBOCYTOPENIA AND PLATELET TRANSFUSION

29. A 39-week-gestation, appropriately grown male neonate is noted to have petechiae shortly after birth. The platelet count is 9000/μL, and the MPV is 8.2 fL. The remainder of the CBC is normal. Appropriate actions include which of the following?
   - Repeat the platelet count, and examine the blood film to obtain an estimimate of whether the platelets are abnormally small, normal in size, or abnormally large.

- Order a platelet transfusion, and obtain a repeat platelet count after the transfusion.
- Have a platelet count performed on the mother (if not already done).
- Look for malformations, syndromes, and evidence of congenital infection.

All the preceding steps can be appropriate depending on the circumstances.

Repeating an abnormal platelet count is generally wise because artifactually low platelet counts can occur with platelet clumping, as sometimes happens in a difficult and slowly oozing capillary draw, where platelets can aggregate at the wound edge and render the platelet count artifactually low. However, the presence of petechiae in this case strongly suggests that the platelet count is indeed pathologically low; do not let repeating the count delay your other orders.

In a neonate with severe congenital thrombocytopenia, an estimate of the platelet size can be an important diagnostic aid. Very small platelets in a male can suggest Wiscott–Aldrich syndrome (OMIM #301000, Xp11.23) or X-linked thrombocytopenia (OMIM #313900, Xp11.22). Very large platelets can suggest accelerated platelet destruction (as with neonatal alloimmune thrombocytopenia), a familial macrothrombocytopenia such as Bernard–Soulier syndrome (OMIM # 231200), or the MHY9-related disorders.

Ordering a platelet transfusion for this patient would be in keeping with usual practice in the United States. In a recent survey more than 90% of neonatologists in the United States and Canada would order a platelet transfusion for a neonate with a platelet count below 10,000/μL on the day of birth, even if no clinical bleeding manifestations (other than petechiae) were identified. Measuring the platelet count after (within 30 minutes) completing the platelet transfusion can help you determine whether the thrombocytopenia is the result of reduced platelet production (adequate rise with transfusion) or accelerated destruction (poor rise with transfusion).

A low platelet count in the mother could be an important diagnostic finding, suggesting an immunologic basis for the low platelets in both mother and neonate. Idiopathic thrombocytopenic purpura, systemic lupus erythematosis, or any maternal autoimmune disorder could be responsible, but the platelet count of 9000/μL in this patient is very low for maternal autoimmune thrombocytopenia.

Most neonates whose mothers have autoimmune thrombocytopenia do not have platelet counts below 30,000 or 40,000/μL. Also, a variety of familial thrombocytopenias might be found in the mother, and the platelet size in these cases can be either normal or large. Familial thrombocytopenia with normal-size platelets include Paris–Trousseau syndrome (11q23 deletion), RUNX1 mutation, and the ANKRD26 mutation.

Thrombocytopenia is part of many syndromes. For instance, neonates with trisomy 13 and 18 are almost always thrombocytopenic. However, the platelet counts in most syndromes with dysmorphia rarely have platelet counts this low, generally not below 40,000/μL. Severe thrombocytopenia, as observed in this case, can be seen with TAR syndrome (thrombocytopenia and absent radii), but the patient must have short forearms with normal-looking thumbs for TAR to be a consideration. Another syndrome associated with severe thrombocytopenia is ATRUS (amegakaryocytic thrombocytopenia with radioulnar synostosis) and should be expected if the forearms look normal but radioulnar rotation is severely limited (you are unable to supinate and pronate the forearm). Another is CAMT (congenital amegakaryocytic thrombocytopenia), which generally occurs with no other malformations but rarely can accompany other conditions, such as Noonan syndrome.

Congenital infections (e.g., TORCH) can be associated with thrombocytopenia, and some cases result in values as low as seen in this patient. The kinetic mechanism for this variety of neonatal thrombocytopenia is often a mixture of reduced production and accelerated destruction.

The prinicipal considerations for this appropriately grown, 37-week-gestation, otherwise healthy-appearing neonate with a platelet count of 9000/μL (if the MPV is normal or slightly increased, perhaps approximately 11 or 12 fL) include neonatal alloimmune thrombocytopenia, congenital infection, CAMT, and ATRUS.

In this case, an x-ray (Figure 12-12) of the forearms showed radioulnar synostosis, making ATRUS the likely diagnosis (a mutation in *HOXA11* mapping to 7p15). ATRUS is an autosomal dominant condition, but neonates can be much more severely affected than their affected parent. Generally, the affected parent has radioulnar synostosis with limited forearm pronation and supination, but his or her platelet counts tend to be only moderately low (50,000/μL) with minimal clinical bleeding problems. Neonates with ATRUS are likely to be dependent on platelet transfusion, and marrow or cord blood transplantation is the only known curative procedure.

Strauss RG. Platelet transfusions in neonates: questions and answers. Expert Rev Hematol 2010;3:7–9.

30. **What is the expected rise in platelet count after a platelet transfusion? What is the average survival time of transfused platelets in a neonate?**
A transfusion of 15 mL donor platelets per kg will generally increase the recipient's platelet count by 70,000 to 100,000/μL. The life span of normal platelets *in vivo* is approximately 10 days. Therefore, when platelets are harvested from a donor, about 10% of these are newly formed and might survive in the recipient for up to 10 days. However, about 10% are effete and will not survive at all in the recipient. On average the donor platelets will decay after transfusion with a half-life of between 1 and 2 days. Thus in 3 or 4 days most (>75%) of the transfused platelets will be gone, and by 5 or 6 days essentially all the transfused platelet will be gone.

In cases of ATRUS, the rise in platelet count following transfusion and the disappearance of the transfused platelets should conform to these principles, because the kinetic mechanism responsible for the thrombocytopenia is reduced platelet production. However, in cases of neonatal thrombocytopenia caused by a platelet consumptive process, such as DIC, a propagating thrombus, or

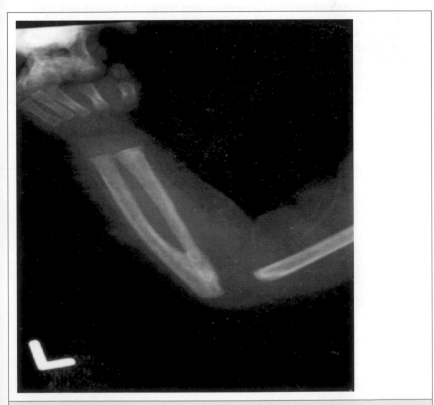

Figure 12-12. An x-ray of the forearm of a 37-weeks'-gestation female infant who, shortly after birth, was noted to have scattered petechiae and a platelet count of 9000/μL. She was otherwise well-appearing and in no distress. Fusion of the proximal radius and ulna is seen. This is a case of ATRUS (**A**megakaryocytic **T**hrombocytopenia with **R**adio**U**lnar **S**ynostosis) (From Sola, et al. J Perinatol 2004;24:528–530.)

immune-mediated thrombocytopenia, the platelet count will not increase by the expected amount after transfusion and will fall much more rapidly than previously described.

Christensen RD. Platelet transfusion in the neonatal intensive care unit: benefits, risks, alternatives. Neonatology 2011;100:311–8.

31. What product is recommended for platelet transfusion in the NICU?
According to a recent survey of neonatologists in North America, about half of the respondents routinely order a platelet transfusion volume of 10 mL/kg and about half order 10 to 15 mL/kg. Because every platelet transfusion given results in another donor exposure, one larger transfusion might offer an advantage over two smaller ones (each from a different donor). On that basis the author recommends a volume of 15 mL/kg. About half of respondents use single-donor platelets, about 10% use platelets pooled from 2 to 3 donors, and about 25% use apheresis-prepared platelets. Pooling donors results in more donor exposures, and the volume reduction needed after pooling reduces platelet viability. The Intermountain Healthcare NICUs (where the author works) use apheresis-prepared platelets exclusively. Between 60% and 70% of respondents use only irradiated platelets for all neonatal platelet transfusions.

REFERENCE RANGES FOR NEUTROPHIL COUNTS AND NEUTROPENIA

32. Why are neutrophil counts of neonates much higher at high altitude? Is the difference of any clinical significance?
Newborn nurseries in Colorado, New Mexico, and Utah, 4000 to 5500 feet above sea level, have reported much higher reference ranges for blood neutrophil concentrations during the first 3 days after birth than nurseries at or near sea level. It is curious that hematocrit/Hgb levels and NRBC/μL are not higher at the high-altitude hospitals; the mechanism explaining the difference in neutrophil counts is not known. Figure 12-13 shows the reference ranges for high-altitude and sea-level centers superimposed. One value in recognizing that these differences exist is that NICUs at high altitude

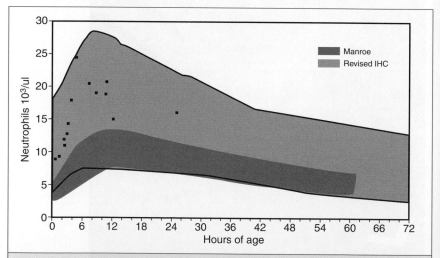

Figure 12-13. Reference ranges are shown for blood neutrophil counts during the first 3 days after birth. The *light-gray scale* indicates the reference range for neutrophil counts obtained from neonates at high altitude (identified as *Revised IHC*). The *dark-gray scale* indicates the reference range for counts obtained from neonates near sea-level (identified as *Manroe*). The *black dots* represent 14 healthy term neonates in Utah who would have been termed "neutrophilic" according to the Manroe chart but were seen to be well within the high-altitude reference ranges. (From Lambert, et al. J Perinatol 2009;29:822–825.)

can falsely label neonates as neutrophilic if the sea-level range is used. Perhaps the opposite is also true; neonates at sea level could have the diagnosis of neutrophilia missed if the reference range for high-altitude centers is used.

33. A neonate delivered at 29 weeks' gestation is unstable on a mechanical ventilator, and the first blood gas reading indicates severe metabolic acidosis. Hypotension and poor perfusion are present. The infant is small for gestational age with asymmetric growth retardation; birth weight is below 5th percentile, length is at the 20th percentile, and the occipital-frontal circumference falls at the 40th percentile. His mother has been diagnosed with pregnancy-induced hypertension (PIH). The first CBC, obtained on the neonate just after birth, shows neutropenia, with 750 neutrophil/μL and a marked left shift, with 1% polymorphonuclear neutrophil, 21% band neutrophils and 4% metamyelocytes. A senior neonatologist notes that the neutropenia in this patient is the very common variety seen in small-for-gestational-age neonates born after PIH; that this variety is transient, resulting from reduced neutrophil production that will improve in the next day or two; and that antibiotic treatment is not needed. What do you think about this advice?

Neutropenia is indeed common in neonates born after PIH, particularly if the neonate is preterm and small for gestational age. However, the marked "left shift" is not typical of that variety of neutopenia. It is important to consider that the hypotension, metabolic acidosis, and respiratory distress accompanying the neutropenia and left shift are manifestations of sepsis. Therefore it would be unwise to withhold antibiotic treatment for this patient under the possibly erroneous assumption that the baby has neutropenia associated with PIH and being small for gestational age.

34. A well-appearing term neonate has a screening CBC performed as part of a protocol for asymptomatic neonates delivered to women testing positive for Group B Streptococcus who did not receive intrapartum antibiotics. The CBC is normal, with the exception of a neutrophil count of 550/μL. No band forms were seen, and the platelet count is normal. The baby has no dysmorphic features and appears totally healthy. Which of the following steps would be appropriate for evaluating the neutropenia in this neonate?

   ▪ Repeat the CBC, and examine the blood film to estimate whether the neutrophil count indeed appears low on the smear and whether the neutrophils appear morphologically normal.
   ▪ Examine the neonate carefully to ensure that no subtle or early signs of infection are present, such as respiratory distress, tachycardia, and poor perfusion.
   ▪ Have a CBC performed on the mother (if not already done), and inquire whether she has a past history of neutropenia or an autoimmune disorder (e.g., systemic lupus erythematosus) and whether neonatal neutropenia was recognized in any of her other children.

All the preceding actions are appropriate.

35. The repeat CBC on the healthy term baby described in Question 34 is similar to the first. The pathologist reports that the neutrophil concentration on the blood film is indeed low, that the rare neutrophils present appear mature and morphologically normal, and that the other leukocytes and the erythrocytes and platelets also appear normal. You find that the mother had a normal CBC before delivery. She never had a diagnosis of neutropenia or an autoimmune disorder, and her two previous children were healthy with no known medical problems. The next morning the CBC on this neonate is essentially unchanged, with an absolute neutrophil count of 490/μL. He still appears to be healthy and is breastfeeding well. Can you construct a reasonable differential diagnosis for this variety of neonatal neutropenia?

Table 12-1 categorizes neonatal neutropenia into subtypes. Some of these varieties are very common, and others are exceedingly rare. Some are the result of reduced neutrophil production, and

CATEGORY	COMMON OR RARE?	AGE OF DETECTION	IS THE ANC GENERALLY <500/µL OR >500/µL	LARGE LEFT SHIFT PRESENT?	USUAL DURATION OF NEUTORPENIA	IS RG-CSF TREATMENT EFFECTIVE AND RECOMMENDED?
Severe congenital	Very rare; (1 in 200,000)	Birth	<500; many times <250	No (unless infected)	Lifelong	Yes
PIH/SGA	Very common	Birth	Can be <500 but usually <2 to 4 days	No	2 to 4 days	No
Sepsis	Common	During infection	Can be <500	Yes	<1 day	No
Neonatal alloimmune	Fairly common	Birth	Can be <500	No	Up to several months	Yes, if severe and prolonged
Maternal autoimmune	Fairly common	Birth	Generally >500	No	Days to weeks	No
Neonatal autoimmune	Rare	Birth	Generally >500	No	Up to many months	Yes, if severe and prolonged
Chronic idiopathic of prematurity	Fairly common	Generally after 3 to 4 weeks	Generally >500	No	Perhaps 2 to 4 weeks	No

TABLE 12–1. AN INITIAL APPROACH TO A NEONATE WITH NEUTROPENIA

ANC, Absolute neutrophil count; PIH, pregnancy-induced hypertension; RG-CSF, recombinant granulocyte colony-stimulating factor; SGA, small for gestational age.

others the result of accelerated neutrophil utilization (sepsis) or destruction (immune mediated). Although this could be one of the subtypes of severe congenital neutropenia, those are extremely rare. Given that the patient is not ill and has no left shift, this is not the neutropenia of overwhelming sepsis. Because this infant is not small for gestational age and the mother did not have PIH, it is not that variety. Most likely this is a case of alloimmune neonatal neutropenia (ANN), wherein the mother has immunoglobulin G antibody against a neutrophil antigen she lacks but that is expressed by father and fetus.

Maheshwari A, Christensen RD, Calhoun DA. Immune neutropenia in the neonate. Adv Pediatr 2002;49:317–39.

36. **Because ANN is high on the list of possibilities, what can you cite about the pathogenesis, diagnostic tests, natural history, and treatment options for that condition?**

ANN is a common variety of severe congenital neutropenia, with a prevalence estimated to be as high as one to two per thousand births.

ANN is a potentially critical disorder, with a mortality rate estimated to be as high as 5%, on the basis of acquiring a significant infection during a period of severe neutropenia.

The pathogenesis of ANN involves the passive transfer of neutrophil-specific maternal immunoglobulin G antibodies across the placenta. The antibodies bind to fetal neutrophils, which express an antigen inherited from the father that is absent in the mother. These maternal immunoglobulin G antibodies can result in severe neutropenia before and after birth. Neutrophil-specific antibodies directed against the human neutrophil antigens (HNAs) HNA-1a, HNA-1b and HNA-2a, are detected in more than 50% of ANN cases. Antibodies to HNA-1c, HNA-3a, and HNA-4a are occasionally identified.

A reference laboratory skilled in the diagnosis of ANN is required to ensure an accurate diagnosis. One such outstanding laboratory is the American Red Cross North Central Blood Services in St. Paul, Minnesota. Simply looking for maternal antineutrophil antibodies is not always sufficient. Generally, the evaluation begins using the mother's serum and granulocyte agglutination (GA) or granulocyte immunofluorescence (GIF) assays. If maternal antineutrophil antibodies are identified, neutrophil genotyping can be performed on whole blood collected from the father and the mother to identify the HNA involved.

Work with your pediatric hematology consultant to decide whether to treat the neonate with ANN with recombinant granulocyte colony-stimulating factor. We generally do so if the neutropenia is severe (<500/µL) for several days, if it is in the range of 500 to 999/µL for approximately 1 week, or if the patient has a bacterial infection. A dose of 10 µg/kg given subcutaneously once daily for about 3 days will usually result in an absolute neutrophil count greater than 1000/µL. Subsequent doses may be needed to keep the absolute neutrophil count above 1000/µL. The duration of the condition roughly corresponds to the disappearance of maternal antineutrophil antibody from the neonate, which sometimes takes up to 2 months or so.

37. **What is the *ELANE* gene, and how is it involved in severe congenital neutropenia?**

ELANE (**ELA**stase, **N**eutrophil **E**xpressed) is the gene encoding neutrophil elastase and is located at 19p13.3. Most cases of severe congential neutropenia (excluding cases of severe alloimmune neutropenia) are the result of *ELANE* mutations. Severe congenital neutropenia type 1 (OMIM #202700) is an autosomal dominant disorder. More that 70 different *ELANE* mutations have been identified that result in type 1 severe congenital neutropenia. These mutations each produce a gene product that folds into an incorrect three-dimensional shape. The abnormal neutrophil elastase protein accumulates in neutrophils and damages or kills these cells before they are fully mature.

Other *ELANE* mutations result in cyclic neutropenia, which can also be categorized as a type of severe congenital neutropenia, wherein cyclic drops in the absolute neutrophil count occur on an every-3-to-4-week cycle. The *ELANE* mutations causing cyclic neutropenia are generally single nucleotide substitutions that produce a defective neutrophil elastase protein retaining some level of function.

Maheshwari A, Christensen RD, Calhoun DA. Immune neutropenia in the neonate. Adv Pediatr 2002;49:317–39.

Boztug K, Klein C. Genetic etiologies of severe congenital neutropenia. Curr Opin Pediatr 2011;23:21–6.

38. **Is Kostmann syndrome the same as severe congenital neutropenia type 1?**

No. The Swedish kindred described by Dr. Kostmann in 1956 was an autosomal recessive disorder. The phenotype of Kostmann syndrome is similar to that of severe congenital neutropenia type 1 but is more clinically heterogenous. The OMIM number for Kostmann syndrome is 610738, and it is currently termed severe congenital neutropenia type 3. The condition results from mutations in the *HAX1* gene, located at 1q21. *HAX1* encodes a mitochondrial-associated protein involved in neutrophil signal transduction and cytoskeletal regulation. Patients with severe congenital neutropenia type 3 can be either homozygous for the mutation or compound heterozygotes, meaning that they inherited one mutation in *HAX1* from one parent and a different *HAX1* mutation from the other parent.

EOSINOPHILIA

39. **The CBC of a newborn infant admitted to the NICU after birth at 33 weeks' gestation has an eosinophil count (WBCs multiplied by the percentage of eosinophils) of 1000/μL. Is that value high, or is it within the expected (normal) reference range?**

Expected values, also called reference ranges, for eosinophil counts on the day of birth are a function of gestational age, increasing gradually through the second and third trimesters. Reference ranges for eosniophil counts at birth are shown in Figure 12-14. The 95th percentile value (the highest expected limit) at 34 weeks is about 1100/μL. Thus a value of 1000/μL is normal.

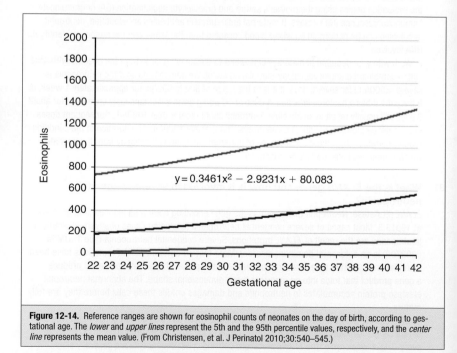

$$y = 0.3461x^2 - 2.9231x + 80.083$$

Figure 12-14. Reference ranges are shown for eosinophil counts of neonates on the day of birth, according to gestational age. The *lower* and *upper lines* represent the 5th and the 95th percentile values, respectively, and the *center line* represents the mean value. (From Christensen, et al. J Perinatol 2010;30:540–545.)

Christensen RD, Jensen J, Maheshwari A, et al. Reference ranges for blood concentrations of eosinophils and monocytes during the neonatal period defined from over 63,000 records in a multihospital health-care system. J Perinatol 2010;30:540–5.

40. **The CBC of the neonate in discussed in Question 39 is now 27 days old. The infant is about to be discharged home. The eosinophil count is now 1500/μL. Is that value high, or is it within the expected (normal) reference range?**

    Although the eosinophil count has increased significantly from that measured on the day of birth, the value is within the expected range. The reference range for blood eosinophil concentration during the first 28 days after birth is shown in Figure 12-15.

41. **If the eosinophil count of the neonate discussed in Questions 39 and 40 were 3500/μL, the term *eosinophilia* would properly apply. What are the more common conditions that might be associated with such a high eosinophil count in this neonate?**

    Eosinophils are effector cells involved in allergic and nonallergic inflammatory conditions. Circulating eosinophils are derived from myelocytic progenitors within the marrow and within extramedullary sites as well. After exiting the site of production and entering the blood, eosinophils circulate for approximately 1 day (T½ 18 hours), after which they transmigrate to tissues, primarily in the gastro-intestinal tract, where they produce cytokines and chemokines. Several pathologic conditions in neonates are associated with eosinophilic tissue infiltration, and these conditions are often accompanied by blood eosinophilia. The conditions include erythema toxicum, neonatal eosinophilic pustulosis, and bronchopulmonary dysplasia. Other inflammatory conditions associated with eosinophilia are neonatal eosinophilic esophagitis, eosinophilic colitis, subcutaneous fat necrosis with eosinophilic granules, a variety of infectious diseases, and necrotizing enterocolitis after erythrocyte transfusion. A slight increase can occasionally be expected in preterm infants corresponding to the time weight gain is established.

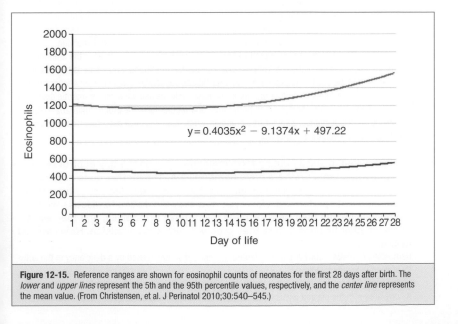

Figure 12-15. Reference ranges are shown for eosinophil counts of neonates for the first 28 days after birth. The *lower* and *upper lines* represent the 5th and the 95th percentile values, respectively, and the *center line* represents the mean value. (From Christensen, et al. J Perinatol 2010;30:540–545.)

COAGULATION

42. **You are asked to see a healthy term female newborn shortly after birth because the mother has von Willebrand disease. The parents want to discuss with you the possibility that the child might also have this condition. What facts would be helpful for you to give them?**

First, you might inquire if the mother knows the type of von Willebrand disease that she has. You should also find out if she had any bleeding problems as a baby and about her own bleeding history. Perhaps the parents already know that von Willebrand disease is the most common inherited disorder of coagulation, with a prevalence as high as 1% of the general population. They might also already know that von Willebrand disease is not a single disorder and that the most common variety, type 1 (the most likely type the baby may have inherited from mother), is hardly ever problematic during the newborn period. Only type 3, a very rare autosomal recessive variety completely lacking von Willebrand factor antigen and activity, is likely to result in excessive bleeding in infants. Table 12-2 reviews the features of von Willebrand subtypes.

Saxonhouse MA, Manco-Johnson MJ. The evaluation and management of neonatal coagulation disorders. Semin Perinatol 2009;33:52–65.

43. **You are asked to see a healthy term female newborn shortly after birth because the mother has the factor V Leiden mutation. The parents want to discuss with you the possibility that the child might also have this condition. What facts would be helpful for you to give them?**

The factor V Leiden mutation and the prothrombin 20210 mutation are so commonly found in women (men, too, for that matter) that this specific question of neonatal risk with an affected parent comes up regularly in NICU practice.

Up to 10% of people of Northern European ancestry carry one copy of the factor V Leiden mutation (OMIM #188055), which is a single nucleotide substitution (R506Q) in the *F5* gene on 1q24.2. This variation results in activated factor V that is resistant to inactivation by its physiologic regulator, activated protein C. In the very rare instance when both parents carry the factor V Leiden mutation, one in four of their offspring can inherit both defective genes in a homozygous fashion, and the neonate can indeed be at high risk for neonatal thrombosis. However, neonates with a single copy of the factor V Leiden mutation (heterozygote) appear to be at no increased risk for neonatal thrombosis. Thrombotic risks similar to that of the affected parent will be present during adolescence and adult life.

Up to 2% of Caucasians carry the prothrombin 20210 mutation, which increases the amount of prothrombin in the circulation by 15% to 30%. The human prothrombin *(F2)* gene is located at 11p11-q12, and the 20210 mutation is a single nucleotide substitution. Neonates who inherit this mutation from their father or mother are not at increased risk, as neonates, for thrombotic disorders. However, in the very rare instance when both father and mother have the prothrombin 20210 mutation, the fetus can be homozygous for this mutation. Such neonates have been reported to have a significant risk of neonatal thrombosis.

44. **You are asked to see a healthy term male newborn on the day of birth because two of the mother's brothers have hemophilia A. The mother does not know whether she is a hemophilia carrier, and the parents elected not to have fetal diagnostic tests performed. However, now they would like to discuss with you the possibility that their newborn son might have hemophilia, and they want to know whether he does before they proceed with a circumcision. How can you help them?**

Hemophilia A (OMIM # 306700) is an X-linked recessive disorder caused by a deficiency in the activity of coagulation factor VIII.

The gene *F8* encoding factor VIII is located at Xq28. Bleeding severity in patients with hemophilia A correlates with the plasma levels of factor VIII. Patients are expected to have "mild" bleeding

TABLE 12-2. TYPES OF VON WILLEBRAND DISEASE, GENERALLY THE RESULT OF MUTATIONS AFFECTING THE QUALITY OR QUANTITY OF VWF PROTEIN.

TYPE (OMIM #)	EXPLANATION	PREVALENCE	INHERITANCE	GENE	SEVERITY	OTHER FEATRUES
Type 1 193400	Low levels of VWF (20% to 40% of normal)	60% to 80% of all cases	Autosomal dominant	12p13.31	Usually mild mucocutaneous bleeding or asymptomatic	Treatment usually not needed; severe bleeding sometimes treated with dDAVP*
Type 2 613554	All type 2 subtypes have VWF that functions poorly	10% to 30% of all cases	Usually autosomal dominamt	12p13.31	Mild to moderate mucocutaneous bleeding	Can be treated with dDAVP*, which raises the level of factor VIII/VWF in plasma
Type 2A	Low, medium, and high molecular weight VWF multimers		Autosomal dominamt	12p13.31		
Type 2B	"Gain of function" caused by large VWF multimers, leading to rapid clearance		Autosomal dominamt	12p13.31		May have mild thrombocytopenia; 2B is the only variety of type 2 that should not be treated with dDAVP
Type 2M	Normal antigen levels but decreased function		Usually autosomal dominamt	12p13.31		
Type 2 Normany	Abnormal binding site for factor VIII		Usually autosomal dominamt	12p13.31	Can be moderately severe	Sometimes confused with hemophilia A
Type 3 277480	homozygous or compound heterozygous mutation; no VWF activity	1 or 2 per million births	Autosomal recessive	12p13.31	Generally the most severe form	Can develop anti-VWF antibodies after exposure to VWF concentrates
Platelet type also known as pseudo von Willebrand disease 177820	Mutation in the GP1BA gene resulting in abnormal (avid) binding of VWF to platelets, with rapid clearance	More common than type 2B (the other type with low platelets)	Autosomal dominant	17p13.2	Frequent and severe nosebleeds and excessive bleeding after tooth extraction	Has caused neonatal thrombocytopenia; usual treatments that increase VWF (infusion or dDAVP) actually make the platelet count fall further

VWF, Von Willebrand factor.
*dDAVP (1-deamino-8-D-arginine vasopressin) is not commonly used in the neonatal period because of the risks of hyponatremia and edema.

problems with levels in the range of 6% to 30% of normal, "moderate" with levels 2% to 5% of normal, and "severe" with levels less than 1% of normal.

Hemophilia B (OMIM # 306900) is also an X-linked recessive disorder but is caused by a deficiency in the activity of coagulation factor IX. The gene *F9* encoding factor IX is located at Xq27.1.

The parents of this boy are wise to determine whether their son has hemophilia before a circumcision is done. In fact, the CDC recommends that a baby who might have hemophilia (born to a known carrier, or to a mother with brothers known to have hemophilia) should avoid circumcision. However, if parents of such a neonate insist that a circumcision is performed, the Centers for Disease Control and Prevention recommend that a pediatric hematologist be consulted before the procedure to ensure that the child receives proper treatment to prevent excessive bleeding. Many neonates with mild or moderate hemophilia have been circumcised with little or no abnormal bleeding, but it is unwise to proceed with circumcision given this family history without first making a diagnosis and without involving a hematologist.

It is helpful for parents who are planning to deliver a son with a risk of hemophilia (based on the family history) to inform you before the delivery. This knowledge will allow you to obtain the necessary tests from fetal blood drawn from the placental end of the umbilical vein immediately after placental delivery. This method does not require blood to be drawn from the neonate for diagnostic testing.

Using umbilical cord (fetal) plasma, you can quantify factor VIII and factor IX and obtain a prothrombin time (PT) and activated partial thromboplastin time (aPTT). You can also order a CBC from the umbilical cord blood so that you are aware of the initial platelet count and Hgb level. Because factor IX is a vitamin K–dependent factor, normal levels are relatively low at birth. Therefore mild hemophilia B is difficult to confirm at times, based on low factor IX levels, for the first month or so. However, factor VIII plasma levels should be at adult levels even in the cord blood. Thus a diagnosis of hemophilia A can be made using umbilical cord blood.

45. **An ill 32-week-gestation male newborn, approximately 24 hours old, is being managed with mechanical ventilation for severe respiratory distress and is being treated with dopamine because of hypotension. He is also receiving antibiotics because of the possibility of bacterial sepsis. You notice a rather sudden appearance of bright red blood in the endotracheal tube, and you see oozing around the umbilical catheters and at venipuncture sites. You suspect the patient has developed DIC. How do you proceed?**

DIC in a neonate is actually more of a clinical than a laboratory diagnosis—bleeding at multiple sites with hypotension. Laboratory confirmation includes thrombocytopenia, or at least a falling platelet count, along with a low fibrinogen or at least a falling fibrinogen level, and elevated or rising D-dimers. Prolongation in the PT and aPTT also support the diagnosis. No single test is sufficient to unequivocally diagnose DIC in a neonate.

Acute bleeding as a result of liver failure is rare in neonates but can present much like DIC. This condition, largely the result of poor production of procoagulant factors by damaged or abnormal hepatocytes, can be distinguished from DIC by the factor VIII level. Factor VIII is not made by hepatocytes but by endothelial cells, and plasma levels increase in liver failure but fall in DIC.

The only treatment for DIC in neonates that works reliably is to reverse the DIC triggers: sepsis, hypoxia, acidosis, hypotension. The nonintuitive treatment of anticoagulation has not been adequately tested in hemorrhaging neonates. It sometimes seems to work, but it is best left to the rare cases of DIC that present with multiple thrombotic sites, such as purpura fulminans.

Transfusing fresh frozen plasma and platelets has been said to exacerbate DIC, but when the bleeding is severe and difficult to control and all else is failing, these transfusions probably have a place.

In case reports recombinant factor VIIa has been used successfully to treat life-threatening bleeding in neonates with DIC. Also, activated protein C is under investigation as an adjunctive treatment for neonates with DIC, but the risks of either of these potential treatments are great, and risk-to-benefit evaluations are needed.

✓ KEY POINTS

1. The presence of Barts Hgb on a Hgb electrophoresis (a gamma chain tetramer) is indicative of alpha-thalassemia trait. These infants commonly have microcytic red blood cells.

2. The lowest limit for Hgb concentration in a term infant is 14 g/dL.

3. Subgaleal hemorrhages can result hypovolemia and shock, whereas cephalohematomas will not.

4. The viscosity of blood in a neonate does not change significantly with white blood counts >100,000/µL.

5. In a neonate with physiologic disturbances (e.g., findings related to the central nervous system) and a hematocrit >70% from a non-capillary peripheral vein, a reduction transfusion is indicated.

6. A platelet transfusion of 15 mL/kg will increase the recipient's platelet count by 70,000-100,000/µL.

7. The neutropenia observed in infants born to women with pregnancy induced hypertension is not usually accompanied by a "left shift."

8. Neonates with a single mutation in factor V Leiden are not at increased risk for thrombosis.

9. The only reliable treatment for disseminated intravascular coagulation is to reverse the triggers (i.e., treat the underlying disorder).

CHAPTER 13

INFECTION AND IMMUNITY

Beatriz Larru, MD, PhD, and Theoklis E. Zaoutis, MD, MSCE

DEVELOPMENTAL IMMUNOLOGY

1. **In which way is the immune response of the neonate unique?**

   Except in the case of congenital infection, all pathogen encounters in the neonatal period are first-time encounters. For those first-time exposures to pathogens, neonates are dependent on the innate immune system. The innate immune system comprises cells and mechanisms that defend in a nonspecific manner. T- and B-cell responses are part of the specific (adaptive) immune system. The adaptive immune response allows the immune system to remember specific pathogens.

Maródi L. Innate cellular immune responses in newborns. Clin Immunol 2006 Feb;118(2-3):137–44.

Burgio GR, Hanson LA, Ugazio AG, editors. Immunology of the neonate. 1st ed. Berlin: Springer; 2012.

Dzwonek AB, Neth OW, Thiébaut R, et al. The role of mannose-binding lectin in susceptibility to infection in preterm neonates. Pediatr Res 2008;63(6):680–5.

2. **Does the immune system of the fetus and newborn prefer T_h1 or T_h2 immune responses?**

   There are two types of effector CD4+ helper cells: T_h1 and T_h2. Each of these is responsible for eliminating a specific kind of pathogen. The T_h1 response leads to cell-mediated immunity (important defense against viruses and intracellular pathogens.) T_h1 responses are considered proinflammatory. T_h2 responses activate B cells to make antibodies, leading to humoral immunity (important defense against extracellular bacteria, parasites, and toxins). T_h2 responses are antiinflammatory. T_h2 inflammatory responses are favored in the fetus, dampening the fetal immune response and preventing alloimmune reactions between mother and fetus (e.g., miscarriage). Decreased production of T_h1 cytokines increases the susceptibility to infection and contributes to the poor response to vaccines.

Strunk T, Burgner D. Genetic susceptibility to neonatal infection. Curr Opin Infect Dis 2006;19(3):259–63.

3. **What are the components of the innate immune system?**

   The nonspecific innate immune system includes host defense mechanisms that operate effectively without prior exposure. It includes the following:
   - Physical barriers; intact skin and mucosal membranes
   - Mononuclear inflammatory cells; particularly mast cells and tissue macrophages
   - Soluble plasma proteins; such as cytokines and complement components

Nussbaum C, Sperandio M. Innate immune cell recruitment in the fetus and neonate. J Reprod Immunol 2011;90(1):74–81.

4. **How does the skin of a neonate protect against invasive infections?**

   The vernix caseosa is a waxy coating in newborns that is secreted by fetal sebaceous glands. It contains antimicrobial peptides that act as a microbicidal shield. The lipids and acid pH of the neonatal skin inhibit microbial growth and reach maturity by week 2 to 4 in term neonates (later in premature infants). Small breaks in the integrity of the skin can serve as entry points for infection.

Levy O. Innate immunity of the newborn: basic mechanisms and clinical correlates. Nat Rev Immunol 2007;7(5):379–90.

Härtel C, Osthues I, Rupp J, et al. Characterisation of the host inflammatory response to *Staphylococcus epidermidis* in neonatal whole blood. Arch Dis Child Fetal Neonatal Ed. 2008;93(2):F140–5.

Strunk T, Richmond P, Simmer K, et al. Neonatal immune responses to coagulase-negative staphylococci. Curr Opin Infect Dis. 2007;20(4):370–5.

5. **What are the levels of serum complement at birth relative to the adult?**

   Complement components are synthesized as early as 6 to 14 weeks of gestation. However, neonatal plasma concentrations of complement components are diminished, ranging from 10% to 70% of adult levels. A relative deficiency in complement might contribute to the inability of newborns to limit the replication of many bacterial strains in the blood because opsonization is impaired; these differences are greater in preterm than in term neonates.

   Overall activity and components of the alternative pathway are more consistently decreased than those of the classical pathway. This finding is especially problematic for neonates who are exposed to organisms with polysaccharide capsules, such as *Escherichia coli* K1 and group B *Streptococcus* (GBS) and who cannot rely on classical pathway activation owing to the lack of specific antibodies.

Remington JS, Klein JO, Wilson CB, et al. Infectious diseases of the fetus and newborn: expert consult—online and print. 7th ed. Philadelphia: Saunders; 2010.

6. **Can neonates produce C-reactive protein (CRP)?**

   CRP is a soluble protein that facilitates clearance of infected cells and microorganisms by phagocytes. It is produced by the liver and is part of the acute-phase response. It does not cross the placenta. Neonates can produce CRP, and levels reach concentration similar to that of adults in the first days of life in term neonates.

7. **When do the cells of the immune system develop?**

   The pluripotent hematopoietic stem cells are generated from embryonic para-aortic tissue, fetal liver (by 4 weeks' gestation) and bone marrow (by 11 weeks' gestation). The yolk site is a major site of production of erythrocytes and phagocytes (by 3 weeks' gestation). Liver hematopoiesis ceases by week 20 and continues only in bone marrow. All major lineages of the hematopoietic cells that are part of the immune system are present in the fetus by the beginning of the second trimester (Fig. 13-1).

Nussbaum C, Sperandio M. Innate immune cell recruitment in the fetus and neonate. J Reprod Immunol 2011;90(1):74–81.
   Yang KD, Hill HR. Granulocyte function disorders: aspects of development, genetics and management. Pediatr Infect Dis J 2001;20(9):889–900.

8. **How are monocytes and macrophages in a neonate different from those in an adult?**

   Circulating monocytes first appear in the fetal blood at 18 to 20 weeks' gestation; by week 30 they increase to 3% to 7% of the circulating formed blood cells. By birth values exceed $500/mm^3$, which is higher than in most adults. Monocytes undergo tissue-specific differentation into mononuclear macrophages, which utilize a respiratory burst (biosynthesis of O_2^- and H_2O_2) to kill organisms.

   The microbicidal activity of macrophages can be regulated by cytokines (interferon gamma [IFN-gamma], granulocyte-macrophage colony-stimulating factor [GM-CSF], and tumor necrosis factor alpha [TNF-alpha]). The ability of mononuclear phagocytes to generate reactive oxygen intermediates is normal in neonates. However, IFN-gamma production and response to exogenous IFN-gamma are diminished in newborns.

Strunk T, Currie A, Richmond P, et al. Innate immunity in human newborn infants: prematurity means more than immaturity. J Matern Fetal Neonatal Med 2011;24(1):25–31.

9. **What are the stages of development of T cells?**

   T-cell precursors differentiate into immunocompetent T cells within the thymus. Before entering the thymus, stem cells lack antigen receptors and do not express CD3, CD4, or CD8 on their surface. Prothymocytes do not initially express CD4 or CD8 (double negatives); however, during the process of differentialtion they express both CD4 and CD8 (double positives) and then proceed to express either CD4 or CD8. A double-positive cell will differentiate into a CD4-positive one if it comes into contact with a cell bearing class II major histocompatibility complex (MHC) proteins but will differentiate into a CD8-positive cell if it comes into contact with a cell bearing class I MHC proteins.

   The double-negative and double-positive cells are located in the cortex of the thymus, whereas the single-positive cells are located in the medulla, from which they migrate out of the thymus into the

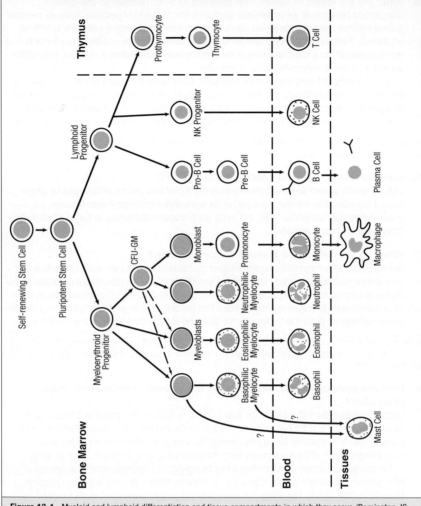

Figure 13-1. Myeloid and lymphoid differentiation and tissue compartments in which they occur. (Remington JS, Klein JO, Wilson CB, et al. Infectious diseases of the fetus and newborn infant. 7th ed. Philadelphia: Saunders; 2011. p. 88.)

blood. The thymic education of T cells includes negative selection; self-reactive cells are removed to prevent autoimmune reactions and positive selection; CD4-positive and CD8-positive cells bearing antigen receptors that do not react with self MHC proteins are eliminated.

10. **What is the clinical relevance of neonatal eosinophilia?**
   In healthy neonates the number of eosinophils increases postnatally, reaching a maximum at 3 to 4 weeks, when it represents a larger percentage (10% to 20%) of total granulocytes than in adults. This physiologic eosinophilia does not suggest the presence of allergic diseases or helminthic infections as strongly as they do in adults and is not associated with increased amounts of circulating immunoglobulin (Ig) E.

Remington JS, Klein JO, Wilson CB, et al. Infectious diseases of the fetus and newborn: expert consult—online and print. 7th ed. Philadelphia: Saunders; 2010.

11. **When does cell-mediated immunity mature in the fetus?**

By week 12 of gestation, lymphocytes obtained from the human thymus respond to mitogens and foreign histocompatibility antigens. Furthermore, fetal cells stimulated with alloantigens exhibit normal antigen-specific cytotoxicity. In contrast, the phenotypic appearance and proportion of circulating cells are diminished, and the production of some cytokines such as interleukin (IL)-12 is reduced in neonates. The most significant defect appears to be a deficiency of memory T cells, which may be responsible for the deficient production of IFN-gamma in the neonate. The mother does not transfer T-cell–specific immunity to the fetus.

Marchant A, Goldman M. T cell-mediated immune responses in human newborns: ready to learn? Clin Exp Immunol 2005;141(1):10–8.

12. **Why is neutropenia commonly observed in neonatal sepsis?**

Immature polymorphonuclear neuthrophils (PMNs) (metamyelocytes and band forms) and mature bone marrow PMNs constitute a reserve pool of cells that may be rapidly mobilized into the circulation in response to inflammation. The rate of proliferation of neuthrophil precursors in the human neonate seems to be near maximal, and therefore their capacity to increase numbers in response to infection might be limited. As a result, rather than develop neutrophilia, as might occur in the septic adult, the neonate will rapidly develop neutropenia as a result of exhaustion or depletion of the storage pools.

van den Berg JM, Kuijpers TW. Educational paper: defects in number and function of neutrophilic granulocytes causing primary immunodeficiency. Eur J Pediatr 2011;170(11):1369–76.

13. **How do neutrophils in a neonate differ from those in an adult?**

Circulating PMNs increase dramatically after birth, peak at 12 to 24 hours, and then decline slowly by 72 hours in a neonate without complications. The fraction of immature forms remains constant at about 15%. A limited ability to accelerate neutrophil production in response to infection and impaired migration of PMNs to areas of microbial invasion in tissues contribute to the higher risk of developing overwhelming sepsis in neonates (especially premature infants). However, phagocytosis and microbial killing by PMNs seem not to be greatly impaired unless the neonates are critically ill.

Clapp DW. Developmental regulation of the immune system. Semin Perinatol 2006;30(2):69–72.

14. **What is the maternal contribution of Ig to the newborn? How long do maternal Igs last?**

The IgG content of the fetus and the newborn infant is mainly maternal in origin and is predominantly transferred during the latter third of pregnancy. Levels of all classes of IgG fall rapidly after birth, and the respective concentrations derived from maternal placental transfer and active production by the young infant are approximately equal by 2 months' postnatal age. By 10 to 12 months of age, catabolism of passively acquired IgG is complete, and the infant produces all the circulating IgG (Fig. 13-2).

15. **Why do newborn infants respond poorly to polysaccharide vaccines or encapsulated bacteria such as GBS?**

In humans the antigens can be divided into three groups depending on the nature of the immune response: (1) thymus-dependent (TD) antigens, which include most protein antigens; (2) thymus-independent type 1 (TI-1) antigens, which bind directly to B lymphocytes and do not require T cells for antibody production; and (3) thymus-independent type 2 (TI-2) antigens, which are mostly polysaccharides composed of multiple identical subunits and require small numbers of T lymphocytes for antibody production to occur. The response to TI-2 antigens appears last chronologically at approximately 6 months of age, accounting for the poor neonatal response to polysaccharide vaccines and to the higher risk of infection with encapsulated organisms such as GBS.

Philbin VJ, Levy O. Developmental biology of the innate immune response: implications for neonatal and infant vaccine development. Pediatr Res 2009;65(5 Pt 2):98R–105R.

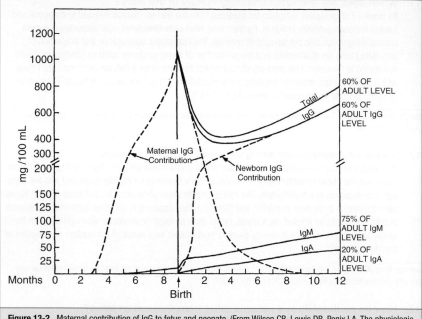

Figure 13-2. Maternal contribution of IgG to fetus and neonate. (From Wilson CB, Lewis DB, Penix LA. The physiologic immunodeficiency of immaturity. In Stiehm R, editor. Immunologic disorders in infants and children. 4th ed. Philadelphia: Saunders; 1996. p. 253–295.)

16. **Why are neonates particularly susceptible to infection with viruses such as herpes simplex?**

The defenses against viral infections involve numerous mechanisms, including antibody neutralization of extracellular virus, direct cytolysis of infected cells by natural killer (NK) cells, antibody-dependent cellular cytotoxicity and specific cell-mediated cytotoxicity through T lymphocytes. Neonates have deficits in virtually all of these components. Infants infected with herpes simplex virus (HSV) at the time of delivery depend on the presence of passively acquired maternal antibodies, which are low in mothers with primary infection. This is the scenario in which the most severe neonatal infection occurs.

NK cells appear early in gestation and reach normal numbers by mid to late gestation; however, they are largely immature in phenotype, consisting of 50% CD56-negative cells. These cells are deficient in their ability to kill virus-infected cells and to produce critical cytokines such as IFN-gamma. Furthermore, virus-specific T-cell–mediated immunity is also diminished or delayed in the neonates with decreased T-cell killing and production of IFN-gamma. Consequently, infection with HSV in the neonate can result in a rapidly progressive, fulminant, and often fatal infection.

Kimberlin DW. Neonatal herpes simplex infection. Clin Microbiol Rev 2004;17(1):1–13.

17. **When should the clinician suspect a granulocyte disorder in a neonate?**

An unusually severe course of infection or an unusual pathogen, recurrent pyogenic infections, and recurrent upper and lower respiratory tract infections might be caused by immunodeficiency resulting from a congenital neutropenia or dysfunctional neutrophils. A summary of the most important diseases is shown in Table 13-1.

Townshend J, Clark J, Cant A, et al. Congenital neutropenia. Arch Dis Child Educ Pract Ed 2008;93(1):14–8.

TABLE 13-1. SUMMARY OF THE PRINCIPAL GRANULOCYTE DISORDERS IN NEONATES

CATEGORY	SUBGROUP	DIAGNOSIS/PATHOGENESIS
Neutropenia	Iatrogenic/toxic (steroids)	Effect of cessation of drug. Steroids primarily affect PMN migration.
	Immune mediated	Detection of auto or alloantibodies (benign neutropenia of infancy)
	Related infections	CMV, EBV, parvovirus B19…
	Genetic (Kostmann syndrome)	AR mutations in the G-CSF receptor
Decreased motility: adhesion, rolling, migration	Leukocyte adhesion deficiencies (LAD1, LAD2, LAD 3)	LAD 1: Mutations in the beta 2 integrin gene. Delayed separation of umbilical cord, impaired lymphocytic function, and virtual absence of neutrophils in inflammatory exudates despite marked elevations of peripheral blood leukocyte counts. LAD 2: Absence of SLeX oligosaccharide. Mental retardation and periodontitis. LAD 3: Mutations in *FERMT3* gene (LAD 3). Mild LAD phenotype and platelet dysfunction.
Decreased "sensing danger"	Toll-like receptor deficiencies (IRAK 4 deficiency, MyD88 deficiency)	Recurrent pyogenic infections. Failure to activate nuclear factor kappa-light-chain-enhancer of activated B cells impeding secretion of interleukin-1 beta and tumor necrosis factor alpha.
Impaired killing mechanisms	NADPH oxidase dysfunction (chronic granulomatous disease)	Fulminant bacterial (catalase positive) and fungi infections and chronic granulation formation. Mutations of *CYBB* gene (X-linked CGD) or mutation in other NADPH oxidase components (AR). Altered microtubule formation.
	Impaired granule formation (Chédiak–Higashi syndrome, specific granule deficiency)	

AR, Autosomal recessive; CGD, chronic granulomatous disease; CMV, cytomegalovirus; EBV, Epstein–Barr virus; G-CSF, granulocyte colony-stimulating factor; IL, interleukin; PMN, polymorphonuclear neutrophils; TNF, tumor necrosis factor.

NEONATAL SEPSIS EPIDEMIOLOGY

18. **How do we define early-onset sepsis?**

    Early-onset sepsis begins at 3 days of age (or even sooner) when organisms ascend from the birth canal after overt or occult rupture of membranes. Early-onset sepsis usually manifests as fulminant systemic illness and is associated with mortality rates of 3% to 50% (highest in premature infants). Infection with gram-negative pathogens and low-birth-weight infants are at higher risk of mortality.

Randis TM, Polin RA. Early-onset group B Streptococcal sepsis: new recommendations from the Centres for Disease Control and Prevention. Arch Dis Child Fetal Neonatal Ed. 2012;97(4):F291–4.

Polin RA, Committee on Fetus and Newborn. Management of neonates with suspected or proven early-onset bacterial sepsis. Pediatrics 2012;129(5):1006–15.

19. **How has the use of maternal intrapartum antibiotics altered the incidence of early-onset neonatal sepsis?**

    Since consensus guidelines were developed in 1996 and subsequently revised in 2002 and 2010, the incidence of early-onset *Streptococcus agalactiae* (GBS) infections has declined from 1.7 in

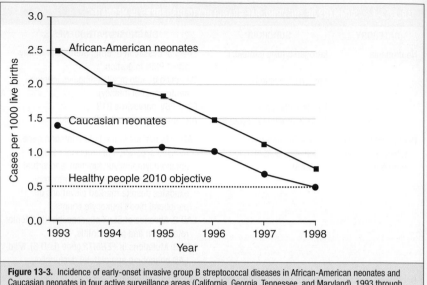

Figure 13-3. Incidence of early-onset invasive group B streptococcal diseases in African-American neonates and Caucasian neonates in four active surveillance areas (California, Georgia, Tennessee, and Maryland), 1993 through 1998. (From Schrag SJ, Phil D, Zywicki S, et al. Group B streptococcal diseases in the era of intrapartum antibiotic prophylaxis. N Engl J Med 2000;342:17.)

1000 live births to 0.28 in 1000 live births, a 70% reduction in the incidence of early-onset GBS sepsis. During the same period, however, intrapartum antibiotic administration has been associated with an increased incidence of drug-resistant neonatal sepsis, particularly ampicillin-resistant gram-negative disease in very-low-birth-weight (VLBW) infants (<1500 g) (Fig. 13-3). Whether the increase in gram-negative sepsis is due to intrapartum antibiotic prophylaxis remains controversial.

Eberly MD, Rajnik M. The effect of universal maternal screening on the incidence of neonatal early-onset group B strepto-coccal disease. Clin Pediatr (Phila) 2009;48(4):369–75.

Sakata H. Evaluation of intrapartum antibiotic prophylaxis for the prevention of early-onset group B streptococcal infection. J Infect Chemother 2012;18(6):853–857.

20. **How has the epidemiology of early-onset sepsis changed in VLBW infants (<1500 g)?**
    Among VLBW infants the incidence of early-onset sepsis increases with decreasing gestational age (15 cases in 1000 live births for preterm versus 2.5 cases in 1000 live births for term infants). Compared with data derived before the inception of guidelines for the prevention of GBS disease, there has been a significant reduction in early-onset GBS disease, from 5.9 to 1.7 cases per 1000 live births, with a concomitant increase in *E. coli* sepsis from 3.2 to 6.8 per 1000 live births. Approximately 85% of the *E. coli* isolates have been resistant to ampicillin. When the years 1991 through 1993 were compared with 1998 through 2000, there was also an increase in the incidence of early-onset fungal disease, from 0.1 to 0.4 per 1000 live births.

Randis TM, Polin RA. Early-onset group B Streptococcal sepsis: new recommendations from the Centres for Disease Control and Prevention. Arch Dis Child Fetal Neonatal Ed 2012;97(4):F291–4.

Stoll BJ, Hansen N, Fanaroff AA, et al. Changes in pathogens causing early-onset sepsis in very-low-birth-weight infants. N Engl J Med 2002;347(4):240–7.

21. **What are the main risk factors for maternal chorioamnionitis?**
    Low parity, spontaneous labor, longer length of labor and membrane rupture, multiple digital examinations, meconium-stained fluid, internal fetal or uterine monitoring, and presence

of genital tract infections. The incidence of chorioamnionitis is inversely related with gestational age.

Schuchat A, Zywicki SS, Dinsmoor MJ, et al. Risk factors and opportunities for prevention of early-onset neonatal sepsis: a multicenter case-control study. Pediatrics 2000;105(1 Pt 1):21–6.

22. **Which maternal and neonatal factors increase the risk of early-onset disease?**
    The major risk factors for early-onset neonatal sepsis are preterm birth (the factor most closely associated with early-onset neonatal sepsis), maternal colonization with GBS, prolonged rupture of membranes (>18 hours before labor), and maternal signs or symptoms of chorioamnionitis. Other variables include ethnicity (e.g., African-American women have higher rates of colonization with GBS), low socioeconomic status, male sex, and low Apgar scores. Infant birth weight is inversely related to risk of early-onset sepsis (Table 13-2).

    The presence of any of these factors alone is not an indication for a complete sepsis work-up and antibiotic therapy; however, combinations of risk factors are clearly cumulative and should give rise to the suspicion of sepsis.

Hyde TB, Hilger TM, Reingold A, et al. Trends in incidence and antimicrobial resistance of early-onset sepsis: population-based surveillance in San Francisco and Atlanta. Pediatrics 2002;110(4):690–5.

23. **What is the attack rate for neonatal sepsis in the presence of the aforementioned risk factors?**
    As a general rule, presence of a major risk factor (e.g., premature rupture of fetal membranes or maternal GBS colonization) leads to an attack rate of about 1% for proven sepsis or 2% for proven or highly suspected sepsis. If a second risk factor is present, the attack rate rises to 4% to 6% for proven and 10% for proven or highly suspected sepsis. Further risk factors are additive; the presence of three risk factors raises the sepsis risk 25-fold over baseline.

24. **What is the distribution of pathogens among term and preterm neonates with sepsis?**
    The pathogenesis of early-onset sepsis has changed over the last decades as intrapartum antibiotic prophylaxis protocols have become widely used. GBS and gram-negative enteric bacilli, predominantly *E. coli,* are the most common pathogens for early-onset disease. In preterm infants who weigh less than

TABLE 13-2. RISK FACTORS FOR PERINATALLY ACQUIRED NEONATAL BACTERIAL INFECTION

From Polin R, Spitzer A. Fetal and neonatal secrets. 1st ed. Philadelphia: Hanley & Belfus; 2001. p. 266.

MATERNAL	NEONATAL
Prolonged rupture of membranes >18-24 hours	Prematurity
Premature rupture of membranes (<37 weeks)	Low birth weight (<2500 gm)
Maternal fever ≥100.4°F	Male gender
Maternal chorioamnionitis	5-minute Apgar score <6
Maternal colonization with GBS	
GBS bacteriuria	
Previous infant with invasive GBS disease	
Maternal urinary tract infection at delivery	
Multiple gestation	
GBS, Group B streptococci.	

1500 grams, *E. coli* is more common than GBS. Coagulase-negative staphylococci (CoNS); *Staphylococcus aureus; Enterococcus, Klebsiella,* and *Enterobacter* species; *Pseudomonas aeruginosa*; and fungi (especially *Candida albicans*) are the major pathogens for late-onset diseases (onset after 72 hours).

Remington JS, Klein JO, Wilson CB, et al. Infectious diseases of the fetus and newborn: expert consult—online and print. 7th ed. Philadelphia: Saunders; 2010.

Stoll BJ, Hansen N, Fanaroff AA, et al. Changes in pathogens causing early-onset sepsis in very-low-birth-weight infants. N Engl J Med 2002;347(4):240–7.

Lin F-YC, Weisman LE, Troendle J, et al. Prematurity is the major risk factor for late-onset group B streptococcus disease. J Infect Dis 2003;188(2):267–71.

25. Why has infection with CoNS become a common pathogen in the NICU?

CoNS have increased as pathogens in the NICU as the survival of extremely-low-birth-weight infants (<1000 grams) has improved. CoNS bacteremia is associated with indwelling vascular lines. CoNS produce a biofilm that facilitates adherence to the catheter and protects them from antibiotic and host immune responses.

Healy CM, Baker CJ, Palazzi DL, et al. Distinguishing true coagulase-negative Staphylococcus infections from contaminants in the neonatal intensive care unit. J Perinatol 2013;33(1):52–58.

26. What are the clinical differences between GBS early-onset sepsis and late or very late-onset sepsis?

Clinical manifestations of GBS late-onset neonatal sepsis are more insidious, and meningitis is frequently part of the clinical picture. Late-onset disease is associated with GBS serotype III and has a lower mortality rate than early sepsis. With increase survival of extremely-low-birth-weight neonates, very-late-onset disease (>98 days) has also been described (Table 13-3).

27. What are the adverse consequences of late-onset infections among VLBW infants?

- Patent ductus arteriosus
- Prolonged need for mechanical ventilation
- Prolonged duration of total parenteral nutrition and need for indwelling catheters
- Necrotizing enterocolitis
- Prolonged length of hospitalization
- Increased cost of care
- Increased risk of death

Wynn JL, Wong HR. Pathophysiology and treatment of septic shock in neonates. Clin Perinatol 2010;37(2):439–79.

TABLE 13-3. CHARACTERISTICS OF EARLY AND LATER-ONSET INFECTIONS

From Polin R, Spitzer A. Fetal and neonatal secrets. 1st ed. Philadelphia: Hanley & Belfus; 2001. p. 267.

CHARACTERISTIC	EARLY-ONSET	LATE-ONSET	LATE, LATE-ONSET
Age at onset	Birth to 7 days	7–30 days	>30 days
Maternal obstetric	Common	Uncommon	Complications vary
Prematurity	Frequent	Varies	Usual, especially if birth weight is <1000 gm
Source of organism	Maternal genital tract	Maternal genital tract or environment	Environment/community
Clinical presentation	Multisystem	Multisystem or focal	Multisystem or focal
Mortality rate	10–20%	5–10%	<5%

28. **What are the major risk factors for late-onset neonatal sepsis?**
    See Table 13-4.

DIAGNOSIS OF NEONATAL SEPSIS

29. **How sensitive is the clinical diagnosis of chorioamnionitis?**
    The most sensitive criteria for the clinical diagnosis of chorioamnionitis is maternal fever higher than 38° C (100.4° F). The presence of two or more of the following criteria also supports the diagnosis; maternal leukocytosis (>15000 cells/mm^3), maternal tachycardia (> 100 bpm), fetal tachycardia (>160 bpm), uterine tenderness, and foul odor of the amniotic fluid. If maternal fever and two or more of the criteria are present, there is a significant sepsis risk for the neonate, with reported attack rates ranging from 6% to 20%. This issue is further confounded by the use of epidural anesthesia, which is associated with a fourfold increased incidence of maternal fever without increasing the neonatal sepsis rate.

Polin RA, Committee on Fetus and Newborn. Management of neonates with suspected or proven early-onset bacterial sepsis. Pediatrics 2012;129(5):1006–15.

30. **What are the presenting signs and symptoms of neonatal sepsis?**
    The clinical diagnosis of sepsis in the neonate is difficult because many of the signs are nonspecific. They include fever, respiratory distress, jaundice, lethargy, irritability, anorexia or vomiting, hypotonia, "not looking well," abdominal distention, hypothermia, hypoglycemia, apnea, seizures, shock, petechiae, and purpura. There is considerable overlap with noninfectious conditions,

TABLE 13-4.   RISK FACTORS FOR LATE-ONSET NEONATAL SEPSIS

From Polin R, Spitzer A. Fetal and neonatal secrets. 1st ed. Philadelphia: Hanley & Belfus; 2001. p. 268.

RISK FACTOR	COMMENTS
Prematurity, low birth weight	Risk of infection is inversely related to gestational age and birth weight.
Intravascular catheters	Intravascular catheters provide a portal of entry for infectious organisms, and risk of infection is directly related to the number of catheter days.
Total parenteral nutrition (TPN)	TPN requires vascular access, which increases risk; intralipids enhance the growth of lipophilic organisms, particularly coagulase-negative staphylococci and *Malassezia furfur*.
Enteral nutrition	Human milk decreases and formula feeding increases risk.
Intubation, ventilation	Endotracheal intubation provides a portal of entry for colonization infection with potential pathogens.
Invasive procedures	These provide a portal of entry for organisms by breaking the skin and mucous membrane barriers.
Medications	Dexamethasone and H_2 blocker use increase risk of infection; widespread and prolonged use of broad-spectrum antibiotics may predispose to infections caused by resistant organisms and fungi.
Hospitalization	Prolonged length of stay increases risk of exposure to hospital pathogens.
Overcrowding, understaffing	These increase the likelihood of poor infection-control practices (especially poor hand-washing), which increase the risk of infection.

and some infants may exhibit transiently abnormal clinical signs during the transition to postnatal life.

31. **Are neonates with fever always febrile?**

The temperature of a neonate with sepsis might be elevated; depressed; or, as is frequently observed, within normal limits. Term infants are more likely to have fever than premature infants, whereas the latter are more prone to exhibit hypothermia. Fever is generally considered as a rectal temperature higher than 38° C (100.4° F). Fever can also be due to many other noninfectious causes, such as elevation in ambient temperature.

32. **How can laboratory data assist in the diagnosis of neonatal sepsis?**

Diagnostic testing can assist with the decision to discontinue treatment. Isolation of the microorganism from a sterile site, such as blood or cerebrospinal fluid (CSF) remains the most valid method of diagnosis of bacterial sepsis.

Jordan JA. Molecular diagnosis of neonatal sepsis. Clin Perinatol 2010;37(2):411–9.

Escobar GJ, Li DK, Armstrong MA, et al. Neonatal sepsis workups in infants >/=2000 grams at birth: a population-based study. Pediatrics 2000;106(2 Pt 1):256–63.

33. **Are body surfaces useful to establish the diagnosis of sepsis?**

Body surface cultures have very limited sensitivity, specificity, and predictive value and do not establish invasive systemic infection. They reveal only colonization and are poorly correlated with pathogens isolated from blood.

34. **How reliable is blood culture in the diagnosis of neonatal sepsis?**

In studies of neonates who died, the postmortem diagnosis of sepsis was confirmed by antemortem blood cultures in only 80% of cases. The current extensive use of maternal antibiotics further confounds the reliability of the newborn blood culture.

Remington JS, Klein JO, Wilson CB, et al. Infectious diseases of the fetus and newborn: expert consult—online and print. 7th ed.Philadelphia: Saunders; 2010.

35. **How much volume of blood should be drawn in neonatal blood culture?**

A minimum of 1 mL of blood should be drawn to establish the diagnosis of bacteremia when a single pediatric blood culture bottle is used. Dividing the specimen in half and inoculating the aerobic and anaerobic bottles is likely to reduce sensitivity (0.5 mL of blood will not reliably detect 4 colonyforming units/mL) and is not recommended.

36. **Should a urine culture be part of the work-up for sepsis in the newborn infant?**

In early-onset sepsis, positive urine cultures are attributable to seeding of the kidneys during an episode of bacteremia unlike the urinary tract infections (UTIs) in older infants, which are usually ascending infections. Therefore urine cultures yield very limited information about the source of infection in early sepsis and should not be part of the sepsis work-up. However, suprapubic aspiration or bladder catheterization should be performed in all infants in whom late-onset sepsis is suspected.

Polin RA, Committee on Fetus and Newborn. Management of neonates with suspected or proven early-onset bacterial sepsis. Pediatrics 2012;129(5):1006–15.

Stoll BJ, Hansen N, Fanaroff AA, et al. Changes in pathogens causing early-onset sepsis in very-low-birth-weight infants. N Engl J Med 2002;347(4):240–7.

Lieberman E, Lang J, Richardson DK, et al. Intrapartum maternal fever and neonatal outcome. Pediatrics 2000;105(1 Pt 1):8–13.

✓ KEY POINTS: DIAGNOSIS OF NEONATAL INFECTION

1. The sensitivity of blood cultures increases with increasing volume.

2. Meningitis may occur in the absence of a positive blood culture.

3. Urine culture specimens should be obtained in all infants in whom late-onset sepsis is suspected.

4. No single laboratory test or combination of test is 100% sensitive or specific for diagnosing infection.

37. **When should a lumbar puncture be performed?**
    The decision to perform a lumbar puncture in neonates with suspected early-onset sepsis remains controversial. Infants with clinical signs that can be attributed to noninfectious conditions such as respiratory distress syndrome have a very low likelihood of meningitis. However, up to 23% of infants with bacteremia have concomitant meningitis and often have no clinical signs directly referable to the central nervous system (CNS). Furthermore, up to 38% of infants with meningitis have a negative blood culture. Therefore the presence of a positive blood culture cannot serve as indication to do a lumbar puncture.

    Because neonatal meningitis is a low-incidence disease (0.25 in 1000 live births), an informal meta-analysis of published reports showed that it would be necessary to do at least 1000 lumbar punctures to diagnose one case that would be missed by lack of symptoms or a negative blood culture result. A rational approach would be to perform a lumbar puncture in infants with positive blood cultures, those who deteriorate with antimicrobial treatment, and those whose clinical or laboratory data strongly suggest bacterial sepsis if they do not have any contraindication for the procedure.

38. **Can we interpret the cell content and chemistry of neonatal CSF with the same parameters used in older children?**
    The cell content and chemistry of neonatal CSF differs from those of older infants. The cell content of CSF particularly in the first week is higher, and polymorphonuclear leukocytes are often present in CSF of normal newborns. In a recent study the upper reference limit of the CSF white blood cell (WBC) count was 12 cells/mm^3 in preterm infants and 14 cells/mm^3 in term infants. Most well infants will have cell counts lower than 10 cells/mm^3. Adjusting the cell count for the number of red cells does not improve its diagnostic utility. Preterm infants have protein concentrations that are inversely correlated with their gestational age. Uninfected term newborns have protein concentrations in the CSF lower than 100 mg/dL, with a physiologic decline with postnatal age reaching values of healthy older infants before the third month of life. CSF glucose concentrations in normoglycemic uninfected neonates are similar to those of older infants (70% to 80% of a simultaneous peripheral blood glucose). Meningitis can occur in neonates with completely normal CSF values.

Srinivasan L, Shah SS, Padula MA, et al. Cerebrospinal fluid reference ranges in term and preterm infants in the neonatal intensive care unit. J Pediatr 2012;161(4):729–34.

39. **How can a WBC count aid in the diagnosis of early-onset sepsis?**
    Elevated WBC counts or abnormal neutrophil indices (low absolute neutrophil counts [neutropenia], elevated band counts, and high immature-to-total neutrophil [I/T] ratios) have a poor positive predictive value for the diagnosis of early-onset sepsis. They are useful for excluding infants without infections rather than identifying infected ones. Neutropenia is the index with the best specificity. The definition of neutropenia changes with age, type of delivery, site of sampling, and altitude; peak values are reached 6 to 8 hours after delivery. A recent study suggested that the lower limits of normal WBCs at that time should be 7500/mm^3 for infants born at more than 36 weeks' gestation, 3500/mm^3 for those between 28 and 36 weeks' gestation, and 1500/mm^3 for less than 28 weeks' gestation.

40. **What is the relevance of CRP in the diagnosis of neonatal sepsis?**
   The sensitivity of CRP at birth is low because it requires an inflammatory response to increase (with the release of IL-6). Its sensitivity improves dramatically if the determination is made 6 to 12 hours later. Two normal CRP determinations (8 to 24 hours after birth and 24 hours later) have a negative predictive accuracy of 99.7% for proven neonatal sepsis.

41. **Are cytokine determinations helpful in the diagnosis of early-onset neonatal sepsis?**
   A number of inflammatory mediators have been investigated as possible diagnostic tests for neonatal sepsis. IL-6, IL-8, and IL-10 have been found to have a critical role in the inflammatory response during neonatal sepsis; however, none of these mediators has sufficient sensitivity or specificity for the diagnosis of infection in this population. These mediators are currently not available for routine clinical purposes.

Venkatesh M, Flores A, Luna RA, et al. Molecular microbiological methods in the diagnosis of neonatal sepsis. Expert Rev Anti Infect Ther 2010 Sep;8(9):1037–48.

ANTIBIOTIC TREATMENT

42. **What is the recommended initial treatment for early-onset sepsis?**
   Once sepsis is suspected in a neonate, antimicrobial treatment should be promptly begun after cultures have been obtained, even when there are no obvious risk factors for sepsis. Because GBS and *E. coli* are the most common pathogens of early-onset sepsis in the United States, a synergistic combination of ampicillin and an aminoglycoside (usually gentamicin) is suitable for the initial treatment of early-onset sepsis. Ampicillin is the antimicrobial of choice for treatment of GBS, *Listeria monocytogenes,* and most enterococci. Once the pathogen is identified, antimicrobial therapy should be narrowed (unless synergism is needed).

Muller-Pebody B, Johnson AP, Heath PT, et al. Empirical treatment of neonatal sepsis: are the current guidelines adequate? Arch Dis Child Fetal Neonatal Ed 2011;96(1):F4–8.

43. **Is cefotaxime an acceptable alternative to gentamicin?**
   Third-generation cephalosporins such as cefotaxime are associated with rapid development of drug-resistant bacteria in nurseries, and extensive use has been reported to be a risk factor for invasive candidiasis. Furthermore, the third-generation cephalosporins are not active against *Listeria* and *Enterococcus* species. Because of its excellent CSF penetration, the use of cefotaxime should be restricted for infants with meningitis attributable to gram-negative organisms.

Hyde TB, Hilger TM, Reingold A, et al. Trends in incidence and antimicrobial resistance of early-onset sepsis: population-based surveillance in San Francisco and Atlanta. Pediatrics 2002;110(4):690–5.

44. **Why should ceftriaxone *not* be used in neonates?**
   Ceftriaxone can displace bilirubin from albumin and may increase the risk of kernicterus in a jaundiced infant.

45. **Should antibiotic treatment be stopped if cultures remain negative after 48 hours?**
   Stopping treatment for bacteremia without an identifiable focus of infection remains controversial, and the final decision requires consideration of antibiotic use during labor and the infant's clinical course. Three recent observational studies have demonstrated an association between antibiotic use for longer than 5 days in infants with suspected early-onset sepsis (and negative blood cultures) with death and necrotizing enterocolitis. Therefore in a well-appearing infant antibiotics should not be continued for more than 48 hours (72 hours in certain cases).

TABLE 13-5.	MAJOR ADVERSE REACTIONS TO ANTIMICROBIALS COMMONLY USED IN NEONATES

From Polin R, Spitzer A. Fetal and neonatal secrets. 1st ed. Philadelphia: Hanley & Belfus; 2001. p. 272–73.

ANTIBIOTIC	ADVERSE EFFECTS
Ampicillin	Rare hypersensitivity reactions*
Amphotericin B	Hypokalemia Reversible nephrotoxicity caused by reduced glomerular filtration rate
Acyclovir	Reversible renal dysfunction caused by the formation of acyclovir crystals in renal tubules†
Cefotaxime	Rare, occasional leukopenia
Ceftriaxone	Displaces bilirubin from albumin, resulting in higher bilirubin concentrations Gallbladder sludging
Gentamicin	Irreversible ototoxicity and reversible nephrotoxicity
Vancomycin	Rare nephrotoxicity, enhanced by combination with an aminoglycoside Red man syndrome (rash and hypotension)‡

*Hypersensitivity reactions are not commonly seen in the neonatal period.
†Adequate hydration helps prevent this complication.
‡Appears rapidly and resolves within minutes to hours. Lengthening infusion time usually eliminates risk for subsequent doses.

46. **Is there any role for adjunctive therapy with intravenous Ig in neonatal sepsis?**
A recent double-blind control trial of adjunctive therapy with intravenous Ig showed no effect on the outcomes (death and major disability at 2 years) of suspected or proven neonatal sepsis.

INIS Collaborative Group, Brocklehurst P, Farrell B, et al. Treatment of neonatal sepsis with intravenous immune globulin. N Engl J Med 2011;365(13):1201–11.

47. **What is acceptable empiric therapy for late-onset sepsis?**
Because *Staphylococcus epidermidis* is the most common cause of nosocomial sepsis in neonates, empiric therapy should include vancomycin. This antibiotic is generally paired with an aminoglycoside antibiotic to cover gram-negative organisms.

48. **What are the major adverse reactions to antimicrobials commonly used in neonates?**
See Table 13-5.

49. **Do twins have a higher risk of sepsis if one of them is infected?**
Some studies have shown a higher risk for contracting ascending intrauterine infection in the first twin born, but this risk is modified by delivery mode and other obstetric variables. More intriguing is the observation of simultaneous occurrence of late-onset sepsis among twins, which warrants close observation and consideration of cultures in the asymptomatic twin.

NEONATAL MENINGITIS

50. **What are the mechanisms of brain injury in meningitis?**
- Vascular infarcts (vasospasm/thrombosis)
- Reactive oxygen species
- Excitotoxic amino acids
- Alterations in cerebral blood flow

TABLE 13-6. FACTORS THAT INFLUENCE ANTIBIOTIC CONCENTRATIONS IN CEREBROSPINAL FLUID

From Polin R, Spitzer A. Fetal and neonatal secrets. 1st ed. Philadelphia: Hanley & Belfus; 2001. p. 201.

VARIABLE	EFFECT ON CNS PENETRATION	EXAMPLE
High degree of protein binding	Reduced	Ceftriaxone
Lipid solubility	Enhanced	Rifampin
High degree of ionization	Reduced	Beta-lactams
Active transport system	Enhanced	Penicillin
Meningeal inflammation	Enhanced*	Beta-lactams, vancomycin

CNS, Central nervous system.
*Meningeal inflammation only influences penetration of hydrophilic antibiotics.

51. **What factors influence antibiotic concentrations in CSF?**
See Table 13-6.

52. **What are the recommendations for initial empiric therapy of meningitis in the neonate?**
A regimen of ampicillin and cefotaxime is recommended for initial empiric therapy. Treatment should be modified according to microbiology results. Meropenem or ceftazidime should be reserved for infections caused by resistant microorganisms.

53. **How should gram-positive and gram-negative meningitis be treated during the neonatal period?**
- Treatment of meningitis caused by enteric organisms: Cefotaxime is preferred and is often paired with an aminoglycoside. Gram-negative meningitis usually is treated for at least 3 weeks.
- Treatment of meningitis caused by gram-positive organisms: Because there is synergism between ampicillin and aminoglycosides for most GBS, *L. monocytogenes,* and enterococci, combination therapy is recommended until the CSF is sterilized. If the GBS is determined to be a tolerant organism, combination therapy should be used for the duration of treatment (approximately 14 days).

Remington JS, Klein JO, Wilson CB, et al. Infectious diseases of the fetus and newborn: expert consult—online and print. 7th ed. Philadelphia: Saunders; 2010.

54. **What else should we include in the differential diagnosis for an infant with clinical signs of meningitis or sepsis whose bacterial culture results remain negative?**
Two viral infections must be considered. The first is disseminated HSV with CNS involvement. One helpful diagnostic clue is the development of skin vesicles, which can also be used as a source from which to isolate virus for diagnosis. However, about 20% of infants with this form of HSV never develop skin vesicles. Other sources for detection of the virus include respiratory secretions, blood, and CSF. If infection with HSV is strongly suspected, therapy with acyclovir should begin while viral polymerase chain reaction (PCR) and cultures remain pending. The other viral infections associated with a severe neonatal sepsis syndrome are enteroviral infections (especially Coxsackievirus).

GROUP B STREPTOCOCCAL (GBS) INFECTIONS

55. **What are the patterns of GBS colonization during pregnancy?**
Between 10% and 30% of women are colonized with GBS in their birth canal. Chronic, intermittent, or transient patterns of GBS colonization have been described. Pregnant woman with GBS colonization are 25 times more likely to deliver an infant with early-onset GBS sepsis than women whose cultures are negative (though infants with early-onset GBS have been born to women with negative antenatal

cultures). Affected infants became infected during labor and delivery. In the absence of intrapartum prophylaxis, 2% of infants will develop early-onset GBS sepsis.

Remington JS, Klein JO, Wilson CB, et al. Infectious diseases of the fetus and newborn: expert consult—online and print. 7th ed. Philadelphia: Saunders; 2010.

56. When should women be screened to detect GBS colonization?

Universal screening of all pregnant women at 35 to 37 weeks' gestation has been recommended since 2002. Specimens should be obtained from the lower rectum and vagina and placed in a selective broth media. This enrichment step significantly increases the sensitivity of the test with at least a twofold greater yield of positive culture results than nonselective methods. On the other hand, standard laboratory methods for the isolation of GBS from blood and spinal fluid are fully adequate.

Nucleic acid amplification tests (NAATs), including PCR, for GBS can be used to screen women at term with no other risk factors but should not replace traditional antenatal cultures because they have lower sensitivity. Chromogenic media can facilitate the detection of beta-hemolytic GBS, but may not detect nonhemolytic strains.

Faro J, Katz A, Bishop K, et al. Rapid diagnostic test for identifying group B streptococcus. Am J Perinatol 2011;28(10):811–4.

de Zoysa A, Edwards K, Gharbia S, et al. Non-culture detection of Streptococcus agalactiae (Lancefield group B Streptococcus) in clinical samples by real-time PCR. J Med Microbiol 2012;61(Pt 8):1086–90.

Schrag SJ, Zell ER, Lynfield R, et al. A population-based comparison of strategies to prevent early-onset group B streptococcal disease in neonates. N Engl J Med 2002;347(4):233–9.

57. How many serotypes of GBS have been identified? What is the clinical and immunologic significance of the serotypes?

Ten serotypes have been identified on the basis of capsular polysaccharide antigens. Early studies of GBS disease in North America demonstrated a predominance of the type III serotype, thought also to be the most virulent serotype. Currently, type III accounts for approximately 70% of isolates from infants with meningitis and is isolated in almost two thirds of infants with late-onset diseases. Since the 1970s there has been a progressive change in the predominant serotypes, with type Ia now the leading cause of early-onset infection. Types VI, VII, VIII, and IX rarely cause human diseases in the United Kingdom or the United States, but worldwide its distribution varies (e.g., types VI and VIII are the most common isolates from healthy Japanese women). From an immunologic and public health perspective, the recognition of multiple new serotypes has confounded the efforts of investigators to develop an effective multivalent vaccine to prevent this disease in newborns.

Remington JS, Klein JO, Wilson CB, et al. Infectious diseases of the fetus and newborn: expert consult - online and print. 7th ed. Philadelphia: Saunders; 2010.

58. What antibiotic should be used for intrapartum prophylaxis?

Penicillin (3 g [5 million units] intravenously followed by 1.5 to 1.8 g [2.5 to 3 million units] every 4 hours administered at least 4 hours before delivery) is the first-line agent for prevention of early onset GBS disease. Ampicillin is an effective alternative. Cefazolin (first-generation cephalosporin) is preferred for penicillin-allergic women at low risk for anaphylaxis.

Stafford IA, Stewart RD, Sheffield JS, et al. Efficacy of maternal and neonatal chemoprophylaxis for early-onset group B streptococcal disease. Obstet Gynecol 2012;120(1):123–9.

59. Can clindamycin be used for intrapartum antibiotic prophylaxis (IAP) in women with penicillin allergy?

The mother's strain should be tested for sensitivity to clindamycin and inducible resistance (D-zone test) because 25% of GBS strains are resistant to clindamycin. If the test is not available, clindamycin should not be used. Erythromycin should also not be used for IAP. Vancomycin is the recommended drug for women with severe allergic reactions if the strain has not been tested for susceptibility to clindamycin. IAP with vancomycin is probably effective but is considered inadequate (in terms of neonatal management) because of the lack of efficacy data.

60. **Which women should receive IAP to prevent early-onset sepsis?**

    According to the American College of Obstetrics and Gynecology (ACOG) the following women should receive antibiotic prophylaxis:

    ■ Antenatal colonization with GBS (except for women who have cesarean delivery without labor or membrane rupture)

    ■ Unknown GBS colonization status and any of the following: preterm labor, maternal fever (38° C or higher), prolonged rupture of membranes (18 hours or longer), or an intrapartum NAAT positive for GBS

    ■ GBS bacteriuria during pregnancy (10^4 or more colony-forming units/mL)

    ■ Prior delivery of neonate with invasive GBS

    Committee on Infectious Diseases, Committee on Fetus and Newborn, Baker CJ, et al. Policy statement—recommendations for the prevention of perinatal group B streptococcal (GBS) disease. Pediatrics 2011;128(3):611–6.

✓ KEY POINTS: CURRENT APPROACH TO GBS

1. In the absence of intrapartum prophylaxis, 2% of infants will develop early-onset GBS sepsis.

2. Screen all pregnant women between 35 and 37 weeks' gestation for GBS colonization.

3. Administer intrapartum antibiotic prophylaxis to women with antenatal colonization with GBS, women delivering a previously infected infant, women with positive GBS bacteriuria, and high-risk mothers with unknown GBS colonization status.

61. **What are the pros and cons of IAP?**

    Pros: IAP has resulted in a dramatic reduction in incidence of early-onset disease. Figure 13-4 illustrates the decline in incidence of early-onset GBS disease over the past decade as IAP programs were implemented. The graph is based on composite data from surveillance centers of the Centers for Disease Control and Prevention (CDC), a National Institute of Child Health and Development multicenter study reviewing disease rates from 1992 to 1997, and ongoing surveillance at the author's center. The incidences of disease from 1990 to 1993 represent the pre-IAP era, whereas data from

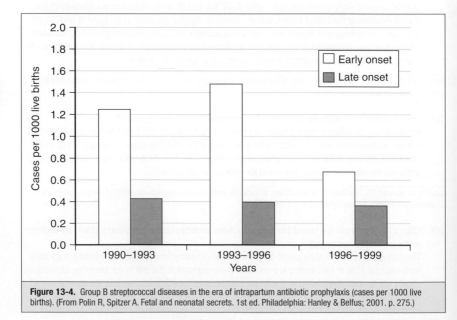

Figure 13-4. Group B streptococcal diseases in the era of intrapartum antibiotic prophylaxis (cases per 1000 live births). (From Polin R, Spitzer A. Fetal and neonatal secrets. 1st ed. Philadelphia: Hanley & Belfus; 2001. p. 275.)

1993 to 1996 followed the ACOG and American Academy of Pediatrics (AAP) recommendations published in 1993. The third data set reflects the impact of the CDC recommendations published in 1996.
Cons:
- Risk of maternal anaphylaxis
- IAP is not 100% effective; 20% of cases occurred despite intrapartum antibiotics
- Screening-based strategy identifies only maximum of 85% to 90% of affected infants' mothers
- Emergence of resistant organisms in mothers and infants (i.e. *E. coli*, *Enterococcus* species)
- Increasing resistance of GBS to clindamycin and erythromycin
- Does not address other adverse outcomes of GBS infection in pregnancy (i.e. early fetal loss, preterm labor, premature rupture of fetal membranes)

Cagno CK, Pettit JM, Weiss BD. Prevention of perinatal group B streptococcal disease: updated CDC guideline. Am Fam Physician 2012;86(1):59–65.
    Schrag SJ, Zywicki S, Farley MM, et al. Group B streptococcal disease in the era of intrapartum antibiotic prophylaxis. N Engl J Med 2000;342(1):15–20.

62. **What are the new CDC recommendations for management of newborns?**
    In 2010 the CDC published new guidelines for prevention of early-onset GBS sepsis (http://www.cdc.gov/groupbstrep/guidelines/index.html). These are summarized in Figure 13-5.

63. **Is late maternal colonization responsible for the high number of negative GBS screens among women who subsequently deliver infants with early-onset GBS infection?**
    A recent retrospective analysis revealed that women undergoing GBS screening at the time of labor were as likely to have false-negative cultures as those undergoing screening between 35 and 37 weeks' gestation. This study claimed that the majority of false-negative screens result from inappropriate collection or processing of specimens. Another ongoing challenge is clinical adherence to current guidelines; missed opportunities for GBS prevention happen frequently, particularly among women delivering preterm infants.

64. **What is the natural history of nosocomial acquisition of GBS in late-onset disease?**
    Most infants who contract late-onset disease acquire the organism outside the hospital. Mothers of these infants may have no history of genital colonization with GBS during pregnancy.

Sass L. Group B streptococcal infections. Pediatr Rev 2012;33(5):219–24–quiz224–5.

STAPHYLOCOCCUS EPIDERMIDIS

65. **Are CoNS common pathogens in the NICU?**
    CoNS are commensal skin and mucosal flora. Nearly 99% of healthy neonates will have positive nose or umbilicus swabs for CoNS by day 4 of life. However, these organisms also account for up to one half of reported bloodstream infections in VLBW (<1500 g) infants.

Kilbride HW, Wirtschafter DD, Powers RJ, et al. Implementation of evidence-based potentially better practices to decrease nosocomial infections. Pediatrics 2003;111(4 Pt 2):e519–33.

66. **Why has awareness of CoNS in the NICU increased over the last decades?**
    Improved survival rates of VLBW infants have resulted in an increased risk for sepsis because of the many invasive therapies required for management, such as central venous catheters. Central lines are associated with an increased risk of CoNS bacteremia. Colonization precedes infection with this species. Therefore CoNS infections present a particular dilemma because their isolation from a single blood culture in a neonate can either reflect contamination or true bacteremia. A suggested algorithm for interpreting blood cultures caused by CoNS is shown in Figure 13-6.

Craft A, Finer N. Nosocomial coagulase negative staphylococcal (CoNS) catheter-related sepsis in preterm infants: definition, diagnosis, prophylaxis, and prevention. J Perinatol 2001;21(3):186–92.

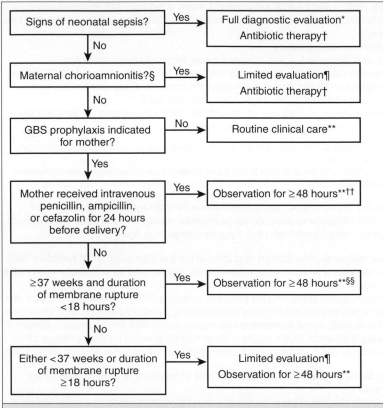

Figure 13-5. Algorithm for secondary prevention of early-onset of group B streptococcal diseases among newborns. (Randis TM, Polin RA. Early-Onset group B Streptococcal sepsis: new recommendations from the Centres for Diseases Control and Prevention. Arch Dis Child Fetal Neonatal Ed 2012;97(4):F291–4.)
*Full diagnostic evaluation includes a blood culture, a complete blood count (CBC) including white blood cell differential and platelet counts, chest radiograph (if respiratory abnormalities are present), and lumbar puncture (if patient is stable enough to tolerate procedure and sepsis is suspected).
†Antibiotic therapy should be directed toward the most common causes of neonatal sepsis, including intravenous ampicillin for GBS and coverage for other organisms (including *Escherichia coli* and other gram-negative pathogens) and should take into account local antibiotic resistance patterns.
§Consultation with obstetric providers is important to determine the level of clinical suspicion for chorioamnionitis. Chorioamnionitis is diagnosed clinically and some of the signs are nonspecific.
¶Limited evaluation includes blood culture (at birth) and CBC with differential and platelets (at birth and/or at 6–12 hours of life).
**If signs of sepsis develop, a full diagnostic evaluation should be conducted and antibiotic therapy initiated.
††If ≥37 weeks' gestation, observation may occur at home after 24 hours if other discharge criteria have been met, access to medical care is readily available, and a person who is able to comply fully with instructions for home observation will be present. If any of these conditions is not met, the infant should be observed in the hospital for at least 48 hours and until discharge criteria are achieved.
§§Some experts recommend a CBC with differential and platelets at age 6–12 hours.

67. Are blood cultures taken from intravascular catheters easy to interpret?

Umbilical vessels and intravascular catheters are essential in the NICU, and results of blood cultures can yield ambiguous interpretations (e.g., contamination versus catheter colonization versus systemic infection). Some microbiological features can be useful assisting this decision, such as time to growth (the longer the time elapsed between obtaining the blood culture and its growth, the

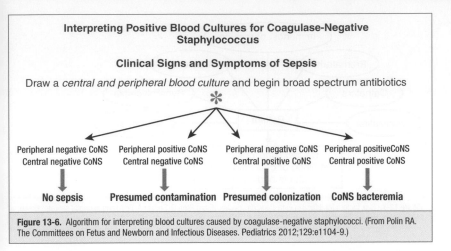

Figure 13-6. Algorithm for interpreting blood cultures caused by coagulase-negative staphylococci. (From Polin RA. The Committees on Fetus and Newborn and Infectious Diseases. Pediatrics 2012;129:e1104-9.)

more likely it is it represents a contaminant), number of positive cultures (especially if obtained from different sources; peripheral and central), the organisms' isolates (contamination is more likely when multiple specimens grow), and clinical signs.

Healy CM, Baker CJ, Palazzi DL, et al. Distinguishing true coagulase-negative Staphylococcus infections from contaminants in the neonatal intensive care unit. J Perinatol 2013;33(1):52–8.

Struthers S, Underhill H, Albersheim S, et al. A comparison of two versus one blood culture in the diagnosis and treatment of coagulase-negative staphylococcus in the neonatal intensive care unit. J Perinatol 2002;22(7):547–9.

68. **The most common manifestation of CoNS infection is bacteremia and sepsis, but what are the focal complications of persistent bacteremia with CoNS?**
   - Endocarditis: particularly if prolonged central catheter bacteremia or congenital heart disease is present
   - Soft-tissue infections: pustulosis, breast infections, omphalitis
   - Pneumonia
   - Meningitis, brain abscess: particularly if ventriculoperitoneal shunts are placed
   - Necrotizing enterocolitis

Isaacs D, Australasian Study Group for Neonatal Infections. A ten year, multicentre study of coagulase negative staphylococcal infections in Australasian neonatal units. Arch Dis Child Fetal Neonatal Ed 2003;88(2):F89–93.

69. **What is the recommended therapy for CoNS infection?**
   The initial recommended therapy is vancomycin, which may be modified once the isolate susceptibility is known. In cases of persistent bacteremia, a combination of vancomycin and rifampin may increase efficacy.
   When an indwelling catheter must be left in place, antibiotic therapy should be administered through the catheter. Removal of the catheter may be necessary if the culture remains positive. The same applies for other medical devices, such as meningitis resulting from an infected ventriculoperitoneal shunt.

70. **Should vancomycin prophylaxis be used to prevent neonatal nosocomial CoNS sepsis?**
   Because of concerns regarding the emergence of vancomycin-resistant organisms, routine use of prophylactic vancomycin for all neonates at risk of CoNS bacteremia is not currently recommended.

Kilbride HW, Powers R, Wirtschafter DD, et al. Evaluation and development of potentially better practices to prevent neonatal nosocomial bacteremia. Pediatrics 2003;111(4 Pt 2):e504–18.

Karlowicz MG, Buescher ES, Surka AE. Fulminant late-onset sepsis in a neonatal intensive care unit, 1988-1997, and the impact of avoiding empiric vancomycin therapy. Pediatrics 2000;106(6):1387–90.

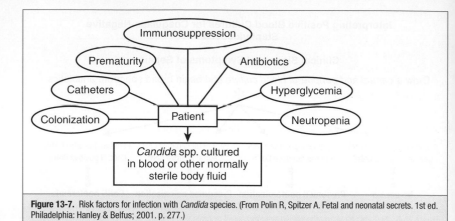

Figure 13-7. Risk factors for infection with *Candida* species. (From Polin R, Spitzer A. Fetal and neonatal secrets. 1st ed. Philadelphia: Hanley & Belfus; 2001. p. 277.)

CANDIDA

71. **What are the most important risk factors for neonatal systemic candidiasis?**
    - Prematurity: The incidence of systemic candidiasis, particularly in the VLBW infant, has increased significantly over the past decades, with a mortality rate approaching 30%. Significant neurodevelopmental sequelae are common among survivors.
    - Long-term use of broad-spectrum antibiotics (cephalosporin or carbapenems), use of gastric-acid inhibitors (H$_2$ blockers): Suppression of normal gastrointestinal flora enhances *Candida* species overgrowth.
    - Central intravenous catheterization and parenteral nutrition: These allow a portal of entry for the organism into the bloodstream.
    - Prolonged steroid use: This may impair neutrophil function (Figure 13-7).

Robinson JA, Pham HD, Bloom BT, et al. Risk factors for persistent candidemia infection in a neonatal intensive care unit and its effect on mortality and length of hospitalization. J Perinatol 2012;32(8):621–5.

Benjamin DK, Ross K, McKinney RE, et al. When to suspect fungal infection in neonates: a clinical comparison of *Candida albicans* and *Candida parapsilosis* fungemia with coagulase-negative staphylococcal bacteremia. Pediatrics 2000;106(4):712–8.

Chitnis AS, Magill SS, Edwards JR, et al. Trends in Candida central line-associated bloodstream infections among NICUs, 1999-2009. Pediatrics 2012;130(1):e46–52.

✓ KEY POINTS: *CANDIDA* DISEASES IN PREMATURE INFANTS

1. Risk factors for invasive candidiasis are prematurity, long-term use of broad-spectrum antibiotics, central intravenous catheterization, parenteral nutrition, and prolonged use of steroids.

2. Congenital candidiasis diseases almost always involve the skin and may infect the respiratory tract, leading to significant lung diseases that worsen the prognosis.

3. Fluconazole prophylaxis can reduce these infections among preterm infants, with the highest efficacy among very-low-birth-weight infants and those weighing 750 g or less.

4. Infants with candidemia should be evaluated for involvement of end organs, including eyes, kidneys, meninges, lungs, and heart.

5. Amphotericin is well tolerated in neonates. If urine tract involvement is excluded, the lipid formulation of amphotericin B can be used.

72. How common are invasive *Candida* infections (ICIs) in the neonatal intensive care units?

Approximately 1.4% of early-onset neonatal infections result from *Candida* species (mainly *Candida albicans* but increasingly from other species, such as *Candida parapsilosis* and *Candida glabrata*). For late-onset sepsis the incidence varies from 2.6% to 16.7% among VLBW infants and up to 20% for extremely-low-birth-weight infants. There is a marked inverse correlation between mortality caused by *Candida* species and neonatal weight; a recent analysis reported an all-cause mortality rate of 26% in infants weighing less than 1000 g with candidiasis compared with 13% in infants without candidiasis.

Miranda LDN, Rodrigues ECA, Costa SF, et al. Candida parapsilosis candidemia in a neonatal unit over 7 years: a case series study. BMJ Open 2012;2(4).

Ali GY, Algohary EHSS, Rashed KA, et al. Prevalence of Candida colonization in preterm newborns and VLBW in neonatal intensive care unit: role of maternal colonization as a risk factor in transmission of disease. J Matern Fetal Neonatal Med 2012;25(6):789–95.

73. What is the spectrum of *Candida* infection among neonates?

Early-onset candidal disease, or congenital candidiasis, arises from exposure of the infant to organisms colonizing the maternal genital tract. Cutaneous findings are the hallmark of the disease, but the association with pulmonary disease conveys a poor prognosis despite systemic antifungal therapy. On the other hand, catheter-associated fungemia generally arises from organisms on the skin or within the gastrointestinal tract.

Candida infections acquired after the first week of life might be limited to the bloodstream, urine, or CSF or may disseminate to involve one or many organ systems. Fungal abscesses may be found in the heart, bones, kidneys, bladder, eyes, or brain. The medical literature concerning end-organ evaluation after neonatal candidemia is heterogeneous; however, a retrospective study suggested potential damage from the following sources: endophthalmitis (median, 3%), meningitis (15%), brain abscess or ventriculitis (4%), endocarditis (5%), positive renal ultrasound (5%), and positive urine culture (61%).

Benjamin DK, Poole C, Steinbach WJ, et al. Neonatal candidemia and end-organ damage: a critical appraisal of the literature using meta-analytic techniques. Pediatrics. 2003;112(3 Pt 1):634–40.

Karlowicz MG, Giannone PJ, Pestian J, et al. Does candidemia predict threshold retinopathy of prematurity in extremely low birth weight (</=1000 g) neonates? Pediatrics 2000 May;105(5):1036–40.

74. How can ICI be prevented in preterm infants?

The highest risk period for ICIs in preterm neonates occurs during the first 4 to 8 weeks of life. Several studies have shown that fluconazole prophylaxis can reduce those infections among preterm infants, with highest efficacy among VLBW infants and those weighing 750 g or less. The pros and cons of antifungal prophylaxis are summarized in Table 13-7.

Kaufman DA, Manzoni P. Strategies to prevent invasive candidal infection in extremely preterm infants. Clin Peritanol 2010;37(3):611–28.

75. What antifungal should be used for prophylaxis among neonates whose birth weight is below 1000 g?

Studies in more than 4000 neonates have demonstrated efficacy and safety with fluconazole prophylaxis in extremely preterm neonates, with an overall reduction of 83%. No significant increases in azole-resistant strains have been documented. Enteral fluconazole is 90% absorbed; therefore once neonates achieve enteral feeding, the dosing can be switched from intravenous to oral administration to complete 4 to 6 weeks of prophylaxis.

Leibovitz E. Strategies for the prevention of neonatal candidiasis. Pediatr Neonatal 2012;53(2):83–9.

76. Is nystatin an alternative to fluconazole for prophylaxis of ICI among high-risk neonates?

A randomized control trial of infants with birth weight below 1500 g compared oral fluconazole to oral nystatin prophylaxis started in the first 7 days of life and continued until enteral feeding was

TABLE 13-7. PROS AND CONS OF ANTIFUNGAL PROPHYLAXIS FOR ELBW INFANTS

From Kaufman D, Manzoni P. Strategies to prevent invasive Candida *infection in extremely preterm infants. Clin Perinatol 2012;37:611–628.*

	PROS	CONS
Efficacy	>80% efficacy for fluconazole prophylaxis in reducing ICI. >50% efficacy for nystatin prophylaxis. Infection, death, and neurodevelopmental impairment could be prevented even if rates are low (2% or less). A unified approach, as with GBS prophylaxis, has the most benefit.	Rates vary by country and NICU.
ICI mortality	Multicenter data report >20% mortality in ELBWs (A-II)	Some single-center studies report no mortality (B-II). Empiric therapy could eliminate mortality (B-11). Appropriate treatment of documented infections could eliminate mortality.
NDI in survivors	57% NDI in infants weighing <1000 g (A-II) Neither CVC removal nor empiric therapy improved NDI (A-11)	Optimal treatment with CVC removal or empiric therapy in all patients may improve outcomes (further study needed).
ICI rate	5%-10% in infants weighing <1000 g when all ICI (BSI, UTI, meningitis, peritonitis) included (A-II) 20% for infants 23 to 24 weeks' GA (A-II)	Some NICUs report lower rates of 2% to 3% in infants <1000 g using only BSI and meningitis (B-II).
Cost	Fluconazole is inexpensive. ICI increases hospital costs (A-II); >$500,000 decreased costs over 18 months in one NICU.	Some infection-control measures are inexpensive (B-II).
Safety	All RCTs showed safety with no increase in liver function tests and no adverse effects; >4100 infants from all FP studies.	One retrospective study reported increased cholestasis with FP, though no significant difference at discharge. Possible concern with osmolarity of nystatin and NEC in extremely preterm infants.
Azole resistance	RCTs have not demonstrated increased azole resistance. Amphotericin (or a nonazole) is used for treating suspected or documented ICI. This appropriately treats ICI if resistance would occur and places less azole pressure on fungi to become resistant if exposed to high-dose fluconazole for treatment.	There is concern that resistance may still occur over time.
Alternative approaches	Empiric therapy and infection-control measures are not subjected to RCTs, and impact is unknown.	Other approaches (empiric therapy, infection control measures) might be efficacious.

BSI, Bloodstream infection; CVC, central venous catheter; FP, fluconazole prophylaxis; GA, gestational age; GBS, group B streptococci; ICI, invasive Candida infections; NDI, neurodevelopmental impairment; NNT, number needed to treat; UTI, urinary tract infection.

achieved. ICIs occurred in 5.3% of fluconazole-treated patients compared with 14.3% of nystatin-treated infants. The study also raised the question of safety of enteral nystatin in extremely premature infants when they were not receiving full enteral feedings. The oral nystatin suspension contains a high concentration of sucrose and is highly osmolar. This raises a theoretical concern of bacterial translocation and increased risk of necrotizing enterocolitis. Other advantages of fluconazole over nystatin are lower cost, administration twice-weekly compared with thrice daily, and ability to administer the drug intravenously when the infant is not receiving anything by mouth.

Kaufman D, Boyle R, Hazen KC, et al. Fluconazole prophylaxis against fungal colonization and infection in preterm infants. N Engl J Med 2001;345(23):1660–6.

77. What are the advantages of prophylaxis over empiric treatment?

Although empiric or prompt standardized treatment (including prompt removal of central venous catheters) may reduce *Candida*-related deaths, neurodevelopmental impairment may still occur in the survivors, particularly in those weighing less than 1000 g. Strategies to reduce morbidity and mortality in NICUs are summarized in Table 13-8.

Kaufman DA, Manzoni P. Strategies to prevent invasive candidal infection in extremely preterm infants. Clinics in Perinatology 2010;37(3):611–28.
Hsieh E, Smith PB, Jacqz-Aigrain E, et al. Neonatal fungal infections: when to treat? Early Hum Dev 2012;88 Suppl 2:S6–S10.
Greenberg RG, Benjamin DK, Gantz MG, et al. Empiric antifungal therapy and outcomes in extremely low birth weight infants with invasive candidiasis. J Pediatr 2012;161(2):264–9.

78. What is the recommended treatment of neonatal systemic *Candida* infection?

According to the Infectious Diseases Society of America Guidelines published in 2009, amphotericin B deoxycholate remains the mainstay of therapy (dose is 1 mg/kg/day). Although side effects include nephrotoxicity, hypokalemia, hepatotoxicity, and bone marrow suppression, the drug appears to be well tolerated in neonates. If urinary tract involvement is excluded, the lipid formulation of amphotericin B (3 to 5 mg/kg/day) can be used. Fluconazole at 12 mg/kg/day is a reasonable alternative.

TABLE 13-8.   STRATEGIES TO REDUCE ICI MORTALITY AND MORBIDITY AMONG NICUs

From Kaufman D, Manzoni P. Strategies to prevent invasive Candida *infection in extremely preterm infants. Clin Perinatol 2012(37);611–628.*

1. Use antifungal prophylaxis (IV fluconazole) while IV access is in use (central or peripheral) for infants with birth weight less than 1000 g and/or 27 weeks' gestational age or less (A-I)*
   - There is B-I and B-II evidence for antifungal prophylaxis with nystatin but limited data in infants <750 g and <26 weeks gestation. Because fluconazole prophylaxis has greater efficacy compared with nystatin, efficacy in the most immature patients is less expensive and can be given to infants not feeding; the evidence currently would favor fluconazole prophylaxis in preterm infants.

2. Start treatment of documented infections with appropriate antifungal dosing and prompt catheter removal for candidal BSI (A-II).

3. Decrease broad-spectrum antibiotic use (B-II).
   Restrict third- and fourth-generation cephalosporins and carbapenems to treatment of proven gram-negative infections.

4. Decrease H₂ blocker and proton-pump inhibitor use (B-II).
   Use only for proven gastritis, and restrict use to 3 days or until symptoms resolved.

5. Decrease postnatal dexamethasone use (B-II).Use only for severe lung disease.

U.S. Public Health Service Grading System for ranking recommendations in clinical guidelines: Strength of recommendation and levels of evidence. *A,* Good evidence; *B,* moderate evidence; *C,* poor evidence; *I,* at least one randomized clinical trial; *II,* at least one well-designed but nonrandomized trial; *III,* expert opinions based on experience or limited clinical reports.

The recommended length of treatment is 3 weeks. Echinocandins (e.g., caspofungin) should be used with caution among neonates and are usually reserved for situations in which resistance or toxicity precludes the use of fluconazole or amphotericin.

Manzoni P, Benjamin DK, Franco C, et al. Echinocandins for the nursery: an update. Curr Drug Metab 2013;14(2):203–207.
Ascher SB, Smith PB, Watt K, et al. Antifungal therapy and outcomes in infants with invasive Candida infections. Pediatr Infect Dis J 2012;31(5):439–43.

79. **What complementary investigations should be performed in a neonate with an invasive candidal infection?**
    A lumbar puncture and dilated retinal examination are recommended in neonates with sterile body fluid or urine cultures positive for *Candida* species. Imaging of the kidney and heart should be performed if the results of sterile body fluid cultures are positive.

80. **Has late-onset *Candida* disease been described?**
    The recurrence of *Candida* disease has been described in four immunocompetent infants after a prolonged period of latency (up to 1 year). All the infants presenting with *Candida* arthritis and osteomyelitis were born prematurely, had received parenteral nutrition through indwelling catheters, and had a history of systemic candidiasis during the newborn period. The pathogenesis of these latent infections remains unknown.

Harris MC, Pereira GR, Myers MD, et al. Candidal arthritis in infants previously treated for systemic candidiasis during the newborn period: report of three cases. Pediatr Emerg Care 2000;16(4):249–51.

INFECTION CONTROL

81. **What is the difference between incidence rate and prevalence rate?**
    Incidence rate is the number of new cases of a disease that occur during a specific period of time in a population at risk for developing the disease (i.e., number of cases of bacteremia per 1000 catheter-days). Prevalence is the number of affected persons present in the population at a specific time divided by the number of persons in the population at the time (i.e., proportion of pneumonia cases in a neonatal unit on a particular day).

82. **What is the difference between endemic and epidemic nosocomial infections?**
    Endemic infections represent the bulk of nosocomial infections and are the usual level of infection expected during a given period for a given population. Epidemic infections are marked by an unusual increase in the incidence of disease entity.

83. **Are health care–associated infections (HAIs) common in nurseries?**
    Neonates, especially if premature, require intensive medical care and are among the patients at highest risk for HAIs. Some series have reported that more than 20% of critically ill neonates who survive longer than 48 hours acquire a HAI, with a significant worsening of their prognosis and excessive direct health costs.

Clark R, Powers R, White R, et al. Nosocomial infection in the NICU: a medical complication or unavoidable problem? J Perinatol 2004;24(6):382–8.

84. **What are the routes of transmission of HAIs among neonates?**
    Nonmaternal routes of transmission (generally accepted when symptoms start 3 days or longer after admission) can be categorized as follows:
    - Contact: Direct or indirect; from an infected person or a contaminated source. Transmission by the hands of health care workers is the most important route.
    - Droplet: Large respiratory droplets that travel 3 feet or less (e.g., pertussis).
    - Airborne: Smaller particles that can travel longer distances (e.g., varicella).

Specific microorganisms can be spread by more than one route, but in most cases one mechanism predominates. Most of the HAIs are caused by the infant's own flora.

Polin RA, Denson S, Brady MT, et al. Epidemiology and diagnosis of health care-associated infections in the NICU. Pediatrics 2012;129(4):e1104–9.

85. **Which kinds of patients need to be isolated in negative-pressure rooms?**
    Patients suspected of having tuberculosis, varicella, or measles must be placed on airborne precautions in negative-pressure rooms to prevent aerosol spread of their infection. It is important to assess the family members of such patients because they might be potential sources of the infection as well.

Remington JS, Klein JO, Wilson CB, et al. Infectious diseases of the fetus and newborn: expert consult - online and print. 7th ed. Philadelphia: Saunders; 2010.

86. **A nurse tells you that she has just been exposed to varicella, and she never had it as a child. What do you tell her about the period of isolation?**
    Patients (or nonimmune staff or visitors) must be isolated from day 8 to day 21 after documented exposure to a person with active varicella zoster virus (VZV) infection. If a patient has received varicella-zoster immune globulin (VZIG), the incubation period is extended to 28 days. Varicella immunization is recommended for people without evidence of immunity, provided there are no contraindications for vaccine use.

87. **What is contact isolation?**
    Contact precautions involve the use of barriers to prevent transmission of organisms by direct or indirect contact with the patient or contaminated objects in the patient's immediate environment. Ideally, patients should be placed in private rooms. Cohorting of patients infected with the same microorganisms can be a safe and effective alternative. Health care workers should wash hands when entering and leaving the room and wear clean nonsterile gloves and a cover gown when entering the room.

88. **Which diseases require contact isolation?**
    The following diseases require contact isolation:
    - *Clostridium difficile*
    - Rotavirus
    - Respiratory syncytial virus
    - Croup
    - Mucocutaneous herpes simplex
    - Resistant organisms, including methicillin-resistant *S. aureus* (MRSA) and vancomycin-resistant enterococci

89. **What are droplet precautions?**
    Droplet precautions are intended to reduce the risk of transmission of infected agents by large-particle droplets from an infected person. Such transmission usually occurs when an infected person generates droplets while coughing, sneezing, or talking and during procedures such as suctioning.
    Patients should be placed in private rooms, and staff should wear masks when working within 3 feet of the patient. Examples of conditions that necessitate droplet precautions include influenza virus, adenovirus, parvovirus, rubella, pertussis, and meningitis caused by *Haemophilus influenzae* or *Neisseria meningitidis*.

90. **What are universal or standard precautions?**
    Standard precautions are designed to reduce the risk of transmission of microorganisms from recognized and unrecognized sources and are to be followed for the care of all patients, including neonates. They apply to blood; all body fluids, secretions, and excretions except sweat; nonintact mucous membranes; and skin.
    Components of standard precautions include performing proper hand hygiene and wearing gloves, gowns, masks, and other forms of eye protection.

91. **What are the most frequently cited reasons that nursery personnel do not wash their hands (all invalid)?**
    - Hand-washing takes too much time.
    - There is a lack of soap (54%) and lack of towels (65%).
    - One thorough wash per day is sufficient (26%).
    - Gloves can substitute for hand-washing (25%, including 50% of physicians).
    - Hand-washing is not important if an infant is receiving antibiotics (10%).

92. **What are the current recommendations for hand hygiene in the NICU?**
    - Most experts recommend removal of hand and wrist jewelry. CDC guidelines state that staff who have direct contact with infants in NICU should not wear artificial fingernails or nail extenders. Nails should be kept less than ¼ inch long. Clear nail polish is acceptable but not nail polish with colors.
    - The minimum initial wash should be long enough to ensure thorough washing and rinsing of all parts of the hands and forearms (3-minute scrub without a brush to the elbow).
    - At least a 15-second scrub should be performed before and after handling of each infant.
    - An alcohol-based hand gel should be used before and after handling infants.

93. **Do careful hand hygiene practices reduce the incidence of nosocomial infection?**
    Hand hygiene plays a key role for caregivers in the reduction of HAIs for patients.

94. **When should health care workers wash their hands with water and soap?**
    Soap and water should be used when hands are visibly soiled or contaminated with proteinaceous materials, blood, or body fluids and after using the restroom.

95. **What is the advantage of alcohol-based hand rubs?**
    When hands are not visibly soiled, alcohol-based hand rubs, foams, or gels are important tools for hand hygiene. Compared with washing with soap and water, use of alcohol-based products is at least as effective against a variety of pathogens and requires less time. Furthermore, these agents are less damaging to skin.

96. **What is the preferred method for hand disinfection in the NICU?**
    Hand disinfection with an alcohol-based hand rub is the preferred method because of its rapid action and effectiveness. In addition, alcohol-based rubs contain emollients that serve as dermal protectors and decrease bacterial dispersal. In contrast, antiseptic skin washes can damage the skin barrier and offer no advantages.

Polin RA, Denson S, Brady MT, et al. Strategies for prevention of health care-associated infections in the NICU. Pediatrics 2012;129(4):e1085–93.

97. **Do health care workers need to wear gowns for routine patient contact?**
    CDC guidelines recommend nonsterile, fluid-resistant gowns to be worn as protection when soiling of clothing is anticipated and in performing procedures likely to result in splashing or spraying of body substances.

98. **When should the health care worker wear gloves?**
    Gloves should be worn whenever contact with blood, body fluids, secretions, excretions, and contaminated items are anticipated. Wearing gloves is not a substitute for hand hygiene. Hand hygiene should be performed immediately after glove removal.

99. **Should visitors be allowed in the NICU?**
    The principles of family-centered care encourage liberal visitation policies in neonatal units (well-infant nurseries and NICUs). Parents and siblings should be allowed liberal visitation. Written policies should

TABLE 13-9. CAUSES OF NEONATAL CONJUNCTIVITIS AND TIME OF ONSET

From Polin R, Spitzer A. Fetal and neonatal secrets. 1st ed. Philadelphia: Hanley & Belfus; 2001. p. 283–84.

ETIOLOGY	USUAL TIME OF ONSET AFTER BIRTH
Chemical (with silver nitrate prophylaxis)	6 to 24 hours
Chlamydia trachomatis	5 to 14 days
Neisseria gonorrhoeae	2 to 5 days

Other bacterial etiology:
  Staphylococcus aureus
  Haemophilus species
  Streptococcus pneumoniae
  Enterococcus species
	>5 days

Herpes simplex	5 to 14 days

be in place to guide siblings' visits, and parents should be encouraged to share the responsibility of protecting the newborn from contagious illness.

Remington JS, Klein JO, Wilson CB, et al. Infectious diseases of the fetus and newborn: expert consult—online and print. 7th ed. Philadelphia: Saunders; 2010.

CONJUNTIVITIS

100. What are the common causes of neonatal conjunctivitis, and when do they present?
Ophthalmia neonatorum is a conjunctivitis that occurs within the first 4 weeks of life. It has been associated with a variety of organisms, which have changed in their relative importance and geographic distribution over a period of years. The introduction of neonatal ocular prophylaxis and routine screening and treatment of maternal gonorrhea and more recently *Chlamydia trachomatis* infection have altered the epidemiology of ophthalmia neonatorum. In the United States *C. trachomatis* is likely the most common cause of conjunctivitis in neonates.

In addition to *C. trachomatis* and *Neisseria gonorrhoeae*, *S. aureus* and various gram-negative bacteria such as *E. coli*, *Klebsiella* species, and rarely *Pseudomonas* species have also been associated with neonatal conjunctivitis.

Viral causes of conjunctivitis are rare during the first month; however, 70% of cases with viral etiology are due to HSV, which may also cause severe systemic disease.

The age at onset may suggest a specific etiology; however, there is substantial overlap among the various causes depending on obstetric factors such as prolonged rupture of membranes (Table 13-9).

Darville T. Chlamydia trachomatis infections in neonates and young children. Semin Pediatr Infect Dis 2005;16(4):235–44.
Shah S. Pediatric practice infectious diseases. 1st ed. Pennsylvania: McGraw-Hill Professional; 2009.

101. A 5-day-old term baby presents in the emergency room with purulent material coming from one eye. What work-up should you do?
The first step should be a Gram stain of the conjunctiva exudate. If it shows gram-negative intracellular bean-shaped diplococci, *Neisseria gonorrhoeae* (or other *Neisseria* species) should be assumed to be the cause of the eye discharge, and the infant should be admitted for urgent systemic treatment. If treatment is delayed, the infection could spread to the cornea leading to ulcerations and ultimately loss of vision. Note that the eye discharge seen in gonococcal ophthalmia is often thick, copious, and golden-yellow in color. Cultures of blood, eye discharge, and other potential sites of

infection, such as CSF, should be performed to confirm the diagnosis and determine antimicrobial susceptibility. Testing for concomitant infection with *C. trachomatis, Treponema pallidum,* and human immunodeficiency virus (HIV) should also be done, as well as a review of hepatitis B status in the mother.

NAATs are highly sensitive and specific, but only a few are approved by the U.S. Food and Drug Administration (FDA) for conjunctival specimens; therefore the diagnosis still relies on culture. A combined DNA probe for the detection of both *N. gonorrhoeae* and *C. trachomatis* is also commercially available. Remember that *C. trachomatis* is an obligate intracellular organism, so the collection swab must be scraped across the conjunctiva or nasopharynx to ensure that there are adequate cells for detection. In the eye the pus should be wiped away before the conjunctiva scrapings are obtained. If herpes conjunctivitis is suspected, a PCR test for herpes simplex or culture should also be done. The identification of *C. trachomatis* or *N. gonorrhoeae* in a newborn infant indicates untreated infection in the parents.

Pickering LK, Baker CJ, Kimberlin DW, Long SS, editors. Red Book Report of the Committee on Infectious Diseases. 29th ed. American Academy of Pediatrics; 2012.

102. What is the treatment for conjunctivitis?

Nondisseminated gonococcal neonatal infections such as ophthalmia neonatorum should be treated with ceftriaxone, at a dose of 25 to 50 mg/kg administered intravenously or intramuscularly given once, not to exceed 125 mg. Additional topical therapy is not needed when ceftriaxone is used; however, the infant's eyes should be irrigated with normal saline frequently until the discharge has resolved.

Infants with chlamydial conjunctivitis are treated with oral erythromycin (50 mg/kg/day divided into four equal doses) for 14 days. Additional topical therapy is not needed. Because the efficacy of erythromycin is only 80%, a second course may be required, and follow-up of infants is recommended. Limited data suggest that azithromycin at an oral dose of 20 mg/kg given once a day for 3 days may be effective. Herpes conjunctivitis is rare and is almost always accompanied by other systemic manifestations of neonatal herpes. The treatment for neonatal herpes conjunctivitis is parenteral acyclovir plus topical therapy with 1% trifluridine solution, 0.1% iododeoxyuridine, or 3% vidarabine applied to the eye every 2 hours for 7 days or until the cornea has re-epithelialized.

Thordsen JE, Harris L, Hubbard GB. Pediatric endophthalmitis. A 10-year consecutive series. Retina (Philadelphia, Pa.) 2008;28(3 Suppl):S3–7.

103. Why does conjunctivitis caused by *C. trachomatis* not cause blindness in neonates when it causes so many cases of blindness in third-world countries?

The visual loss associated with trachoma is caused by irreversible corneal damage resulting from chronic folliculitis owing to repeated chronic infections. Because of their immature immune systems, newborns lack the requisite lymphoid tissue in their conjunctiva to mount such an inflammatory response. The length of infection also makes a difference. Even older children do not develop folliculitis until the infection has been present for at least 1 to 2 months; newborn conjunctivitis caused by *C. trachomatis* usually clears by 2 months even without antibiotic treatment, so it rarely results in long-term sequelae. Another important factor may be that the serotypes of *C. trachomatis* that cause endocervical infections in women and conjunctivitis in neonates (types D through K) differ from the serotypes that cause blinding trachoma (types A through C).

104. Does the use of antibiotic eye prophylaxis at birth decrease the incidence of neonatal conjunctivitis resulting from *C. trachomatis*?

No. Topical silver nitrate, tetracycline, and erythromycin given at birth are equally effective in preventing gonococcal ophthalmia neonatorum, but none of these agents significantly decreases the incidence of chlamydial conjunctivitis. The only way to prevent *Chlamydia* infections in the newborn is by treating infected mothers before delivery.

CHLAMYDIAL INFECTIONS

105. Does *C. trachomatis* infection in pregnant women cause complications other than neonatal infection?

C. trachomatis is the most common sexually transmitted pathogen in Western industrialized countries. Most of the infections in adults are asymptomatic but can cause severe reproductive complications in women; chronic salpingitis caused by *C. trachomatis* can lead to infertility and an increased risk for ectopic pregnancy. This is in contrast with gonococcal infections, in which most infected individuals are symptomatic and therefore present acutely for care. Although studies are conflicting, *C. trachomatis* infection in pregnancy is weakly linked to premature rupture of membranes and premature delivery. Between 10% and 30% of women with chlamydial infections who undergo induced abortions develop late endometritis.

Remington JS, Klein JO, Wilson CB, et al. Infectious diseases of the fetus and newborn: expert consult—online and print. 7th ed. Philadelphia: Saunders; 2010.

Hammerschlag MR. Chlamydial and gonococcal infections in infants and children. Clin Infect Dis 2011;53 (Suppl 3):S99–102.

106. What is the risk of chlamydial infection in infants born to mothers whose endocervical culture result is positive for *C. trachomatis*?

Chlamydia infection can be transmitted from an infected mother to her newborn during delivery, resulting in conjunctivitis, pneumonia, or both.

An infant born to a mother with chlamydial infection of the cervix is at 60% to 70% risk of acquiring the infection during passage through the birth canal. Of exposed infants, 20% to 50% develop conjunctivitis at 5 to 14 days of age and 10% to 20% develop pneumonia between 4 and 12 weeks of life (conjunctivitis is not a prerequisite to develop pneumonia). *In utero* transmission is not known to occur.

The remaining infants develop an apparently asymptomatic colonization of the nasopharynx, rectum, or vagina. These infants can remain colonized for up to 3 years, although most clear the infection even without treatment by 1 year of age. There is no evidence to suggest that infants with chlamydial infections should be isolated. Note that successful treatment of the mother during pregnancy with oral erythromycin or azithromycin prevents most cases of vertical transmission.

Silva MJPM de A, Florêncio GLD, Gabiatti JRE, et al. Perinatal morbidity and mortality associated with chlamydial infection: a meta-analysis study. Braz J Infect Dis 2011;15(6):533–9.

107. Does *Chlamydia pneumoniae* cause pulmonary diseases among neonates?

C. pneumoniae is a common cause of atypical pneumonia in school-age children and young adults; along with *Mycoplasma* species. It is not known to cause pulmonary diseases in newborns.

108. What procedures are used to diagnose *C. trachomatis* infection in infants?

Chlamydia culture of the conjunctiva (for conjunctivitis) or nasopharynx (for pneumonia) remains the gold standard for diagnosis. However, cultures have many disadvantages; specimens require special handling, which can make transport to the laboratory challenging and generally require 3 to 7 days for processing, which may delay treatment. NAATs have largely replaced tissue culture isolation and nonamplified direct detection methods (e.g., DNA probe, direct fluorescent antibody [DFA] test or enzyme immunoassays [EIA]) because of their better sensibility and specificity.

NAATs have FDA approval for cervical swabs from women, urethral swabs for men, and urine from women and men. Published evidence of NAATs on conjunctival specimens or nasopharyngeal samples is limited, but preliminary results show that their sensitivity and specificity is as high as with culture. Serologic diagnosis of chlamydial infections are difficult to interpret and only done in a few clinical laboratories

109. What is the proper treatment for *C. trachomatis* infections in adults?

Mothers with positive endocervical cultures should be treated during pregnancy to prevent vertical transmission. The recommended treatment for pregnant women is azithromycin (1 g orally as single dose) or amoxicillin (1.5 g/day in 3 divided daily doses for 7 days). Repeated testing (preferably NAATs) is recommended in pregnant women 3 weeks after treatment to determine whether treatment has been successful; if not, a second course of treatment may be indicated. Sexual partners of positive women must be treated as well. Chlamydia infection in both male and female genital tracts can be asymptomatic, which is why routine screening in pregnancy is warranted.

Pickering I K, Baker CJ, Kimberlin DW, Long SS, editors. Red Book Report of the Committee on Infectious Diseases. 29th ed. American Academy of Pediatrics; 2012.

110. What is the proper treatment for *C. trachomatis* infections in infants?

Until recently, the AAP recommended that babies born to mothers with untreated chlamydial cervical infections receive oral erythromycin (50 mg/kg per day in four divided doses) for 14 days, starting on the first day of life. However, the efficacy of prophylactic treatment is unknown; moreover, reports of an association between the use of oral erythromycin for pertussis and infantile hypertrophic pyloric stenosis have appeared. The AAP now recommends that treatment be reserved for infants with actual infection and not for prophylaxis.

Neonates with chlamydial conjunctivitis or pneumonia should receive oral erythromycin base or ethylsuccinate, 50 mg/kg/day in four divided doses, for 14 days. The efficacy of erythromycin is approximately 80%; therefore a second course may be required, and follow-up of infants is recommended. Limited data on azithromycin for treatment of chlamydial infection in infants suggest that dosing of 20 mg/kg as a single dose for 3 days may be effective. Its shorter treatment course and less severe gastrointestinal side effects could improve treatment compliance.

Pickering LK, Baker CJ, Kimberlin DW, Long SS, editors. Red Book Report of the Committee on Infectious Diseases. 29th ed. American Academy of Pediatrics; 2012.

111. What are the characteristics of *C. trachomatis* pneumonia?

The onset of *C. trachomatis* pneumonia usually occurs between 4 and 12 weeks of age (a few cases present as early as 2 weeks, but none has been reported beyond 4 months). Most infants have a prodromal period of approximately 1 week's duration that involves nasal obstruction or discharge without fever and a persistent paroxysmal staccato cough that can lead to respiratory distress. Expiratory wheezing occurs in fewer than 25% of infants with the disease; 60% have abnormal eardrum findings. Although a severe illness is relatively rare, affected infants appear irritable, eat poorly, and cough often.

The chest x-ray shows hyperinflation of the lungs with bilateral diffuse nonspecific infiltrates. Possible laboratory findings include a distinctive peripheral eosinophilia (>300 to $400/mm^3$), mild arterial hypoxemia, and elevated serum immunoglobulins.

Without treatment, symptoms last an average of 6 weeks. Treatment of any previous conjunctivitis with oral erythromycin seems to prevent pneumonia, although there are case reports of treatment failures. Approximately 50% of the infants with chlamydial pneumonia do not have a history of previous conjunctivitis.

Bellulo S, Bosdure E, David M, et al. Chlamydia trachomatis pneumonia: two atypical case reports. Arch Pediatr 2012;19(2):142–5.
Horvat JC, Starkey MR, Kim RY, et al. Early-life chlamydial lung infection enhances allergic airways disease through age-dependent differences in immunopathology. J Allergy Clin Immunol 2010;125(3):617–25.

OSTEOMYELITIS AND SEPTIC ARTHRITIS

112. What pathogens cause neonatal osteomyelitis?

Because most cases of neonatal osteomyelitis arise as a consequence of bacteremia, the organisms responsible for causing osteomyelitis reflect the changing trends in the ethology of neonatal sepsis as well as the different likelihood of osteoarticular shedding within pathogens.

- S. *aureus;* predominant organism, with increasing MRSA isolates
- GBS: second most important cause
- Gram-negative enteric bacilli (i.e., *E. coli, Klebsiella* species, *Pseudomonas* species, *Proteus* species, *Enterobacter, Serratia marcescens,* and *Salmonella* species): uncommon despite the frequency of neonatal bacteremia caused by these agents
- *Candida* species: particularly in premature infants
- *Mycoplasma hominis* and *Ureaplasma urealyticum:* rare
- *T. pallidum:* largely eliminated thanks to antenatal maternal screening and treatment.

Long SS, Pickering LK, Prober CG. Principles and practice of pediatric infectious diseases: expert consult—online and print. 4th ed. Philadelphia: Saunders; 2012.

Zhang J, Lee BH, Chen C. Gram-negative neonatal osteomyelitis: two case reports. Neonatal Netw 2011;30(2):81–7.

113. What is the incidence of osteomyelitis in the neonate?

Although osteomyelitis was rare in the past, recent studies suggest that it might be increasing in neonates. The overall rate of nosocomial bone and joint infections is approximately 1 or 2 in 1000 admissions.

114. What is the pathogenesis of osteomyelitis in the newborn?

Hematogenous dissemination is responsible for most cases; however, skeletal infections can also result from the following:

- Extension from infection in surrounding tissues (e.g., an infected cephalohematoma spreading to the parietal bone)
- Direct inoculation after heel-stick capillary blood sampling or fetal scalp monitoring
- Maternal bacteremia with transplacental infection and fetal sepsis (i.e., syphilis)

Remington JS, Klein JO, Wilson CB, et al. Infectious diseases of the fetus and newborn: expert consult—online and print. 7th ed. Philadelphia: Saunders; 2010.

115. What distinct anatomic and physiologic features place the newborn infant at risk for osteomyelitis and septic arthritis?

Hematogenous infection of long bones is initiated in dilated capillary loops of the metaphysis, adjacent to the cartilaginous growth plate (physis), where blood flow slows, providing pathogenic bacteria with an ideal environment to multiply. In neonates there is an anatomic communication between the circulatory systems of the metaphysis and epiphysis (transphyseal vessels) that can lead to severe damage of the cartilage cells on the epiphyseal side of the growth plate when infection occurs. This damage is generally irreversible and results in abnormal growth of the bone. The vascular connection is obliterated at 8 to 18 months of age when the epiphyseal and metaphyseal become totally separated.

Decompression of the primary metaphyseal abscess through the adjacent cortex also permits entrance of pus into the articular space of the bones whose metaphyses lie within the articular capsule of the joint. Suppurative arthritis of hips, shoulders, elbows, and knees is frequently seen in osteomyelitis of the humerus or the femur (Fig. 13-8).

116. Why do neonates not exhibit many of the features of chronic osteomyelitis seen in older children and adults?

On account of a relatively thin cortex, the abscess usually spreads into the subperiosteal space and rapidly involves the entire circumference and length of the bone. This free communication between the original site of osteomyelitis and the subperiosteal space prevents the necrosis and cortical sequestra that happens in older children and adults. The efficient vasculature and fertility of the inner layer of the periosteum encourage early development of new bone formation (involucrum), permitting remodeling of bone within a very short time after the infectious process has been controlled.

117. What are the manifestations of osteomyelitis in neonates?

- Systemic signs are usually absent in neonatal osteomyelitis but occasionally are present.

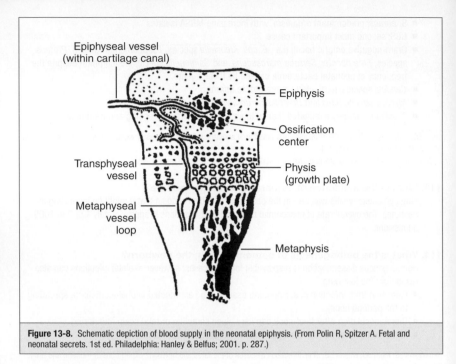

Figure 13-8. Schematic depiction of blood supply in the neonatal epiphysis. (From Polin R, Spitzer A. Fetal and neonatal secrets. 1st ed. Philadelphia: Hanley & Belfus; 2001. p. 287.)

- In most infants the earliest presenting signs are pain, limitation of motion (pseudoparalysis), and swelling. Discoloration and increased warmth may accompany the swelling.
- Feeding and weight gain are usually undisturbed if only local symptoms are present, leading to a delay in the diagnosis while bone destruction progresses.
- The distribution of bone involvement is as follows:
  - Femur (39%)
  - Humerus (18%)
  - Tibia (14%)
  - Fibula (10%)
  - Radius (5%)
  - Maxilla (4%)
  - Ulna (3%)
  - Clavicle (2%)
  - Tarsal bones (2%)
  - Ribs (2%)
  - Vertebrae (1%)

118. **How often are bacterial culture results positive in neonatalosteomyelitis and septic arthritis?**
- Up to 60% of blood cultures can be positive.
- Approximately 60% to 70% of joint and bone aspirates are positive, but previous antibiotic therapy may decrease this percentage.

119. **Is the erythrocyte sedimentation rate (ESR) or CRP helpful in the management of osteomyelitis?**
In most studies the ESR is significantly elevated on days 2 through 5. ESR values slowly return to normal within 3 weeks of therapy. In contrast, CRP rises within 6 to 12 hours of a triggering

stimulus and returns to normal within 1 week of therapy. A secondary rise in either ESR or CRP could be a sign of recrudescence. Neither CRP nor ESR can be used to rule out osteomyelitis when normal.

Dessì A, Crisafulli M, Accossu S, et al. Osteo-articular infections in newborns: diagnosis and treatment. J Chemother 2008;20(5):542–50.

120. How common is fungal septic arthritis?

Candida species have become a more frequent cause of bone and joint infection. Some studies report that approximately 17% of septic arthritis in premature infants is caused by *Candida* species.

121. What are the unique features of *Candida* bone infections?

- Unlike bacterial infections, inflammatory signs other than edema of the extremity are generally lacking.
- Radiographs demonstrate "punched-out" metaphyseal lucencies that appear less aggressive than staphylococcal osteomyelitis.
- Affected infants often have a history of central line–related fungemia.
- Fungal septic arthritis can appear as late as 1 year after a treated fungal infection.
- Fluconazole may be a good alternative to amphotericin B because of its good joint penetration.

122. What is the first line of management for a suspected septic arthritis in a newborn infant?

Joint aspiration with incision and drainage is appropriate whenever there is a significant collection of pus in the soft tissues. Often, surgical drainage is indicated for relief of intraarticular pressure when the hip or shoulder is affected.

123. What radiologic studies are helpful in the diagnosis of osteomyelitis?

See Table 13-10.

124. What is the presentation of maxillary osteomyelitis?

Neonatal osteomyelitis of the maxilla is a distinct clinical entity usually caused by *S. aureus*. The clinical course of this condition begins with acute onset of fever and nonspecific systemic symptoms that shortly after are accompanied by the following:

- Early edema and redness of the cheeks
- Unilateral nasal discharge
- Swelling of the eyelid with conjunctivitis

This entity can be confused with orbital cellulitis or dacryocystitis.

125. What are the initial antibiotics used for the treatment of osteomyelitis?

Once cultures are obtained, the initial choice of antimicrobial agents must be based on the presumptive bacteriologic diagnosis. Penicillinase-resistant penicillins (i.e., oxacillin) are effective against methicillin-sensitive *S. aureus,* group A streptococci, and GBS. Vancomycin should be used if MRSA or CoNS infection is suspected. Osteomyelitis caused by enteric organisms is sufficiently common in neonates to justify adding an aminoglycoside to the initial regimen.

If the organism is identified and antibiotic sensitivities have been determined, treatment should be changed to the safest and most effective drug. Therapy should be continued for a minimum of 4 to 6 weeks. In the neonatal age group, orally administered antibiotics are not used because there are insufficient data regarding their absorption and efficacy.

Ecury-Goosssen GM, Huysman MA, Verhallen-Dantuma JCTM, et al. Sequential intravenous-oral antibiotic therapy for neonatal osteomyelitis. Pediat Infect Dis J 2009;28(1):72–3.

TABLE 13–10. RADIOLOGIC STUDIES FOR THE DIAGNOSIS OF OSTEOMYELITIS

From Polin R, Spitzer A. Fetal and neonatal secrets. 1st ed. Philadelphia: Hanley & Belfus; 2001. p. 288.

TEST	PROS	CONS
Skeletal x-rays	Eventually, bony changes will be seen (i.e., punched-out lytic lesions, osseous lucencies, and periosteal elevation). Multiple sites of involvement can eventually be seen. Trauma (i.e., fracture) as a cause of swelling or pseudoparalysis can be ruled out.	X-ray changes do not occur for 7 to 12 days. Conventional radiographs are insensitive to the destruction of <30% of the bone matrix.
^{99m}Tc	Osteomyelitis can be detected earlier than on traditional skeletal surveys. With the higher-resolution gamma cameras used today, multiple sites of infection are often noted.	Patient is exposed to radiation. False-negative studies have been reported. False-positive results result from increased metabolic bone activity.
Gallium bone	In equivocal ^{99m}Tc bone scans, gallium might be useful.	The radiation scan dose is significantly higher than in ^{99m}Tc bone scan.
Sonography	Most useful as a tool for guiding needle aspiration of fluid collections in joints or adjacent to bone. It is inexpensive. There is no radiation exposure.	An experienced sonographer is required. Accuracy is variable in neonates.
MRI	Can detect inflammatory intramedullary diseases and gives excellent anatomic details in the early stages.	Requires general anesthesia
CT	Provides good definition of cortical bone and is sensitive for foe early detection of bone destruction, periosteal reaction and sequestra.	Requires anesthesia, radiation and lack of detection of intramedullary diseases (not however involvement of marrow compartment is uncommon in neonates)

^{99m}Tc, ^{99m}Technetium; CT, computed tomography; MRI, magnetic resonance imaging.

PYELONEPHRITIS AND URINARY TRACT INFECTION

126. **A 10-day-old male infant presents with a 2-day history of fever, vomiting, lethargy, and jaundice. Examination reveals a temperature of 39° C, a blood pressure measurement of 65/40, and a pulse of 170 bpm; there are no focal abnormal physical findings. Laboratory data include the following levels: bilirubin, 7 mg/dL (direct, 2 mg/dL); creatinine, 0.2 mg/dL; WBC count, 20,000 cells/mm³; and urinalysis 60 WBCs per high-power field. What is the most likely diagnosis?**

The signs and symptoms suggest an acute infectious process. The urinalysis is consistent with a diagnosis of acute pyelonephritis (assuming that the specimen has been properly obtained). The incidence of UTI in infants during the first month of life varies between 0.1% to 1% depending on the population studied. Unlike the distinction of cystitis and pyelonephritis in older infants and children, infection of the urinary tract in the neonate often involves the kidney.

127. What is the incidence of asymptomatic bacteriuria in neonates?

Asymptomatic bacteriuria occurs in 2% of healthy term neonates and up to 10% of premature infants. Males are affected more often than females in the neonatal period, and uncircumcised males are even more susceptible, with a threefold to sevenfold increased risk.

128. What is the pathogenesis of UTI in the neonate?

Unlike in older infants, hematogenous spread of infection is more common in neonates than ascending infection. Anatomic or physiologic abnormalities of the urinary tract, such as obstructive uropathy, are also common underlying factors. Urinary tract anomalies have been detected in 30% to 55% of infants with UTI younger than 2 months of age.

129. What are the signs and symptoms of UTI in the neonate?

The symptoms of UTI are varied and nonspecific. UTI can present as an insidious illness with failure to thrive and low-grade fever or simply as a fever without apparent source or septicemia. Jaundice is an important feature of UTI; it usually occurs suddenly and clears rapidly after adequate treatment has been started. Many infants with UTIs and jaundice have positive blood cultures.

130. How is the diagnosis of a UTI in the neonate made?

The definitive diagnosis is made by positive culture of urine that is obtained by percutaneus aspiration or urethral catheterization of the bladder. Urine from bags and other nonsterile materials should not be used because false-positive results are very common. The yield of urine culture in neonates younger than 3 days of age is poor.

Urinalysis is not very helpful insofar as neither the presence nor absence of pyuria is completely reliable evidence for or against UTI. However, an enhanced urinalysis (leukocytes measured in unspun urine by a hemocytometer) has been shown to be a sensitive marker of UTI when more than 10 WBC/mm^3 are found. A dipstick test for leukocyte sterase and nitrite is inadequate to exclude UTIs in neonates.

131. What are the common organisms responsible for UTI in newborn infants?

The most common organism causing UTI in neonates is *E. coli,* which accounts for 91% of community-acquired infection in children younger than 8 weeks of age. Other organisms include *Proteus, Pseudomonas, Klebsiella,* and *Enterococcus* species or *S. aureus*, which may be associated with localized suppurative lesions in the urinary tract. With prolonged hospitalization, CoNS and *Candida* species can also cause UTIs in patients with or without urinary catheters. Candidiasis can be associated with fungal balls in the kidney and renal pelvis, which can lead to obstruction.

Remington JS, Klein JO, Wilson CB, et al. Infectious diseases of the fetus and newborn: expert consult - online and print. 7th ed. Philadelphia: Saunders; 2010.

132. How should pyelonephritis be treated?

Parenteral antibiotics are used to treat pyelonephritis, usually a combination of a penicillin and an aminoglycoside. The clinician should try to obtain a urine culture before initiating antibiotic treatment and then modify the treatment once culture results and sensitivities are known. For suspected staphylococcal infection, a penicillinase-resistant penicillin or vancomycin should be considered. Amphotericin is used for *Candida* species infection. For an uncomplicated UTI the duration of therapy is usually 10 to 14 days. The transition to an oral regimen depends on the clinical and microbiological response and the presence of bacteremia or anatomic abnormalities. A second urine sample is often obtained after 48 hours to ensure clearance of the organisms from the urinary tract.

In the past, prophylactic antibiotics were often used for structural anomalies of the urinary tract or vesicoureteral reflux. However, a systematic review of randomized controlled trials revealed limited evidence for its efficacy. Moreover, antibiotic prophylaxis may increase the risk of a subsequent UTI by a resistant microrganism.

Long SS, Pickering LK, Prober CG. Principles and practice of pediatric infectious diseases: expert consult—online and print. 4th ed. Philadelphia: Saunders; 2012.

Montini G, Rigon L, Zucchetta P, et al. Prophylaxis after first febrile urinary tract infection in children? A multicenter, randomized, controlled, noninferiority trial. Pediatrics 2008;122(5):1064–71.

133. In addition to urinalysis and urine culture, what other tests are indicated in the treatment of an infant with possible UTI?

A UTI is generally a bloodborne disease; however, some neonates may have associated meningitis and septicemia. Therefore, in addition to urinalysis and urine culture, neonates should have blood and CSF culture specimens drawn before the initiation of antibiotics.

In addition to diagnosing UTI, it is also important to evaluate the urinary tract for underlying structural or functional abnormalities that may predispose the infant to recurrent UTIs. Abdominal ultrasound is a safe and noninvasive method of evaluating structural abnormalities of the urinary tract and is the initial imaging test of choice. Intravenous pyelography can be useful in assessing the function of the kidneys. Radionuclide scans such as dimercaptosuccinic acid scans can also be used to evaluate function and structural abnormalities, specifically renal scars following UTI. Vesicoureterography to evaluate the presence or absence of vesicoureteric reflux should be performed after completion of treatment of the UTI, because transient vesicoureteral reflux commonly occurs with the acute infection.

Beetz R. Evaluation and management of urinary tract infections in the neonate. Curr Opin Pediatr 2012;24(2):205–11.

OMPHALITIS

134. What are the presenting signs of omphalitis in neonates?
- Foul-smelling discharge from the umbilicus
- Periumbilical erythematous streaking, induration, and tenderness to palpation
- Purulent or serosanguinous discharge
- May be accompanied by signs of a systemic infection if infection progresses

135. What is the incidence of omphalitis?
In hospitalized infants the incidence is approximately 2%. In infants delivered at home the incidence may be as high as 21%.

136. What are the predisposing factors for omphalitis?
- Prematurity
- Complicated delivery
- Improper care of the umbilical cord
- Poor hygienic practices during the neonatal period

Mullany LC, Saha SK, Shah R, et al. Impact of 4.0% chlorhexidine cord cleansing on the bacteriological profile of the newborn umbilical stump in rural Sylhet District, Bangladesh: a community-based, cluster-randomized trial. Pediatr Infect Dis J 2012;31(5):444–450.

137. Which bacteria cause omphalitis?
- *S. aureus*
- *Streptococcus pyogenes* (group A streptococcal infections may result in a wet, malodorous stump with only mild evidence of inflammation)
- Gram-negative organisms (i.e., *E. coli, Klebsiella* species)

Shah S. Pediatric practice infectious diseases. 1st ed. Pennsylvania: McGraw-Hill Professional; 2009.

138. **What are the noninfectious causes of increased umbilical drainage?**

Serosanguinous drainage may be seen with a patent urachus or omphalomesenteric duct.

139. **What are the major complications of omphalitis?**

- Septic umbilical arteritis
- Suppurative thrombophlebitis of the umbilical or portal veins (resulting in portal vein thrombosis and portal hypertension)
- Liver abscess
- Endocarditis
- Abdominal wall necrotizing fasciitis
- Peritonitis
- Intestinal gangrene
- Pyourachus (infection of the urachal remnant)

140. **How should infants with omphalitis be treated?**

First-line treatment includes a penicillinase-resistant penicillin and an aminoglycoside antibiotic. If MRSA is suspected, vancomycin should be considered.

141. **What syndrome can be associated with chronic omphalitis or delayed separation of the umbilical cord?**

Leukocyte adhesion deficiency is a life-threatening, autosomal-recessive inherited deficiency of cell adhesion molecules associated with chronic omphalitis or delayed separation of the umbilical cord. The hallmark of leukocyte adhesion deficiency is the absence of granulocytes at the site of infection.

142. **You are informed that a newborn is suspected to have funisitis. Where should you look for that infection?**

Funisitis is a mild inflammation of the umbilical stump with minimal drainage and erythema in the surrounding tissue. It is a local noninvasive infection that may become invasive and lead to a severe abdominal wall inflammation associated with necrotizing fasciitis.

Remington JS, Klein JO, Wilson CB, et al. Infectious diseases of the fetus and newborn: expert consult—online and print. 7th ed. Philadelphia: Saunders; 2010.

LISTERIOSIS

143. **Is *L. monocytogenes* still a significant pathogen to consider when evaluating sepsis in neonates?**

Listeriosis causes an estimated 2500 serious illness and 500 deaths annually in the United States. The incidence is highest among newborns: 2 to 13 cases per 100,000 live births, representing 30% to 40% of the total cases in humans. Pregnant women along with elderly adults and those with immunodeficiencies are also at-risk groups. Pregnant women account for about 27% of cases, with the highest incidence in the third trimester. Fecal carriage in pregnant women may lead to vaginal colonization and can be responsible for late-onset infections in infants born of healthy mothers. The frequent presence of chorioamnionitis in the absence of ruptured membranes supports the hypothesis that *Listeria* infection can occur through a transplacental route.

144. **How do mothers acquire *L. monocytogenes*?**

Listeria species organisms are ubiquitous in nature. Although direct transmission to humans from infected animals has been reported, most human infections are acquired through ingestion of contaminated food. The relative resistance of *Listeria* organisms to high temperatures and their ability to multiply at low temperatures provide opportunities for heavy colonization of dairy products if pasteurization has been improperly carried out. Outbreaks are commonly associated with prepared meat products and seafood products. Although *L. monocytogenes* is probably ingested frequently, the incidence of clinical diseases in humans is relatively low, suggesting that the organism has a relatively low virulence. This is supported by the large inoculum required to cause infection in normal hosts. Nevertheless, listeriosis represents the leading cause of death from foodborne diseases in the United States.

Taillefer C, Boucher M, Laferrière C, et al. Perinatal listeriosis: Canada's 2008 outbreaks. J Obstet Gynaecol Can 2010;32(1):45–8.

Jackson KA, Iwamoto M, Swerdlow D. Pregnancy-associated listeriosis. Epidemiol Infect 2010;138(10):1503–9.

145. What are the clinical manifestations of listeriosis during pregnancy?

After ingestion of the microorganism, the incubation period for *L. monocytogenes* is less than 24 hours, but it can range from 6 hours up to 3 weeks. Invasion of the intestinal mucosal barrier leads to bacteremia, resulting in a flulike illness with fever, chills, myalgia, arthralgia, headache, and backache. Premature labor in pregnant women with listeriosis is common in approximately 70% of cases. The neonatal mortality rate, including stillbirth and abortion, is 40% to 50%. Often the placenta becomes a reservoir for bacterial proliferation, resulting in amnionitis with persistence of maternal symptoms until abortion or delivery occurs. Symptoms in the mother usually subside with or without antibiotic treatment soon after delivery. If the infection is recognized promptly, the mother may be treated effectively, preserving the pregnancy.

Jackson KA, Iwamoto M, Swerdlow D. Pregnancy-associated listeriosis. Epidemiol Infect 2010;138(10):1503–9.

Lamont RF, Sobel J, Mazaki-Tovi S, et al. Listeriosis in human pregnancy: a systematic review. J Perinat Med 2011;39(3):227–36.

146. How does listeriosis present in neonates?

Similar to GBS, neonatal listeriosis is divided into two clinical forms defined by age: early onset (≤1 week) and late onset (>1 week). Evidence of preceding maternal illness is often described in infants with early-onset disease, and most cases are clinically apparent at delivery with meconium-stained fluid, septicemia, and pneumonia. In severe infections a granulomatous rash—called granulomatosis infantiseptica—has been described with microabscesses throughout the body but particularly on the the liver and spleen. Blood cultures are positive in 75% of cases, and death might occur within a few hours in up to 25% of infected newborns, particularly if premature.

Late-onset neonatal listeriosis commonly presents as meningitis. Affected infants may not appear particularly ill and might elude diagnosis for several days. A striking predominance of boys has been noticed in most series. Other clinical forms of diseases at this age include colitis with associated diarrhea and sepsis without meningitis. Gram stain of the CSF does not always yield the correct diagnosis because variable decoloration results in organisms that appear as either gram-negative rods or gram-positive cocci. The mortality risk of late-onset disease is generally low if treatment is started promptly.

Remington JS, Klein JO, Wilson CB. Infectious diseases of the fetus and newborn: expert consult—online and print. 7th ed. Philadelphia: Saunders; 2010

Le Monnier A, Abachin E, Beretti J-L, et al. Diagnosis of Listeria monocytogenes meningoencephalitis by real-time PCR for the hly gene. J Clin Microbiol 2011;49(11):3917–23.

Jiao Y, Zhang W, Ma J, et al. Early onset of neonatal listeriosis. Pediatr Int 2011;53(6):1034–7.

147. What is the pathogenesis of *L. monocytogenes* infection, and why does insufficiency of cellular immunity in particular contribute to the development of disease?

L. monocytogenes is an intracellular, facultative anaerobic, non–spore-forming, motile gram-positive bacillus that multiplies intracellularly. Once phagocytized, invasive *L. monocytogenes* replicates rapidly within the cytosol, thanks to its major virulence factor, listeriolysin O. Using the cell's own cytoskeletal actin polymerization mechanism, *L. monocytogenes* pushes outward on the host cell's membrane, forming filopods, which are then injected into neighboring cells. Cell-to-cell transmission spreads rapidly without exposure to extracellular host defenses such as antibodies or neutrophils. T-lymphocytes therefore provide the only natural recognition and immunity toward *L. monocytogenes,* although macrophage killing (probably using nitric oxide) may also occur. Because cellular immunity is suppressed during pregnancy and is naturally deficient during early neonatal life, *L. monocytogenes* enjoys an advantage during these host-vulnerable periods. In hosts with adequate cellular responses, symptomatic infection is rare and self-limited.

Long SS, Pickering LK, Prober CG. Principles and practice of pediatric infectious diseases: expert consult—online and print. 4th ed. Philadelphia: Saunders; 2012.

148. How is listeriosis treated in a neonate?

L. monocytogenes remains sensitive to ampicillin. Adding an aminoglycoside, usually gentamicin, is recommended for severe infections because of synergism with ampicillin. Because of the organism's tendency to hide in tissue reservoirs, higher doses of ampicillin are usually recommended for extended durations (10 to 14 days for invasive infections and 14 to 21 days for meningitis). Longer courses might be necessary for patients who are severely ill or have endocarditis or rhombencephalitis (brainstem encephalitis).

Trimethoprim-sulfamethoxazole (TMP-SMX) can be considered for mothers who are sensitive to penicillin. Cephalosporins are not active against listeriosis. Iron therapy for anemia should be withheld during treatment of listeriosis because iron enhances the organism's growth *in vitro* and is therefore a virulence factor, contributing to the host's susceptibility to infection. Listeriosis is a notifiable disease in the United States.

Pickering LK, Baker CJ, Kimberlin DW, Long SS, editors. Red Book Report of the Committee on Infectious Diseases. 29th ed. American Academy of Pediatrics; 2012.

SYPHILIS

149. How has the incidence of congenital syphilis in United States changed?

The changing incidence of congenital syphilis over the years follows the trend of acquired syphilis in women. After a major public success in early 1990, with the lowest rates since reporting began in 1941 (10.5 cases/100,000 live births), the incidence of primary and secondary syphilis has increased since 2005, particularly in large urban areas and in the southern United States. Insufficient public health resources, use of illegal drugs (particularly crack cocaine), and coinfection with HIV are factors implicated in this increase. The World Health Organization (WHO) estimates that 1 million pregnancies are affected by syphilis worldwide.

Remington JS, Klein JO, Wilson CB, et al. Infectious diseases of the fetus and newborn: expert consult - online and print. 7th ed. Philadelphia: Saunders; 2010.

150. How does *T. pallidum* infect neonates?

Congenital syphilis starts with *T. pallidum* crossing the placenta from mother to fetus. Fetal infection can occur as early as at 9 to 10 weeks' gestation, but infection can occur any time after that, including at birth because of contact with maternal lesions. Transmission *in utero* causes the wide dissemination of the spirochetes in the fetus, analogous to secondary-acquired syphilis. Untreated congenital syphilis can progress through the same stages as postnatally acquired syphilis (except for the absence of a primary stage or chancre).The likelihood of vertical transmission is directly related to the maternal stage of syphilis: 60% to 100% during primary and secondary syphilis, 40% in early latent infection, and 8% with late latent infection.

151. Are all infected newborns symptomatic at birth?

Syphilis has commonly been described as the "great imitator" because of the variety of clinical manifestations; approximately two thirds of infected newborns are asymptomatic at birth, but later (even decades later) manifestations are not uncommon. Clinical manifestations appearing within the first

TABLE 13-11. CLINICAL MANIFESTATIONS OF CONGENITAL SYPHILIS

EARLY CONGENITAL SYPHILIS		LATE CONGENITAL SYPHILIS
Hepatosplenomegaly	Dentition	Hutchinson teeth (i.e., peg-shaped,
Snuffles, hemorrhagic rhinitis	Eyes	notched central incisors)
Condylomata lata	Ears	Interstitial keratitis (5 to 20 years of age)
Osteochondritis, periostitis	Nose and face	Eighth nerve deafness (10 to 14 years
Mucocutaneous lesions (bullous,	Skin	of age)
palmar, and plantar rash)	Central nervous system	Saddle nose, protuberant mandible
Jaundice	Bones and joints	Rhagades (perioral fissures)
Nonimmune hydrops fetalis		Mental retardation, convulsive disorders
Hemolytic anemia, coagulopathy,		Saber shins, Clutton joints (symmetric
thrombocytopenia		painless swelling of the knees),
Pneumonitis		olympian brow (frontal bossing)
Nephrotic syndrome		
Intrauterine growth retardation		

2 years of life are considered early congenital syphilis, and manifestations occurring after this time are considered late congenital syphilis (Table 13-11).

Remington JS, Klein JO, Wilson CB, et al. Infectious diseases of the fetus and newborn: expert consult - online and print. 7th ed. Philadelphia: Saunders; 2010.

152. What is pneumonia alba?

Pneumonia alba, a fibrosing pneumonitis, is characterized by yellow-white, heavy, grossly enlarged lungs. There is a marked increase in the amount of connective tissue in the interalveolar septa and interstitium histologically, with loss of alveolar spaces and obliterative fibrosis. The classic radiographic appearance is one of complete opacification of both lung fields. This may lead to a chronic pulmonary disease in 10% of cases.

153. What is the Hutchinson triad?

The findings of Hutchinson teeth, interstitial keratitis, and eighth nerve deafness constitute Hutchinson triad and are virtually pathognomonic for late congenital syphilis.

Long SS, Pickering LK, Prober CG. Principles and practice of pediatric infectious diseases: expert consult—online and print. 4th ed. Philadelphia: Saunders; 2012.

154. Which infants should be evaluated for congenital syphilis?

All women should be screened for syphilis during pregnancy with a nontreponemal test, and no neonate should leave the hospital without determination of the mother's status at least once during pregnancy and close to delivery in high-risk populations.

155. How useful are treponemal antibody tests in the diagnosis of congenital syphilis?

Nontreponemal tests for syphilis include the Venereal Diseases Research Laboratory (VDRL) test and the rapid plasma regain (RPR) test. These tests are inexpensive and rapid, so they are used mainly for screening. Quantitative results can assist in monitoring disease activity or response to treatment (preferably if performed in the same laboratory). They can be falsely negative in early primary syphilis and late congenital syphilis. Any reactive nontreponemal test needs to be confirmed with a specific treponemal test to exclude a false-positive reading, but treatment should not be delayed if the patient is symptomatic or at high risk for infection. A positive VDRL in CSF is highly specific for neurosyphilis but is insensitive. Treponemal tests include fluorescent treponemal antibody absorption (FTA-ABS) and *T. pallidum* particle agglutination (TP-PA). These tests will remain reactive for life even after successful treatment, and they correlate poorly with disease activity.

Pickering LK, Baker CJ, Kimberlin DW, Long SS, editors. Red Book Report of the Committee on Infectious Diseases. 29th ed. American Academy of Pediatrics; 2012.

156. What is the prozone phenomenon?
Occasionally, a nontreponemal test performed on serum samples containing high concentrations of antibodies against *T. pallidum* can be weakly positive or falsely negative. Diluting the serum results in a positive test.

157. Which infants should be treated for congenital syphilis?
Even if the evaluation is normal, all infants born to mothers who are untreated or who have been treated less than 4 weeks before delivery, *or* have received a nonpenicillin drug, *or* who have evidence of relapse or re-infection should be evaluated at delivery.

Infants should be treated if they have the following:
- Any evidence of active disease (abnormal complete blood count [CBC], physical examination findings, or x-ray)
- A reactive CSF VDRL
- An abnormal CSF finding, regardless of serology
- Quantitative nontreponemal antibody titers that are at least four times greater than maternal titers
Aqueous crystalline penicillin G intravenous for 10 days is the regimen of choice for congenital syphilis.

Pickering LK, Baker CJ, Kimberlin DW, Long SS, editors. Red Book Report of the Committee on Infectious Diseases. 29th ed. American Academy of Pediatrics; 2012.

158. Should neonates with a reactive serologic test for syphilis be followed in infancy?
All infants with reactive serologic tests for syphilis or born from mothers who were seroreactive at delivery should receive careful follow-up with repeated nontreponemal testing every 2 or 3 months until they become nonreactive or the titer has decreased at least fourfold. Nontreponemal tests should decrease by 3 months and should be nonreactive by 6 months if the infant was adequately treated or the elevated titers resulted from transplacentally acquired maternal antibodies. The serologic response might be slower for infants treated after the neonatal period.

HUMAN IMMUNODEFICIENCY VIRUS

159. Does the HIV prevalence among children vary worldwide?
Pediatric acquired immunodeficiency syndrome (AIDS) cases account for less than 1% of all reported cases of AIDS in the United States, and the CDC estimates that each year 215 to 370 infants acquire HIV in the United States, mainly as a consequence of missed prevention opportunities. The rate of vertical transmission has decreased to below 2% in the United States and Europe.

This scenario is drastically different in resource-limited countries where the prevention of mother-to-child transmission is a major public health challenge. Despite knowing the routes of transmission of the virus, approximately 500,000 children worldwide acquire the infection each year, primarily through mother-to-child transmission. Children still represent 14% of new HIV infections worldwide and almost one fifth of annual HIV-related deaths.

Fauci AS, Folkers GK. Toward an AIDS-free generation. JAMA 2012;308(4):343–4.

160. What is the risk of transmission of HIV infection to newborns?
The risk of infection for an infant born to an HIV-infected mother without an intervention to prevent transmission is estimated to range between 12% and 40%. Dramatic declines in the number of HIV-infected children, to less than 2%, have been observed after the introduction of universal antenatal HIV testing, combination antiretroviral treatment during pregnancy, elective cesarean section, and avoidance of breastfeeding.

161. **What factors are associated with an increased risk of perinatal transmission of HIV?**
   - Maternal AIDS diagnosis
   - CD4 count less than 200/mm^3
   - High maternal viral load
   - Breastfeeding
   - Preterm delivery
   - Chorioamnionitis
   - Prolonged rupture of membranes
   - Vaginal delivery versus cesarean section

162. **When during the perinatal period is HIV transmitted?**
   HIV infection may be transmitted *in utero,* intrapartum, or after birth through breastfeeding. In the absence of breastfeeding, it is believed that approximately 20% to 30% of perinatal infections occur *in utero,* with the remaining 70% to 80% occurring during the intrapartum period. If an infant escapes infection *in utero* and during delivery but is then breastfed, the risk for HIV transmission is approximately 15% when breastfeeding is continued for at least 6 months.

Nielsen-Saines K, Watts DH, Veloso VG, et al. Three postpartum antiretroviral regimens to prevent intrapartum HIV infection. N Engl J Med 2012;366(25):2368–79.

163. **Which pregnant women should be offered HIV testing?**
   Every woman worldwide should be tested at least once for HIV during pregnancy. Because risk factor assessments fail to detect more than 40% of HIV-infected pregnant women, the AAP and ACOG both recommend routine HIV counseling to all pregnant women, with universal voluntary HIV testing.

164. **Why is the enzyme-linked immunosorbent assay (ELISA) HIV antibody screening test not useful for the diagnosis of HIV-exposed neonates?**
   The ELISA measures IgG anti-HIV antibodies, which readily cross the placenta in the third trimester; therefore antibody assays are not informative for diagnosis of infection in children younger than 18 months of age unless assay results are negative.

165. **What is the best diagnostic test for defining HIV infections in infants, and when should it be ordered?**
   The preferred test for diagnosis of HIV infection in infants is the HIV DNA PCR assay, which can detect 1 to 10 copies of proviral DNA in peripheral mononuclear cells. Plasma HIV RNA assays also have been used to diagnose HIV infection, but false-positive results might occur in infants receiving antiretroviral prophylaxis.

   All HIV-exposed infants should have an HIV PCR-DNA assay performed at 14 to 21 days of age; if results are negative, it should be repeated at 1 to 2 months of age and again at 4 to 6 months of age. An infant is considered infected if two separate samples test positive for DNA or RNA PCR.

Pickering LK, Baker CJ, Kimberlin DW, Long SS, editors. Red Book Report of the Committee on Infectious Diseases. 29th ed. American Academy of Pediatrics; 2012.

✓ KEY POINTS: PREVENTION AND TESTING OF HIV

1. Every woman worldwide should be tested at least once for HIV during pregnancy.

2. All HIV-exposed infants should have an HIV PCR-DNA assay performed at 14 to 21 days of age. If results are negative, the test should be repeated at 1 to 2 months of age and again at 4 to 6 months of age.

3. Updates on recommendations for vertical prophylaxis are available at http://www.aidsinfo.nih.gov.

166. **What tests are used to monitor immune dysfunction in HIV-infected neonates?**
The CD4+ T-lymphocyte percentage and the absolute CD4+ T-lymphocyte count are used to monitor immunogenic function in HIV-infected individuals. Remember that normal CD4+ counts for infants and children are much higher than those found in adults (a normal infant CD4 count is 2500 to 3500/mL^3, and normal adult values are 700 to 1000/mL^3). The risk of opportunistic infections correlates with the CD4+ T-lymphocyte count.

167. **What treatments are recommended for pregnant HIV-infected women?**
Close prenatal monitoring, attention to nutritional status, antiretroviral therapy, and elective cesarean sections are all recommended for infected pregnant women. Current guidelines recommend cesarean delivery for HIV-infected women if the viral load is above 1000 copies/mL or unknown at the time of delivery.

168. **What factors are used to decide when to initiate antiretroviral treatment in children?**
Starting antiretroviral treatment in an infant depends on virologic, clinical, and immunologic parameters. Recommendations change with time, and consultation with a pediatric HIV expert is advised. Current guidelines are available online at http://www.aidsinfo.nih.gov.

169. **What are the major HIV-related complications seen in HIV-infected infants?**
Pneumocystis jiroveci pneumonia (PCP) is the most common serious HIV-related infection in infancy. The peak age of onset is 3 to 9 months, and it carries a 50% mortality rate. Fortunately, PCP can be prevented by TMP-SMX prophylaxis. All exposed infants should start PCP prophylaxis at 6 weeks of age and continue until HIV infection is definitively excluded. Growth failure (i.e., failure to thrive) and a progressive encephalopathy are other common serious complications of HIV infection in the first year of life.

CYTOMEGALOVIRUS (CMV)

170. **What is the most common congenital viral infection in the United States?**
Congenital CMV infection occurs in 1% to 2% of all live births. It is transmitted transplacentally and is 40% more common after primary infections in the mother during the first half of the pregnancy than in those who have serologic evidence of previous CMV infection. Approximately 90% of infants with congenital CMV infection are asymptomatic at birth. The major concern in these babies is the 5% to 10% risk of developing hearing loss during the preschool years.

Nassetta L, Kimberlin D, Whitley R. Treatment of congenital cytomegalovirus infection: implications for future therapeutic strategies. J Antimicrob Chemother 2009;63(5):862–7.

171. **How do infants acquire CMV infection?**
Vertical transmission can occur *in utero* by transplacental passage of the virus, at birth by passage through an infected birth canal, or postnatally by infected breast milk.

172. **What are the most common manifestations of congenital CMV infection in neonates?**
Approximately 10% of infected babies have symptoms at birth. Manifestations include the following:
- Petechiae, purpura
- Intrauterine growth restriction
- Hepatosplenomegaly
- Jaundice
- Microcephaly, intracranial calcifications
- Retinitis

173. **What are the most reliable methods for diagnosing congenital CMV infection?**
The diagnosis of congenital CMV is challenging because of the ubiquity of the virus. Isolation of CMV from urine during the first 2 to 4 weeks of life is the most reliable method for diagnosing congenital infection. Detection of strongly positive IgM antibodies to CMV in serum obtained within the first few days after birth is highly suggestive of congenital infection, but different assays vary in accuracy for identification of primary infection.

Bradford RD, Cloud G, Lakeman AD, et al. Detection of cytomegalovirus (CMV) DNA by polymerase chain reaction is associated with hearing loss in newborns with symptomatic congenital CMV infection involving the central nervous system. J Infect Dis 2005;191(2):227–33.

174. **What methods are available to prevent the transmission of CMV to neonates through blood products?**
Transmission of CMV to neonates by blood transfusion can be prevented by using blood that is obtained from seronegative donors, frozen in glycerol, or depleted of WBCs.

175. **What is the frequency of hearing loss in infants with congenital CMV infection?**
Sensorineural hearing loss (SNHL) can be unilateral or bilateral. It varies in severity and can be progressive up to 7 years of age. Half of babies with SNHL and CMV infection identified at birth will have no other finding of CMV. SNHL is delayed in onset in approximately 20% of infants and progressive in 50% of cases. By 5 years of age, SNHL can be observed in about one third of those babies with abnormal physical findings at birth and about 10% of those with no manifestations at birth.

176. **What is the relationship between neonatal clinical signs and neurologic outcome in congenital CMV infection?**
Long-term neurologic disability (excluding SNHL) has been reported in approximately 50% of those with manifestations and less than 5% of those without manifestations at birth.

Oliver SE, Cloud GA, Sanchez PJ, et al. Neurodevelopmental outcomes following ganciclovir therapy in symptomatic congenital cytomegalovirus infections involving the central nervous system. J Clin Virol 2009;46(Suppl 4):S22–6.

177. **Is there a treatment available that improves neurologic outcome?**
Data in infants with symptomatic congenital CMV involving the CNS suggest that the prognosis at 1 to 2 years of age may be improved if infected infants are treated with parenteral ganciclovir for 6 weeks. Valganciclovir given orally provides the same systemic levels of intravenous ganciclovir.

Kimberlin DW, Lin C-Y, Sanchez PJ, et al. Effect of ganciclovir therapy on hearing in symptomatic congenital cytomegalovirus disease involving the central nervous system: a randomized, controlled trial. J Pediatr 2003;143(1):16–25.
Kimberlin DW, Acosta EP, Sanchez PJ, et al. Pharmacokinetic and pharmacodynamic assessment of oral valganciclovir in the treatment of symptomatic congenital cytomegalovirus disease. J Infect Dis 2008;197(6):836–45.

178. **What are the side effects of ganciclovir treatment?**
Patients treated with ganciclovir need to have their absolute neutrophil count monitored closely because as many as 60% of patients will develop significant neutropenia. If neutropenia is evident, the dose should be reduced by 50%; if neutropenia persists, the therapy should be discontinued.

Kimberlin DW, Lin C-Y, Sanchez PJ, et al. Effect of ganciclovir therapy on hearing in symptomatic congenital cytomegalovirus disease involving the central nervous system: a randomized, controlled trial. J Pediatr 2003;143(1):16–25.

HERPES SIMPLEX VIRUS

179. **What should be done when a baby develops skin vesicles in the neonatal period?**
Newborns with skin vesicles should be rapidly evaluated for the possibility of neonatal HSV infection. HSV PCR is the diagnostic method of choice, especially with CNS involvement (a reported sensitivity

of 75% to 100% with CSF). HSV PCR can also be used to test serum; however, the test is not as reliable when serum is used. HSV grows readily in cultures. Babies in whom the diagnosis is established or who are strongly suspected of having neonatal HSV should be further evaluated for the possibility of disseminated infection and involvement of the CNS. Usually this means obtaining liver function tests, an ophthalmologic examination, lumbar puncture, and magnetic resonance imaging (MRI) or computed tomography (CT) scan.

Kimberlin DW. Herpes simplex virus infections in neonates and early childhood. Semin Pediatr Infect Dis 2005;16(4):271–81.
  Kimberlin DW. Herpes simplex virus infections of the newborn. Semin Perinatol 2007;31(1):19–25.

180. How should women with a history of genital herpes be screened during pregnancy?

Until fairly recently, it was thought that women with frequent reactivation episodes of genital HSV were at greatest risk to deliver an infected infant. Prospective studies, however, indicate that the infant at greatest risk of developing neonatal HSV is born to a woman with a primary asymptomatic genital HSV infection. The risk of infection is only about 2% in infants born to mothers with recurrent HSV but 25% to 60% in infants born to women with a primary HSV at term. All women need to be examined for the presence of active lesions; however, even this will miss asymptomatic infections. The best screening test for prevention of severe neonatal HSV is a high index of suspicion when an infant develops vesicular skin lesions because more than three quarters of vertically infected infants are born from mothers with no history or clinical findings suggestive of HSV. ACOG recommends that women with active recurrent genital herpes be offered suppressive viral therapy at or beyond 36 weeks' gestation to delivery. Universal screening is not recommended.

Pickering LK, Baker CJ, Kimberlin DW, Long SS, editors. Red Book Report of the Committee on Infectious Diseases. 29th ed. American Academy of Pediatrics; 2012.

181. How is neonatal HSV classified? What is the importance of the classification with regard to prognosis?

Clinically, HSV infection in newborns can manifest in the following ways: (1) disease localized to the skin, eye, or mouth in 45% of cases; (2) disseminated infection involving multiple organs, especially the liver and lungs in 25% of cases; and (3) CNS involvement with or without skin involvement in 30% of cases.

Even with appropriate antiviral therapy, the prognosis for infants with disseminated HSV and CNS disease is much poorer than that for infants who have infection confined to the skin, eye, and mouth. It is believed that administering early therapy with acyclovir to infants with disease localized to the skin, eye, or mouth can decrease the incidence of disseminated and CNS disease. Therefore it is recommended that all infants with skin lesions caused by HSV, even if they are otherwise well, should be treated with acyclovir.

182. When do the manifestations of HSV occur in the neonate?

Initial signs can occur at any time between birth and 6 weeks of age, although most infected infants exhibit symptoms within the first month of life. Infants with disseminated disease and involvement of the skin, eye, and mouth present earlier, usually between the first and second week of life; infants with CNS involvement usually present later, between the second and third week of life.

183. What is the pathogenesis of HSV infections that present in the newborn?

Most often, the virus multiplies on the mucosa of the maternal genital tract, and the baby is infected during vaginal delivery. In only about 5% of infections the virus crosses the placenta to cause congenital, rather than neonatal, infection. If the diagnosis of maternal primary HSV is known at delivery and the membranes are not ruptured, infection of the newborn infant can be prevented by performing

✓ KEY POINTS: CLINICAL PRESENTATION OF HSV

1. Disseminated diseases and skin-eye-mouth (SEM) diseases typically present in neonates between the first and second weeks of life.

2. Infants with CNS diseases usually have a later age of onset (i.e., between the second and third weeks of life).

3. Approximately 25% of cases of neonatal HSV manifest as disseminated diseases, 30% as CNS diseases, and 45% as SEM diseases.

4. Skin lesions might not be present at the time of presentation of CNS or disseminated diseases.

5. Acyclovir should be started promptly if any type of HSV infection is suspected.

a cesarean section. The risk that the infant will be infected is increased if the skin is broken for any reason (e.g., from a scalp monitor). Infants also can be infected with HSV type 1 if a mother has primary active HSV-1 infection, usually in the throat and mouth, at delivery. Furthermore, infants can become infected by nursing on an infected breast. Transmission from care providers, fathers, and grandparents has also been demonstrated.

Remington JS, Klein JO, Wilson CB, et al. Infectious diseases of the fetus and newborn: expert consult—online and print. 7th ed. Philadelphia: Saunders; 2010.

184. What is the treatment for neonatal HSV?

The treatment is administration of intravenous acyclovir to all infants in whom the diagnosis of neonatal HSV is either established or suspected pending diagnostic studies. Acyclovir is an antiviral drug that interferes with the replication of HSV DNA by acting as a chain terminator and interfering with the action of DNA polymerase. Because its action occurs mainly in infected cells, it is very well tolerated. Early therapy with acyclovir has decreased mortality and morbidity resulting from serious HSV infections by 30% to 50%. Acyclovir is usually administered at a dosage of 60 mg/kg/day intravenously for 14 to 21 days, depending on the condition of the infant.

Kimberlin DW, Whitley RJ, Wan W, et al. Oral acyclovir suppression and neurodevelopment after neonatal herpes. N Engl J Med 2011;365(14):1284–92.

185. How should infants with neonatal HSV be followed up after treatment?

Approximately 50% of infants who survive neonatal HSV experience cutaneous recurrences. Use of oral acyclovir suppressive therapy for 6 months after treatment of acute neonatal HSV diseases has been shown to improve neurodevelopmental outcomes in infants with HSV CNS involvement and to prevent skin recurrences in all infants infected with HSV regardless of their neonatal manifestations. Neutrophil counts should be monitored at 2 and 4 weeks after initiation of therapy and then monthly during the acyclovir treatment. The rate of severe neutropenia (<500 cells/mL) ranges from 20% to 25% while on acyclovir suppressive therapy; in every instance, the neutropenia was reversible and no infants had associated complications.

Pickering LK, Baker CJ, Kimberlin DW, Long SS, editors. Red Book Report of the Committee on Infectious Diseases. 29th ed. American Academy of Pediatrics; 2012.

186. How should infants born to women with active recurrent genital HSV infection be managed?

Cesarean section is recommended for mothers who have active genital lesions and a suspected primary infection. Infants born to mothers with active genital HSV disease should be isolated from other infants and evaluated with "surface cultures" at 24 to 48 hours of life. Those infants born to mothers with primary disease might benefit from empiric parenteral acyclovir treatment after obtaining "surface cultures." However, virtually no experts recommend treatment for infants born from mothers with active recurrent disease. If "surfaces cultures" are positive, the infant should be evaluated for HSV disease and should be treated to prevent progression to HSV disease. The duration of treatment is controversial.

Pinninti SG, Angara R, Feja KN, et al. Neonatal herpes disease following maternal antenatal antiviral suppressive therapy: a multicenter case series. J Pediatr 2012;161(1):134–8.

187. Are antibody titers useful for diagnosis of HSV? What are their limitations?

Antibody titers are of little use in the diagnosis of HSV because it takes at least several days after infection for antibodies to rise. Therefore it is preferable to demonstrate the presence of virus, viral antigens, or DNA in tissues for diagnosis. Antibody titers may be useful to differentiate between maternal first infections versus recurrence because many primary infections are asymptomatic.

Kimberlin DW. Diagnosis of herpes simplex virus in the era of polymerase chain reaction. Pediatr Infect Dis J 2006;25(9):841–2.

VARICELLA ZOSTER VIRUS

188. What is congenital varicella syndrome?

Congenital varicella syndrome is usually associated with maternal varicella during the first or early second trimester of pregnancy. Transmission of VZV from mother to infant occurs in 25% to 50% of cases of infected mothers. However, congenital varicella syndrome occurs in fewer than 2% of cases of maternal chickenpox before week 20 of gestation. Common manifestations of the syndrome include skin scarring (either generalized or localized in a dermatomal distribution), limb deformities (e.g., hypoplasia, missing digits), eye abnormalities (e.g., chorioretinitis, cataract, nystagmus, hypoplasia), low birth weight, and mental retardation.

Reactivation of VZV acquired *in utero* is common. Thus zoster develops in approximately 15% of infants with the congenital syndrome, usually in the first few years of life.

Mandelbrot L. Fetal varicella—diagnosis, management, and outcome. Prenat Diagn 2012;32(6):511–8.

189. What is the appropriate management of an infant born to a woman with varicella at term delivery?

Infants whose mothers have the onset of the rash of varicella within 5 days before delivery to 2 days postpartum are at high risk of developing varicella because of insufficient transfer of maternal antibodies and the immature cellular immunity of the neonate. In as many as 30% of infants who are untreated, the varicella may be disseminated and even fatal. This form of varicella resembles that seen in other immunocompromised patients, such as children with leukemia receiving chemotherapy.

It is possible to prevent this severe form of infant varicella by administering VZIG to the baby as soon as possible after birth. Rarely, VZIG may be ineffective in infants, so babies given this prophylaxis warrant close follow-up. Many will develop a mild form of clinical varicella with fewer than 100 skin vesicles despite VZIG. Indications for adding antiviral therapy (acyclovir) are extensive skin lesions and development of pneumonia, which suggests severe varicella. Hospitalized preterm infants exposed to VZV should receive VZIG if they are older than 28 weeks' gestation and have mothers who lack immunity against VZV or if they are younger than 28 weeks' gestation regardless of maternal immunity status.

Pickering LK, Baker CJ, Kimberlin DW, Long SS, editors. Red Book Report of the Committee on Infectious Diseases. 29th ed. American Academy of Pediatrics; 2012.

190. Are all newborns candidates for VZIG?

Infants whose mothers develop varicella more than 48 hours postpartum are at significantly less risk from varicella and do not require VZIG, although some physicians may elect to administer it in infants exposed to VZV during the first 2 weeks of life whose mothers lack immunity. In this case, infection of the infant would not result from exposure to VZV *in utero* but rather from postpartum exposure.

Infants whose mothers had the onset of varicella more than 5 days before delivery do not need to receive VZIG because they will have developed sufficient transplacental VZV antibodies by that time.

191. What isolation measures are indicated in infants with a perinatal VZV exposure?

With regard to isolation of infants perinatally exposed to VZV, there are two points to consider:
1. The incubation period can be as short as 10 days and is counted from the time of onset of maternal rash.
2. Infants are contagious only around the time when rash is expected to occur.

The Red Book recommends airborne and contact precautions for neonates born to women with varicella, and if the neonate is still hospitalized, the isolation should be continued until 21 or 28 days of age after exposure for those who received VZIG or intravenous Ig.

Remington JS, Klein JO, Wilson CB, et al. Infectious diseases of the fetus and newborn: expert consult—online and print. 7th ed. Philadelphia: Saunders; 2010.

Kellie SM, Makvandi M, Muller ML. Management and outcome of a varicella exposure in a neonatal intensive care unit: lessons for the vaccine era. Am J Infect Control 2011;39(10):844–8.

192. What is the appropriate management of an infant born to a woman with zoster at term?

Women with zoster have high antibody titers to VZV, and their infants are well protected from the virus by transplacental antibodies. Therefore no special management is required. VZIG is not indicated for neonates whose mothers have zoster.

193. When is it appropriate to administer acyclovir to a pregnant woman with chickenpox?

Varicella in adults tends to be more severe than in children. Although the data are not conclusive, most experts believe that varicella in pregnant women is likely to be more severe than in non-pregnant women, especially in the third trimester of pregnancy. Therefore pregnant women with varicella should be closely observed, particularly for development of primary pneumonia. Pneumonia usually presents with fever, cough, dyspnea, and bilateral fluffy interstitial infiltrates on chest x-ray. Pregnant women with varicella pneumonia or even suspected varicella pneumonia should be treated with intravenous acyclovir for 7 days. Maternal acyclovir therapy has not been associated with fetal malformations, so most physicians will treat women who developed varicella or zoster within 1 day of the onset of varicella and 3 days of the onset of zoster.

MacMahon E. Investigating the pregnant woman exposed to a child with a rash. BMJ 2012;344:e1790.

194. When can a mother be immunized?

Varicella vaccine should not be administered to pregnant women because it contains a live virus. However, no cases of congenital varicella syndrome have been reported in women who inadvertently received the vaccine. Pregnancy is not a contraindication to immunizing children in the household. If a woman lacks VZV immunity after delivery, the varicella vaccine should be administered; there is no evidence of transmission of vaccine strain through breast milk.

Pickering LK, Baker CJ, Kimberlin DW, Long SS, editors. Red Book Report of the Committee on Infectious Diseases. 29th ed. American Academy of Pediatrics; 2012.

TOXOPLASMOSIS

195. How is the infection acquired in the mother?

Toxoplasma gondii is a protozoan and obligate intracellular parasite that exists in three developmental stages: tachyzoite (in acute infections), tissue cyst containing bradyzoites in chronic latent infection, and oocyst containing sporozoites in the intestines of cats. Once infected with the tachyzoite, the organism may encyst, commonly in the skeletal muscles. Infection occurs in multiple animal species, but the cat appears to be the definitive host, and the parasite replicates sexually in the feline small intestine. Cats excrete millions of oocysts in their stool after primary infection. Oocysts must mature or sporulate in the soil (which takes at least 24 hours) before they are infectious. Sporulated oocysts can survive for a long time.

Therefore *Toxoplasma* infection is acquired through the ingestion of undercooked or raw meat (containing tissue cysts) or water or other foods contaminated by oocysts that have been excreted in the feces of infected domestic animals. It is possible to become infected through exposure to soil contaminated with cat feces.

Kaye A. Toxoplasmosis: diagnosis, treatment, and prevention in congenitally exposed infants. J Pediatr Health Care 2011;25(6):355–64.

Montoya JG, Liesenfeld O. Toxoplasmosis. Lancet 2004;363(9425):1965–76.

196. How common is congenital toxoplasmosis?

The incidence of congenital toxoplasmosis in the United States is estimated to be between 1 in 1000 and 1 in 10,000 live births. Congenital infection is associated with maternal primary infection in pregnancy. Transmission rates to the fetus depend on the stage of the pregnancy and treatment during pregnancy, but approximately one third of infected women will have an infected fetus. Transmission during the first trimester tends to produce a more severe disease. Maternal treatment with spiramycin may decrease the severity of sequelae in the fetus once congenital toxoplasmosis has occurred.

Olariu TR, Remington JS, McLeod R, et al. Severe congenital toxoplasmosis in the United States: clinical and serologic findings in untreated infants. Pediatr Infect Dis J 2011;30(12):1056–61.

197. What are the clinical manifestations of congenital toxoplasmosis?

Most infected newborns are asymptomatic at birth (70% to 90%), although a large proportion of them will have visual or hearing impairment, learning difficulties, seizure disorders, or mental retardation later in life. The classic triad of chorioretinitis, hydrocephalus resulting from aqueduct stenosis, and intracranial calcifications is very suggestive of congenital toxoplasmosis. Other features include maculopapular rash, petechial purpura, lymphadenopathies, hepatosplenomegaly, CSF pleocytosis, thrombocytopenia, eosinophilia, and metaphyseal bone lucencies.

198. What is the treatment of congenital toxoplasmosis for neonates?

When there is clear evidence of congenital infection in the newborn, pyrimethamine combined with sulfadiazine and supplemented with folinic acid is recommended as initial therapy. The treatment is continued for approximately 12 to 14 months (consult an expert on infectious diseases for confirmation regarding a specific case). For mild congenital toxoplasmosis many experts will alternate the previous combination with spiramycin during months 7 through 12 of treatment, but severe cases should receive combined pyrimethamine-sulfadiazine for the entire 12 months.

The dosage should be adjusted weekly. In addition, a CBC with differential should be performed by finger stick twice weekly to measure the absolute neutrophil count. Remember that pyrimethamine is a folic acid antagonist and therefore may cause thrombocytopenia, granulocytopenia, and anemia resulting from bone marrow suppression. The use of folinic acid can counteract this side effect.

SYROCOT (Systematic Review on Congenital Toxoplasmosis) study group, Thiébaut R, Leproust S, et al. Effectiveness of prenatal treatment for congenital toxoplasmosis: a meta-analysis of individual patients' data. Lancet 2007;369(9556):115–22.

Pickering LK, Baker CJ, Kimberlin DW, Long SS, editors. Red Book Report of the Committee on Infectious Diseases. 29th ed. American Academy of Pediatrics; 2012.

199. If maternal infection is suspected but full evaluation for toxoplasmosis in the newborn is negative except for *T. gondii*–specific IgG antibodies, what should be done?

In this case, transfer of maternal antibodies may be suspected as the reason for the presence of IgG antibodies. A continuous decrease in transplacental IgG antibody should be observed, with the antibody becoming undetectable by 6 to 12 months of age. The diagnosis of congenital toxoplasmosis is complex, and consultation with an infectious disease specialist is recommended.

UREAPLASMA UREALITYCUM

200. What is the carriage rate of *Ureaplasma urealyticum* in the female lower genital tract?
Ureaplasma can be isolated from the genital tract of 40% to 80% of sexually active asymptomatic women. Colonization has been linked to younger age, lower socioeconomic status, multiple sexual partners, oral contraceptive use, recent antibiotic treatment, and African-American ethnicity.

Remington JS, Klein JO, Wilson CB, et al. Infectious diseases of the fetus and newborn: expert consult—online and print. 7th ed. Philadelphia: Saunders; 2010.

201. What is the rate of vertical transmission for *U. urealyticum*, and what factors influence that rate?
The vertical transmission rate ranges from 25% to 60%. Transmission occurs *in utero* by ascending infection or during delivery through an infected birth canal. Preterm and VLBW infants are more likely to acquire *U. urealyticum* in the lower respiratory tract. The mode of delivery does not influence the rate of transmission, but it increases in the presence of chorioamnionitis or prolonged rupture of membranes. Neonatal colonization can last for several months, so a positive culture does not confirm causality in infections.

Fonseca LT, Silveira RC, Procianoy RS. Ureaplasma bacteremia in very low birth weight infants in Brazil. Pediatr Infect Dis J 2011;30(12):1052–5.

202. What are the clinical manifestations of *U. urealyticum* infection?
- Isolation of the organism in the amniotic fluid has been associated with histologic evidence of chorioamnionitis, even among asymptomatic women.
- Postpartum fever, septic abortion, fetal loss, and preterm birth have been associated with *Ureaplasma* infection.
- Several case reports suggest that *U. urealyticum* causes pneumonia in the newborn, though its role in chronic lung disease in prematurity remains controversial.
- *U. urealyticum* has been isolated from CSF of newborns with meningitis, intraventricular hemorrhage, and hydrocephalus. Although several case reports describe a clinical response to treatment, its role remains unclear.

Kafetzis DA, Skevaki CL, Skouteri V, et al. Maternal genital colonization with Ureaplasma urealyticum promotes preterm delivery: association of the respiratory colonization of premature infants with chronic lung disease and increased mortality. Clinical Infectious Diseases 2004;39(8):1113–22.

Kasper DC, Mechtler TP, Böhm J, et al. In utero exposure to Ureaplasma spp. is associated with increased rate of bronchopulmonary dysplasia and intraventricular hemorrhage in preterm infants. J Perinatol Med 2011;39(3):331–6.

203. How is U. *urealyticum* diagnosed?
Although usually limited to research settings, PCR techniques are available and have greater sensitivity than culture. The organism is fastidious, so specimens should be transported to the laboratory in special transport media and refrigerated if transport is not immediately possible. Serologic tests are not useful.

204. Does treatment of *U. urealyticum* prevent chronic lung disease?
Causation has not been fully established for chronic lung disease and *Ureaplasma*. Furthermore, organisms are often present in healthy infants and can spontaneously disappear without treatment. Small randomized, controlled trials have not shown any benefit of treatment of *U. urealyticum* to prevent chronic lung disease.

INFECTIOUS HEPATITIS

205. What are the common causes of infectious hepatitis in the neonate?

Several infectious agents can cause hepatitis in neonates and infants, including the TORCH pathogens: *T. gondii*, **O**ther infectious etiologies (i.e., syphilis; hepatitis B, C, and D; and, rarely, hepatitis A virus), **R**ubella, **C**MV, and **H**erpes simplex. Additional etiologies in this age group include adenovirus, coxsackievirus, enterovirus, Epstein–Barr virus, HIV, and VZV.

Long SS, Pickering LK, Prober CG. Principles and practice of pediatric infectious diseases: expert consult—online and print. 4th ed. Philadelphia: Saunders; 2012.

206. How is hepatitis B virus (HBV) transmitted?

HBV is transmitted by infected blood or body fluids. Perinatal transmission occurs from exposure to blood during labor and delivery. Only a small proportion of infections occur *in utero*. With no postexposure prophylaxis the risk that an infant will acquire HBV from an infected mother is 70% to 90% if the mother is positive for hepatitis B e antigen (HBeAg) and hepatitis B surface antigen (HBsAg). The risk is lower (5% to 20%) for infants born from mothers who are HBsAg positive but HBeAg negative.

207. What are the best ways to prevent transmission of HBV from an infected mother to a newborn?

- Perform universal screening of pregnant women for HBV.
- Provide active immunization with HBV vaccine and passive immunization with hepatitis B immunoglobulin within 12 hours of birth, including those infants weighing less than 2000 g. Breastfeeding is not associated with increased risk.
- Perform routine immunization of all children.

Tran TT. Hepatitis B: treatment to prevent perinatal transmission. Clin Obstet Gynecol 2012;55(2):541–9.

208. What are the complications of HBV?

Age at infection is the main determinant of risk for progression to chronic disease. As many as 90% of infected newborns or infants younger than 1 year of age will develop chronic infection; 25% to 50% will develop chronic infection if the infection occurs between 1 and 5 years of age; and 5% to 10% will develop chronic infection when infection happens in older children or adults. In the absence of treatment, up to 25% of infants and children who have chronic hepatitis B will die as a result of hepatocellular carcinoma or cirrhosis.

Pickering LK, Baker CJ, Kimberlin DW, Long SS, editors. Red Book Report of the Committee on Infectious Diseases. 29th ed. American Academy of Pediatrics; 2012.

209. How is hepatitis C virus (HCV) transmitted?

Hepatitis C is transmitted mainly by parenteral exposure to blood and blood products from a HCV-infected person. Approximately 5% of infected women transmit HCV to their neonates; however, transmission occurs only if the mother is HCV RNA positive at the time of delivery. Maternal coinfection with HIV has been associated with increased risk for perinatal transmission of HCV. Breastfeeding has not been shown to be a risk factor for transmission.

210. What are the clinical manifestation of HCV in the neonate?

Signs and symptoms of HCV are similar to those of hepatitis A virus and HBV, although acute disease tends to be milder, with fewer occurrences of jaundice or elevated liver transaminases. However, 80% of infected children with HCV develop persistent infection, as many as 70% develop chronic hepatitis, and 20% develop cirrhosis that may progress to hepatocellular carcinoma.

211. How is HCV infection diagnosed in a neonate after *in utero* exposure?

Maternal HCV IgG antibody can persist in a neonate for up to 18 months. Therefore diagnosis in a neonate can be made only by using reverse transcriptase PCR assays for HCV RNA, which can be detected within

1 to 2 weeks of exposure. However, because false-negative and false-positive results can occur with PCR tests, a single result is not conclusive. It is therefore recommended that infants born to infected mothers be tested at or after the first well-baby visit at 1 or 2 months of age and then undergo repeat testing. Children with persistence of HCV RNA beyond 6 months' duration are assumed to have chronic infection.

Pickering LK, Baker CJ, Kimberlin DW, Long SS, editors. Red Book Report of the Committee on Infectious Diseases. 29th ed. American Academy of Pediatrics; 2012.

PARVOVIRUS

212. What percentage of women of child-bearing age are immune to parvovirus B19?
Parvovirus B19 is highly contagious, and almost 60% of adults are seropositive. Transmission occurs from person to person by droplets from oral secretions. Women who are not immune have a fivefold increased risk for parvovirus B19 if they have occupational daily contact with school-age children. In epidemic periods 1% to 4% of susceptible women become infected during pregnancy.

213. If parvovirus B19 infection occurs during pregnancy, what is the risk for an adverse fetal outcome (i.e., nonimmune hydrops fetalis or fetal demise)?
The risk of fetal death is between 2% and 6% when infection occurs during pregnancy. The greatest risk appears to occur during the first half of pregnancy.

Dijkmans AC, de Jong EP, Dijkmans BAC, et al. Parvovirus B19 in pregnancy: prenatal diagnosis and management of fetal complications. Curr Opin Obstet Gynecol 2012;24(2):95–101.

214. You receive a call from a worried mother of a 2-year-old patient. The family puppy was just diagnosed with parvovirus hemorrhagic colitis. The mother is concerned about possible transmission to her toddler or herself (she is 3 months pregnant). What advice do you give?
She need not worry. Canine parvovirus is not a human pathogen.

215. Parvovirus B19 is the cause of erythema infectiosum (EI). How often do children or adults infected with parvovirus B19 develop classic EI?
Classic EI with "slapped cheeks" appearance followed by a characteristic lacy or reticular rash on the trunk and limbs is fairly easy to diagnose clinically. Unfortunately, most adults infected with parvovirus B19 do not develop classic signs. In adults, especially women, joint symptoms occur in 60% to 80% of cases; knees are frequently involved in children, whereas fingers are commonly involved in women. The joint symptoms of parvovirus B19 infection usually manifest as the sudden onset of a symmetric peripheral polyarthropathy and might persist long enough to satisfy clinical diagnosis criteria for rheumatoid arthritis.

216. Why does parvovirus B19 infection cause aplastic anemia in patients with hemolytic anemia?
Parvoviruses require actively dividing cells to replicate. Therefore it preferentially infects red blood cell (RBC) precursors. In patients with hemolytic anemia and a high RBC turnover, the viral cytopathic effect destroys bone marrow RBC precursors, resulting in reticulocytopenia. The transient arrest of erythrocyte production results in profound anemia in persons with a shortened RBC survival, such as patients with hemolytic anemia. In fetuses shortened RBC survival (60 to 80 days versus 110 to 120 days in adults) also contributes to the severity of anemia.

Remington JS, Klein JO, Wilson CB, et al. Infectious diseases of the fetus and newborn: expert consult—online and print. 7th ed. Philadelphia: Saunders; 2

CHAPTER 14

NEUROLOGY

Courtney J. Wusthoff, MD, and Robert Ryan Clancy, MD

NEUROLOGIC EXAMINATION OF THE NEWBORN INFANT

✓ KEY POINTS: BASIC ELEMENTS OF THE NEONATAL NEUROLOGIC EXAMINATION

1. Mental status (level of alertness)

2. Eyes and other cranial nerves

3. Primitive (neonatal) reflexes

4. Motor and sensory function

5. Deep tendon reflexes

1. **What are a normal baby's biobehavioral states?**
   - Crying, inconsolable
   - Alert and irritable, possibly tremulous or jittery
   - Awake, alert, calm
   - Drowsy
   - Sleeping (dream, or rapid-eye-movement, sleep makes up a high percentage of a neonate's total sleep time)

   The ideal state for a neurologic examination, state 3, is usually achieved 1 to 2 hours after feeding or, conversely, 1 to 2 hours before the next feed.

   Prechtl HFR. Continuity of neonatal function from prenatal to postnatal life. Oxford, England: Spastics International Medical; 1984.

2. **What is acute neonatal encephalopathy?**
   Acute neonatal encephalopathy (ANE) refers to the clinical syndrome of global brain dysfunction in the newborn, diagnosed through the history and examination. Babies with ANE have depression at birth, impaired mental status (lethargy or coma), hypotonia, inactivity, disordered sucking and swallowing, diminished primitive and postural reflexes, and reduced or absent deep tendon reflexes. Many, but not all, have clinical or subclinical seizures. ANE has numerous potential etiologies, such as acquired brain injury (e.g., hypoxic-ischemic encephalopathy, trauma, stroke, hemorrhage); infection; metabolic disease; or even severe, catastrophic types of neonatal epilepsy, which will be discussed later. Neonatal encephalopathy must always be distinguished from the term *hypoxic-ischemic encephalopathy (HIE),* which specifically refers to the clinical syndrome of acute encephalopathy in a newborn owing to hypoxic ischemia. The majority of neonates with ANE do not have HIE.

3. **What are the developmental reflexes, and when do they extinguish?**
   Developmental reflexes include both primitive and postural reflexes. *Primitive* reflexes are patterns of behavioral responses to stimulation that arise and extinguish at predictable ages in healthy newborns

and infants. The familiar Moro reflex is elicited by sudden extension of the head in relation to the body, as with a light drop of the head (Fig. 14-1). A newborn will respond by opening the hands and abducting and extending the arms and legs, followed by flexion. The Moro reflex is abnormal if asymmetric or depressed. Other examples of primitive reflexes include the palmar grasp, plantar grasp, glabellar, root, and suck reflexes. *Postural* reflexes determine the distribution of flexion or extension tone in the trunk and limb muscles depending on the orientation of the head and neck in space. The familiar "fencing posture" arises from the asymmetric tonic neck reflex, which is elicited by turning and holding the supine baby's head to the left or right side for several seconds. The newborn reflexively responds by extending the arm and leg (by way of increased extension tone) on the side to which the face is pointing, while the other arm and leg flexes (by way of increased flexion tone) (Table 14-1).

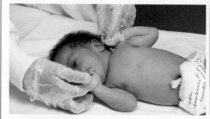

A, Palmar grasp

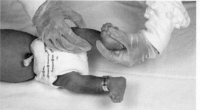

B, Plantar grasp

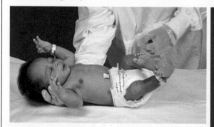

C, Moro

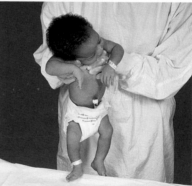

D, Placing

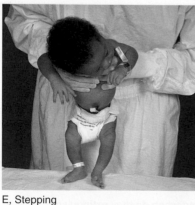

E, Stepping

F, Asymmetric tonic neck or "fencing"

Figure 14-1. Examples of normal primitive and postural reflexes in the newborn.

4. **What is the scarf maneuver? How is it helpful? (Fig. 14-2)**

The maneuver is performed by grasping the baby's hand and trying to bring the baby's elbow across the midline. In a healthy term infant the elbow can be brought no further than the midclavicular line on the same side. In the case of prematurity, hypotonia, or brachial plexus injury, the elbow is easily brought past the midline, like a scarf.

The New Ballard Score. Scarf sign. <http://www.ballardscore.com/Pages/mono_neuro_scarf.aspx>; 2013 [accessed 17.06.13].

5. **Is a Babinski sign (up-turning toe or extensor plantar response) present in a normal neonate?**

The plantar response is extensor (upward response of the hallux) in most neonates for at least the first month up through the first year of life. A flexor response (toes turning down and inward, with foot everting) is also normal and not of concern. A definite and reproducible assymetry could be abnormal.

6. **How are the eyes examined?**

The term newborn should be able to follow an object both horizontally and vertically with the eyes. This may be assessed using a picture with contrasting black and white lines (e.g., Teller acuity targets); an object of a single bright color; or the examiner's face, at about 10 inches from the baby. The examiner

TABLE 14-1.

REFLEX	AGE AT APPEARANCE	AGE AT DISAPPEARANCE
Moro	30-34 weeks PMA	3-6 months
Palmar grasp	28-32 weeks PMA	3-6 months
ATNR	35 weeks PMA	3 months
ATNR, Asymmetric tonic neck reflex; PMA, postmenstrual age.		

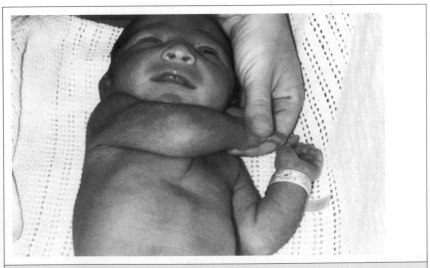

Figure 14-2. Scarf sign. The elbow cannot be drawn, with gentle traction on the upper extremity, across this term infant's chest. This is in contrast to the marked flexibility of a preterm infant of 29 weeks' gestation.

can move the object slowly across the field of vision to assess if eye movements are full and conjugate. Another method is to use a striped cloth or drum to elicit opticokinetic response and determine that eye movements are symmetric. Pupillary constriction responses to light develop between 30 and 32 weeks.

Ricci D, Cesarini L, Groppo M, et al. Early assessment of visual function in full term newborns. Early Hum Dev 2008;84(2):107–113.

7. **How are the rest of the cranial nerves examined?**
The glabellar tap is performed by tapping between the eyes to elicit bilateral blinking. It is a "poor man's" corneal reflex that tests the afferent loop (cranial nerve V) and the efferent loop (cranial nerve VII). The same goal may be accomplished by stroking the eyelashes to elicit a blink. Facial nerve function is evident with good bilateral eye closure and symmetry of the face during crying. Auditory function is tested by behavioral responses to sound. A coordinated sucking and swallowing reflex should develop at approximately 35 weeks' gestation, and poor sucking in a term newborn is of concern. Observe the tongue for fasciculations. Listen to the cry. An encephalopathic neonate may have a characteristic cry that is shorter and higher pitched. An infant who has been intubated may be hoarse; however, one with laryngeal palsy can be stridorous or hoarse. An infant with neuromuscular weakness may make the facial grimace of a cry, but be unable to generate sound.

8. **In newborns with facial paralysis, how is peripheral nerve involvement distinguished from a central etiology?**
A central facial paralysis (or "central seventh") is caused by a lesion in the brain somewhere in the pathway from the primary motor cortex down to the nucleus of the seventh cranial nerve. A central facial palsy (i.e., central seven palsy) produces a *gradation* of weakness, which affects the lower face and mouth much more severely than the forehead muscles, which are less weak. Central facial paralysis may also have an associated hemiplegia. A peripheral facial palsy is caused by a lesion in the facial nerve nucleus or anywhere along the nerve's track. A peripheral facial palsy affects the upper and lower face equally. For example, a "10%" injury of the peripheral 7th nerve will cause an equal 10% weakness of the forehead muscles, nasolabial fold, and lower mouth muscles.

Sometimes confused for a true facial palsy is an absence or hypoplasia of the left or right "depressor anguli oris" muscles. These muscles insert on the angle of the mouth and pull down or depress the corners of the mouth when an infant is crying. If the muscle from one side is missing or underdeveloped, that side of the mouth does not pull down as far during crying. To those not aware of this condition, this may be misinterpreted as "facial drooping" or weakness on the good side. Of course, without crying, the two sides of the mouth appear even. This condition is occasionally associated with congenital heart disease.

9. **How is the motor examination performed?**
First, observe the position of the baby and the spontaneous movements. Observe the quantity and quality of the movements. Examine the tone by gentle flexion and extension of the limbs. Is there an associated paucity of movement of an arm or leg? Observe the rebound of the extremity; the rate at which a limb returns to its original position is helpful in gauging tone (Fig. 14-3). Measuring the popliteal angle (which may be as great as 180 degrees at 28 weeks' gestation but decreases to 110 degrees at term) allows for objective interobserver comparison of lower extremity tone. Head control can be gauged by either sitting the infant in the neutral position with good shoulder girdle support or pulling the baby off the surface of a bed (traction maneuver).

Ballard JL, Khoury JC, Wedig K, et al. New Ballard Score, expanded to include premature infants. J Pediatr 1991;119:417–23.
Dubowitz L, Ricci D, Mercuri E. The Dubowitz neurological examination of the full-term newborn. Ment Retard Dev Disabil Res Rev 2005;11:52–60.

10. **When do the tendon stretch reflexes develop?**
The deep tendon reflexes develop, as does tone, several weeks earlier in the legs than in the arms, and the patellar and Achilles responses are attainable by 33 weeks' gestation in most neonates.

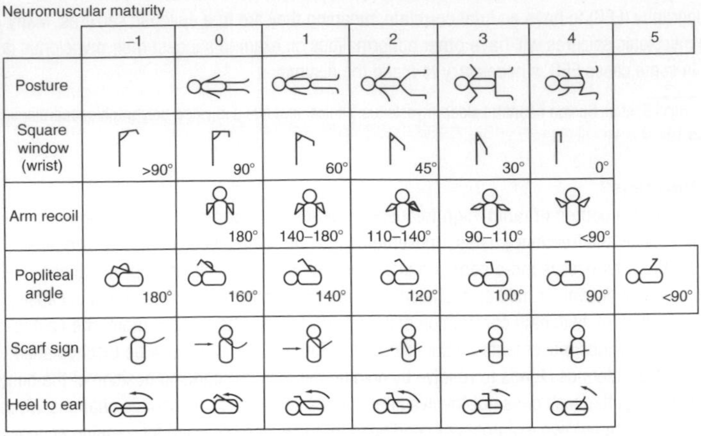

Neuromuscular maturity

	−1	0	1	2	3	4	5
Posture							
Square window (wrist)	>90°	90°	60°	45°	30°	0°	
Arm recoil		180°	140–180°	110–140°	90–110°	<90°	
Popliteal angle	180°	160°	140°	120°	100°	90°	<90°
Scarf sign							
Heel to ear							

Physical maturity

								Maturity rating	
Skin	Sticky friable, transparent	Gelatinous, red, translucent	Smooth, pink, visible veins	Superficial peeling &/or rash, few veins	Cracking, pale areas, rare veins	Parchment, deep cracking, no vessels	Leathery, cracked, wrinkled	Score	Weeks
								−10	20
Lanugo	None	Sparse	Abundant	Thinning	Bald areas	Mostly bald		−5	22
								0	24
Plantar surface	Heel–toe 40–50 mm: −1 <40 mm: −2	>50 mm no crease	Faint red marks	Anterior transverse crease only	Creases ant. 2/3	Creases over entire sole		5	26
								10	28
Breast	Imperceptible	Barely perceptible	Flat areola, no bud	Stippled areola, 1–2 mm bud	Raised areola, 3–4 mm bud	Full areola, 5–10 mm bud		15	30
								20	32
Eye/ear	Lids fused loosely: −1 tightly: −2	Lids open pinna flat stays folded	Sl.curved pinna: soft: slow recoil	Well-curve pinna; soft but ready recoil	Formed & firm, instant recoil	Thick cartilage, ear stiff		25	34
								30	36
Genitals male	Scrotum flat, smooth	Scrotum empty, faint rugae	Testes in upper canal, rare rugae	Testes descending, few rugae	Testes down, good rugae	Testes pendulous, deep rugae		35	38
								40	40
Genitals female	Clitoris prominent, labia flat	Prominent clitoris, small labia minora	Prominent clitoris, enlarging minora	Majora & minora equally prominent	Majora large, minora small	Majora cover clitoris & minora		45	42
								50	44

Figure 14-3. The Ballard scoring system. (From Ballard JL, Khoury JC, Wedig K, et al. New Ballard Score, expanded to include extremely premature infants. J Pediatr 1991;119:417–423.)

Note that when a knee-jerk response is obtained, a crossed adductor response may also occur as a normal variant up through 6 months of age.

11. **Is ankle clonus normal in a newborn infant?**
Bilateral ankle clonus of 3 to 5 beats may be a normal finding, especially in infants who are crying, hungry, or jittery. Sustained ankle clonus is abnormal.

12. **What is myoclonus? When is it normal or abnormal?**
Myoclonus is a brief, involuntary twitch or jerk of a muscle or group of muscles. It is frequently seen in healthy newborns, particularly when they are drowsy or sleeping. Benign neonatal myoclonus is very common, may persist for several weeks, and does not indicate a brain abnormality. Much less

common are myoclonic seizures in newborns; these are myoclonic jerks that are shown on electroencephalography (EEG) to have an ictal correlate, meaning they are true epileptic seizures. Many
babies with myoclonic seizures will have other abnormalities on exam to suggest their myoclonus is
not benign; in some cases EEG is necessary to make the distinction.

Di Capua M, Fusco L, Ricci S, et al. Benign neonatal sleep myoclonus: clinical features and video-polygraphic recordings.
Mov Disord 1993;8(2):191–4.

13. **What is jitteriness?**

Jitteriness describes a pattern of rapid, high frequency, vibratory, shaking movements that may
fluctuate in amplitude and frequency. These movements may be spontaneous or may be triggered
by touch or startle. Jitteriness is more common in babies with hypoglycemia or other metabolic
disturbance, drug withdrawal, or mild encephalopathy. Jitteriness differs from myoclonus because
myoclonus is a very brief, twitching contraction of muscles, whereas jitteriness is more often a sustained pattern of tremulous movements lasting seconds or longer. Jitteriness may be distinguished
from seizures in that jitteriness tends to resolve by holding the baby or changing position of the baby
or limb. Furthermore, jitteriness does not involve altered consciousness or autonomic changes. Myoclonus and jitteriness are but two examples of conditions that could be confused for genuine epileptic
seizures in the neonate.

Laux L, Nordli D Jr. Neonatal nonepileptic events. In: Kaplan PW, Fisher RS, editors. Imitators of epilepsy. 2nd ed. New York:
Demos Medical Publishing; 2005.
Clancy R. Imitators of epileptic seizures specific to neonates and infants. In: Panayiotopoulos CP, editor. The atlas of
epilepsies. London: Springer; 2010.

✓ KEY POINTS: SIGNS AND SYMPTOMS OF DRUG WITHDRAWAL

1. W = Wakefulness

2. I = Irritability

3. T = Tremulousness, temperature variation, tachypnea

4. H = Hyperactivity, high-pitched cry, hyperacusis, hyperreflexia, hypertonus

5. D = Diarrhea, diaphoresis, disorganized sucking

6. R = Rub marks, respiratory distress, rhinorrhea

7. A = Apneic attacks, autonomic dysfunction

8. W = Weight loss or poor weight gain

9. A = Alkalosis (respiratory)

10. L = Lacrimation

THE SKULL, SPINE, AND BRACHIAL PLEXUS

14. **What is the normal head circumference in a term neonate?**

The 50th percentile is 35 cm. Normal head circumference involves approximately 2 cm growth per
month for 3 months, 1 cm growth per month for 3 more months, and then roughly 0.5 cm growth per
month for the next 6 months, for a total of 12 cm in the first 12 months after birth. Premature infants
should attain the head circumference of a healthy term infant, but illness and nutritional factors may
slow the rate of growth. Relative to term infants, the head circumference of an otherwise healthy

TABLE 14-2. NORMAL HEAD CIRCUMFERENCE BY GESTATIONAL AGE

Fenton TR. A new growth chart for preterm babies: Babson and Benda's chart updated with recent data and a new format. BMC Pediatr 2003;3:13.

GESTATIONAL AGE (Weeks)	HEAD CIRCUMFERENCE (Cm)
28	26
32	30
36	33
40	35

preterm infant may even be greater for the first 5 postnatal months, after which differences are less pronounced (Table 14-2).

15. **How is head circumference affected in symmetric and asymmetric intrauterine growth restriction (IUGR)?**
Asymmetric IUGR is restricted growth affecting weight and sometimes length but with normal head growth ("head sparing"). This is thought to reflect a protective mechanism in the face of extrinsic factors, by which the developing fetal brain is spared at the cost of other aspects of growth. *Symmetric IUGR* refers to restricted growth in all dimensions of growth, including head circumference, and carries a more worrisome neurologic prognosis.

16. **How is the examination of the anterior fontanel useful?**
The examination of the anterior fontanel is somewhat subjective and inexact, but it is useful nonetheless. The anterior fontanel should be slightly depressed and pulsatile when a neonate is sleeping comfortably. Sitting the baby up should depress the fontanel further in a normal newborn. A sunken anterior fontanel suggests dehydration. When the anterior fontanel is bulging, increased intracranial pressure may be a cause of concern. The normal anterior fontanel should remain open for at least the first 6 months. Premature closure is a concern for craniosynostosis.

17. **What are signs of increased intracranial pressure (ICP) in the neonate?**
The neonate with increased ICP may show poor feeding, lethargy, and irritability. Vomiting may increase or become more forceful. Bulging of the anterior fontanel, particularly while the baby is calm, is worrisome because ICP may be increased. With progression there may be bulging at the posterior fontanel or separation of the cranial sutures. Changes in pupils, eye movements, and autonomic function are late signs of increased ICP in the neonate. Although the open anterior fontanel may offer a limited outlet for increased ICP (when bulging), neonates can incur permanent injury or death from increased ICP.

18. **What is craniosynostosis? What are the different variations of this problem?**
Craniosynostosis is the result of premature closure of a cranial suture. Normal cranial sutures are shown in Figure 14-4. Premature closure results in the arrest of growth perpendicular to the affected suture. Types of craniosynostosis and their appearance are illustrated in Figure 14-5. They involve the following:
- Dolichocephaly: sagittal synostosis (long, narrow head)
- Brachycephaly: coronal synostosis (wide head)
- Acrocephaly: coronal, sagittal, and lambdoidal
- Synostosis (tower head)
- Trigonocephaly: Metopic synostosis (pointed front of the head)

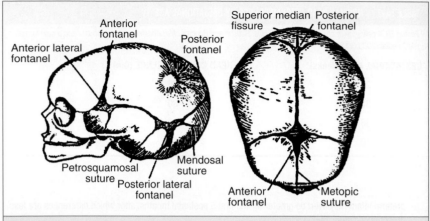

Figure 14-4. Normal cranial sutures. (From Silverman FN, Kuhn JP, editors. Caffey's pediatric x-ray diagnosis. 9th ed. St. Louis: Mosby; 1993. p. 5.)

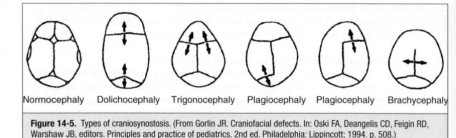

Normocephaly   Dolichocephaly   Trigonocephaly   Plagiocephaly   Plagiocephaly   Brachycephaly

Figure 14-5. Types of craniosynostosis. (From Gorlin JR. Craniofacial defects. In: Oski FA, Deangelis CD, Feigin RD, Warshaw JB, editors. Principles and practice of pediatrics. 2nd ed. Philadelphia: Lippincott; 1994. p. 508.)

19. **What are the normal cerebrospinal fluid (CSF) values for healthy neonates?**
    - More than 15 cells in a CSF sample should be considered suspect for meninigitis and more than 20 cells elevated.
    - The CSF glucose concentration should be 70% to 80% of the blood glucose concentration.
    - Protein concentrations in excess of 100 mg/dL in a nontraumatic tap from a term infant should be considered suspect.
    - There is an inverse correlation between the protein concentration in CSF and gestational age. See Table 14-3.

20. **What are two devastating spinal cord injuries that can occur in the neonatal period?**
    Fortunately, spinal cord injury is uncommon in neonates. One instance in which it can occur, however, is when excessive traction is applied to the neck during a difficult delivery, especially if there is shoulder dystocia. The resulting cord injury causes a flaccid quadriplegia with sparing of the face and cranial nerves. Secondly, an indwelling umbilical arterial catheter misplaced at T11 can obstruct the artery of Adamkiewicz, which feeds the anterior spinal artery. The resulting cord ischemia causes an irreversible paraplegia.

TABLE 14-3. NORMAL CEREBROSPINAL FLUID VALUES IN HEALTHY TERM AND PRETERM INFANTS

*	CELL COUNT (Mean)	PROTEIN (Mg/Dl)
Ahmed (Term)	7.3 (90th percentile 11)	64 ± 24
Bonadio (Term)	11 (90th percentile 22)	84 ± 45.1
Martin–Ancel (Term)	1 (range 0-5)	No data
Nascimento–Carvalho: Term[†] :Preterm[†]	4.5 (95th percentile 11.7) 5.1 (95th percentile 16.7)	77.6 ± 31.5 101.2 ± 45.7
Kestenbaum (Term and preterm [n=142])	9.2 (95th percentile 19)	No data

*All studies excluded traumatic lumbar puncture and were sterile; Ahmed and Bonadio did viral cultures. Excluded enteroviruses, herpes simplex virus, syphilis, seizures, non–central nervous system bacterial infection, and traumatic lumbar puncture (<500 red blood cells)
[†]Cisternal puncture.

TABLE 14-4. MAJOR PATTERN OF WEAKNESS WITH ERB (UPPER) BRACHIAL PLEXUS PALSY

WEAK MOVEMENT	SPINAL CORD SEGMENT	RESULTING POSITION
Shoulder abduction	C5	Adducted
Shoulder external rotation	C5	Internally rotated
Elbow flexion	C5, C6	Extended
Supination	C5, C6	Pronated
Wrist extension	C6, C7	Flexed
Finger extension	C6, C7	Flexed
Diaphragmatic descent	C4, C5	Elevated

21. **How is Erb palsy diagnosed? What is the most common cause in the newborn?**

Erb palsy is an injury to the brachial plexus, particularly the upper trunk. This causes weakness in flexion at the shoulder and elbow. At rest, the arm of a baby with Erb palsy hangs by the side and is internally rotated, and there are limited or no spontaneous movements of the hand. The most common cause is injury to the brachial plexus during delivery, particularly in babies who are large for gestational age, or in cases of shoulder dystocia (Table 14-4).

22. **What is the prognosis of obstetric brachial plexus injury?**

Most babies with brachial plexus injury recover well, although this may take as long as 6 months. As many as 30% of cases may have lasting deficits or will require intervention. In the initial weeks and months, physiotherapy may be useful. If problems persist, nerve and muscle transfer surgery may be warranted.

Malessy MJ, Pondaag W. Obstetric brachial plexus injuries. Neurosurg Clin N Am 2009;20(1):1–14.

MALFORMATIONS OF THE CENTRAL NERVOUS SYSTEM

 KEY POINTS: MAJOR EVENTS IN HUMAN BRAIN DEVELOPMENT AND PEAK TIMES OF OCCURRENCE

1. Primary neurulation at 3 to 4 weeks' gestation

2. Prosencephalic development at 2 to 3 months' gestation

3. Neuronal proliferation at 2 to 4 months' gestation

4. Neuronal migration at 3 to 5 months' gestation

5. Organization at 5 months' gestation through early life

6. Myelination from 8 months' gestation through early life

23. **How do meningocele, meningomyelocele, and spina bifida occulta differ?**
    A meningocele is the protrusion of only the meninges through a bony defect in the spine, whereas in meningomyelocele, both meninges and spinal cord protrude through bone. Spina bifida occulta is a vertebral cleft without spinal cord or meningeal herniation; it is a frequent incidental finding when neuroimaging the lumbar spinal region.

24. **What is the incidence of meningomyelocele, and what is the best way to prevent its occurrence?**
    The incidence of meningomyelocele is approximately 0.5 to 1 per 1000 live births. Prophylaxis is accomplished in most cases by the intake of 0.4 mg of folic acid daily, starting, if possible, before the pregnancy begins. If the parents have had a previous child with spina bifida, 4 mg/day is recommended. With supplementation there has been a significant decrease in neural tube defects in the United States.

25. **If the diagnosis of meningomyelocele is made prenatally, what treatment options can be considered?**
    Until recently, standard treatment for meningomyelocele was surgery after birth. However, a randomized trial showed that prenatal surgery (i.e., fetal surgery performed before 26 weeks of gestation) led to a reduction in the need for CSF shunt in the first year and improved motor outcomes at 30 months. Because of the maternal and fetal risks of this operation, treatment is now available only at highly specialized fetal surgery centers.

Adzick NS, Thom EA, Spong CY, et al. A randomized trial of prenatal versus postnatal repair of myelomeningocele. N Engl J Med 2011;364(11):993–1004.

26. **Which congenital cerebral disorders are associated with meningomyelocele?**
    The Arnold–Chiari type II (ACTII) malformation is frequently associated with meningomyelocele. ACTII consists of a low-lying cerebellar vermis and a ventral medulla that often protrudes into the foramen magnum. By obstructing the flow of CSF, it leads to hydrocephalus. Aqueductal stenosis may be found with ACTII malformation or in isolation, again leading to CSF flow obstruction. Agenesis of the corpus callosum can also be associated with meningomyelocele.

27. **What is the prognosis for cognitive development in children with meningomyelocele?**
    Many factors should be considered in formulating a neurologic prognosis. In general, the lower the level of the lesion, the better the prognosis. However, the presence and degree of hydrocephalus present at birth, in addition to the need for and any complications in shunting procedures (e.g., infection), also significantly affect outcomes. Any associated central nervous system (CNS)

malformations, including agenesis of the corpus callosum, also contribute to morbidity. A child with a relatively low-lying lesion with an ACTII lesion and who has hydrocephalus is likely to have cognitive development in the normal range if there are no complications related to the shunting procedure.

Fobe JL, Rizzo AM, Silva IM. IQ in hydrocephalus and meningomyelocele: implications of surgical treatment. Arch Neuropsychiatr 1999;57:44–50.

28. **In an infant born with meningomyelocele, how does the cord level of the lesion on initial evaluation predict long-term ambulation?**
    This assessment is accomplished by determining motor level and reflex level on examination (Table 14-5). Sensory level assessment is less reliable in the newborn.

29. **What is a tethered cord? Why is it clinically important?**
    A tethered cord is a low-lying lumbosacral cord anchored posteriorly by a thickened filum terminale. It can occur in association with meningomyelocele or with other lumbosacral abnormalities such as lipomeningocele. It may be overlain by a dermal defect such as a hair tuft or sacral dimple. The lesion may be asymptomatic, but with growth it may lead to problems with sphincter control and walking and may also cause lumbar back pain. When a newborn has a sacral tuft or dimple suspicious for underlying cord abnormality, ultrasound is often used for immediate assessment, and magnetic resonance imaging (MRI) provides a definitive diagnosis.

✓ KEY POINTS: DORSAL MIDLINE FEATURES SUGGESTING SPINAL DYSRAPHISM

1. An abnormal collection of hair is present.

2. Cutaneous abnormalities (e.g., hemangioma or pigmented nevi) occur.

3. Cutaneous dimples or tracts or a subcutaneous mass on the lower back appear.

4. In 80% to 90% of cases, there is an associated vertebral abnormality.

5. The diagnosis should also be suspected in patients with symptoms of progressive lower extremity weakness or sensory loss, gait abnormalities, foot deformities, or neurogenic bowel and bladder problems.

6. Spinal dysraphism is associated with Chiari hindbrain malformations, syringomyelia, and tethered cord.

30. **What is the Dandy–Walker malformation? What are the associated abnormalities and treatment?**
    The components of the Dandy–Walker malformation are cystic dilation of the fourth ventricle, partial or complete agenesis of the cerebellar vermis, and enlargement of the posterior fossa with a high

TABLE 14-5. SPINAL LEVELS: MOTOR, REFLEXES, AND AMBULATION*		
LEVEL	**MOTOR FUNCTION**	**AMBULATION**
T-L2	None or hip flexion only	None
L3-L4	Knee extension, hip adduction	In 50%, with braces or other devices
L5-S1	Knee flexion, ankle flexion	In 50%, some unaided
S2-S4	Bowel and bladder	Almost all unaided
*S2-S4 levels have only bladder and bowel abnormalities, as do all higher levels.		

attachment of the tentorium cerebelli. The Dandy–Walker malformation is frequently associated with hydrocephalus, which may not be present at birth but develops in the first year of life. Agenesis of the corpus callosum or cortical migrational defects (or both) coexist in many cases and increase the risk for intellectual disability when present. Treatment consists of observation and shunting of the ventricles. Sometimes the cyst itself needs to be shunted.

31. **What is the distinction between porencephaly and schizencephaly?**
Porencephaly is an acquired abnormality that is seen as CSF-filled cysts at the site of injury, often adjacent to or connecting with the ventricular system. It usually is the result of an early parenchymal bleed, infarction, or infection. Schizencephaly represents a "split" or "cleft" in the cortex resulting from a congenital migrational defect and appears in one or both hemispheres from the surface of the brain down to the ventricular surface. In schizencephaly the walls of the cleft are lined with abnormal cortex (e.g., polymicrogyria), further distinguishing it from porencephaly.

32. **What is lissencephaly?**
Lissencephaly means "smooth brain." With this condition there are few if any gyri formed on the brain's surface. Lissencephaly is a severe migrational disorder of genetic etiology. There are two basic types. Type I is characterized by diffuse failure of migration on histology. These infants have an initially normal head size, but they also have hypotonia and seizures. A majority of these cases are caused by mutations affecting the genes *LIS1*, *XLIS*, or *DCX*. Type II lissencephaly is characterized by a "bumpy" or "pebbly" brain surface on pathology and is associated with congenital muscular dystrophy.

33. **What are the types of holoprosencephaly and their common associations?**
Holoprosencephaly reflects an early failure of the rudimentary forebrain to divide into two halves, resulting in various kinds of single-ventricle anomalies. These range in severity from alobar, in which there are no distinct cerebral hemispheres, to lobar variants, in which division between cerebral lobes is incomplete. The alobar form is particularly severe in terms of neurologic dysfunction, may result in a wide spectrum of facial abnormalities, and may be observed in infants with trisomy 13 or 18 syndrome.

Patterson MC. Holoprosencephaly: the face predicts the brain—the image predicts its function. Neurology 2002;59:1833–1834.

34. **How is hydrocephalus classified?**
Hydrocephalus is a build-up of CSF, usually owing to obstruction in the outflow of the CSF pathways. By conventional definitions, the obstruction can be "communicating," in which the block is outside the ventricular system, or "noncommunicating," in which the block is within the ventricular system. Choroid plexus papillomas (90% benign) are a rare cause of nonobstructive hydrocephalus; these tumors *oversecrete* CSF and lead to hydrocephalus that is often present at birth.

35. **What are main causes of intrauterine (fetal) hydrocephalus?**
Structural malformations, such as aqueductal stenosis and ACTII malformation (usually associated with meningomyelocele and the Dandy–Walker malformation), are the most common causes of fetal hydrocephalus (Table 14-6).

36. **What is the distinction between hydrocephalus and ventriculomegaly?**
With hydrocephalus the CSF is under pressure, causing a dilation of the ventricles proximal to the cause of obstruction. This condition will often worsen until surgical correction of the obstruction or placement of a CSF shunt. Ventriculomegaly, in contrast, occurs when ventricles are of a larger size than normal, but no evidence of increased CSF pressure exists. In cases of ventriculomegaly the cause is an underlying difference in brain development, and surgery is not indicated.

TABLE 14-6. MAJOR CAUSES OF HYDROCEPHALUS OVERT AT BIRTH IN 127 CASES	
Data from Mealey J Jr, Gilmor RL, Bubb MP. The prognosis of hydrocephalus overt at birth. J Neurosurg 1973:39:348–55; and McCullough DC, Balzer-Martin LA. Current prognosis in overt neonatal hydrocephalus. J Neurosurg 1982;57:378–83.	
CAUSE	**PERCENTAGE (%)**
Aqueductal stenosis	33
Myelomeningocele: Chiari type II malformation	28
"Communicating" hydrocephalus	22
Dandy–Walker malformation	7
Other	10

37. **What are the principal causes of hydrocephalus acquired in the newborn period?**
    Posthemorrhagic hydrocephalus resulting from intraventricular hemorrhage (IVH) is by far the most frequent cause of acquired hydrocephalus in the neonatal period. Other causes of hydrocephalus include blocked reabsorption of CSF by the meninges, as occurs with inflammation associated with subarachnoid hemorrhage or meningitis.

38. **How does a vein of Galen malformation usually present in the newborn period?**
    The vein of Galen malformation is rare overall, but it accounts for 30% of intracranial pediatric vascular abnormalities. A characteristic feature of the malformation is the presence of an arteriovenous shunt, which typically presents as high-output congestive heart failure in the neonatal period. There may be a bruit, sometimes quite loud, best heard over the posterior aspect of the newborn's head. Sometimes there is head enlargement caused by an extrinsic aqueductal stenosis produced in the pons and midbrain by the bulk of the malformation. Only very rarely do these malformations present as bleeds at birth. Diagnosis is through neuroimaging (color Doppler and MRI and magnetic resonance angiography); ultimate treatment is through intravascular embolization or neurosurgery.

    Heuer GG, Gabel B, Beslow LA, et al. Diagnosis and treatment of vein of Galen aneurysmal malformations. Childs Nerv Syst 2010;26:879–887.

NEUROCUTANEOUS SYNDROMES

39. **What is a phakomatosis?**
    The term *phakomatosis* is derived from the Greek *phakos,* meaning "lentil" or "lens," and refers to the patchy, circumscribed dermatologic lesions that are their hallmark. Because both skin and CNS tissue arise from the same ectodermal precursors, conditions that affect the CNS may have pathognomonic skin features. In addition to dermatologic features, these syndromes have hamartomata (errors in development) with involvement of multiple tissues. More commonly, the term *neurocutaneous syndrome* is used when referring to this group of diseases.

40. **What are the two most common neurocutaneous syndromes?**
    Neurofibromatosis (NF) and tuberous sclerosis complex (TSC) are both autosomal dominant conditions; the majority are sporadic. The prevalence of NF1 is about 1 in 3000 live births, and the incidence of NF2 is 1 in 100,000 live births. The prevalence of TSC is 1 in 6000.

41. **How common are café-au-lait spots at birth?**
    Café-au-lait spots are present in as many as 2% of infants; these vary in prevalence and are not always indicative of NF. Children with NF1 may have few or no café-au-lait spots at birth; these may become more

obvious within the first year. Because of the high spontaneous mutation rate for this autosomal dominant disease, only about 50% of newly diagnosed cases of NF1 are associated with a positive family history.

Hurwitz S. Neurofibromatosis. Clinical pediatric dermatology. 2nd ed. Philadelphia: Saunders; 1993. p. 624–629.
National NF Foundation. <http://www.nf.org>; [accessed 24.08.12].

42. What is NF1?

NF1 is an autosomal dominant disorder of a tumor-suppressor gene located on chromosome 17q11.2 that encodes neurofibromin, a negative regulator of the Ras oncogene. Characteristic café-au-lait-spots may appear at birth. Osseous lesions are usually apparent within the first year of life, and tumors of the optic chiasm present relatively early in life. Axillary freckling and peripheral, spinal, or central nerve NFs may develop in later childhood. Early ascertainment is difficult, and almost half of infants younger than 1 year of age do not fulfill the full criteria for this disorder.

DeBella K, Szudek J, Friedman JM. Use of the National Institutes of Health criteria for diagnosis of neurofibromatosis 1 in children. Pediatrics 2000;105:608–614.

43. What is the spectrum of TSC?

TSC is characterized by multiple and variable organ involvement. Commonly recognized clinical features include hypomelanotic skin macules, facial angiofibromas, periungual fibromas, delayed development, epilepsy, and autism. The kidney, heart, and retina are among other commonly affected organs. Abnormalities on brain imaging include subependymal nodules, cortical tubers, radial white matter lines, and subependymal giant cell astrocytomas (SEGAs). In 2010 everolimus was approved for the nonsurgical treatment of SEGAs (U.S. Food and Drug Administration Bulletin 2010). Sometimes computed tomography (CT) may be superior to MRI in detecting *calcified* cortical tubers. Seizures may begin in the neonatal period and are one example of a "well baby with seizures." At the same time, symptoms for a given individual may be subtle; it is possible for a parent to have undiagnosed TSC come to light only when their affected baby is born.

44. What is the significance of facial port-wine stains?

Port-wine stains can occur as isolated cutaneous birthmarks or in association with structural abnormalities

---

✓ KEY POINTS: PRIMARY CLINICAL DIAGNOSTIC FEATURES OF TUBEROUS SCLEROSIS COMPLEX IN THE NEONATAL PERIOD

1. Cardiac hamartomas (may be diagnosed *in utero* before developing neurologic and skin symptoms)

2. Subependymal nodules or giant cell astrocytomas

3. Multiple calcified subependymal nodules protruding into the ventricle

4. Multiple retinal astrocytomas

5. Skin lesions (uncommon in the neonate); hypopigmented macules and café-au-lait spots possibly observed

---

of choroidal vessels of the eye leading to glaucoma and of the leptomeningeal vessels in the brain leading to seizures (Sturge–Weber syndrome). Almost invariably, the hemangioma in Sturge–Weber syndrome involves the trigeminal V1 area or is bilaterally distributed. Ophthalmologic assessment and radiologic studies (CT or MRI) are indicated for children who exhibit hemangiomas in the upper eyelid or forehead. This neurocutaneous syndrome arises sporadically and is not known to result from a specific genetic mutation.

The Sturge-Weber Foundation. <http://www.sturge-weber.com>; [accessed 24.08.12].

45. **What is incontinentia pigmenti?**

Incontinentia pigmenti, or Bloch–Sulzberger syndrome, is an X-linked dominant disorder characterized by abnormalities of skin, teeth, hair, and eyes; mental retardation; seizures; skewed X-inactivation; and recurrent miscarriages of male fetuses. The first stage (i.e., vesicular stage) is characterized by lines of blisters, particularly on the extremities in newborns, that disappear in weeks or months. This is followed by stage 2 (i.e., verrucous stage), in which lesions develop at approximately age 3 to 7 months that are brown and hyperkeratotic, resembling warts. The final stage, stage 3 (i.e., pigmented stage), is characterized by whorled, swirling (marble cake–like) macular hyperpigmented lines that may fade with time. Rarely, neonatal seizures have been reported in this condition.

Porksen G, Pfeiffer C, Hahn G, et al. Neonatal seizures in two sisters with incontinentia pigmenti. Neuropediatrics 2004 Apr;35(2):139–42.

46. **What is hypomelanosis of Ito?**

Hypomelanosis of Ito was originally described as a purely cutaneous disease with a swirling pigmentary pattern, sometimes visible in the neonatal period, but subsequent reports have included a frequent association with multiple extracutaneous manifestations, mostly of the central nervous and musculoskeletal systems. Neurologic complications include mental retardation, autism, brain malformations, microcephaly, and epilepsy. When associated with structural brain malformations such as hemimegalencephaly, neonatal seizures may arise. Miscellaneous chromosomal mosaicisms have been demonstrated in some but not all affected persons. Additional associated abnormalities include limb length discrepancies, facial hemiatrophy, scoliosis, sternal abnormalities, dysmorphic facies, and genitourinary and cardiac abnormalities.

INTRACRANIAL HEMORRHAGE

47. **What are the three major forms of extracranial hemorrhage that can occur after a difficult delivery?**

- Caput succedaneum involves hemorrhagic edema of the presenting portion of the scalp and is common in vacuum extractions.
- Cephalohematoma involves hemorrhage that is confined by the periosteum and therefore respects the sutures. Cephalohematomas sometimes calcify and may produce a cosmetic deformity.
- Subgaleal hemorrhage involves the area under the epicranial aponeurosis and may become large and pitting, even dissecting into the neck. This has the potential to cause clinically significant blood loss in the neonate. It is also associated with vacuum extractions (Fig. 14-6).

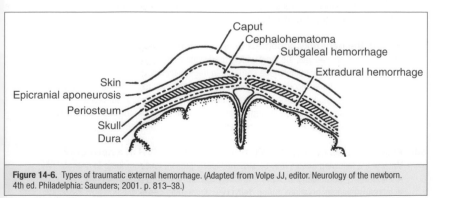

Figure 14-6. Types of traumatic external hemorrhage. (Adapted from Volpe JJ, editor. Neurology of the newborn. 4th ed. Philadelphia: Saunders; 2001. p. 813–38.)

48. **What are the major forms of intracranial hemorrhage?**
    - Subdural hemorrhage (SDH) occurs in term infants with vaginal deliveries, more often with forceps or vacuum extraction, leading to bleeding in the subdural space where bridging veins can tear. Although more common supratentorially, SDH can occur beneath the tentorium cerebelli.
    - IVH is most common in very-low-birth-weight (VLBW) preterm babies because of the fragility of blood vessels in the germinal matrix, adjacent to the lateral ventricle. IVH has also been described in term newborns, particularly those with HIE. IVH in a term infant typically results from vasodilation and rupture of arteries within the choroid plexus.
    - Intraparenchymal hemorrhage occurs in the brain substance of neonates usually as a result of vascular malformation, arterial infarction, or venous thrombosis.

    It is important to note that a small intracranial hemorrhage is a common and often asymptomatic finding. In one series of neonates with MRI in the first 3 weeks, more than 50% of those born vaginally had some degree of intracranial hemorrhage. Therefore such findings on MRI should be interpreted with caution.

Gupta SN, Kechi AM, Kanamalla US. Intracranial hemorrhage in term newborns: management and outcomes. Pediatr Neurol 2009;40(1):1–12.

Tavani F, Zimmerman RA, Clancy RR, et al. Incidental intracranial hemorrhage after uncomplicated birth: MRI before and after neonatal heart surgery. Neuroradiology 2003;45(4):253–8.

49. **What are the symptoms, signs, diagnostic aids, and treatment of supratentorial SDH?**
    Most SDHs are asymptomatic and are usually identified as incidental findings on CT and MRI scans. They may not be visible on ultrasound scans. When caused by a tentorial or a falx tear, a newborn's condition can rapidly deteriorate as a result of blood loss and brainstem herniation. More often, an infant with symptomatic subdurals will be lethargic and may have seizures. Examination may reveal an enlarged head; bulging fontanel; excessive retinal hemorrhages; and focal weakness in the face, leg, or arm on one side of the body. Diagnosis is made by CT scan that shows a bright signal (i.e., blood) over one or both hemispheres, or by MRI. Treatment consists of watchful waiting most of the time. On occasion, sequential subdural taps may be necessary. Only rarely is surgical evacuation or a subdural-peritoneal shunting required.

50. **What are the principal sites of origin of IVH in the newborn?**
    The subependymal germinal matrix is the most common site for IVH in VLBW babies; venous hemorrhagic infarction of the white matter, which shares some of the pathogenesis with germinal matrix hemorrhage, may contribute to the injury. In term infants bleeding usually originates in the choroid plexus of the lateral ventricle.

51. **What is the procedure of choice for the diagnosis of IVH?**
    Cranial ultrasound is a reliable, portable, safe, and cost-effective method for evaluating infants for IVH. It allows for visualization of the subependymal germinal matrix, which is the most common site for IVH in VLBW babies. Cranial ultrasound can be performed at the bedside with minimal disturbance of the infant and is the study of choice.

52. **What is the generally accepted classification of IVH?**
    Although there are variants, the most widely used systems group IVH into four categories.
    - Grade I hemorrhage: hemorrhage confined to the subependymal germinal matrix only
    - Grade II hemorrhage: blood extending into the ventricle(s) without ventricular enlargement
    - Grade III hemorrhage: ventricular dilation in addition to intraventricular blood
    - Grade IV hemorrhage: grade III hemorrhage accompanied by hemorrhagic parenchymal infarction (formerly described by the misnomer "parenchymal extension")

53. **What variables contribute to the development of IVH in a newborn?**
    Many of the following factors may be simultaneously present and contribute to neonatal IVH:
    - Prematurity, particularly VLBW or extremely-low-birth-weight (ELBW) infants
    - Increased venous pressure during delivery or fluctuating cerebral blood flow associated with mechanical ventilation

- Increased cerebral blood flow associated with systemic hypertension or hypercarbia
- Hypotension followed by rapid volume expansion
- Coagulopathy caused by clotting factor deficiencies, thrombocytopenia, or platelet dysfunction (or a combination)
- The immature, delicate, friable microvascular network in the germinal matrix
- An inflammatory response with cytokine and immunomodulator production, most often from prenatal maternal infection, or infection or systemic inflammatory response in the neonate.

54. What are the major courses of progression of posthemorrhagic ventricular dilation and their rates of occurrence?

- Slowly progressive ventricular dilation (SPVD) with spontaneous arrest (<4 weeks)—65%
- Persistent SPVD (>4 weeks)—30%
- Rapidly progressive ventricular dilation—5%

Of the persistent SPVD group, approximately 67% will have a spontaneous arrest, whereas 33% will continue to progress. In the spontaneous arrest group, 5% will have late progressive dilation.

Volpe JJ, editor. Neurology of the newborn. 4th ed. Philadelphia: Saunders; 2001.

55. What are some of the various treatment options for IVH and SVPD?

- Close observation: This is the first step in managing the conditions. The infant's clinical condition and head circumference should be closely followed. Head growth that exceeds 1 cm per week should be monitored with serial ultrasound scans documenting ventricular size.
- Trial of serial lumbar punctures: This controversial and unproven approach is considered by some to be the initial procedure when progressive ventricular dilation does not resolve spontaneously. An ultrasound scan should be obtained after 10 to 15 mL of CSF are withdrawn to see whether the procedure has been helpful in reducing ventricular size. Although this technique is widely used, clinical trials of serial lumbar puncture show no benefit in preventing later CSF shunt placement.
- Carbonic anhydrase inhibitors: Although sometimes still used, acetazolamide (up to a high dose 100 mg/kg/day) combined with furosemide (1 to 2 mg/kg/day) has no clear benefit and increases the risk of nephrocalcinosis.
- Ventricular drainage: This can be accomplished in numerous ways: direct external drainage, via an indwelling subcutaneous Ommaya reservoir, or by ventriculosubgaleal shunting. These are most often temporizing measures until an infant is able to undergo a more permanent procedure, usually a ventriculoperitoneal shunt. The smaller the infant, the greater the likelihood of obstruction or infection (i.e., ventriculitis) by a shunting procedure.

de Vries LS, Liem KD, van Dikj K, et al. Early versus late treatment of posthemorrhagic ventricular dilatation: results of a retrospective study from five neonatal studies in the Netherlands. Acta Pediatr 2002;91:212–7.

Fulmer BB, Grabb PA, Oakew WJ, et al. Neonatal ventriculosubgaleal shunts. Neurosurgery 2000;47:80–4.

Kennedy CR, Ayers S, Campbell MJ, et al. Randomized, controlled trial of acetazolamide and furosemide in posthemorrhagic ventricular dilation in infancy: follow-up at 1 year. Pediatrics 2001;108:569–607.

56. What is the incidence of long-term neurologic sequelae in children with IVH?

The incidence of neurologic sequelae is linked not only to the grade of hemorrhage but also to gestational age of the patient and the degree of parenchymal insult resulting from infarction and periventricular leukomalacia (PVL). Some series have shown a 5% incidence of neurologic sequelae (e.g., intellectual disability, spastic diplegia, and seizures) for grade I IVH, 15% for grade II, 33% for grade III, and almost 90% for grade IV with large infarction. However, long-term studies have demonstrated that at least 50% of ELBW and VLBW babies go on to have scholastic and behavioral abnormalities, with IVH being only one contributor to adverse outcomes. Recent data indicate that IVH that is not accompanied by white-matter injury has a better prognosis.

Hack M, Flannery DJ, Schluchter M, et al. Outcomes in young, very low-birth-weight infants. N Engl J Med 2002;346:149–57.

Ment LR, Vohr B, Allan W. Change in cognitive function over time in very low-birth-weight infants. JAMA 2003;289:705–11.

Roland EH, Hill A. Germinal matrix-intraventricular hemorrhage in the premature newborn: management and outcome. Neurol Clin 2003;21:833–51.

O'Shea MT, Allred EN, Kuban KC, et al. Intraventricular hemorrage and developmental outcomes at 24 months of age in extremely preterm infants. J Child Neurol 2012;27:22–9.

PRETERM BRAIN DEVELOPMENT AND PERIVENTRICULAR LEUKOMALACIA

57. **What factors influence neurodevelopmental outcome after prematurity?**

Gestational age significantly affects later prognosis. Overall, infants born extremely premature (22 to 25 weeks) are at a higher risk (50% to 75%) for death or neurodevelopmental impairments, including moderate or severe cerebral palsy (CP), bilateral blindness, and lower cognitive performance at age two. However, these risks are influenced not only by gestational age but also by sex, exposure to antenatal corticosteroids, twin or other multiple gestation, and birth weight. The EPICure study found fewer than half (41%) of children with a history of extreme prematurity (<26 weeks' gestation) when tested at age 6 years were cognitively impaired compared with their classmates. The rates of severe, moderate, and mild disability were 22%, 24%, and 34%, respectively. Disabling CP was present in 12% (Fig. 14-7).

Although prognosis is much more optimistic for infants born late preterm, some increased risk of learning or behavior problems remains. One recent study found the risk of developmental delay or disability was increased by 36% among babies born between 34 and 36 weeks' gestation compared with those born at term.

Tyson JE, Parikh NA, Laner J, et al. Intensive care for extreme prematurity—moving beyond gestational age. New Engl J Med 2008;358:1672–81.

Morse SB, Zheng H, Tang Y, et al. Early school-age outcomes of late preterm infants. Pediatrics 2009;123:e622–e629.

Marlow N, Wolke D, Bracewell MA, et al. EPICure Study Group: Neurologic and developmental disability at six years of age after extremely preterm birth. N Engl J Med 2005;352:9–19.

58. **What is PVL, and where is it localized?**

Periventricular leukomalacia (PVL) is white matter necrosis, seen mostly in preterm babies. This white matter necrosis surrounding the ventricular walls may be cystic (with fluid-filled cavities) or noncystic. However, white matter injury can extend far beyond the periventricular region; the anterior and posterior periventricular regions are most commonly affected. The former region is where white matter fibers pass to the legs, accounting for subsequent leg spasticity, and the latter, posterior area is responsible for the visual abnormalities of PVL.

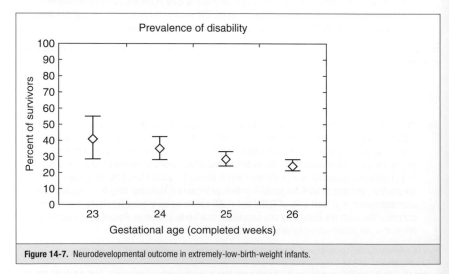

Figure 14-7. Neurodevelopmental outcome in extremely-low-birth-weight infants.

59. **How can white matter development be affected in preterm babies without PVL?**

Underdevelopment of the white matter and hypomyelination are seen at term in 50% of VLBW survivors as diffuse excessive high signal intensity (DEHSI) in the centrum semiovale of the white matter on T2 MRI sequences. As injured white matter fails to grow, ex vacuo ventriculomegaly becomes visible on ultrasound, CT, and MRI scans. Even in the absence of marked ventriculomegaly, many premature infants will demonstrate overall loss of white matter volume.

60. **What is the current thinking about the pathogenesis of PVL?**

The two most common factors that may increase the risk of white matter injury in the preterm infant are hypoxia-ischemia and infection. However, PVL can definitely occur in the absence of either documented hypoxia-ischemia or infection.

- Hypoxia-ischemia: The blood vessels supplying the white matter surrounding the lateral ventricles are arrayed radially, thus creating vascular end zones. In sick preterm infants autoregulation may be blunted or absent. Thus systemic hypotension can result in low cerebral blood flow and poor perfusion to the deep periventricular vascular regions. Low cerebral blood flow may lead to brain tissue hypoxia followed by glutamate and free radical damage to the preoligodendrocytes, the precursor cells to the oligodendrocytes that form the white matter.
- Maternal or fetal infections: Infection can produce cytokines that may cross the blood–brain barrier of the fetus. The cytokines set off an inflammatory cascade and activate white matter microglia that secrete products that damage those same preoligodendrocytes.

Volpe JJ. Cerebral white matter injury of the premature infant: more common than you think. Pediatrics 2003;112:176–80.

O Khwaja, JJ Volpe. Pathogenesis of cerebral white matter injury of prematurity. Arch Dis Child Fetal Neonatal Edition 2008;93(2):F153–F161.

61. **What are the neuroimaging correlates of PVL in VLBW babies?**

In the first days and weeks after injury, PVL may appear as a bright "periventricular flare." Approximately 2 to 3 weeks later, some infants may exhibit cystic changes which can be detected on cranial ultrasound. When VLBW babies reach term gestation, DEHSI and ventriculomegaly can be observed on T2 MRI images, in addition to the aforementioned cysts and infarcts. After 6 months to 2 years, the MRI will demonstrate periventricular hypomyelination and white matter scarring (particularly, but not exclusively, in the frontal and posterior periventricular areas), ventriculomegaly, ventricular wall scalloping and irregularity, thinning of the corpus callosum, and brain atrophy. In the setting of PVL, volumetric MRI studies also commonly show shrinkage of gray matter in the cortex and the deep lentiform nuclei.

Counsell SJ, Allsop JM, Harrison MC. Diffusion weighted imaging of the brain in preterm infants with focal and diffuse white matter abnormality. Pediatrics 2003;112:1–7.

62. **What are the common neurologic sequelae of PVL?**

The principal sequelae include spastic diplegia and visual and cognitive deficits.

63. **Name the primary visual deficits related to PVL.**

- Poor visual acuity
- Delayed visual maturation
- Strabismus

HYPOXIC ISCHEMIC ENCEPHALOPATHY (HIE)

64. **What is HIE?**

Recall first that the syndrome of ANE (see Question 3) is not synonomous with HIE. HIE is a specific neurologic syndrome in the newborn infant that results from low oxygen and blood delivery to the brain. For an intrapartum event to contribute to neonatal brain injury, the following should be present: (1) a history of intrauterine distress, (2) depression at birth, and (3) an obvious neonatal neurologic syndrome in the immediate postnatal period.

American College of Obstetricians and Gynecologists and American Academy of Pediatrics, editors. Neonatal encephalopathy and cerebral palsy: defining the pathogenesis and pathophysiology. Washington, DC: ACOG and AAP; 2003.

65. **What are the American College of Obstetricians and Gynecologists (ACOG) and American Academy of Pediatrics (AAP) criteria to define an intrapartum event sufficient to cause CP?**
Essential criteria (must meet all four):
- Evidence of a metabolic acidosis in fetal umbilical cord arterial blood obtained at delivery (pH <7 and base deficit ≥12 mmol/L)
- Early onset of severe or moderate neonatal encephalopathy in infants born at 34 or more weeks of gestation
- Resulting CP of the spastic quadriplegic or dyskinetic type
- Exclusion of other identifiable etiologies, such as trauma, coagulation disorders, infectious conditions, or genetic disorders

Criteria that collectively suggest an intrapartum timing (within close proximity to labor and delivery, [e.g., 0–48 hours]) but are nonspecific to asphyxial insults:
- A sentinel (signal) hypoxic event occurring immediately before or during labor
- A sudden and sustained fetal bradycardia or the absence of fetal heart rate variability in the presence of persistent, late, or variable decelerations, usually after a hypoxic sentinel event when the pattern was previously normal
- Apgar scale score of 0 to 3 beyond 5 minutes
- Onset of multisystem involvement within 72 hours of birth
- Early imaging study showing evidence of acute nonfocal cerebral abnormality

66. **How often is neonatal encephalopathy caused by intrapartum asphyxia?**
Although definitions and methods of study vary, most research suggests that ANE is *not* usually the result of isolated intrapartum HIE. For example, one case-control study identified numerous risk factors for ANE, such as maternal infertility treatment, maternal thyroid disease, and severe preeclampsia, all of which were antenatal. Similarly, a Scottish neuropathology study examined the brains of infants with ANE who died soon after delivery. Among 53 neonates initially thought clinically to have "birth asphyxia," the majority had histopathologic evidence of brain injury that could have only predated labor and delivery.

Badawi N, Kurinczuk JJ, Keogh JM, et al. Antepartum risk factors for newborn encephalopathy: the Western Austrialian case-control study. BMJ 1998;317(7172):1549–53.

Becher JC, Bell JE, Keeling JW, et al. The Scottish perinatal neuropathology study: clinicopathological correlation in early neonatal deaths. Arch Dis Child Fetal Neonatal Ed 2004;89:F399–F407.

67. **What factors would suggest hypoxia-ischemia that predates delivery?**
Some babies with ANE have evidence of hypoxic-ischemic injury that started before labor and delivery. For example, one retrospective series of babies with ANE found that at initial presentation to the hospital 70% already had absent fetal movements and nonreactive fetal heart rate tracings (absence of spontaneous cardiac accelerations), and many had chronic meconium staining. This constellation of findings is consistent with a prior hypoxic-ischemic event. Additional evidence has recently emerged that babies with an admission history of "reduced fetal movements" had already sustained a brain injury; these patients may not benefit from therapeutic hypothermia and may show a "subacute" injury pattern on MRI.

Phelan JP, Ahn MO. Perinatal observations in forty-eight neurologically impaired infants. Am J Obstetrics and Gynecology 1994;171(2):424–31.

Bonifacio SI, Glass HC, Vanderpluym J, et al. Perinatal events and magnetic resonance imaging in therapeutic hypothermia. J Pediatr 2011;158:360–5.

TABLE 14-7.	MANIFESTATIONS OF ORGAN INJURY IN TERM ASPHYXIATED INFANTS*

Data from Perlman JM, Tack ED, Martin T, et al. Acute systemic organ injury in term infants after asphyxia. Am J Dis Child 1989;143:617–20; and Martin–Ancel A, Garcia–Alix A, Gaya F, et al. Multiple organ involvement in perinatal asphyxia. J Pediatr 1995;127:786–93.

ORGAN	PERCENTAGE OF TOTAL
None	22%
CNS only	16%
CNS and one or more other organs	46%
Other organ(s), no CNS	16%

CNS, Central nervous system.
*Cumulative total of 107 term infants; definition of asphyxia in both series included umbilical cord arterial pH <7.2.

68. **What are the Sarnat encephalopathy stages, and how are they clinically useful?**
    - Stage 1: Mild encephalopathy in a newborn infant who is hyperalert, irritable, and oversensitive to stimulation. There is evidence of sympathetic overstimulation with tachycardia, dilated pupils, and jitteriness.
    - Stage 2: Moderate encephalopathy with the newborn displaying lethargy, hypotonia, and proximal weakness. There is parasympathetic overstimulation with low resting heart rate, small pupils, and copious secretions. The EEG is abnormal, and 70% of infants will have seizures.
    - Stage 3: Severe encephalopathy with a stuporous, flaccid newborn and absent reflexes. The newborn may have seizures and has an abnormal EEG with decreased background activity, voltage suppression, or both.

    The use of the Sarnat scoring system gives clinicians a shorthand method to categorize the severity of infants' ANE.

69. **Which other markers support a hypoxic-ischemic basis for neonatal encephalopathy?**
    When hypoxia-ischemia does produce ANE, it is typically expected that other body organs and systems are also affected, although this does not occur in every case. This could clinically include (1) hypoxic-ischemic depression of the myocardium (hypotension requiring volume expanders and pressor support); (2) acute renal failure (low urine output, hematuria, and climbing creatinine values); (3) hepatopathy with elevated liver enzymes and sometimes coagulopathy owing to multiple clotting factor deficiencies; (4) necrotizing enterocolitis; and (5) muscle ischemia resulting in excessively elevated serum creatine kinase. Multisystem dysfunction is not unique to HIE, however, and can be seen in other conditions, such as septic shock (Table 14-7).

70. **Why and how is brain monitoring performed on a baby with HIE?**
    Brain monitoring is the only direct way to measure the function of the brain after HIE or any cause of ANE. The gold standard for neonatal brain monitoring is continuous video-EEG recording. This allows the most accurate description of the EEG background, a sensitive and specific tool to formulate a neurologic prognosis. It is also the most objective method to diagnose and accurately quantify electrographic seizures, which occur in up to two of every three neonates after HIE. When continuous video-EEG monitoring is unavailable, amplitude-integrated EEG ([aEEG], popularly called cerebral function monitoring) or a series of routine EEG examinations are also very useful.

Shellhaas RA, Chang T, Tsuchida T, et al. The American Clincial Neurophysiology Society's guideline on continuous electroencephalography monitoring in neonates. J Clin Neurophys 2011;28(6):611–7.

71. **Which areas of the CNS are injured by HIE in a term newborn, and why?**
    The patterns of brain injury vary with gestational age and the duration and severity of the asphyxia event (Table 14-8).

TABLE 14-8. SITES OF PREDILECTION FOR THE DIFFUSE FORM OF HYPOXIC-ISCHEMIC SELECTIVE NEURONAL INJURY IN PREMATURE AND TERM NEWBORNS*

BRAIN REGION	PREMATURE	TERM NEWBORN
Cerebral neocortex		+
Hippocampus		
Sommer sector		+
Subiculum	+	
Deep nuclear structures		
Caudate–putamen	+	+
Globus pallidus	+	+
Thalamus	+	+
Brainstem		
Cranial nerve nuclei	+	+
Pons (ventral)	+	+
Inferior olivary nuclei	+	+
Cerebellum		
Purkinje cells		+
Granule cells (internal, external)	±	±
Spinal cord		
Anterior horn cells (alone)		±
Anterior horn cells and contiguous cells (? infarction)	±	

*See text for references.
+, Common; ±, less common.

There are several different HIE pathways, which are associated with their own distinctive pattern of neonatal brain injury. In acute, profound, near total asphyxia, the hypoxia-ischemia is actually caused by an abrupt prolonged terminal bradycardia. Prolonged terminal bradycaria results from a uterine rupture, cord prolapse, sudden total placental abruption, or maternal cardiac arrest, among other conditions. In acute, near total asphyxia, brain injury is mostly confined to the deep gray structures (globus pallidus, caudate, putamen, and thalami) and sometimes the gray and white matter of the bilateral perirolandic regions. A different type of injury is seen in partial prolonged asphyxia owing to a progressive but more gradual loss of brain oxygenation and perfusion. Slowly progressive placental abruption is an example of one condition that leads to a partial prolonged type of asphyxia causing a watershed brain injury pattern with prominent edema of the deep white matter, creating slitlike lateral ventricles. These patterns of insult are not mutually exclusive, and some babies show both watershed and deep gray lesions. There is growing evidence that maternal–fetal inflammation or infection may predispose the fetus to hypoxic-ischemic injury. Furthermore, maternal–fetal infection or inflammation can produce a clinical syndrome and MRI pattern that closely mimic genuine HIE.

Roland EH, Poskitt K, Rodriguez E, et al. Perinatal hypoxic-ischemic thalamic injury: clinical features and neuroimaging. Ann Neurol 1998;44:161–6.

Pasternak JF, Gorey MT. The syndrome of acute near-total intrauterine asphyxia in the term infant. Pediatr Neurol 1998;18:391–8.

TABLE 14-9. OUTCOME OF TERM INFANTS WITH HYPOXIC-ISCHEMIC ENCEPHALOPATHY AS A FUNCTION OF SEVERITY OF NEONATAL NEUROLOGICAL SYNDROME*

Data from Robertson C, Finer N. Term infants with hypoxic-ischemic encephalopathy: outcome at 3.5 years. Dev Med Child Neurol 1985;27:473–84; and Thornberg E, Thiringer K, Odeback A, et al. Birth asphyxia: incidence, clinical course and outcome in a Swedish population. Acta Paediatr 1995;84:927–32.

SEVERITY OF NEONATAL SYNDROME	NO. OF PATIENTS	DEATHS	PERCENTAGE OF TOTAL NEUROLOGICAL SEQUELAE	NORMAL
Mild	115	0%	0%	100%
Moderate	136	5%	24%	71%
Severe	40	80%	20%	0%
All	291	13%	14%	73%

*Derived from 291 full-term infants with hypoxic-ischemic encephalopathy.

Myers RE. Two patterns of perinatal brain damage and their conditions of occurrence. Am J Obstet Gynecol 1972;112:246–76.

Eklind S, Mallard C, Leverin A, et al. Bacterial endotoxin sensitizes the immature brain to hypoxic-ischemic injury. Eur J Neurosci 2001;13:1101–6.

72. **What is the pathogenesis of HIE at the cellular level?**
The initial deprivation of oxygen causes swelling and necrotic cell death in the susceptible areas described previously. Thus early on an area of necrosis appears, surrounded by a penumbral area of brain in which reperfusion and reoxygenation takes place. In this area further cellular damage is created by glutamate release, which in turns leads to free radical and calpain (apoptotic death factor) release that causes programmed cell death. This is a secondary process that may go on for days to weeks after the initial asphyxial insult. Treatments for HIE target these elements of "secondary energy failure" in the days after the acute event.

73. **What are currently the most useful clinical and laboratory tools when estimating the prognosis in cases of HIE?**
Clinically, judicious use of the previously discussed Sarnat scoring method is helpful. Newborns with stage I generally do well. Surviving stage III newborns are at very high risk for spastic quadriplegia, intellectual disability, and seizures. Outcomes after Sarnat stage II are the most difficult to predict, and additional investigations may be very useful to refine the neurologic prognosis (Table 14-9). An initial cord pH below 7, elevated serum lactate levels, evidence of multisystem involvement, and increased creatine kinase values in blood also have been correlated to guarded prognosis.

74. **What are currently the most useful neurodiagnostic laboratory tools in estimating prognosis in cases of HIE?**
The EEG may be very useful. A normal EEG background in the first 3 days has 90% to 100% specificity for a good outcome. Interictal EEG patterns of burst suppression and inactive low-voltage background have extremely guarded prognoses. This is particularly true when still present 24 hours after birth. MRI may also be helpful. Abnormalities appear early on diffusion-weighted images in 3 to 6 hours, and then 2 to 3 days later on T1- and T2-weighted sequences. An abnormal signal in the posterior limb of the internal capsule has a positive predictive value for motor impairment of nearly 100% when performed in infants of term equivalent age. Magnetic resonance spectroscopy (MRS) may also help define functional abnormality.

Rutherford M, Ward P, Allsop J, et al. Magnetic resonance imaging in neonatal encephalopathy. Early Hum Dev 2005;81:13–25.

Nash KB, Bonifacio SL, Glass HC, et al. Video-EEG monitoring in newborns with hypoxic-ischemic encephalopathy treated with hypothermia. Neurology 2011;76:556–82.

75. Are there objective markers of cerebral injury on MRI and MRS?

Apparent diffusion coefficient values from the posterior limb of the internal capsule are significantly greater in term infants with HIE who ultimately survive. Among survivors a reduced apparent diffusion coefficient value in the posterior limb on the internal capsule is associated with a greater probability of an abnormal neuromotor outcome. In contrast, an elevated N-acetylaspartate–to–total–creatine ratio is associated with a higher likelihood of a normal outcome at 18 months. Most important, the presence of an abnormal lactate peak predicts an abnormal outcome with a sensitivity of 100% and a specificity of 80%.

Barkovich AJ, Baranski K, Vigneron D, et al. Proton MR spectroscopy for the evaluation of brain injury in asphyxiated, term neonates. AJNR Am J Neuroradiol 1999;20:1399–1405.

Hunt RW, Neil JJ, Coleman LT, et al. Apparent diffusion coefficient in the posterior limb of the internal capsule predicts outcome after perinatal asphyxia. Pediatrics 2004;114:999–1003.

Wolf RL, Haselgrove JH, Clancy RR, et al. Quantitative apparent diffusion coefficient measurements in term neonates for early detection of hypoxic-ischemic brain injury: initial experience. Radiology 2001;218:825–33.

76. What treatment exists for HIE?

Multiple large, randomized, controlled trials have now shown therapeutic hypothermia is efficacious in reducing neurodevelopmental disability after HIE (Fig. 14-8). Therapeutic hypothermia (or "cooling") must be initiated within 6 hours of birth and continued for 72 hours to lower the neonate's body temperature to a target of 33.5° to 35° centigrade. Cooling may either be implemented through cooling blankets or selective head-cooling devices.

All affected newborns require supportive treatment. This includes maintenance of cardiorespiratory function, including ventilation when needed. Newborns with HIE require careful fluid, glucose, and electrolyte management, and the clinician must remember that the asphyxial insult may involve myocardium, kidneys, liver, and gastrointestinal tract. Finally, there must be a high suspicion for, and appropriate treatment of, seizures.

Gluckman PD, Wyatt JS, Azzopardi D, et al. Selective head cooling with mild systemic hypothermia after neonatal encephalopathy: multicentre randomised trial. Lancet 2005;365:663–70.

Shankaran S, Laptook AR, Ehrenkranz RA, et al. Whole-body hypothermia for neonates with hypoxic-ischemic encephalopathy. N Engl J Med 2005;353(15):1574–84.

Azzopardi DV, Strohm B, Edwards AD, et al. Moderate hypothermia to treat perinatal asphyxial encephalopathy. N Engl J Med 2009;361(14):1349–58.

Hypothermia and other treatment options for neonatal encephalopathy: an executive summary of the Eunice Kennedy Shriver NICHD Workshop. J Pediatr 2011;159(5):851–8.

AD Edwards, et al. Neurological outcomes at 18 months of age after moderate hypothermia for perinatal hypoxic ischaemic encephalopathy: synthesis and meta-analysis of trial data. BMJ 2010;340:c363.

Study or subgroup	Hypothermia		Normothermia		Risk ratio (95% CI)	Weight (%)	Risk ratio (95% CI)
	Events	Total	Events	Total			
TOBY	74	163	86	162		39.0	0.86 (0.68 to 1.07)
NICHD	45	102	64	106		28.3	0.73 (0.56 to 0.95)
CoolCap	59	116	73	118		32.7	0.82 (0.65 to 1.03)
Total (95% CI)		381		386		100.00	0.81 (0.71 to 0.93)
Total events	178		223				

0.2 0.5 1 2 5
Favors hypothermia   Favors normothermia

Figure 14-8. Summary of meta-analysis demonstrating beneficial effect of hypothermia on outcomes following neonatal HIE. (Edwards AD, Brocklehurst P, Gunn AJ, et al. Neurological outcomes at 18 months of age after moderate hypothermia for perinatal hypoxic ischaemic encephalopathy: synthesis and meta-analysis of trial data. BMJ 2010;340:c363.)

STROKE

77. What is the study of choice to diagnose neonatal stroke?

In any sick newborn with seizures or a focal neurologic abnormality, the suspicion for an underlying structural lesion should be high. Ultrasound examination may be useful at the bedside for detecting strokes, though sensitivity is highly user dependent. CT scans are superior to ultrasound in the acute setting; however, they lack the detail of MRI and expose the infant to radiation. MRI is thus the diagnostic test of choice. Diffusion-weighted images can detect recent strokes from as little as 6 hours to 7 days after the event. Traditional MRI sequences (T1 and T2) are adequate for more remote strokes.

Cowan FM, Pennock JM, Hanrahan JD, et al. Early detection of cerebral infarction and hypoxic ischemic encephalopathy in neonates using diffusion-weighted magnetic resonance imaging. Neuropediatrics 1994;25:172–5.

78. What is the further diagnostic work-up of perinatal stroke?
(Table 14-10)

Once stroke is diagnosed, an etiologic work-up should be undertaken, along with evaluation for comorbidities. The placenta should undergo a careful histopathologic examnination because it is a likely source for emboli. Infants with stroke should undergo a complete blood count to rule out polycythemia; lupus anticoagulant and protein C, protein S, and antithrombin III levels should be measured. Genetic tests looking for factor V Leiden mutation, MTHFR mutation, and prothrombin 20210G mutation are indicated. An echocardiogram to rule out a cardiac source of emboli should also be done, particularly if any cardiac signs are present or if the infant has experienced a multifocal stroke. An EEG might demonstrate electrographic seizures, slowing, or attenuation. Magnetic resonance angiography and venography help visualize the cerebral vessels to rule out pathology.

Nelson KB, Lynch KB. Stroke in newborn infants. Lancet Neurol 2004;3:150–6.

79. What is the therapy and outcome of perinatal stroke?

Initial management includes general medical support and administration of antiseizure medications if the child has seizures. Anticoagulation is controversial and is probably not indicated unless an active source of emboli is apparent. In a recent review of outcomes in infants with strokes in the perinatal period, 40% of infants were judged to be normal, 57% were neurologically or cognitively abnormal, and 3% died.

TABLE 14-10. SUGGESTED DIAGNOSTIC WORK-UP OF NEONATAL STROKE	
HISTORY	**FACTORS NOTED IN TABLE 7-2**
Radiologic examination	Cranial ultrasound, magnetic resonance imaging/angiography/venography with diffusion-weighted imaging If appropriate, echocardiography, ultrasound of neck vessels or indwelling catheters
Laboratory examination*	Coagulopathy work-up: proteins C and S, antithrombin III, factor V Leiden, anticardiolipin Ab, lupus anticoagulant/antiphospholipid Ab, fasting homocysteine, methylene tetrahydrofolate reductase C 677T mutation, prothrombin 20210 variant, lipoprotein (a), fibrinogen, plasminogen, factor VIIIC
Placental evaluation	Complete pathologic examination of placenta

*There is no consensus regarding the number of these tests that should be performed in cases of ischemic perinatal stroke.

Lynch JK, Nelson KB Epidemiology of perinatal stroke. Curr Opin Pediatr 2001;13:499–505.

Mercuri E, Rutherford M, Cowan F, et al. Early prognostic indicators of outcome in infants with neonatal cerebral infarction: a clinical, electroencephalogram, and magnetic resonance imaging study. Pediatrics 1999;103:39–46.

80. **When is sinovenous thrombosis most likely to occur?**

    Sinovenous thrombosis has been increasingly recognized, and its true incidence likely exceeds early estimates of 1 per 100,000. Identifiable causes are those that would increase the overall risk of thrombosis in a newborn. They include dehydration, extracorporeal membrane oxygenation (ECMO), and congenital heart disease. Similarly, genetic thrombophilias are a risk factor. Many cases are multifactorial. Newborns have a higher risk for sinovenous thrombosis than members of any other age group.

Wu YW, Miller SP, Chin K, et al. Multiple risk factors in neonatal sinovenous thrombosis. Neurology 2002;3:438–40.

81. **How does sinovenous thrombosis present? How is diagnosis confirmed?**

    The clinical presentation is usually nonspecific; lethargy and poor feeding are the most common signs. Seizures are another initial early sign. Neuroimaging is required for diagnosis. Although thrombus may be directly visualized on MRI, other supportive findings are absence of Doppler flow through the affected vein on cranial ultrasound and decreased flow on magnetic resonance venography. The straight sinus and superior sagittal sinus are most often involved, although multiple sinuses are often affected. The diagnosis may be difficult because deeper thrombosis is harder to visualize.

Kersbergen KJ, Groenendaal F, Benders MJNL, de Vries LS. Neonatal cerebral sinovenous thrombosis: neuroimaging and long-term follow-up. J Child Neurol 2011;26:1111–20.

Florieke JB, Kersbergen KJ, van Ommen CH, et al. Neonatal cerebral sinovenous thrombosis from symptom to outcome. Stroke 2010;41:1382–8.

82. **How are hemorrhagic infarcts related to sinovenous thrombosis?**

    Some cases of sinovenous thrombosis disrupt blood flow out of parenchymal tissue such that there is a resulting blockade of arteriolar blood perfusing that tissue. This disruption of blood flow can cause brain infarction and secondary hemorrhagic transformation. Venous infarction is often distinguished from arterial infarction on MRI by its distribution. Arterial infarction more likely appears as a wedge-shaped stroke in an arterial vascular distribution, whereas venous infarction arises in the context of sinovenous thrombosis and is more likely to result in hemorrhage.

83. **How do outcomes of sinovenous thrombosis compare with those of arterial strokes?**

    Although the location and size of injury play important roles in shaping outcomes, prognosis after sinovenous thrombosis is generally worse than that after arterial stroke. One prospective study of 104 newborns found 61% at follow-up had either died or experienced a disability, including epilepsy, moderate to severe language deficits, and CP.

Moharir MD, Shroff M, Pontigon AM, et al. A prospective outcome study of neonatal cerebral sinovenous thrombosis. J Child Neruol 2011;26:1137–44.

PERINATAL ILLNESS AND LATER CP

84. **What is CP, and how does it relate to neonatal factors?**

    CP is a nonprogressive disorder of motor function ("a palsy") of CNS ("cerebral") origin occurring usually *in utero* or early in life (up to age 2 years). Intellectual deficit is not implicit in CP, although it accompanies the motor disability in a high percentage of cases. The overall prevalence of CP is 1.7 to 2 of 1000 among survivors at the age of 1 year. Premature infants have the highest incidence of CP, although most infants with CP have birth weights greater than 2500 g. The lower the birth weight and gestational age, the greater chance for the child to develop CP. Although the CNS injury that leads to CP usually occurs in the perinatal period, the signs of CP may not be obvious until after the first year.

United Cerebral Palsy. <http://www.ucp.org>; [accessed 27.08.12].

85. **Why is CP difficult to diagnose clinically in the first year of life?**
In a very broad sense, all healthy neonates show motor signs similar to those of CP. All healthy neonates lack purposeful, voluntary movements, and their motor activities are dominated by developmental reflexes. They have reflex overflow of deep tendon reflexes, clonus (unsustained), and Babinski signs. As they age and mature, they become able to subjugate their involuntary reflexes and gain mastery and control over their motor systems. Consequently, the neonate with damaged motor systems may not look entirely different from a healthy baby during examination. Keep in mind that in babies with CP, the following is true:
- Hypotonia is more common than hypertonia and spasticity in the first year.
- Infants have a limited variety of volitional movements for evaluation.
- Substantial myelination takes months to evolve and may delay the clinical picture of abnormal tone and increased deep tendon reflexes.
- Choreoathetosis (e.g., that resulting from acute kernicterus) often is not obvious before the first birthday.

86. **How does maternal infection affect the incidence of CP in term children of normal birth weight?**
Maternal temperature above 38° C (100.4° F) during labor or a clinical diagnosis of chorioamnionitis is associated with a markedly (ninefold) increased risk of CP, especially spastic quadriplegic CP (19-fold increase). Remember that approximately 50% of maternal cases of chorioamnionitis are subclinical.

Neufeld MD, Frigon C, Graham AS, et al. Maternal infection and risk of cerebral palsy in term and preterm infants. J Perinatol 2005;2:108–13.
Wu YW, Escobar GJ, Grether JK, et al. Chorioamnionitis and cerebral palsy in term and near-term infants. JAMA 2003;290:2677–84.

87. **What is the evidence to suggest that inflammatory cytokines are associated with prematurity and development of CP?**
The inflammatory response to infection activates a number of cytokines and chemokines, which in turn may trigger preterm contractions, cervical ripening, rupture of the membranes, and prematurity. The levels of interleukin (IL)-1, IL-8, IL-9, and tumor necrosis factor are independent risk factors for the subsequent development of CP at the age of 3 years.

Hagberg H, Mallard C, Jacobsson B. Role of cytokines in preterm labour and brain injury. BJOG 2005;112(Suppl 1):16–8.
Yoon BH, Park CW, Chaiworapongsa T. Intrauterine infection and the development of cerebral palsy. BJOG 2003;110(Suppl 20):124–7.

88. **How has the prevalence of CP changed since the advent of neonatal intensive care in the 1960s?**
The prevalence rose approximately 20% from the early 1960s to the late 1980s, almost entirely because of increased survival of low-birth-weight and VLBW infants. Since the 1980s there has been no significant change.

NEONATAL SEIZURES

89. **What are neonatal seizures?**
There are two ways to define neonatal seizures: electrographically and clinically. EEG seizures are defined as a sudden (paroxysmal) attack of abnormal, hypersynchronous electrical discharges in the brain. Clinical seizures are a sudden (paroxysmal) attack of abnormal-appearing movements,

behaviors, or autonomic functions. There is a very imperfect overlap between clinical and EEG seizures. Clinical seizures that are specifically linked to simultaneous EEG seizures are called electroclinical. Abnormal-appearing clinical seizures that occur without simultaneous EEG seizures are classified as non-epileptic seizures. EEG seizures that do not provoke any outwardly visible motor or autonomic signs are called subclinical, silent, or occult seizures.

90. **What clinical signs may be evident during seizures?**
   - Autonomic changes: Sudden, unexplained autonomic signs such as apnea, episodic hypertension or tachycardia, flushing, tearing, or salivation may be the only outward manifestation of a seizure.
   - Clonic seizures: These are characterized by sustained, repetitive, rhythmic jerking movements of a muscle group. Clonic seizures may be focal or multifocal, involving several body parts, often in a migrating fashion.
   - Focal tonic seizures: These are characterized by abrupt changes in muscle *tone*. Sustained changes in muscle tone modify the body's posture. Focal tonic seizures may produce posturing of an arm or leg or the extraocular muscles, leading to a sustained, unnatural deviation of both eyes to one side.

91. **How often are seizures subtle, or subclinical?**
   Multiple studies have shown that upward of 80% of confirmed EEG seizures in the neonate are invisible to the naked eye and have no outward signs detectable by bedside caregivers. Accurate detection and diagnosis of neonatal seizures therefore requires EEG monitoring.

Murray DM, Boylan GB, Ali I, et al. Defining the gap between electrographic seizure burden, clinical expression, and staff recognition of neonatal seizures. Arch Dis Child Fetal Neonatal Ed 2008;93:F187–191.

92. **How does aEEG compare with conventional EEG monitoring for detection of seizures?**
   The sensitivity of aEEG for seizure detection depends in part on the experience of the user in interpreting these recordings. Although experts have reported theoretical sensitivity of approximately 80%, most users correctly identify fewer than half of seizures using aEEG alone.

Shah DK, Mackay MT, Lavery S, et al. Accuracy of bedside electroencephalographic monitoring in comparison with simultaneous continuous conventional electroencephalography for seizure detection in term infants. Pediatrics 2008;121(6):1146–54.

93. **What is the incidence of neonatal seizures?**
   Seizures are the most common clinical sign of neonatal cerebral dysfunction and may occur in up to 1% of all newborns. The reported incidence of neonatal seizures, however, varies with the population studied, gestational age, and risk status. It also depends on the standard used to diagnose seizures.

94. **What are the common causes of neonatal seizures?**
   Most neonatal seizures are symptomatic of an acute illness. ANE is the most frequent cause of neonatal seizures. HIE is but one specific type of ANE. Other common causes of brain injury include stroke, hemorrhage, infection, cerebral malformation, drug withdrawal, and metabolic causes. The latter include hypoglycemia and electrolyte abnormalities, hyponatremia, hypocalcemia, hypomagnesemia, and inborn errors of metabolism (e.g., urea cycle defects, phenylketonuria, maple syrup urine disease, lactic and organic acidurias, and nonketotic hyperglycinemia). A small percentage of unprovoked neonatal seizures are caused by specific genetic disorders.

95. **What are the vitamin-responsive causes of neonatal seizures?**
   Vitamin-responsive neonatal seizures, especially vitamin B_6 dependency, should always be considered in seizures refractory to treatment, particularly without a clear symptomatic etiology. Other vitamin and cofactor deficiencies with the potential to cause seizures include molybdenum, pyridoxal phosphate, and folinic acid.

Pearl PL. New treatment paradigms in the metabolic epilepsies. J Inherit Metab Dis 2009;32(2):204–13.

96. **What are other causes of refractory or malignant neonatal seizures and epilepsy?**

There are increasing numbers of recognized malignant epilepsy syndromes with onset in the neonatal period. Many of these are characterized by refractory seizures, a characteristic EEG pattern, and a poor prognosis. Examples include early infantile epileptic encephalopathy with burst-suppression (Ohtahara syndrome) and early myoclonic epilepsy. Some of these syndromes are now understood to have multiple underlying causes, including structural lesions, metabolic disease, and genetic mutations. A malignant epilepsy syndrome should be suspected when no symptomatic cause for seizures can be found and when seizures remain refractory to initial treatment.

Deprez L, Weckhuysen S, Holmgren P. Clinical spectrum of early-onset epileptic encephalopathies associated with STXBP1 mutations. Neurology 2010;75:1159–65.

Yamamoto H, Okumura A, Fukuda M. Epilepsies and epileptic syndromes starting in the neonatal period. Brain Dev 2011;33:213–20.

Ficicioglu C, Bearden D. Isolated neonatal seizures: when to suspect inborn errors of metabolism. Pediatr Neurol 2011 Nov;45(5):283–91.

97. **What are the more benign causes of neonatal seizures?**

Seizures in a "well baby" may be caused by simple hypocalcemia or hypoglycemia or may be the first sign of a *benign neonatal epilepsy*. Hypocalcemia and hypocalcemic tetany resulting from milks with a high phosphate load are now rarely seen in the United States. Benign neonatal epilepsy syndromes have been described and have a relatively good prognosis for seizure remission and development. The familial syndromes are associated with genetic mutations in sodium or potassium channels.

Berkovic SF, Heron SE, Giordano L, et al. Benign familial neonatal-infantile seizures: characterization of a new sodium channelopathy. Ann Neurol 2004;55:550–7.

98. **How are neonatal seizures evaluated?**

The work-up should include a bedside glucose measurement followed by a laboratory glucose measurement and determination of calcium, magnesium, sodium, and acid–base status. A blood culture and lumbar puncture should be performed. A cranial ultrasound scan may confirm suspected hemorrhage and hydrocephalus, but MRI is best to evaluate for malformations of cortical development and the extent of any acquired injury such as stroke or sinovenous thrombosis. Testing should not delay symptomatic treatment of seizures.

99. **Once a diagnosis is confirmed, is the EEG helpful in the management of neonatal seizures?**

Continuous EEG monitoring is the most accurate and comprehensive method to confirm the diagnosis and measure the abundance and spatial distribution of EEG seizures. It is also useful in monitoring ongoing treatment. Ideally, treatment with antiseizure medications should terminate all EEG seizures, but that is not always the case. When continuous EEG monitoring is not available, aEEG or a series of routine (60 minute duration) EEGs remains very helpful.

100. **What is the treatment of neonatal seizures?**

The initial treatment of neonatal seizures should always be aimed at correcting the underlying disorder and maintaining hemodynamic and respiratory stability. First-line pharmacologic treatment for neonatal seizures is usually phenobarbital, followed by phenytoin. Although their efficacy has never been demonstrated by a randomized, placebo-controlled trial, these drugs have the advantage of having been used for a long time in newborns. Phenobarbital or phenytoin are effective in suppressing seizures in less than half of neonates. When one drug fails, adding a second results in a 70% success rate. Third-line treatments (e.g., benzodiazepenes) are variable (Table 14-11).

Painter MJ, Scher MS, Stein AD, et al. Phenobarbital compared with phenytoin for the treatment of neonatal seizures. N Engl J Med 1999;341:485–9.

Clancy, RR. Summary proceedings from the neurology group on neonatal seizures. Pediatrics 2006;117:S23–S27.

TABLE 14-11. ANTICONVULSANT DRUGS FOR NEONATAL SEIZURES

From van de Bor M. The recognition and management of neonatal seizures. Curr Paediatr 2002;12:382–7.

DRUG*	LOADING DOSE	MAINTENANCE DOSE	WITHDRAWAL	SIDE EFFECTS
Phenobarbital	20 mg/kg IV max: 40 mg/kg	3-5 mg/kg per 24 h IV or PO	Irritability, altered sleep, tremors	Drowsiness
Midazolam	>35 wks GA: 0.05 mg/kg IV (in 10 min)	0.15 mg/kg/h	If seizure free for 24 h	Temporary reduction of blood pressure and cerebral blood flow
Lidocaine	2 mg/kg IV	6 mg/kg/h IV	After 24 h of treatment: 4 mg/kg/hr After 36 h: 2 mg/kg/h After 48 h: stop	Arrhythmia, seizures, hypotension
Clonazepam	0.15 mg/kg IV repeat 1-2 times	0.1 mg/kg per 24 h	If seizure-free for 24 h	
Phenytoin	20 mg/kg IV (infusion rate 1 mg/kg/min)	3-4 mg/kg per 24 h IV	At removal of IV lines	Dysrhythmia
Pyridoxine	50-100 mg	50-100 mg	If no effect: stop	
Thiopental	10 mg/kg IV	Increase dose until EEG shows burst-suppression.	After 24 h	Hypotension

*For each drug, monitoring should include blood pressure, respiratory status, and EEG. For lidocaine, ECG monitoring is a special consideration.
ECG, Electrocardiogram; EEG, electroencephalogram; GA, gestational age; IV, intravenous; PO, by mouth.

101. When is antiseizure medication tapered?

In the well-appearing baby with a normal EEG, early discontinuation of medication is recommended while the neonate is still in the intensive care unit or soon after discharge. Some clinicians prefer to continue treatment for 3 to 6 months after discharge.

102. What is the prognosis of neonates with seizures?

The ultimate prognosis is determined by the severity of the seizures' etiology and if the infant experienced status epilepticus. EEG background activity and MRI and MRS are also useful in predicting prognosis. Depending on etiology, between 25% and 33% of those with neonatal seizures go on to display chronic postnatal epilepsy, including serious conditions such as infantile spasms or the Lennox–Gastaut syndrome.

NEUROMUSCULAR DISORDERS

103. What is meant by central versus peripheral hypotonia?

Central hypotonia results from a CNS lesion—a problem in the brain or spinal cord. Peripheral hypotonia results from a lesion in the peripheral nervous system—the nerves, neuromuscular junction, or

TABLE 14-12.   CEREBRAL (CENTRAL) HYPOTONIA

Chromosomal disorders

Other genetic defects

Acute hemorrhagic and other brain injury

Hypoxic/ischemic encephalopathy

Peroxisomal disorders (e.g., Zellweger syndrome, neonatal adrenoleukodystrophy)

Metabolic defects

Drug intoxication

Benign congenital hypotonia

TABLE 14-13.   ANATOMIC LOCALIZATION OF HYPOTONIC WEAKNESS IN NEWBORN

	CNS LESION	ANT. HORN CELL	NERVE	NMJ	MUSCLE
Distribution	D (SA)	P > D	D	B (P)	P*
Symmetry	A	S	S	S	S
DTRs	Inc, N, Dim	0	0	N	Dim or 0
Face	N or A	N (F)	N	Ptosis 15%	Bifacial
Sensation	N or Dim	N	N or Dim	N	N

A, Asymmetric; ANT., anterior; B, bulbar; D, distal; Dim, diminished; DTRs, deep tendon reflexes; F, tongue fasciculations; Inc, increased; N, normal; NMJ, neuromuscular junction; P, proximal; S, symmetric; SA, shoulder–arm; 0, absent.
*Exception: myotonic dystrophy is D.

muscles. Central should not be confused with axial or "truncal" hypotonia, which describes hypotonia affecting primarily the core trunk muscles. Similarly, peripheral hypotonia should not be confused with "appendicular" hyptonia in the extremities.

104. **What is the differential diagnosis for central hypotonia?**
See Table 14-12.

105. **What are the components of the lower motor neuron? Why is it useful to think in terms of these anatomic entities when evaluating a floppy newborn infant?**
It is useful to think anatomically because clinical localization is facilitated in this way (Table 14-13). The components of the lower motor neuron from the spinal cord to most peripheral part are as follows:
- Anterior horn cell
- Peripheral nerve
- Neuromuscular junction
- Muscle (Table 14-14)

106. **What are the tests to confirm lower motor neuron disease?**
The physical examination shows weakness, atrophy, diminished to absent deep tendon reflexes, and sometimes fasiculations. Ancillary testing includes blood creatine phosphokinase measurement,

TABLE 14-14.	NEUROMUSCULAR DISEASES IN THE HYPOTONIC INFANT AND CHILD
Anterior horn cell or peripheral nerve	Spinal muscular atrophies
	Hypoxic-ischemic myelopathy
	Traumatic myelopathy
	Neurogenic arthrogryposis
	Congenital neuropathies: axonal
	Hypomyelinating
	Dejerine–Sottas disease
	Hereditary sensory and autonomic neuropathy
	Giant axonal neuropathy
	Metabolic inflammatory
Neuromuscular junction	Transient neonatal myasthenia gravis
	Congenital myasthenic syndromes
	Hypermagnesemia
	Aminoglycoside toxicity
	Infantile botulism
Muscle	Congenital muscular dystrophies
	Congenital myotonic dystrophy
	Infantile facioscapulohumeral muscular dystrophy
	Congenital myopathies
	Metabolic myopathies
	Mitochondrial myopathies

serum carnitine measurement, motor nerve conduction velocities, needle electromyography (EMG), DNA testing, and muscle biopsy.

- Elevated serum creatine phosphokinase values beyond the seventh postnatal day suggest active muscle disease, most commonly one of the congenital muscular dystrophies.
- Low carnitine levels either suggest the very rare primary carnitine deficiency or result from fatty acid or organic acid abnormalities.
- Abnormally low nerve conduction velocities suggest a neuropathy but are reported in 30% to 50% of cases of anterior horn cell disease. Needle EMG studies are helpful to distinguish a neuropathic from a myopathic process. Myotonia on insertion is rare in neonatal myotonic dystrophy but is invariably present in Pompe disease (i.e., acid maltase deficiency).
- DNA analysis is useful to confirm specific diseases; spinal muscular atrophy, myotonic dystrophy, and Prader–Willi syndrome are examples of conditions in which genetic diagnosis is possible.
- In some cases muscle biopsy (with both histologic and biochemical analysis) is the only way to make a precise diagnosis.

107. How should infants with hypotonia be evaluated?

Our stepwise approach to the diagnostic investigation of infantile hypotonia is as follows (Figure. 14-9):

- Conduct a detailed history (history of polyhydraminios, intrauterine growth retardation, reduced fetal movement), and physical examination, including tests of muscle stretch reflexes, antigravity limb movements, and contractures.
- Exclude systemic illness and congenital laxity of ligaments.
- If central hypotonia is suspected, conduct MRI or MR spectroscopy studies, metabolic studies, and genetic testing for Prader-Willi syndrome (deletion of 15q11-13) and Down syndrome (trisomy 21). Also test for very–long-chain fatty acids and/or perform other peroxisomal tests.

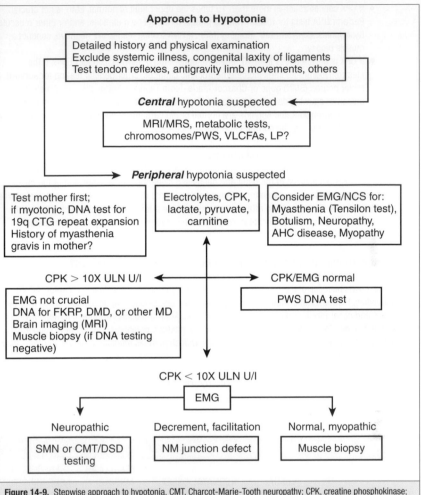

Approach to Hypotonia

Detailed history and physical examination
Exclude systemic illness, congenital laxity of ligaments
Test tendon reflexes, antigravity limb movements, others

Central hypotonia suspected

MRI/MRS, metabolic tests,
chromosomes/PWS, VLCFAs, LP?

Peripheral hypotonia suspected

Test mother first;
if myotonic, DNA test for
19q CTG repeat expansion
History of myasthenia
gravis in mother?

Electrolytes, CPK,
lactate, pyruvate,
carnitine

Consider EMG/NCS for:
Myasthenia (Tensilon test),
Botulism, Neuropathy,
AHC disease, Myopathy

CPK > 10X ULN U/l

CPK/EMG normal

EMG not crucial
DNA for FKRP, DMD, or other MD
Brain imaging (MRI)
Muscle biopsy (if DNA testing
negative)

PWS DNA test

CPK < 10X ULN U/l

EMG

Neuropathic

SMN or CMT/DSD
testing

Decrement, facilitation

NM junction defect

Normal, myopathic

Muscle biopsy

Figure 14-9. Stepwise approach to hypotonia. CMT, Charcot-Marie-Tooth neuropathy; CPK, creatine phosphokinase; DMD, Duchenne muscular dystrophy; EMG, electromyography; FKRP, fukutin-related protein; MD, muscular dystrophy; MRI, magnetic resonance imaging; MRS, magnetic resonance spectroscopy; NCS, nerve conduction study; NM, neuromuscular; SMN, survival motor neuron; VLCFAs, very-long-chain fatty acids.

Consider lumbar puncture for measurement of cerebrospinal fluid lactate, glucose, and protein and, if indicated, cerebrospinal fluid neurotransmitter testing.
- If peripheral hypotonia is suspected, first examine the mother. If she has signs of myotonic dystrophy, perform a DNA test for 19qCTG repeat expansion in the child. Elicit any history of autoimmune myasthenia gravis in the mother.
  □ Consider electromyography and nerve conduction studies to evaluate for myasthenia, botulism, neuropathy or anterior horn cell disease, and myopathy. Consider performing a Tensilon test if myasthenic syndrome is suspected.
  □ Measure the child's electrolytes, CPK, lactate, pyruvate, carnitine, and/or other biochemical markers:
    ● If CPK/EMG results are normal, conduct a DNA test for Prader-Willi syndrome.

- If CPK concentration is more than 10 times the upper limit of normal, EMG is not crucial. Perform DNA tests for fukutin-related protein (FKRP) gene mutations, and/or other muscular dystrophies. Consider brain imaging (MRI). If DNA testing results are negative, conduct a muscle biopsy.
- If CPK is elevated less than 10 times the upper limit of normal, conduct EMG. If the electromyogram findings indicate neurogenic changes, order genetic testing for survival motor neuron (SMN) gene or Charcot-Marie-Tooth/Dejerine-Sottas disease. An electromyogram showing decrement or facilitation indicates a neuromuscular junction defect. If the electromyographic findings are normal or indicate myopathy, conduct a muscle biopsy (EMG findings may be normal in certain myopathies).

108. What can cause ptosis is a newborn?

Unilateral ptosis is most commonly familial. Sometimes it is part of Horner syndrome, which also includes miosis (smallness) of the pupil and decreased sweating on the same side of the face. Neck masses, iatrogenic injury during cardiac surgery, and birth injury to the lower brachial plexus are other causes. Facial swelling after delivery may cause a temporary pseudoptosis. Bilateral ptosis is seen in centronuclear (myotubular) myopathy, myotonic dystrophy, and myasthenic syndromes.

109. What is transient neonatal myasthenia, and how is it diagnosed?

Transient neonatal myasthenia occurs in 15% of deliveries to mothers with autoimmune myasthenia gravis because of the transplacental passage of maternal acetylcholine receptor (AChR) antibodies. Predominant symptoms include respiratory and swallowing difficulties. There may be ptosis and generalized weakness with intact reflexes. AChR antibodies are present. Repetitive stimulation on EMG shows a decrement in muscle amplitude potentials. Treatment is supportive, but supplementation with subcutaneous or oral pyridostigmine is often necessary. Symptoms may persist for 1 to 5 weeks.

110. What are the congenital myasthenic syndromes?

See Table 14-15.

TABLE 14–15. CONGENITAL MYASTHENIC SYNDROMES				
BASIC ABNORMALITY	USUAL INHERITANCE	NEONATAL ONSET COMMON	EXTRAOCULAR MUSCLE WEAKNESS	RESPONSE TO ACHE INHIBITOR COMMON
Presynaptic Abnormalities				
Defects in ACh synthesis	Recessive	+	-	+
Paucity of synaptic vesicles	Recessive	+	-	+
Synaptic Abnormalities				
AChE deficiency	Recessive	+	+	-
Postsynaptic Abnormalities				
ACh receptor deficiency	Recessive	+	+	+
Slow-channel syndrome	Dominant	-	+	-
Postchannel syndrome	Recessive	+	-	?
ACh, Acetylcholine; AChE, acetylcholinesterase.				

111. **What are four characteristics of damage to the anterior horn cell?**
  - Weakness
  - Fasciculations (most easily observed on the tongue in the neonate)
  - Atrophy (difficult to see in the newborn because of adipose tissue surrounding almost all muscles)
  - Hyporeflexia or areflexia

112. **Why is myotonic dystrophy an example of the phenomenon of "anticipation"?**
  Genetic studies have shown that the defect in myotonic dystrophy is an expansion of a trinucleotide (CTG) repeat in a gene on the long arm of chromosome 19 that codes for a protein kinase. In successive generations this repeating sequence has a tendency to increase, sometimes into the thousands (normal is <40 CTG repeats), and the extent of repetition correlates with the severity. Thus an affected mother may have mild or subclinical symptoms, whereas the neonate with increased CTG repeats may be more severely affected.

CHAPTER 15

NEONATAL OPHTHALMOLOGY

Daniel A. Greninger, MD, and Michael F. Chiang, MD

NORMAL VISUAL DEVELOPMENT

1. How well does a normal term newborn see?
Term newborns can often fixate on a target. The ability to track an object, however, does not generally develop until approximately 2 months after birth. Visual acuity, measured with visual evoked potentials, has been estimated around 20/400 at birth. Color vision and contrast sensitivity have only rudimentary function in the newborn. Best-corrected visual acuity gradually improves during early childhood as the brain and retina mature.

2. Does visual development differ in the preterm infant?
The central retina is still actively developing throughout the 20th and 30th weeks of gestation. Myelination of the optic nerves and radiations continues during this time as well. Infants have fused eyelids until 25 weeks' gestational age (GA), and the lids can remain fused in some cases until 30 weeks' GA. The effects of these changes on the development of visual function are still being studied. It is unknown whether earlier exposure to visual stimuli has a positive or negative effect on eventual visual development. However, premature infants may demonstrate delayed visual milestones in early infancy.

3. What type of visual function can be observed in the NICU?
The pupillary light reflex should be observable after 31 weeks' gestational age. A blink reflex to light can often be observed a few days after birth.

Mills MD. The eye in childhood. Am Fam Physician 1999;60(3):907–16.
  Repka MX. Ophthalmological problems of the premature infant. Mental Retardation and Developmental Disabilities Research Reviews 2002;8:249–57.

BASIC OCULAR EXAMINATION

4. What are the basic components of a typical NICU eye examination?
The lids should be examined for any abnormalities, including malformation, swelling, or discharge. Pupils should be examined for signs of irregular shape. The cornea, lens, and retina should be assessed with the red reflex test.

5. How does the red reflex test work? Who should get it?
The red reflex test was well described in a policy statement by the American Academy of Pediatrics in 2008, part of which is included here. The test uses the transmission of light from an ophthalmoscope through all the normally transparent parts of a subject's eye, including the cornea, aqueous humor, lens, and vitreous. The light reflects off the retina and optic nerve, is transmitted back through the optical media and through the aperture of the ophthalmoscope, and is imaged in the eye of the examiner. Any factor that impedes or blocks this optical pathway will result in an abnormality of the red reflex.

  The test is performed by holding an ophthalmoscope close to the examiner's eye with power set at "0" and projecting the light simultaneously onto both eyes of the infant from a distance of approximately 18 inches away in a darkened room. Abnormalities include a diminished reflex, white reflex, or asymmetric reflexes.

Before discharge from the neonatal nursery, all children should have an examination of the red reflex of the eyes performed by a pediatrician or neonatologist. The test is important for the early detection of vision disorders and systemic diseases with eye manifestations. All infants with an abnormal or absent reflex should be referred immediately to an ophthalmologist.

6. Do the eyes need to be dilated to perform the red reflex test?

In general, no. An adequate examination can usually be performed through the undilated pupil. There has been some question as to whether pupil-dilated red reflex examinations improve identification of conditions such as retinoblastoma and congenital cataract, but this has not been definitively established.

7. What is leukocoria?

Leukocoria means "white pupil." Differential diagnosis includes retinoblastoma, retinal detachment, cataract, retinopathy of prematurity (ROP), coloboma, primary persistent hyperplastic vitreous, congenital infection, and vitreous hemorrhage. Prompt ophthalmologic consultation is important in cases of suspected leukocoria.

8. What are some causes of corneal clouding in a newborn?

Sclerocornea, Peters anomaly, forceps trauma, congenital glaucoma, congenital hereditary endothelial dystrophy, mucopolysaccaridoses, and corneal dermoids can result in a white or clouded appearance to the cornea and cause an abnormal red reflex. Prompt ophthalmologic consultation is important in cases of corneal clouding.

9. Does a newborn make tears?

In a term baby tears are produced with crying beginning between month 1 and month 3 of life. Excessive tearing in the early stages of life most often represents congenital nasolacrimal duct obstruction, which is common and spontaneously resolves in approximately 90% of cases within the first year. However, excessive tearing associated with other abnormalities, such as blepharospasm and photophobia (in congenital glaucoma), or periocular erythema and edema (in dacryocystitis), warrants urgent evaluation.

10. What is strabismus?

Strabismus refers to misalignment of the eyes. Intermittent strabismus is often observed in the newborn and tends to resolve. Strabismus that persists beyond the first few months of life should be referred to an ophthalmologist for further evaluation.

Ramasubramanian A, Johnston S. Neonatal eye disorders requiring ophthalmology consultation. NeoReviews 2011;12(4):c216–c222.

Buckley EJ, Ellis GS, Glaser S, for the American Academy of Pediatrics section on ophthalmology. Red reflex examination in neonates infants, and children. Pediatrics 2008;122:1401–1404.

Hoyt CS, Good W, Petersen R. Disorders of the eye. In: Taeusch HW, Ballard RA, Avery ME, editors. Schafer and Avery's diseases of the newborn. 6th ed. Philadelphia: Saunders; 1991.

ROP

11. What does "ROP" stand for?

ROP stands for retinopathy of prematurity. ROP is a vascular disease affecting the developing retina that is a leading cause of childhood blindness in the United States and throughout the world.

12. How does this disease happen?

Retinal vascular development begins during the second trimester of pregnancy, and full maturation typically occurs during or after the third trimester of pregnancy. In premature babies much of this development is taking place *ex utero*. The abnormal retinal development seen in ROP is in response to the artificial environment experienced by the neonate after birth.

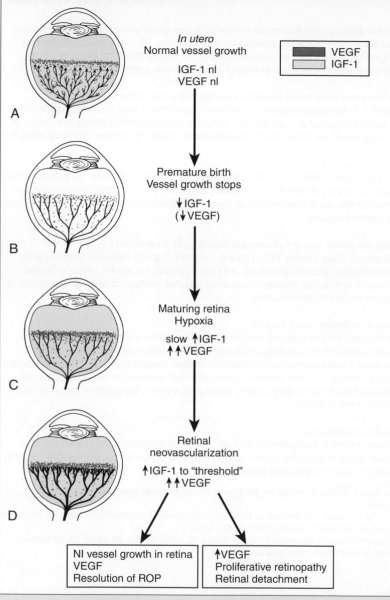

Figure 15-1. Schematic representation of IGF-1/VEGF control of blood vessel development in ROP. **A,** In utero, VEGF is found at the growing front of vessels. IGF-1 is sufficient to allow vessel growth. **B,** With premature birth, IGF-1 is not maintained at in utero levels, and vascular growth ceases despite the presence of VEGF at the growing front of vessels. Both endothelial cell survival (AKT) and proliferation (MAPK) pathways are compromised. With low IGF-1 and cessation of vessel growth, a demarcation line forms at the vascular front. High oxygen exposure (as occurs in animal models and in some premature infants) may also suppress VEGF, further contributing to inhibition of vessel growth. **C,** As the premature infant matures, the developing but nonvascularized retina becomes hypoxic. VEGF increases in retina and vitreous. With maturation, the IGF-1 level slowly increases. **D,** When the IGF-1 level reaches a threshold at 34 weeks' gestation, with high VEGF levels in the vitreous, endothelial cell survival and proliferation driven by VEGF may proceed. Neovascularization ensues at the demarcation line, growing into the vitreous. If VEGF vitreal levels fall, normal retinal vessel growth can proceed. With normal vascular growth and blood flow, oxygen suppresses VEGF expression, so it will no longer be overproduced. If hypoxia (and elevated levels of VEGF) persists, further neovascularization and fibrosis leading to retinal detachment can occur. (Smith LEH. Pathogenesis of retinopathy of prematurity. Semin Neonatol 2003;8:469–73.)

In the first phase of pathogenesis, hyperoxia leads to cessation of the normal vascular development of the peripheral retina. In the second phase increased metabolic demand causes relative hypoxia to the peripheral retina, which leads to increased production of pro-angiogenic growth factors such as vascular endothelial growth factor (VEGF) in the eye. This in turn stimulates abnormal proliferative vascular development. The proliferation can cause traction on the retina and bleeding inside the eye, which leads to vision loss (Fig.15-1).

13. **Which infants are at risk for ROP?**

The "first epidemic" of ROP occurred in the 1950s and involved premature babies exposed to high levels of oxygen after birth. In most developed countries the danger of high levels of oxygen to the neonatal eye is a well-known risk factor. Survival rates of extremely-low-birth-weight (ELBW) infants have increased as neonatal and oxygen management has improved in developed countries, and these ELBW infants are at high risk for ROP ("second epidemic"). In developing countries, where neonatal intensive care is still developing and infants are often exposed to high levels of supplemental oxygen, larger and more mature babies are once again getting ROP. This has been termed a potential "third epidemic" of ROP.

Risk factors for ROP include degree of prematurity; low birth weight; slow weight gain after birth; and general health factors, such as anemia; intraventricular hemorrhage; and acidosis. There may be a genetic predisposition to ROP, and advanced maternal age may also be an independent risk factor.

The frequency of ROP in the United States has been found to be approximately 65% in infants with birth weight below 1251 g. In most cases the disease is mild and spontaneously regresses. A small percentage of these infants will progress to disease requiring treatment, usually between 36 and 40 weeks postmenstrual age.

14. **Who should be screened for ROP, and what does the screening process entail?**

Infants with a birth weight of ≤1500 g or gestational age of 30 weeks or less (as defined by the attending neonatologist), and selected infants with a birth weight between 1500 and 2000 g or gestational age of >30 weeks with an unstable clinical course, should have retinal screening examinations. This examination is to take place either at 31 weeks' GA or 4 weeks after birth, whichever is later.

The examination involves dilating the child's pupils with eyedrops (e.g. Cyclomydril, which is a combination of 1% phenylephrine, a sympathomimetic, and 0.2% cyclopentolate, an anticholinergic). These drops are usually administered in each eye by the nursing staff. During the eye examination the ophthalmologist will typically look at the anterior segment (cornea, iris, and lens) of the eye with a penlight, and then examine the retina using indirect ophthalmoscopy (a headlamp with a handheld lens). The examination may include using a lid speculum to keep the eyelids open during the examination and pressing gently on the sclera using a small rod to view the peripheral retina. If retinopathy is noted, the severity (stage), extent (clock hours), location relative to the central retina (zone), and degree of vascular tortuosity (plus) are recorded. Examinations continue every 1 to 2 weeks until the peripheral retina is fully vascularized or more frequently if warranted by clinical findings (Table 15-1).

15. **When is ROP treated, and what are the treatment options?**

Large, multicenter studies have shown that zone I disease with stage 3 severity, zone I disease in any stage with plus disease, or zone II disease with stage 2 or 3 severity and plus disease warrant prompt treatment. These entities were collectively defined by the Early Treatment for ROP (ETROP) study as "type 1 ROP." Without prompt treatment a significant percentage of these children will progress to severe vision loss. On average, type 1 ROP occurs at 37 weeks' postmenstrual age.

Laser treatment to the peripheral retina is currently the standard of care for the treatment of type 1 ROP. The treatment attempts to halt the production of VEGF by ablating the metabolically active, yet hypoxic peripheral retina. Ophthalmologists are divided regarding whether the infant should be intubated and anesthetized for the laser procedure or whether it may be performed at the NICU bedside with topical anesthesia and intravenous sedation. This varies depending on surgeon preference, extent of treatment, and other systemic comorbidities.

TABLE 15-1.	AGE AND TIMING OF FIRST ROP SCREENING EXAMINATION FOR INFANTS
AGE AT BIRTH	**TIMING OF FIRST ROP EXAMINATION**
24 weeks GA	31 weeks GA
25 weeks GA	31 weeks GA
26 weeks GA	31 weeks GA
27 weeks GA	31 weeks GA
28 weeks GA	32 weeks GA
29 weeks GA	33 weeks GA
30 weeks GA	34 weeks GA
>30 weeks GA	4 weeks after birth

GA, Gestational age; ROP, retinopathy of prematurity.

New data suggest that an injection of anti-VEGF medications such as bevacizumab (Avastin) directly into the vitreous of the eye may be beneficial for treatment of ROP, and the standard of care is still evolving in this area.

If the ROP progresses to the retinal detachment stage, further surgery is often required. This may consist of a vitrectomy (incisional surgery to remove fibrous tissue and flatten retinal detachment) or a scleral buckle (insertion of an encircling band around the eye to flatten retinal detachment).

16. **Does screening hurt the baby?**

Studies have shown that transient, small elevations in both heart rate and blood pressure may occur. These may result from both the administration of the dilating eyedrops and the eye examination itself. There are typically no lasting effects after the examination, but infants should be monitored carefully during ROP examinations.

17. **Is it possible to make a diagnosis with a special photograph? If so, how does this work?**

In some centers bedside photographs of the retina with a specialized handheld camera (RetCam; Clarity Medical Systems, Pleasanton, Calif.) are obtained by trained staff in the NICU and sent electronically to an ophthalmologist for ROP screening and interpretation. This has been used in some areas, particularly where in-person ophthalmologic examination is difficult. The standard of care is still evolving in this area.

18. **Why is outpatient follow-up so important for extremely premature babies?**

Many babies are discharged or transferred from the NICU at just about the time when most type 1 (treatment requiring) ROP will develop: at 37 weeks' GA. It is imperative that the neonatologist, ophthalmologist, and discharge planner communicate and coordinate appropriately regarding discharge and follow-up in children who are high risk. ROP can progress rapidly, and even a short delay in a necessary follow-up ophthalmic examination can be the difference between a lifetime of functional vision and a lifetime of blindness for a premature child. Loss to timely outpatient ophthalmologic follow-up at the time of NICU discharge or transfer has been a common source of both poor visual outcome and malpractice claims against care providers.

19. **If a child does not require treatment for ROP, will the eye still develop normally?**

Usually yes. Although severe complications are less frequent, follow-up with a pediatric ophthalmologist is recommended for infants with ROP who do not require treatment. This is because of the increased prevalence of myopia, strabismus, and astigmatic refractive errors in this population.

Chen J, Stahl A, Hellstrom A, et al. Current update on retinopathy of prematurity: screening and treatment. Curr Opin Pediatr 2011;23(2):173–8.

Mills MD. Evaluating the cryotherapy for retinopathy of prematurity study (CRYO-ROP). Arch Ophthalmol 2007;125(9):1276–81.

Good WV. Final results of the early treatment for retinopathy of prematurity (ETROP) randomized trial. Trans Am Ophthalmol Soc 2004;102:233–50.

Mintz-Hittner HA, Kennedy KA, Chuang AZ for the BEAT-ROP Cooperative Group. Efficacy of intravitreal bevacizumab for stage 3+ retinopathy of prematurity. N Engl J Med 2011;364:603–15.

Darlow BA, Ells AL, Gilvert CE, et al. Are we there yet? Bevacizumab therapy for retinopathy of prematurity. Arch Dis Child Fetal Neonatal Ed 2013;98(2):F170–4

Chiang MF, Melia M, Buffenn AN, et al. Detection of clinically significant retinopathy of prematurity using wide-angle digital retinal photography: a report by the American Academy of Ophthalmology.Ophthalmology 2012;119(6):1272–80.

Richter GM, Williams SL, Starren J, et al. Telemedicine for retinopathy of prematurity diagnosis: evaluation and challenges. Surv Ophthalmol 2009;54:671–85.

Laws DE, Morton C, Weindling M, et al. Systemic effects of screening for retinopathy of prematurity. Br J Ophthalmol 1996;80:425–8.

TORCH COMPLEX

20. What are the most common eye manifestations of the TORCH infections?
See Table 15-2.

21. What is the eye-related finding most characteristic of a prenatal congenital disease?
Chorioretinal scar or active chorioretinitis is most characteristic. This has been reported in congenital toxoplasmosis, syphilis, cytomegalovirus, herpes simplex, lymphocytic choriomeningitis virus, varicella zoster virus, and West Nile virus. Chorioretinitis can be seen at birth but is often not evident until approximately the 10th day of life.

Mets MB, Chhabra MS. Eye manifestations of intrauterine infections and their impact on childhood blindness. Surv Ophthalmol 2008;53(2):95–111.

CATARACT

22. What is a cataract? I thought only old people get cataracts.
A cataract is an opacity of the crystalline intraocular lens. Congenital cataracts can be associated with intrauterine infections, associated syndromes, metabolic disorders, genetic factors, or

TABLE 15-2.	COMMON EYE MANIFESTATIONS OF TORCH INFECTIONS	
NAME	**SYSTEMIC MANIFESTATIONS**	**COMMON EYE MANIFESTATIONS**
Toxoplasma gondii	Hydrocephalus, intracranial calcifications	Chorioretinitis
Rubella	Deafness, heart disease	Cataract, retinopathy, glaucoma
Cytomegalovirus	Most asymptomatic	Chorioretinitis
Herpes simplex virus	Sepsis (natal/postnatal)	Conjunctivitis, chorioretinitis
Syphilis	Hepatosplenomegaly, rash	Interstitial keratitis, cataract, chorioretinitis

other ocular abnormalities. The prevalence is estimated to be between 1 and 13 cases per 10,000 births (Table 15-3).

23. **How do cataracts cause problems in a newborn?**
Cataracts can cause blurring of the images reaching the retina or, in severe cases, block almost all light from reaching the retina. Visual stimuli to the developing retina are important for the early development of visual function in the brain. Lack of stimulation to the visual cortex during this critical developmental period results in decreased vision. Therefore if the retinal image is distorted from a cataract, the child may develop dense amblyopia and never develop normal vision, even if the cataract is removed later in life.

24. **Which cataracts require a systemic workup?**
Bilateral cataracts with no family history should be further evaluated because they are often associated with an underlying etiology. Unilateral cataracts are rarely associated with other disease and generally do not require evaluation beyond clinical examination performed by an ophthalmologist.

25. **How are congenital cataracts treated?**
Surgery is indicated if a congenital cataract is greater than 3 mm in diameter, prevents a good view of the retina, or is associated with either nystagmus or strabismus. Unilateral cataracts are often removed within the first 6 weeks after birth to prevent form-deprivation amblyopia. Bilateral cataracts are often removed within 10 weeks after birth. Postoperative visual rehabilitation often includes aphakic contact lenses, specialized glasses, and patching for an extended period of time.

Krishnamurthy R, Vanderveen DK. Infantile cataracts. Int Ophthalmol Clin 2008;48(2):175–92.

GLAUCOMA

26. **What is glaucoma? Do only old people get glaucoma?**
Glaucoma is a disease of the optic nerve that is associated in most cases with slow, progressive vision loss and elevated intraocular pressure. Congenital glaucoma is a particular subtype of glaucoma that is often caused by structural or developmental abnormalities of the newborn eye. In congenital glaucoma elevated pressure inside the eye can cause rapid loss of vision if left untreated.

27. **What is the classic triad of signs and symptoms in congenital glaucoma?**
Epiphora (excess tearing), blepharospasm (spastic lid closure), and photophobia (light sensitivity) are the classic triad of congenital glaucoma. Other signs and symptoms include buphthalmos

TABLE 15-3. CONGENITAL CATARACT ASSOCIATIONS	
Intrauterine infections	Toxoplasmosis, rubella, CMV, herpes, syphilis
Syndromes	Trisomy 21: bilateral cataract eventually in 13% to 21% of patients, but only 1.4% presenting in neonatal period Lowe syndrome
Genetics	Autosomal dominant in approximately 25% of bilateral congenital cataract, but generally sporadic in unilateral congenital cataract
Other ocular disorders	Aniridia, microphthalmos, anterior segment dysgenesis, persistent fetal vasculature
Metabolic	Galactosemia, hypoparathyroidism, mannosidosis, hypoglycemia
CMV, Cytomegalovirus	

(enlarged eye), corneal clouding (due to elevated intraocular pressure causing corneal edema), and pain.

28. How is congenital glaucoma treated?
In most cases surgery is required. Eyedrops and oral medications such as acetazolamide are often used as adjunctive therapy.

CORTICAL VISUAL IMPAIRMENT

29. What is cortical visual impairment?
Cortical visual impairment describes abnormal vision resulting from brain dysfunction instead of eye dysfunction. Perinatal hypoxic ischemic injury is the most common cause of cortical visual impairment in children. Intracranial hemorrhage and periventricular leukomalacia can also cause cortical visual impairment. Cortical visual impairment is frequently accompanied by neurologic deficits. The eye examination reveals normal anatomy with normal pupil responses.

30. What degree of vision impairment can result?
In severe cases there can be an inability to perceive light (i.e., complete blindness) in both eyes. It may be difficult to assess visual function in affected children in the perinatal period, and follow-up examinations after hospital discharge are needed to fully assess visual potential.

Flanagan C, Kline L, Curè J. Cerebral blindness. Int Ophthalmol Clin 2009;49(3):15–25.

NYSTAGMUS

31. What is nystagmus?
Nystagmus is an involuntary, rhythmic pendular or jerking movement of the eyes.

32. What types of nystagmus can be seen in the early infant period?
Infantile nystagmus syndrome is an ocular motor disorder of unclear etiology, characterized by involuntary oscillations of the eye. These movements are usually horizontal with a small torsional component. Infantile nystagmus syndrome can occur in association with sensory visual defects, or it can be an isolated problem. Nystagmus that is secondary to severe visual loss is typically not observed at birth but instead develops approximately 2 to 3 months after birth.

Although nystagmus can be a sign of neurologic disease, nystagmus in the first 6 months of life is more likely caused by an ocular than by a neurologic disorder. Intermittent strabismus, or misalignment of the eyes, is common in the newborn period and should not be confused with nystagmus.

Children with suspected nystagmus should be referred to an ophthalmologist for further characterization.

Hertle RW. Nystagmus in infancy and childhood. Semin Ophthalmol 2008;23:307–317.

Kline LB, Chair. Section 5: Neuro-ophthalmology. In: Basic and clinical science course 2009–2010. American Academy of Ophthalmology; 2009.

PERIOCULAR PROBLEMS

33. How does nasolacrimal duct obstruction (NLDO) occur in an infant?
Most cases of NLDO in children result from blockage at the valve of Hasner, at the junction of the distal nasolacrimal duct and the inferior meatus of the nose. Excessive tearing and mucoid eye discharge can result. Most cases resolve spontaneously and are managed conservatively with massage

and topical antibiotic eyedrops. However, some cases require probing and intubation of the nasolacrimal system. If infection of the lacrimal sac (dacryocystitis) develops, administration of intravenous antibiotics, surgical intervention, or both may be required.

34. **What is a dacryocystocele? How does this present after birth?**
The nasolacrimal duct can sometimes be obstructed both proximally and distally at birth. Mucus secreted by lacrimal sac tissue is then trapped inside the sac. This causes a bluish discoloration and distention to develop just below the medial canthus, adjacent to the nose. The discoloration and distention caused by dacryocystocele should be differentiated from discoloration and distention above the medial canthus, which is more likely to be caused by a deep hemangioma, meningioencephalocele, or dermoid.

35. **There is a red discoloration of the skin around the eye. What might this be?**
Capillary hemangiomas and port-wine stains can occur on the face and eyelids. Large facial hemangiomas are sometimes associated with the PHACE syndrome (*P*osterior fossa malformation, *H*emangioma, *A*rterial abnormalities, *C*ardiac abnormalities, *E*ye abnormalities) and can also cause ptosis or astigmatism. Port-wine stains on the face can be associated with Sturge–Weber syndrome and warrant a workup for associated ipsilateral glaucoma. Orbital cellulitis can also cause erythema and edema of the eyelid in the newborn, most often in association with a recent upper respiratory infection.

36. **What is congenital ptosis and when should it be treated?**
Congenital ptosis is an inability to raise one or both eyelids. Ptosis can cause significant astigmatism and can also cause form-deprivation amblyopia if the pupil is constantly occluded by the eyelid. A surgical procedure to raise the upper eyelids is often performed if amblyopia is present.

Holds JB, Chair. Section 7: Orbit, eyelids, and lacrimal system. In: Basic and clinical science course 2009–2010. American Academy of Ophthalmology; 2009.

GENETICS

37. **What are some common genetic conditions for which eye examination is often requested in the NICU to assist in diagnosis?**
See Table 15-4.

TABLE 15-4. GENETIC CONDITIONS FOR WHICH EYE EXAMINATION IS COMMONLY REQUESTED IN NICU

CONDITION	EYE FINDINGS
Alagille syndrome	Posterior embryotoxon
PHACE complex	Lid hemangioma, microphthalmia, optic nerve hypoplasia, retinal vascular abnormalities
Down syndrome	Prominent epicanthal folds, upward slanting palpebral fissures, cataract
Aicardi syndrome	Chorioretinal depigmented lesions
CHARGE	Coloboma
Moyamoya disease	Morning Glory syndrome, Coloboma
Septo-optic dysplasia (de Morsier)	Optic nerve hypoplasia

✓ KEY POINTS

1. Every infant should receive a basic eye examination performed by a neonatologist or pediatrician before discharge from the hospital.

2. An abnormal red reflex should prompt further investigation by an ophthalmologist.

3. Infants with a birth weight of ≤1500 g or gestational age of 30 weeks or less (as defined by the attending neonatologist), and selected infants with a birth weight between 1500 and 2000 g or gestational age of >30 weeks with an unstable clinical course, should be screened for retinopathy of prematurity.

4. Intermittent strabismus (eye misalignment) commonly occurs in the newborn period. However, any infant with eye misalignment that persists beyond the 3rd month of life should be referred to an ophthalmologist.

CHAPTER 16

ORTHOPEDICS

Qusai Hammouri, MBBS, MD, and Joshua E. Hyman, MD

1. **What are the components of the newborn orthopedic screening examination?**
   All newborn babies should be examined for evidence of hip dysplasia, spinal dysraphism, and lower and upper extremity deformities.

Blasco PA. Pathology of cerebral palsy. In: Sussman MD, editor. The diplegic child. Rosemont, IL: American Academy of Orthopaedic Surgeons; 1992. p. 3–20.

2. **How do you check for occult spinal dysraphism?**
   Any midline dimple (especially a deep or asymmetric pit), subcutaneous mass, hemangioma, nevus, tuft of hair, or areas of hypopigmentation or hyperpigmentation might indicate occult spinal dysraphism and a tethered cord. Coccygeal pits are generally benign. The presence of two or more midline skin lesions is the strongest predictor of spinal dysraphism. An ultrasound of the spine is indicated whenever occult spinal dysraphism is suspected. Magnetic resonance imaging is an alternative imaging study.

3. **How do you check for extremity deformity?**
   Look at the extremities, and check for asymmetry or an abnormal appearance. Look at the baby when crying to determine if he or she moves all extremities. Gently examine the joints and their range of motion. Finally, stimulating the extremities should result in some kind of response, usually withdrawal.

Blasco PA. Pathology of cerebral palsy. In: Sussman MD, editor. The diplegic child. Rosemont, IL: American Academy of Orthopaedic Surgeons; 1992. p. 3–20.

4. **A premature newborn infant receiving ventilator support in the NICU has decreased movement in the right lower extremity. What diagnostic tests may be appropriate?**
   Neonatal osteomyelitis or fracture need to be ruled out. Baseline laboratory testing should be considered (e.g., complete blood count and C-reactive protein) as part of the evaluation for possible joint infections, which are not uncommon in this setting. If an osteomyelitis is suspected, a blood culture should always be obtained. These tests may not be rewarding because infants may develop infection without abnormalities in laboratory values. Plain radiographs of the entire extremity should be obtained to help detect a subtle fracture that may not be apparent on clinical examination. Radiographs are often normal in the early phases of bone and joint infection. In this setting bone and joint infections most often involve more than one site. Therefore careful clinical assessment to detect subtle joint effusions or swelling over long bones is indicated. Often an ultrasound scan is helpful in confirming a joint effusion in the hip because overlying muscle may mask the usual clinical findings. A technetium-99 bone scan is very useful in detecting other sites of multicentric infection.

Shaw BA, Kasser JR. Acute septic arthritis in infancy and childhood. Clin Orthop Relat Res 1990;257:212–25.

5. **The initial evaluation of a first-born infant reveals multiple stiff joints in both the upper and lower extremities and thin, tapered, and "shiny" fingers. What is the main diagnostic consideration?**
   Arthrogryposis multiplex congenita is a clinical syndrome characterized by poor development of the joints *in utero* leading to multiple contractures. This does not appear to be a hereditary condition,

and there is no increased risk in siblings of the same family. Many mothers report decreased fetal movement *in utero*. On clinical examination the limbs are usually symmetric. Joints may have either flexion or extension contractures. There is decreased active and passive motion of the affected joints. The normal skin creases are usually absent, and the skin is taut and glossy. Dimpling at the joints may be present. There is atrophy of the limbs. Often the hips are dislocated, and clubfoot (i.e., talipes equinovarus) or congenital vertical talus affects the feet. The upper extremities are usually internally rotated at the shoulder, with elbow flexion or extension contractures. There are often radial head dislocations. The forearms are pronated with adduction deformity of the thumbs. Delivery may be difficult as a consequence of the stiff elbow and knee joints. This may result in birth fractures of the humerus and the femur. General health is not affected by this syndrome, although patients often exhibit minor respiratory difficulties and failure to thrive as newborns.

Einhorn T. Orthopaedic Basic Science, Rosemont, IL: American Academy of Orthopaedic Surgery, 2006.
    Morrissy R, Weinstein S, editors. Lovell and Winter's Pediatric Orthopaedics. Philadelphia: Lippincott Williams & Wilkins; 2005. p. 293–296.

6. **What congenital spine malformation is associated with maternal insulin-dependent diabetes?**
Caudal regression syndrome (also known as lumbosacral agenesis) is more common in women with insulin-dependent diabetes. It is characterized by an absence of variable amounts of the sacrum and lumbar spine and the associated neural elements. There may also be concomitant anomalies of the genitourinary and gastrointestinal tracts. The level of the lesion may vary, and this will influence the clinical picture. These lesions are classified into four types according to the Renshaw classification. Depending on the severity of the agenesis, the patient may have variable foot deformities and abnormalities of the hips and knees.

7. **A newborn infant is noted to have external rotation of the lower extremities at rest, with little spontaneous movement and bilateral foot deformities. What radiographs should be ordered?**
Both spine and pelvis radiographs should be ordered. The abnormalities described can result from anomalies of the spine or the lower extremities.

Einhorn T. Orthopaedic Basic Science, Rosemont, IL: American Academy of Orthopaedic Surgery, 2006.
    Morrissy R, Weinstein S, editors. Lovell and Winter's Pediatric Orthopaedics. Philadelphia: Lippincott Williams & Wilkins; 2005. p. 293–296.

8. **A newborn child is suspected of having a genetic skeletal dysplasia. What is the most critical orthopedic radiographic examination?**
The most important radiograph is the lateral cervical spine. More than 150 distinct osteochondrodysplasias have been identified. Each has distinctive features, but many also have similar radiographic findings. One of the most common is agenesis or hypoplasia of the upper cervical spine elements. This can lead to instability and places the child at great risk of spinal cord injury during ordinary handling. Detection of cervical instability is mandatory to allow proper stabilization and protection.

Guille JT, Pizzutillo PD, MacEwen GD. Development dysplasia of the hip from birth to six months. J Am Acad Orthop Surg 2000;8:232–42.

9. **What is developmental dysplasia of the hip (DDH)?**
DDH is a maldevelopment of the hip joint characterized by a spectrum of pathology ranging from instability of the hip to irreducible dislocation.

Guille JT, Pizzutillo PD, MacEwen GD. Development dysplasia of the hip from birth to six months. J Am Acad Orthop Surg 2000;8:232–42.

10. **What is congenital hip dislocation (CDH)?**
CDH is an outdated term; DDH is preferred because it reflects the evolutionary nature of hip problems in infants in the first months of life. The overt pathologic process may not be present at birth, and

periodic examination of the infant's hip is recommended at each routine well-baby visit until the age of 1 year (Fig. 16-1).

Guille JT, Pizzutillo PD, MacEwen GD. Development dysplasia of the hip from birth to six months. J Am Acad Orthop Surg 2000;8:232–42.

11. What are the four examinations that constitute a newborn hip evaluation?
The hip abduction, Ortolani, Barlow, and Galeazzi tests are recommended.

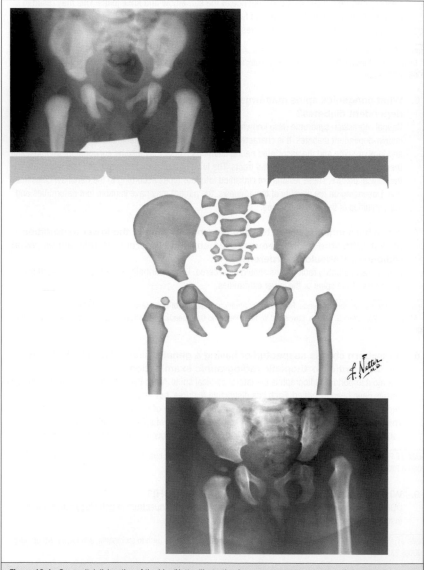

Figure 16-1. Congenital dislocation of the hip. (Netter illustration from www.netterimages.com. © Elsevier Inc. All rights reserved.)

✓ KEY POINTS: DEVELOPMENTAL DYSPLASIA OF THE HIP IN NEWBORNS

1. Every newborn should have a hip examination.

2. The examination consists of the Ortolani, Barlow, and Galeazzi maneuvers.

3. The three main risk factors for DDH are first-born status, female sex, and breech presentation.

Guille JT, Pizzutillo PD, MacEwen GD. Development dysplasia of the hip from birth to six months. J Am Acad Orthop Surg 2000;8:232–42.

12. How do you interpret the hip abduction exam?

Infants should have symmetric hip abduction. Having asymmetry in hip abduction could be a sign of a dislocated hip.

Guille JT, Pizzutillo PD, MacEwen GD. Development dysplasia of the hip from birth to six months. J Am Acad Orthop Surg 2000;8:232–42.

13. How do you perform an Ortolani exam?

It is performed with the child in the supine position. Beginning with the hips flexed 90 degrees and adducted to the midline, the examiner places the index finger on the greater trochanter and the thumb on the inside of the thigh, then gently abducts the hip and lifts up on the greater trochanter. If the hip is dislocated and reducible, a palpable sensation will be felt as the hip reduces into the acetabulum (known as an Ortolani-positive hip) (Fig. 16-2).

Guille JT, Pizzutillo PD, MacEwen GD. Development dysplasia of the hip from birth to six months. J Am Acad Orthop Surg 2000;8:232–42.

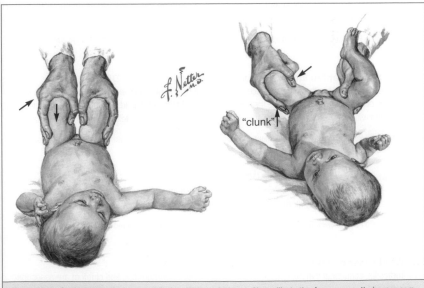

Figure 16-2. Ortolani (reduction) test and Barlow (dislocatable) test. (Netter illustration from www.netterimages.com. © Elsevier Inc. All rights reserved.)

14. **What does it mean to describe a hip as "Ortolani positive"?**
    The Ortolani examination is a reduction maneuver. Therefore an Ortolani-positive hip is a hip that is dislocated in its resting state and reducible with gentle manipulation. A simple way to remember this: Think of the *O* in Ortolani meaning that a hip is "out," or dislocated, when you start the examination.

Guille JT, Pizzutillo PD, MacEwen GD. Development dysplasia of the hip from birth to six months. J Am Acad Orthop Surg 2000;8:232–42.

15. **How do you perform a Barlow examination?**
    It is performed with the child supine on the examination table. The hip is flexed 90 degrees and adducted just beyond midline. Gentle downward pressure is then applied to the hip through the knee. The sensation of the femoral head sliding out of the acetabulum indicates a Barlow-positive hip.

Guille JT, Pizzutillo PD, MacEwen GD. Development dysplasia of the hip from birth to six months. J Am Acad Orthop Surg 2000;8:232–42.

16. **What does it mean to describe a hip as "Barlow positive"?**
    The Barlow examination is a provocative maneuver. A Barlow-positive hip is normally reduced but can be subluxed. A normal hip will not subluxate and is Barlow negative.

Guille JT, Pizzutillo PD, MacEwen GD. Development dysplasia of the hip from birth to six months. J Am Acad Orthop Surg 2000;8:232–242.

17. **How do you perform the Galeazzi examination?**
    It is performed with the child supine. The hips and knees are flexed such that the feet are lying flat on the table. The examiner then looks at the heights of the knees. If there is a difference, there may be a dislocated hip.

Guille JT, Pizzutillo PD, MacEwen GD. Development dysplasia of the hip from birth to six months. J Am Acad Orthop Surg 2000;8:232–42.

18. **What does it mean to have a "Galeazzi-positive" hip?**
    The Galeazzi exam identifies apparent or real shortening of the femur. It could be due to DDH or other congenital anomalies.

Guille JT, Pizzutillo PD, MacEwen GD. Development dysplasia of the hip from birth to six months. J Am Acad Orthop Surg 2000;8:232–42.

19. **What radiographic studies can you order if you suspect DDH?**
    Ultrasound of the hip is the study of choice for suspected DDH in neonates and infants younger than four months of age. In children of this age the ossific nucleus of the femoral head is completely cartilaginous and therefore will not be seen on x-ray. After the infant is four months of age, radiographs should be obtained.

Guille JT, Pizzutillo PD, MacEwen GD. Development dysplasia of the hip from birth to six months. J Am Acad Orthop Surg 2000;8:232–42.

20. **What are the risk factors for DDH?**
    First-born female infants who present in the breech position and have a positive family history of DDH are at a significantly increased risk. A simple mnemonic: First, Female, Family, and Breech

Guille JT, Pizzutillo PD, MacEwen GD. Development dysplasia of the hip from birth to six months. J Am Acad Orthop Surg 2000;8:232–42.

21. **What other conditions are associated with DDH?**
    Torticollis, congenital hyperextension of the knee, metatarsus adductus, and clubfoot are associated with DDH.

Guille JT, Pizzutillo PD, MacEwen GD. Development dysplasia of the hip from birth to six months. J Am Acad Orthop Surg 2000;8:232–42.

22. **How is DDH treated in newborns?**
In a newborn child DDH can be very effectively treated with dynamic splinting in a brace, such as a Pavlik harness. A child in a Pavlik harness will lie with her hips and knees flexed approximately 90 degrees and her hips abducted to 60 degrees. This position is quite comfortable and natural for the infant. In this position the femoral head is deeply seated within the acetabulum. The soft-tissue structures around the hip will then stabilize with the hip in this reduced position.

Roye BD, Hyman JE, Roye DP Jr. Congenital idiopathic talipes equinovarus. Pediatr Rev 2004;25:124–30.

23. **What is clubfoot?**
Clubfoot, (also called talipes equinovarus), is a congenital condition in which the foot points downward and inward. More specifically, the hindfoot is in equinus and varus and the forefoot is in adduction and supination.

Roye BD, Hyman JE, Roye DP Jr. Congenital idiopathic talipes equinovarus. Pediatr Rev 2004;25:124–30.

✓ KEY POINTS: CLUBFOOT

1. Most clubfeet can be treated effectively with manipulation and casting.

2. Treatment should begin as soon as possible after birth.

3. Clubfoot may be associated with other congenital conditions; therefore a thorough evaluation of the entire infant is necessary.

24. **How common is clubfoot?**
The incidence of clubfoot is 1.2 per 1000 live births, although this estimate varies with different ethnic subgroups, ranging from as high as 7 per 1000 in Hawaii to 0.87 in India.

Roye BD, Hyman JE, Roye DP Jr. Congenital idiopathic talipes equinovarus. Pediatr Rev 2004;25:124–130.

25. **Is there a gender difference in the incidence of clubfoot?**
Boys are affected nearly twice as often as girls, and 50% of the patients have bilateral involvement.

Roye BD, Hyman JE, Roye DP Jr. Congenital idiopathic talipes equinovarus. Pediatr Rev 2004;25:124–30.

26. **What are the causes of clubfoot?**
The etiology of clubfoot is unknown. It is seen in conjunction with cerebral palsy, myelomeningocele, arthrogryposis, and other neuromuscular conditions. Most often, however, it occurs as an isolated deformity in an otherwise healthy infant (i.e., it is idiopathic).

Roye BD, Hyman JE, Roye DP Jr. Congenital idiopathic talipes equinovarus. Pediatr Rev 2004;25:124–30.

27. **What is the treatment for clubfoot?**
The initial treatment for clubfoot is weekly manipulation and casting according to the Ponseti method. Approximately 6 to 10 casts are required. A brace is worn for 3 to 4 years to maintain the correct position. With this technique, approximately 80% to 90% of idiopathic clubfeet will be successfully treated. Those feet that cannot be corrected with this method will require surgical correction (Fig. 16-3).

Roye BD, Hyman JE, Roye DP Jr. Congenital idiopathic talipes equinovarus. Pediatr Rev 2004;25:124–130.

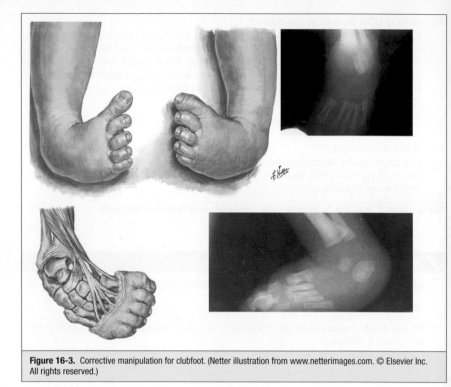

Figure 16-3. Corrective manipulation for clubfoot. (Netter illustration from www.netterimages.com. © Elsevier Inc. All rights reserved.)

28. When should clubfoot treatment be initiated?

As soon as the deformity is recognized, treatment should be started. This can frequently occur in the newborn nursery.

Hyman JE, Roye DP Jr. Torticollis. In: Burg FD, Ingelfinger JR, Polin RA, Gershon AA, editors. Gellis and Kagan's current pediatric therapy. Philadelphia: Saunders; 2002. p. 849–50.

Einhorn T. Orthopaedic Basic Science, Rosemont, IL: American Academy of Orthopaedic Surgery, 2006.

Morrissy R, Weinstein S, editors. Lovell and Winter's Pediatric Orthopaedics. Philadelphia: Lippincott Williams & Wilkins; 2005. p. 332.

29. What is Klippel-Feil syndrome?

A congenital condition characterized by the triad of a short neck, a low posterior hairline, and fusion of elements of the cervical spine. It results in decreased cervical spine motion.

Hyman JE, Roye DP Jr. Torticollis. In: Burg FD, Ingelfinger JR, Polin RA, Gershon AA, editors. Gellis and Kagan's current pediatric therapy. Philadelphia: Saunders; 2002. p. 849–50.

Einhorn T. Orthopaedic Basic Science, Rosemont, IL: American Academy of Orthopaedic Surgery, 2006.

Morrissy R, Weinstein S, editors. Lovell and Winter's Pediatric Orthopaedics. Philadelphia: Lippincott Williams & Wilkins; 2005. p. 889–891.

30. What is the general clinical significance of Klippel-Feil syndrome?

The cervical spine develops embryologically at the same time as the genitourinary and cardiovascular systems. As a result, patients with cervical spine anomalies may also have genitourinary and cardiovascular anomalies. In addition, other fusions and malformations of the spinal column may occur. There may also be abnormalities within the spinal cord, such as syringomyelia and cord tethering.

Hyman JE, Roye DP Jr. Torticollis. In: Burg FD, Ingelfinger JR, Polin RA, Gershon AA, editors. Gellis and Kagan's current pediatric therapy. Philadelphia: Saunders; 2002. p. 849–50.

Einhorn T. Orthopaedic Basic Science, Rosemont, IL: American Academy of Orthopaedic Surgery, 2006.

Morrissy R, Weinstein S, editors. Lovell and Winter's Pediatric Orthopaedics. Philadelphia: Lippincott Williams & Wilkins; 2005. p. 889–891.

31. **What does the evaluation of a child with Klippel–Feil syndrome entail?**
    These children must undergo an abdominal ultrasound scan to evaluate possible genitourinary anomalies. They should have a careful clinical cardiac examination. If the results of this examination are thought to be abnormal, an echocardiogram should be considered. Complete radiographs of the entire spinal column must be obtained to look for other vertebral anomalies. Finally, a thorough neurologic evaluation, including magnetic resonance imaging from the base of the brain to the cauda equina, should be performed.

Shaw BA, Kasser JR. Acute septic arthritis in infancy and childhood. Clin Orthop Relat Res 1990;257:212–225.

✓ KEY POINTS: NEONATAL INFECTIONS

1. Newborn children with a bone or joint infection may present with pseudoparalysis of the affected extremity.

2. A fever is not a prerequisite for a bone or joint infection.

3. Treatment of joint infections requires aspiration and antibiotics.

32. **What are the clinical findings of septic arthritis of the hip in the newborn?**
    The inability of the newborn to communicate makes this diagnosis quite difficult; however, there are some hallmark signs to be aware of. Affected children will appear lethargic and irritable. They will have difficulty feeding and will exhibit pseudoparalysis, or decreased movement, of the affected limb. A fever is not obligatory. The diagnosis is made by joint aspiration and microscopic examination of the fluid.

Shaw BA, Kasser JR. Acute septic arthritis in infancy and childhood. Clin Orthop Relat Res 1990;257:212–25.

33. **What are the consequences of a missed joint infection?**
    Bacteria within the joint will lead to an inflammatory response by the host immune system. The enzymes released (e.g., collagenases, proteases, elastases) by both the leukocytes and bacterial cells cause cartilage damage. Initially, glycosaminoglycans are removed from the cartilage. Over time, there is eventual collagen destruction. This damage is irreversible. In addition, if sufficient pressure develops within the joint, blood flow to the epiphysis will be compromised and may lead to avascular necrosis.

Shaw BA, Kasser JR. Acute septic arthritis in infancy and childhood. Clin Orthop Relat Res 1990;257:212–25.

34. **What are the most common bacterial agents in neonatal osteomyelitis?**
    Staphylococcus aureus; group B streptococci; and *Escherichia coli, Klebsiella, Salmonella,* and *Pseudomonas* species are the most common bacterial agents in neonatal osteomyelitis. As opposed to osteomyelitis with secondary spread to the joint space, isolated septic arthritis is extremely rare. Staphylococci are the most common organisms, but the clinician should always think of gonococci as well with early septic arthritis.

35. **Which bone is most frequently fractured in newborns?**
    The clavicle is most frequently fractured in newborns. This injury, which stems from excessive traction during delivery, generally results in a greenstick fracture. This fracture usually heals quite nicely without any therapy, although the callus formation may be notable.

36. **How long should fractures in neonates be immobilized?**
    Neonatal fractures generally heal more quickly than their counterparts in children or adults. Because of this, and because of the difficulty in casting neonates, some fractures that would be severely

problematic in an adult are barely treated in a neonate. A clavicular fracture will heal within 3 weeks in a newborn infant, as opposed to 6 to 8 weeks in an adult, and does not need to be immobilized in most cases. Femoral fractures, common in premature infants with rickets, are usually well healed within 3 weeks, compared with the 6 to 10 weeks required in an older child or adult with this fracture. Femoral fractures usually are splinted or placed in a Pavlik harness to help healing, but not always if there is minimal displacement.

37. **What are the features of constriction ring syndrome (i.e., Streeter dysplasia).**
    Constriction ring syndrome is a rare syndrome that is characterized by ringlike constriction bands around the upper and lower extremities or the trunk. The etiology is unknown, and it is not hereditary. The extent and depth of the rings vary. The bands may be subcutaneous or may extend down to bone. These bands may interfere with lymphatic and venous return, resulting in edema and enlargement of the distal part with decreased capillary refill. If there is great disruption to the local circulation, the part may undergo autoamputation *in utero*. Often there are other concomitant anomalies of the hand including syndactyly, acrodactyly, hypoplasia, camptodactyly, and symphalangia. Other associated anomalies include cleft palate and lip and talipes equinovarus deformity of the foot.

38. **The foot of a newborn appears to be dorsiflexed such that the top of the foot lies directly against the anterior portion of the lower leg. What are the two diagnostic considerations, and how would you differentiate between the two?**
    Calcaneovalgus foot deformity is the most likely diagnosis. It is believed that there is no intrinsic problem with bone or joint development and that the deformity results from intrauterine positioning. The natural history of the untreated condition is one of spontaneous correction with no long-term sequelae. The second possibility is posteromedial bowing of the distal tibia. The foot is folded on the anterior surface of the leg, but the flexibility of the foot and ankle is normal. There is significant shortening of the affected side and decreased soft tissue. Because the physical findings may be difficult to distinguish from calcaneovalgus foot deformity in the newborn, anteroposterior and lateral radiographs of the leg should be obtained. The deformity improves with time, usually during the first 3 years of life. However, long-term orthopedic care is required because the affected limb always shows significant growth discrepancy and internal tibial torsion at maturity.

39. **What are the orthopedic manifestations of thrombocytopenia with absent radius (TAR) syndrome?**
    TAR syndrome presents with several orthopedic findings. In the upper extremity there is bilateral absence of the radius, usually with all five fingers present. The thumbs may be hypoplastic. Abnormalities of the fingers may include absence of the middle phalanx of the fifth finger, clinodactyly, or partial syndactyly. In almost one half of the patients, shortening or bowing of the ulna with deficiency of the extensor tendons may occur. In addition, the humerus may be short or absent. In almost 40% of patients, there are associated lower extremity anomalies. These mainly involve the knee and include subluxation or dislocation of the patella and hypoplasia of the knee. The most common deformity of the lower extremities is genu varum with a flexion contracture and internal tibial torsion. These patients also may have hip dislocations, varus or valgus deformities of the hips, and shortening of the legs with hypoplastic or absent tibias or fibulas.

40. **A newborn exhibits swelling over the midshaft of the right clavicle. What are the two most common diagnostic considerations?**
    Birth fractures of the clavicle are extremely common but most often are accompanied by pseudoparalysis of the extremity (caused by "splinting" from pain) for at least 3 to 5 days. There is pain with passive movement. Radiographs show the fracture, which usually heals with a massive callus. In the absence of pain, the clinician must consider congenital pseudarthrosis of the clavicle. The pseudarthrosis is fully present at birth. There is no history of birth injury or other trauma. The right

clavicle is almost always affected. At the pseudarthrosis, the clavicular ends are enlarged, and there is painless motion between the two fragments. The etiology remains unknown, but several theories have been proposed, including exaggerated arterial pulsations and pressure on the clavicle by the subclavian artery that is normally more cranial on the right side. In bilateral cases it is thought that an abnormally high subclavian artery is present on both sides. With growth the deformity increases, and the overlying skin becomes thin and atrophic. The affected shoulder often droops, and there is asymmetry between the two shoulders. No functional impairment is noted. Treatment involves resection of the nonunion and internal fixation with bone grafting.

CHAPTER 17

PAIN MANAGEMENT IN THE NEONATE

K.J.S. Anand, MBBS, DPhil, Fabio Savorgnan, MD, and R. Whit Hall, MD

1. **An obstetrician is about to do a circumcision without using analgesia. When you question this practice, he replies that neonates cannot perceive pain. Is this correct?**

   This is not correct. The International Association for the Study of Pain defines pain as "an unpleasant sensory and emotional experience associated with actual or potential tissue damage or described in terms of such damage." The definition further states that although pain is subjective, the inability to communicate verbally does not negate the possibility that an individual is experiencing pain and requires adequate pain-relieving treatment. The issues of pain perception in newborns, its management, and its prevention were neglected for decades. The inability of newborns to "self-report" contributed significantly to the denial of the importance of neonatal pain and the consequences of inadequate treatment. In response to a painful stimulus, all newborns mount acute changes in endocrine, vegetative, immune, and behavioral functions. Multiple lines of evidence show that the pain system is intact and functional in preterm and term neonates, even among the tiniest preterm newborns. Acute pain is processed in the somatosensory cortex, and these responses are altered by the characteristics of neonates, their behavioral state at the time of painful stimulation, the intensity of stimulation, and contextual factors. Such a nuanced response suggests that term and preterm neonates may be capable of conscious sensory perception of acute pain (Fig. 17-1).

Anand KJS, Johnston CC, Oberlander TF, et al. Analgesia and local anesthesia during invasive procedures in the neonate. Clin Ther 2005;27:844–76.

Brady-Fryer B, Wiebe N, Lander JA. Pain relief for neonatal circumcision. Cochrane Database Syst Rev 2004;CD004217.

IASP Pain Terminology, Committee on Taxonomy. International Association for the Study of Pain; 2001. [Accessed 21.05.01] at Anand KJS, Craig KD. New perspectives on the definition of pain. Pain 1996;67:3–6; discussion 209–11.

Anand KJS, Rovnaghi C, Walden M, et al. Consciousness, behavior, and clinical impact of the definition of pain. Pain Forum 1999;8:64–73.

Anand KJS, Hickey PR. Pain and its effects in the human neonate and fetus. N Engl J Med 1987;317:1321–9.

Weber F. Evidence for the need for anaesthesia in the neonate. Best Pract Res Clin Anaesthesiol 2010;24:475–84.

Bouza H. The impact of pain in the immature brain. J Matern Fetal Neonatal Med 2009;22:722–32.

Anand KJS. Clinical importance of pain and stress in preterm neonates. Biol Neonate 1998;73:1–9.

Bartocci M, Bergqvist LL, Lagercrantz H, et al. Pain activates cortical areas in the preterm newborn brain. Pain 2006;122:109–17.

Slater R, Cantarella A, Gallella S, et al. Cortical pain responses in human infants. J Neurosci 2006;26:3662–6.

1a. **How is pain evaluated in the neonate?**

   An ideal pain indicator does not exist for the neonatal period. There are several physiologic (heart rate, respiratory rate, blood pressure, vagal tone, breathing pattern, oxygen saturation, intracranial pressure, palmar sweating, skin color) and behavioral indicators (facial expressions, movements of limbs, crying activity) of pain and a large number of neonatal pain scales have been constructed on the basis of these indicators.

   If pain is prolonged or repetitive, these physiologic and behavioral responses may be muted, transient, or absent. Neonates, especially preterm neonates, have limited energy reserves and cannot mount a prolonged psychophysiologic activation response to pain.

Howard VA, Thurber FW. The interpretation of infant pain: physiological and behavioral indicators used by NICU nurses. J Pediatr Nurs 1998;13:164–74.

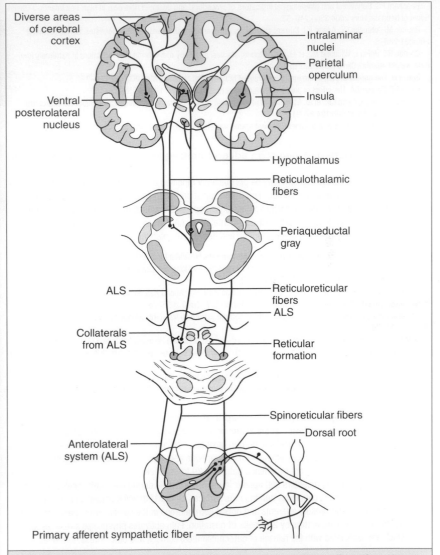

Figure 17-1. Schematic diagram showing the lateral and medial pain systems. Primary afferents from cutaneous, mucosal, visceral, joint and connective tissue, vascular, and other deep-tissue nociceptors enter the spinal cord via A-delta (thinly myelinated)-fibers, C (unmyelinated)-fibers, and sympathetic fibers. These afferents make rich connections in superficial layers of the dorsal horn of the spinal cord (called the substantia gelatinosa). They have direct and indirect links with projection neurons in deeper layers of the dorsal horn that project to the supraspinal pain-processing areas in the brainstem, medial and posterior thalamus, and various areas of the cortex. The lateral pain system mostly transmits somatic and mucosal pain, whereas the medial pain system transmits visceral pain. Cortical areas most closely associated with pain processing include the primary and secondary somatosensory areas, the anterior cingulate cortex, the insula, and parietal association areas. (From Bonaz B. Visceral sensitivity perturbation integration in the brain-gut axis in functional digestive disorders. J Physiol Pharmacol 2003;54[Suppl 4]:27–42.)

Beacham PS. Behavioral and physiological indicators of procedural and postoperative pain in high-risk infants. J Obstet Gynecol Neonatal Nurs 2004;33(2):246–55.

Ranger M, Johnston CC, Anand KJ. Current controversies regarding pain assessment in neonates. Semin Perinatol 2007;31:283–8.

Grunau RE, Holsti L, Whitfield MF, et al. Are twitches, startles, and body movements pain indicators in extremely low birth weight infants? Clin J Pain 2000;16:37–45.

Bouza H. The impact of pain in the immature brain. J Matern Fetal Neonatal Med 2009;22:722–32.

Fuller BF, Conner DA. The effect of pain on infant behaviors. Clin Nurs Res 1995;4:253–73.

Boyle EM, Freer Y, Wong CM, et al. Assessment of persistent pain or distress and adequacy of analgesia in preterm ventilated infants. Pain 2006;124:87–91.

Hummel P, van Dijk M. Pain assessment: current status and challenges. Semin Fetal Neonatal Med 2006;11:237–45.

1b. Are there short- and long-term adverse consequences to pain in the newborn period?

The developing nervous system may be permanently modified after prolonged or repetitive pain, resulting in altered pain processing at the spinal and supraspinal levels. In addition, pain is associated with a number of adverse physiologic responses that include alterations in circulatory (tachycardia, hypertension, vasoconstriction), metabolic (increased catabolism, metabolic acidosis), immunologic (impaired immune response), and hemostatic (platelet activation) systems.

Bouza H. The impact of pain in the immature brain. J Matern Fetal Neonatal Med 2009;22:722–32.

Anand KJS, Grunau RE, Oberlander T. Developmental character and long-term consequences of pain in infants and children. Child Adolesc Psychiatr Clin N Am 1997;6:703–24.

Grunau RE. Long-term consequences of pain in human neonates. In: Anand KJS, Stevens BJ, McGrath PJ, editors. Pain in neonates. 2nd ed. Amsterdam: Elsevier Science Publishers B.V.; 2000. p.55–76.

Whitfield MF, Grunau RE. Behavior, pain perception, and the extremely low-birth weight survivor. Clin Perinatol 2000;27:363–79.

Grunau R. Early pain in preterm infants. A model of long-term effects. Clin Perinatol 2002;29:373–94, vii–viii.

Peters JW, Schouw R, Anand KJS, et al. Does neonatal surgery lead to increased pain sensitivity in later childhood? Pain 2005;114:444–54.

Anand KJS. Clinical importance of pain and stress in preterm neonates. Biol Neonate 1998;73:1–9.

Hall RW, Boyle E, Young T. Do ventilated neonates require pain management? Semin Perinatol 2007;31:289–97.

2. When does pain perception develop in the human fetus?

Neurobiologic studies suggest that the anatomic and physiologic systems for pain perception are sufficiently developed by 20 weeks of human gestation. Thalamocortical projections develop between 16 and 20 weeks of gestation, although misconceptions about brain development have led some to believe that the fetus may not experience pain until 29 to 30 weeks.

Cutaneous sensory receptors first appear in the perioral area during the eighth week of gestation. They are present in all cutaneous and mucous surfaces by the 18th week of gestation. Synapses between peripheral sensory afferents and dorsal horn neurons in the spinal cord appear early in the first trimester and are mature by 20 weeks of gestation. Pain activates physiologic stress responses, which are associated with the release of catecholamines, cortisol, and other stress hormones.

Vanhatalo S, van Nieuwenhuizen O. Fetal pain? Brain Dev 2000;22:145–50.

Anand KJS, Maze M. Fetuses, fentanyl, and the stress response: signals from the beginnings of pain? Anesthesiology 2001;95:823–5.

Fisk NM, Gitau R, Teixeira JM, et al. Effect of direct fetal opioid analgesia on fetal hormonal and hemodynamic stress response to intrauterine needling. Anesthesiology 2001 Oct;95(4):828–35.

Lowery CL, Hardman MP, Manning N, et al. Neurodevelopmental changes of fetal pain. Semin Perinatol 2007;31:275–82.

Anand KJS. Fetal Pain? Pain: Clinical Updates 2006;14:1–4.

Lee SJ, Ralston HJ, Drey EA, et al. Fetal pain: a systematic multidisciplinary review of the evidence. JAMA 2005;294:947–54.

Anand KJS, Hickey PR. Pain and its effects in the human neonate and fetus. N Engl J Med 1987;317:1321–9.

Anand KJS, Rovnaghi C, Walden M, et al. Consciousness, behavior, and clinical impact of the definition of pain. Pain Forum 1999;8:64–73.

Ward-Platt MP, Anand KJS, Aynsley-Green A. The ontogeny of the metabolic and endocrine stress response in the human fetus, neonate and child. Intensive Care Medicine 1989;15(Suppl 1):S44–5.

Giannakoulopoulos X, Sepulveda W, Kourtis P, et al. Fetal plasma cortisol and beta-endorphin response to intrauterine needling. Lancet 1994;344:77–81.

Smith RP, Gitau R, Glover V, et al. Pain and stress in the human fetus. Eur J Obstet Gynecol Reprod Biol 2000;92:161–5.

2b. **What are the stress responses to pain in the fetus, and when do they appear during development?**

Stress responses to a painful stimulation are complex, but they can be detected from the 16th week of gestation. Physiologic stress is different from the pain felt by the more mature fetus, as this stress is mitigated by a pain medication such as fentanyl by 20 to 24 weeks. There is activation of the hypothalamic–pituitary–adrenal axis, autonomic nervous system, and hemodynamic changes in response to fetal pain. In premature infants exposed to pain, there are significant increases of epinephrine, norepinephrine, and cortisol; hemodynamic changes; motor reflexes; and facial reactions.

Partsch CJ, Sippell WG, MacKenzie IZ, et al. The steroid hormonal milieu of the undisturbed human fetus and mother at 16-20 weeks gestation. J Clini Endocrinol Metabol 1991;73:969–74.

3. **Are neonates less sensitive to pain than older children or adults?**

They certainly are not. Developmentally regulated processes and behavioral studies show that pain thresholds increase progressively during late gestation and in the postnatal period. Preterm neonates have much greater sensitivity to pain than term neonates, and they manifest prolonged periods of hyperalgesia after tissue injury. These phenomena were further substantiated in the newborn and infant rat. Central sensitization and immaturity of the pain inhibitory systems are the main neurobiologic explanations for the increased pain sensitivity in newborns.

Anand KJS. Effects of perinatal pain and stress. Prog Brain Res 2000;122:117–29.

Andrews K, Fitzgerald M. Cutaneous flexion reflex in human neonates: a quantitative study of threshold and stimulus-response characteristics after single and repeated stimuli. Dev Med Child Neurol 1999;41:696–703.

Thewissen L, Allegaert K. Analgosedation in neonates: do we still need additional tools after 30 years of clinical research? Arch Dis Child Educ Pract Ed 2011;96:112–8.

Andrews K, Fitzgerald M. Wound sensitivity as a measure of analgesic effects following surgery in human neonates and Infants. Pain 2002;99:185–95.

Taddio A, Shah V, Gilbert-MacLeod C, et al. Conditioning and hyperalgesia in newborns exposed to repeated heel lances. JAMA 2002;288:857–61.

Anand KJS, Coskun V, Thrivikraman KV, et al. Long-term behavioral effects of repetitive pain in neonatal rat pups. Physiol Behav 1999;66:627–37.

Anand KJS, Garg S, Rovnaghi CR, et al. Ketamine reduces the cell death following inflammatory pain in newborn rat brain. Pediatr Res 2007;62:283–90.

Howard RF, Hatch DJ, Cole TJ, et al. Inflammatory pain and hypersensitivity are selectively reversed by epidural bupivacaine and are developmentally regulated. Anesthesiology 2001;95:421–7.

4. **What kind of painful experiences are neonates exposed to in the NICU?**

Neonates admitted to a modern-day NICU are often exposed to acute or prolonged pain from a variety of sources. These include acute pain caused by heel sticks, venipunctures, tracheal suctioning, lumbar punctures, or chest tubes; postoperative pain resulting from circumcision, surgery to repair a hernia or ligate a patent ductus arteriosus; and prolonged pain from necrotizing enterocolitis, meningitis, birth trauma, or ventilation. Even routine care such as diaper changes, daily weighing, removal of adhesive tape, burns from transcutaneous probes, and rectal stimulation will cause low-level noxious stimulation and background excitability in the "pain system." Although there is no definition for chronic pain in newborns, conditions associated with constant prolonged pain may include epidermolysis bullosa, necrotizing enterocolitis, scalded skin syndrome (staphylococcal), septic arthritis, tissue ischemia, and rare congenital conditions such as harlequin-type icthyosis. Identifying chronic pain is clinically relevant because it interferes with the infant's growth, prolongs hospitalization, alters subsequent pain perception, and impairs cognitive and behavioral development (van Ganzewinkel CJ, et al. Unpublished data, 2012).

Carbajal R, Rousset A, Danan C, et al. Epidemiology and treatment of painful procedures in neonates in intensive care units. JAMA 2008;300:60–70.

Losacco V, Cuttini M, Greisen G, et al. Heel blood sampling in European neonatal intensive care units: compliance with pain management guidelines. Arch Dis Child Fetal Neonatal Ed 2011;96:F65–8.

Taylor EM, Boyer K, Campbell FA. Pain in hospitalized children: a prospective cross-sectional survey of pain prevalence, intensity, assessment and management in a Canadian pediatric teaching hospital. Pain Res Manag 2008;13:25–32.

5. **Even if neonates do feel pain, will they ever remember it?**

   Neonatal painful experiences cannot be accessed by conscious recall but may lead to long-term or permanent alterations in brain development that are expressed in unique ways during different stages of development, depending on the type, duration, and severity of neonatal painful stimuli; the neurologic maturity at which pain occurs; and the use of analgesia. Term neonates exposed to acute, short-term pain develop significant degrees of hyperalgesia after tissue injury, which includes the areas where the injury occurred (i.e., primary hyperalgesia) as well as areas adjacent to or remote from the original injury (i.e., secondary hyperalgesia). If pain is prolonged or repetitive, the developing nervous system will be permanently modified, with altered processing at spinal and supraspinal levels. Tissue damage in the early neonatal period causes profound and long-lasting dendritic sprouting of sensory nerve terminals, resulting in hyperinnervation that may continue into childhood and adolescence. Thus repeated heel sticks could lead to gait disorders in childhood, repeated perioral and nasal suctioning may promote oral aversion syndrome, surgical sites may maintain an increased pain sensitivity, and gastric suctioning at birth may increase the likelihood of irritable bowel syndrome or visceral pain in adolescence.

Anand KJS, Hickey PR. Pain and its effects in the human neonate and fetus. N Engl J Med 1987;317:1321–9.

Anand KJS, Grunau RE, Oberlander T. Developmental character and long-term consequences of pain in infants and children. Child Adolesc Psychiatr Clin N Am 1997;6:703–24.

Whitfield MF, Grunau RE. Behavior, pain perception, and the extremely low-birth weight survivor. Clin Perinatol 2000;27:363–79.

Grunau R. Early pain in preterm infants. A model of long-term effects. Clin Perinatol 2002;29:373–94, vii–viii.

Anand KJS, Coskun V, Thrivikraman KV, et al. Long-term behavioral effects of repetitive pain in neonatal rat pups. Physiol Behav 1999;66:627–37.

Anand KJS. Effects of perinatal pain and stress. Prog Brain Res 2000;122:117–29.

Taddio A, Shah V, Gilbert-MacLeod C, et al. Conditioning and hyperalgesia in newborns exposed to repeated heel lances. JAMA 2002;288:857–61.

Fitzgerald M, Millard C, MacIntosh N. Hyperalgesia in premature infants. Lancet 1988;1:292.

Taddio A, Shah V, Atenafu E, et al. Influence of repeated painful procedures and sucrose analgesia on the development of hyperalgesia in newborn infants. Pain 2009;144:43–8.

Liu JG, Rovnaghi CR, Garg S, Anand KJS. Opioid receptor desensitization contributes to thermal hyperalgesia in infant rats. Eur J Pharmacol. May 3 2004;491(2-3):127–136.

Grunau RE. Long-term consequences of pain in human neonates. In: Anand KJS, Stevens BJ, McGrath PJ, editors. Pain in Neonates. 2nd ed. Amsterdam: Elsevier Science Publishers B.V.; 2000. p. 55–76.

Anand KJS, Scalzo FM. Can adverse neonatal experiences alter brain development and subsequent behavior? Biol Neonate 2000;77:69–82.

Anand KJS. Pain, plasticity, and premature birth: a prescription for permanent suffering? Nat Med 2000;6:971–3.

Narsinghani U, Anand KJS. Developmental neurobiology of pain in neonatal rats. Lab Animal 2000;29:27–39.

Peters JW, Schouw R, Anand KJS, et al. Does neonatal surgery lead to increased pain sensitivity in later childhood? Pain 2005;114:444–54.

De Lima J, Alvares D, Hatch DJ, et al. Sensory hyperinnervation after neonatal skin wounding: effect of bupivacaine sciatic nerve block. Br J Anaesth 1999;83:662–4.

Beggs S, Alvares D, Moss A, et al. A role for NT-3 in the hyperinnervation of neonatally wounded skin. Pain 2012;153:2133–9.

Kmita G, Urmanska W, Kiepura E, et al. Feeding behaviour problems in infants born preterm: a psychological perspective. Preliminary report. Med Wieku Rozwoj 2011;15:216–23.

Anand KJS, Runeson B, Jacobson B. Gastric suction at birth associated with long-term risk for functional intestinal disorders in later life. J Pediatr 2004;144:449–54.

6. **What are the experimental data supporting long lasting effects of pain in the newborn period?**

   Twin pairs who were discordant only for the experience of surgery in infancy showed greater signs of attention-deficit/hyperactivity disorder, impulsivity, and socialization problems during early school years in the twin who was exposed to surgery compared with the other twin. Although it was speculated that these individuals may be at increased risk for developing chronic pain syndromes during adulthood, recent epidemiologic data from former preterm young adults suggest that this is not the case.

Former preterm infants exposed to higher numbers of "skin-breaking" procedures in the NICU demonstrate impaired brain and somatic growth, poorer cognitive and motor function, as well as numerous abnormalities in their brain structure (volumetric magnetic resonance imaging [MRI], diffusion tractography), and function (functional MRI, magnetoencephalography). These long-term effects occurred after controlling for illness severity in the NICU, overall morphine therapy, and exposure to postnatal steroids. Other cognitive and behavioral outcomes of former preterm children have been correlated with their cumulative pain experiences or length of NICU stay, but the relative contributions of repetitive pain, early illness severity, or the effects of premature birth itself remain undefined.

Repetitive pain in newborn rats accentuates neuronal excitation and cell death in developmentally regulated cortical and subcortical areas, associated with impaired short-term and long-term memory and altered pain thresholds. Morphine analgesia in newborn rats attenuated the long-term effects of neonatal pain on pain thresholds in adult male rats (but not females), whereas ketamine analgesia mediated similar long-term effects in adult female rats (but not males).

Schultz AH, Jarvik GP, Wernovsky G, et al. Effect of congenital heart disease on neurodevelopmental outcomes within multiple-gestation births. J Thorac Cardiovasc Surg 2005;130:1511–6.

Einaudi MA, Busuttil M, Monnier AS, et al. Neuropsychological screening of a group of preterm twins: comparison with singletons. Childs Nerv Syst 2008;24:225–30.

Littlejohn C, Pang D, Power C, et al. Is there an association between preterm birth or low birthweight and chronic widespread pain? Results from the 1958 Birth Cohort Study. Eur J Pain 2012;16:134–9.

Anand KJS. Pain, plasticity, and premature birth: a prescription for permanent suffering? Nat Med 2000;6:971–3.

Vinall J, Miller SP, Chau V, et al. Neonatal pain in relation to postnatal growth in infants born very preterm. Pain 2012;153:1374–81.

Grunau RE, Whitfield MF, Petrie-Thomas J, et al. Neonatal pain, parenting stress and interaction, in relation to cognitive and motor development at 8 and 18 months in preterm infants. Pain 2009;143:138–46.

Berman JI, Mukherjee P, Partridge SC, et al. Quantitative diffusion tensor MRI fiber tractography of sensorimotor white matter development in premature infants. Neuroimage 2005;27:862–71.

Peterson BS, Vohr B, Staib LH, et al. Regional brain volume abnormalities and long-term cognitive outcome in preterm infants. JAMA 2000;284:1939–47.

Brummelte S, Grunau RE, Chau V, et al. Procedural pain and brain development in premature newborns. Ann Neurol 2012;71:385–96.

Doesburg SM, Ribary U, Herdman AT, et al. Magnetoencephalography reveals slowing of resting peak oscillatory frequency in children born very preterm. Pediatr Res 2011;70:171–5.

Brummelte S, Grunau RE, Zaidman-Zait A, et al. Cortisol levels in relation to maternal interaction and child internalizing behavior in preterm and full-term children at 18 months corrected age. Dev Psychobiol 2011;53:184–95.

Doesburg SM, Ribary U, Herdman AT, et al. Altered long-range alpha-band synchronization during visual short-term memory retention in children born very preterm. Neuroimage 2011;54:2330–9.

Grunau RV, Whitfield MF, Petrie JH. Pain sensitivity and temperament in extremely low-birth-weight premature toddlers and preterm and full-term controls. Pain 1994;58:341–6.

Grunau RV, Whitfield MF, Petrie JH, et al. Early pain experience, child and family factors, as precursors of somatization: a prospective study of extremely premature and fullterm children. Pain 1994;56:353–9.

Grunau RVE, Whitfield MF, Petrie J. Children's judgments about pain at age 8-10 years: do extremely low birthweight (<1000 g) children differ from full birthweight peers. J Child Psychol Psychiatr 1998;39:587–94.

Anand KJS, Coskun V, Thrivikraman KV, et al. Long-term behavioral effects of repetitive pain in neonatal rat pups. Physiol Behav 1999;66:627–37.

Anand KJS, Garg S, Rovnaghi CR, et al. Ketamine reduces the cell death following inflammatory pain in newborn rat brain. Pediatr Res 2007;62:283–90.

Bhutta AT, Rovnaghi CR, Simpson PM, et al. Interactions of inflammatory pain and morphine treatment in infant rats: long-term behavioral effects. Physiol Behav 2001;73:51–8.

8. **Are there any validated methods for pain assessment in neonates?**
    Neonates need to be comfortable and as free of pain as possible to grow and develop normally. Valid, reliable, and regular pain assessments are a major prerequisite for attaining this goal. Behavioral indicators of pain include facial actions, body movements and tone, cry, behavioral state changes,

TABLE 17-1.

PAIN SCALE	AGE	TYPE OF PAIN	PSYCHOMETRIC PROPERTIES
Preterm Infants			
Premature Infant Pain Profile (PIPP)	Preterm and full-term infants (28 to 40 weeks GA)	Acute (procedural) Acute (prolonged)	Interrater reliability Internal consistency Construct validity
Neonatal Infant Pain Scale (NIPS)	Preterm and full-term infants	Acute (procedural)	Interrater reliability Internal consistency Construct validity
Full-term Infants <2 Months			
Neonatal Facial Coding System (NFCS)	Preterm to term and older infants (27 weeks GA up to 2 months PCA)	Acute (procedural pain)	Interrater reliability Construct validity
Full-term Infants <12 Months			
Faces, Legs, Activity, Crying Consolability Scale (FLACC)	Full-term infants up to 2 months	Acute prolonged (postoperative)	Interrater reliability Internal consistency Construct validity
COMFORT Scale	Infants 0 to 12 months (+ children up to 17 years)	Acute (prolonged), chronic, or level of sedation	Interrater reliability Internal consistency Construct validity
Modified Behavioral Pain Scale (MBPS)	Infants 2-6 months	Acute (procedural– immunization)	Interrater reliability Internal consistency Construct validity

sleep patterns, and consolability. Physiologic indicators of pain include increased heart rate, respiratory rate, and blood pressure, as well as decreased heart rate variability and oxygen saturations. Pain assessment in neonates is difficult in neurologically compromised, chemically paralyzed, or nonresponsive infants.

Many methods for measuring the intensity of acute pain in neonates have been validated, but other aspects of painful experiences (e.g., character, location, rhythmicity, duration of pain) have not been routinely assessed in neonates. Very few methods have been validated for the assessment of postoperative pain or chronic pain. The most commonly used methods include the Premature Infant Pain Profile (PIPP), the Neonatal Infant Pain Scale (NIPS), the CRIES score, the Neonatal Pain, Agitation, and Sedation Scale (NPASS), the Neonatal Facial Coding System (NFCS), and the Douleur Aiguë du Nouveau-né (DAN) scale. For acute procedural pain, results using the the NIPS, NFCS, and DAN scales were comparable. A challenge facing clinicians is to develop and validate objective measures of prolonged pain in preterm and term neonates (Table 17-1).

Ranger M, Johnston CC, Anand KJ. Current controversies regarding pain assessment in neonates. Semin Perinatol 2007;31:283–8.

Grunau RE, Holsti L, Whitfield MF, et al. Are twitches, startles, and body movements pain indicators in extremely low birth weight infants? Clin J Pain 2000;16:37–45.

Boyle EM, Freer Y, Wong CM, et al. Assessment of persistent pain or distress and adequacy of analgesia in preterm ventilated infants. Pain 2006;124:87–91.

Thewissen L, Allegaert K. Analgosedation in neonates: do we still need additional tools after 30 years of clinical research? Arch Dis Child Educ Pract Ed 2011;96:112–8.

Stevens BJ, Johnston CC, Grunau RV. Issues of assessment of pain and discomfort in neonates. J Obstet Gynecol Neonatal Nurs 1995;24:849–55.

Fuller BF. Infant behaviors as indicators of established acute pain. J Soc Pediatr Nurs 2001;6:109–15.

Duhn LJ, Medves JM. A systematic integrative review of infant pain assessment tools. Adv Neonatal Care 2004;4:126–40.

Pereira AL, Guinsburg R, de Almeida MF, et al. Validity of behavioral and physiologic parameters for acute pain assessment of term newborn infants. Sao Paulo Med J 1999;117:72–80.

Franck LS, Ridout D, Howard R, et al. A comparison of pain measures in newborn infants after cardiac surgery. Pain 2011;152:1758–65.

Suraseranivongse S, Kaosaard R, Intakong P, et al. A comparison of postoperative pain scales in neonates. Br J Anaesth 2006;97:540–4.

Anand KJS. Pain assessment in preterm neonates. Pediatrics 2007;119:605–7.

Stevens B, Johnston C, Taddio A, et al. The premature infant pain profile: evaluation 13 years after development. Clin J Pain 2010;26:813–30.

Stevens B, Johnston C, Petryshen P, et al. Premature Infant Pain Profile: development and initial validation. Clin J Pain 1996;12:13–22.

McNair C, Ballantyne M, Dionne K, et al. Postoperative pain assessment in the neonatal intensive care unit. Arch Dis Child Fetal Neonatal Ed 2004;89:F537–41.

Lawrence J, Alcock D, McGrath P, et al. The development of a tool to assess neonatal pain. Neonatal Netw 1993;12:59–66.

Krechel SW, Bildner J. CRIES: a new neonatal postoperative pain measurement score. Initial testing of validity and reliability. Paediatr Anaesth 1995;5:53–61.

Hummel P, Lawlor-Klean P, Weiss MG. Validity and reliability of the N-PASS assessment tool with acute pain. J Perinatol 2010;30:474–8.

Hummel P, Puchalski M, Creech SD, et al. Clinical reliability and validity of the N-PASS: neonatal pain, agitation and sedation scale with prolonged pain. J Perinatol 2008;28:55–60.

Uyan ZS, Bilgen H, Topuzoglu A, et al. Comparison of three neonatal pain scales during minor painful procedures. J Matern Fetal Neonatal Med 2008;21:305–8.

Anand KJS, Aranda JV, Berde CB, et al. Summary proceedings from the neonatal pain-control group. Pediatrics 2006;117:S9–S22.

Boyle EM, Freer Y, Wong CM, McIntosh N, Anand KJS. Assessment of persistent pain or distress and adequacy of analgesia in preterm ventilated infants. Pain 2006;124:87–91

Saarenmaa E, Huttunen P, Leppaluoto J, et al. Advantages of fentanyl over morphine in analgesia for ventilated newborn infants after birth: a randomized trial. J Pediatr 1999;134:144–50.

Vaughn PR, Townsend SF, Thilo EH, et al. Comparison of continuous infusion of fentanyl to bolus dosing in neonates after surgery. J Pediatr Surg 1996;31:1616–23.

Guinsburg R, Kopelman BI, Anand KJS, et al. Physiological, hormonal, and behavioral responses to a single fentanyl dose in intubated and ventilated preterm neonates. J Pediatr 1998;132:954–9.

Lago P, Benini F, Agosto C, et al. Randomised controlled trial of low dose fentanyl infusion in preterm infants with hyaline membrane disease. Arch Dis Child Fetal Neonatal Ed 1998;79:F194–7.

Orsini AJ, Leef KH, Costarino A, et al. Routine use of fentanyl infusions for pain and stress reduction in infants with respiratory distress syndrome. J Pediatr 1996;129:140–5.

Anand KJS, Barton BA, McIntosh N, et al. Analgesia and sedation in preterm neonates who require ventilatory support: results from the NOPAIN trial. Neonatal Outcome and Prolonged Analgesia in Neonates. Arch Pediatr Adolesc Med 1999;153:331–8.

Anand KJS, Hall RW, Desai N, et al. Effects of morphine analgesia in ventilated preterm neonates: primary outcomes from the NEOPAIN randomised trial. Lancet 2004;363:1673–82.

Bellu R, de Waal K, Zanini R. Opioids for neonates receiving mechanical ventilation: a systematic review and meta-analysis. Arch Dis Child Fetal Neonatal Ed 2010;95:F241–51.

Dyke MP, Kohan R, Evans S. Morphine increases synchronous ventilation in preterm infants. J PaediatrChild Health 1995;31:176–9.

Lemyre B, Doucette J, Kalyn A, et al. Morphine for elective endotracheal intubation in neonates: a randomized trial [ISRCTN43546373]. BMC Pediatr 2004;4:20.

Simons SH, Anand KJS. Pain control: opioid dosing, population kinetics and side-effects. Semin Fetal Neonatal Med 2006;11:260–7.

Simons SH, van Dijk M, van Lingen RA, et al. Routine morphine infusion in preterm newborns who received ventilatory support: a randomized controlled trial. JAMA 2003;290:2419–27.

9. **What are the clinical effects of continuous morphine or fentanyl infusions in ventilated preterm neonates?**

Randomized placebo-controlled clinical trials have compared the efficacy and safety of intravenous fentanyl or morphine in ventilated preterm neonates. In infants treated with fentanyl, two trials reported lower behavioral stress scores at 16, 24, 48, and 72 hours; a third trial showed reduced pain scores compared with the placebo group. Infants receiving fentanyl had statistically lower heart rate values than the placebo group but required more ventilatory support.

In infants receiving morphine infusions, randomized controlled trials showed lower pain scores but no significant differences in intraventricular hemorrhage (IVH) (relative risk [RR] 1.13; 95% confidence interval [CI], 0.80-1.61), periventricular leukomalacia (RR, 0.81; 95% CI, 0.51-1.29), or mortality (RR, 1.14; 95% CI, 0.81-1.60) between the morphine and placebo groups. Intermittent bolus doses of open-label morphine, however, were associated with hypotension and increased rates of IVH and mortality. Morphine infusions did not improve short-term pulmonary outcomes among ventilated preterm neonates, whereas additional morphine doses were associated with worse respiratory outcomes among preterm neonates with respiratory distress syndrome. Infants receiving morphine spent more days on mechanical ventilation (weighted mean difference [WMD], 0.24 days; 95% CI, 0.11-0.36).

Saarenmaa E, Huttunen P, Leppaluoto J, et al. Advantages of fentanyl over morphine in analgesia for ventilated newborn infants after birth: a randomized trial. Journal of Pediatrics 1999;134:144–50.

Vaughn PR, Townsend SF, Thilo EH, et al. Comparison of continuous infusion of fentanyl to bolus dosing in neonates after surgery. J Pediatr Surg 1996;31:1616–23.

Guinsburg R, Kopelman BI, Anand KJS, et al. Physiological, hormonal, and behavioral responses to a single fentanyl dose in intubated and ventilated preterm neonates. J Pediatr 1998;132:954–9.

Lago P, Benini F, Agosto C, et al. Randomised controlled trial of low dose fentanyl infusion in preterm infants with hyaline membrane disease. Arch Dis Child Fetal Neonatal Ed 1998;79:F194–7.

Orsini AJ, Leef KH, Costarino A, et al. Routine use of fentanyl infusions for pain and stress reduction in infants with respiratory distress syndrome. J Pediatr 1996;129:140–5.

Anand KJS, Barton BA, McIntosh N, et al. Analgesia and sedation in preterm neonates who require ventilatory support: results from the NOPAIN trial. Neonatal Outcome and Prolonged Analgesia in Neonates. Arch Pediatr Adolesc Med 1999;153:331–8.

Anand KJS, Hall RW, Desai N, et al. Effects of morphine analgesia in ventilated preterm neonates: primary outcomes from the NEOPAIN randomised trial. Lancet 2004;363:1673–82.

Bellu R, de Waal K, Zanini R. Opioids for neonates receiving mechanical ventilation: a systematic review and meta-analysis. Arch Dis Child Fetal Neonatal Ed 2010;95:F241–51.

Dyke MP, Kohan R, Evans S. Morphine increases synchronous ventilation in preterm infants. J Paediatr Child Health 1995;31:176–9.

Lemyre B, Doucette J, Kalyn A, et al. Morphine for elective endotracheal intubation in neonates: a randomized trial [ISRCTN43546373]. BMC Pediatr 2004;4:20.

Simons SH, Anand KJS. Pain control: opioid dosing, population kinetics and side-effects. Semin Fetal Neonatal Med 2006;11:260–7.

Simons SH, van Dijk M, van Lingen RA, et al. Routine morphine infusion in preterm newborns who received ventilatory support: a randomized controlled trial. JAMA 2003;290:2419–27.

10. **What are the side effects of using morphine or fentanyl in neonates?**

Opiates have numerous side effects, including respiratory depression, nausea, vomiting, urinary retention, decreased gut motility, and histamine release causing hypotension or bronchospasm. Histamine release occurs more commonly with morphine than with fentanyl. In addition, morphine is associated with greater effects on gut motility, and very high doses may cause biliary spasm or even seizures. Chest wall rigidity or laryngospasm occur more commonly with fentanyl, with the rapid administration of intravenous doses. Fentanyl produces less sedation than morphine but has been associated with greater opioid tolerance because of its shorter duration of action.

Hall RW, Boyle E, Young T. Do ventilated neonates require pain management? Semin Perinatol 2007;31:289–97.

Simons SH, Anand KJS. Pain control: opioid dosing, population kinetics and side-effects. Semin Fetal Neonatal Med 2006;11:260–7.

Kart T, Christrup LL, Rasmussen M. Recommended use of morphine in neonates, infants and children based on a literature review: Part 2—clinical use. Paediatr Anaesth 1997;7:93–101.

Hall RW. Anesthesia and analgesia in the NICU. Clin Perinatol 2012;39:239–54.

Hall RW, Shbarou RM. Drugs of choice for sedation and analgesia in the neonatal ICU. Clin Perinatol 2009;36:15–26.

Semenikhin AA. Etiology of pruritus after epidural administration of narcotic analgesics. Anesteziol Reanimatol 1988:62–4.

Saarenmaa E, Huttunen P, Leppaluoto J, et al. Advantages of fentanyl over morphine in analgesia for ventilated newborn infants after birth: a randomized trial. J Pediatr 1999;134:144–50.

Koren G, Butt W, Pape K, et al. Morphine-induced seizures in newborn infants. Vet Hum Toxicol 1985;27:519–20.

Hall RW, Boyle E, Young T. Do ventilated neonates require pain management? Semin Perinatol 2007;31:289–97.

Fahnenstich H, Steffan J, Kau N, et al. Fentanyl-induced chest wall rigidity and laryngospasm in preterm and term infants. Crit Care Med 2000;28:836–9.

Lindemann R. Respiratory muscle rigidity in a preterm infant after use of fentanyl during Caesarean section. Eur J Pediatr 1998;157:1012–3.

Wells S, Williamson M, Hooker D. Fentanyl-induced chest wall rigidity in a neonate: a case report. Heart Lung 1994;23:196–8.

Anand KJS, Arnold JH. Opioid tolerance and dependence in infants and children. Crit Care Med 1994;22:334–42.

Anand KJS, Willson DF, Berger J, et al. Tolerance and withdrawal from prolonged opioid use in critically ill children. Pediatrics 2010;125:e1208–25.

Menon G, Anand KJS, McIntosh N. Practical approach to analgesia and sedation in the neonatal intensive care unit. Semin Perinatol 1998;22:417–24.

11. What are clinical signs of opioid withdrawal in neonates?

Many of these signs were included in scoring systems designed to quantify opioid withdrawal in neonates born from heroin-addicted mothers. Their applicability to iatrogenic opioid tolerance and withdrawal resulting from prolonged use in the NICU has not been proved. Previous methods included the Neonatal Abstinence Score (NAS) by Finnegan et al. or the Neonatal Narcotic Withdrawal Index (NNWI) by Green and Suffet, but newer methods include the Withdrawal Assessment Tool (WAT-1) and the Sophia Observation Scale (SOS). Signs of opioid withdrawal include the following (Box 17-1):

- Neurologic: high-pitched crying, irritability, increased wakefulness, hyperactive deep tendon reflexes, increased muscle tone, tremors, exaggerated Moro reflex, generalized seizures
- Gastrointestinal: poor feeding, uncoordinated and constant sucking, vomiting, diarrhea, dehydration
- Autonomic signs: increased sweating, nasal congestion, fever, mottling
- Other: poor weight gain, disorganized sleep states, skin excoriation

Finnegan LP. Effects of maternal opiate abuse on the newborn. Fed Proc 1985;44.

Katz R, Kelly HW, Hsi A. Prospective study on the occurrence of withdrawal in critically ill children who receive fentanyl by continuous infusion. Crit Care Med 1994;22:763–7.

Green M, Suffet F. The Neonatal Narcotic Withdrawal Index: a device for the improvement of care in the abstinence syndrome. Am J Drug Alcohol Abuse 1981;8:203–13.

Franck LS, Harris SK, Soetenga DJ, et al. The Withdrawal Assessment Tool-1 (WAT-1): an assessment instrument for monitoring opioid and benzodiazepine withdrawal symptoms in pediatric patients. Pediatr Crit Care Med 2008;9:573–80.

Franck LS, Scoppettuolo LA, Wypij D, et al. Validity and generalizability of the Withdrawal Assessment Tool-1 (WAT-1) for monitoring iatrogenic withdrawal syndrome in pediatric patients. Pain 2012;153:142–8.

Ista E, van Dijk M, Gamel C, et al. Withdrawal symptoms in children after long-term administration of sedatives and/or analgesics: a literature review. Assessment remains troublesome. Intensive Care Med 2007;33:1396–406.

Ista E, van Dijk M, Gamel C, et al. Withdrawal symptoms in critically ill children after long-term administration of sedatives and/or analgesics: a first evaluation. Crit Care Med 2008;36:2427–32.

BOX 17-1   WITHDRAWAL: A MNEMONIC FOR OPIOID WITHDRAWAL COINED BY THE AAP COMMITTEE ON DRUGS, 1983

W: wakefulness

I: irritability

T: tremor, tachypnea, temperature variation

H: hyperactivity, high-pitched cry, hyperreflexia

D: diarrhea, diaphoresis

R: respiratory distress, rhinorrhea

A: apnea, autonomic dysfunction

W: weight loss

A: alkalosis (respiratory)

L: lacrimation

AAP, American Academy of Pediatrics

12. **Can we prevent opioid tolerance in neonates requiring prolonged opioid analgesia?**

Preventing or delaying the onset of opioid tolerance may allow the rapid weaning of opioids, thus reducing the costs and complications of prolonged opioid weaning. Although listed here, the safety and efficacy of these approaches have not been tested in neonates.

- Concomitant infusion of opioid agonists and N-methyl-D-aspartate (NMDA) antagonists such as low-dose ketamine (0.2-0.3 mg/kg/h) can delay the development of opioid tolerance. Opioid drugs such as ketobemidone and methadone also block NMDA receptors and produce less tolerance than morphine or fentanyl.
- Continuous infusion of ultra-low-dose naloxone (0.1-0.5 μg/kg/h) selectively blocks the opioid receptors coupled with stimulatory G_s-proteins, thus blocking the mechanisms for superactivation of the cAMP pathway and inhibiting opioid tolerance.
- Procedural changes in adult or pediatric ICU patients such as the daily interruption of sedatives, nurse-controlled sedation, sequential rotation of analgesics, or the use of neuraxial opioids may also decrease the incidence of opioid tolerance and withdrawal.

Anand KJS, Willson DF, Berger J, et al. Tolerance and withdrawal from prolonged opioid use in critically ill children. Pediatrics 2010;125:e1208–25.

Bell RF. Low-dose subcutaneous ketamine infusion and morphine tolerance. Pain 1999;83:101–3.

Eilers H, Philip LA, Bickler PE, et al. The reversal of fentanyl-induced tolerance by administration of "small-dose" ketamine. Anesth Analg 2001;93:213–4.

Subramaniam K, Subramaniam B, Steinbrook RA. Ketamine as adjuvant analgesic to opioids: a quantitative and qualitative systematic review. Anesth Analg 2004;99:482–95, table of contents.

Anand KJS, Suresh S. Opioid tolerance in neonates: a state-of-the-art review. Paediatr Anaesth 2001;11:511–21.

Chana SK, Anand KJS. Can we use methadone for analgesia in neonates? Arch Dis Child Fetal Neonatal Ed 2001;85:F79–81.

13. **How should opioid withdrawal be treated in newborn infants?**

In addition to supportive therapy and the slow weaning of opioids, some pharmacologic agents with a relatively long half-life can be used to manage opioid withdrawal. The use of drugs such as paregoric, camphorated tincture of opium, phenobarbital, and chlorpromazine are not recommended for opioid withdrawal because of major side effects and lack of standardization. Therapeutic goals are to decrease the severity of withdrawal signs to a tolerable degree, enable regular cycles of sleeping and feeding, and decrease the agitation caused by medical interventions or nursing care.

- Methadone: This opioid agonist and NMDA antagonist has a long half-life (25 to 44 hours in neonates), can be given enterally (oral bioavailability, 80% to 90%), and reverses the tolerance produced by morphine or other opioid drugs. In one clinical study a methadone dose equivalent to 2.5 times the total daily fentanyl dose was effective in minimizing symptoms of opioid withdrawal.
- Buprenorphine: This is a partial μ-opioid agonist, a nociception/orphanin receptor agonist, and delta-opioid antagonist with analgesic effects similar to those of morphine in preterm neonates. Buprenorphine was as potent as high-dose methadone for adult opioid addiction, and its clinical use in opioid-addicted mothers induced significantly less opioid withdrawal in their infants compared with methadone-treated mothers.
- Clonidine: This alpha$_2$-adrenergic receptor agonist has analgesic effects when administered intravenously, intramuscularly, intrathecally, orally, epidurally, or topically. Because the alpha$_2$-adrenergic receptors activate the same inhibitory G_i-proteins, clonidine has been used to treat opioid withdrawal in neonates.
- Benzodiazepines: Benzodiazepines, such as diazepam or lorazepam, may be used for treating the seizures associated with opioid withdrawal, but they are not cross-tolerant with opioids and cannot be used as sole therapy for opioid withdrawal.

Anand KJS, Arnold JH. Opioid tolerance and dependence in infants and children. Crit Care Med 1994;22:334–42.

Anand KJS, Willson DF, Berger J, et al. Tolerance and withdrawal from prolonged opioid use in critically ill children. Pediatrics 2010;125:e1208–25.

Anand KJS, Suresh S. Opioid tolerance in neonates: a state-of-the-art review. Paediatr Anaesth 2001;11:511–21.

Chana SK, Anand KJS. Can we use methadone for analgesia in neonates? Arch Dis Child: Fetal Neonatal Ed 2001;85:F79–81.

Franck L, Vilardi J. Assessment and management of opioid withdrawal in ill neonates. Neonatal Netw 1995;14:39–48.

Siddappa R, Fletcher JE, Heard AM, et al. Methadone dosage for prevention of opioid withdrawal in children. Paediatr Anaesth 2003;13:805–10.

Tobias JD, Schleien CL, Haun SE. Methadone as treatment for iatrogenic narcotic dependency in pediatric intensive care unit patients. Crit Care Med 1990;18:1292–3.

Gowing L, Ali R, White J. Buprenorphine for the management of opioid withdrawal. Cochrane Database Syst Rev 2000:CD002025.

Lacroix I, Berrebi A, Chaumerliac C, et al. Buprenorphine in pregnant opioid-dependent women: first results of a prospective study. Addiction 2004;99:209–14.

O'Connor PG, Fiellin DA. Pharmacologic treatment of heroin-dependent patients. Ann Intern Med 2000;133:40–54.

Gold MS, Pottash AC, Sweeney DR, et al. Opiate withdrawal using clonidine. A safe, effective, and rapid nonopiate treatment. JAMA 1980;243:343–6.

Hoder EL, Leckman JF, Ehrenkranz R, et al. Clonidine in neonatal narcotic-abstinence syndrome. N Engl J Med 1981;305:1284.

Kosten TR, Rounsaville BJ, Kleber HD. Comparison of clinician ratings to self reports of withdrawal during clonidine detoxification of opiate addicts. Am J Drug Alcohol Abuse 1985;11:1–10.

Osborn DA, Jeffery HE, Cole MJ. Sedatives for opiate withdrawal in newborn infants. Cochrane Database Syst Rev 2005:CD002053.

Pohl-Schickinger A, Lemmer J, Hubler M, et al. Intravenous clonidine infusion in infants after cardiovascular surgery. Paediatr Anaesth 2008;18:217–22.

Franck LS, Naughton I, Winter I. Opioid and benzodiazepine withdrawal symptoms in paediatric intensive care patients. Intensive Crit Care Nurs 2004;20:344–51.

Tobias JD. Tolerance, withdrawal, and physical dependency after long-term sedation and analgesia of children in the pediatric intensive care unit. Critical Care Medicine 2000;28:2122–32.

14. What are the methods for treating procedural pain in neonates?

Procedural pain should be prevented whenever possible. Procedural pain can be minimized with an appropriate awareness program involving nursing and respiratory therapy staff members; physicians; and, most important, parents. The most common sources of minor procedural pain are heel sticks and tracheal suctioning. Heel sticks can be treated with 25% sucrose, and tracheal suctioning can be treated with facilitated tucking. More pronounced pain should be treated with opiates. Remifentanyl, for example, is a good choice for short-term procedures such as intubation, whereas more prolonged pain should be treated with a longer-acting opiate such as morphine or fentanyl. Anxiolytics such as midazolam can be used as adjuncts, but they do not treat pain. Circumcision should be performed with sucrose and local anesthetic nerve block before the procedure and acetaminophen after the procedure.

Hall RW. Anesthesia and analgesia in the NICU. Clin Perinatol 2012;39:239–54.

Walter-Nicolet E, Annequin D, Biran V, et al. Pain management in newborns: from prevention to treatment. Paediatr Drugs 2010;12:353–65.

Cignacco EL, Sellam G, Stoffel L, et al. Oral sucrose and "facilitated tucking" for repeated pain relief in preterms: a randomized controlled trial. Pediatrics 2012;129:299–308.

Ward-Larson C, Horn RA, Gosnell F. The efficacy of facilitated tucking for relieving procedural pain of endotracheal suctioning in very low birthweight infants. MCN Am J Matern Child Nurs 2004;29:151–6; quiz 7–8.

Pereira e Silva Y, Gomez RS, Barbosa RF, et al. Remifentanil for sedation and analgesia in a preterm neonate with respiratory distress syndrome. [see comment] Paediatr Anaesth 2005;15:993–6.

Anand KJ, Sippell WG, Aynsley-Green A. Randomised trial of fentanyl anaesthesia in preterm babies undergoing surgery: effects on the stress response. [Republished in Lancet 1987 Jan 31;1(8527):243–8; PMID: 20928962]. Lancet 1987;1:62–6.

Anand KJS, Johnston CC, Oberlander TF, et al. Analgesia and local anesthesia during invasive procedures in the neonate. Clin Ther 2005;27:844–76.

Taddio A, Pollock N, Gilbert-MacLeod C, et al. Combined analgesia and local anesthesia to minimize pain during circumcision. [see comment] Arch Pediatr Adolesc Med 2000;154(6):620–3.

15. Why should EMLA be used with caution in infants?

EMLA is an acronym for eutectic mixture of local anesthetics, containing lidocaine (2.5%) and prilocaine (2.5%). Prilocaine is metabolized to ortho-toluidine, which can oxidize hemoglobin to methemoglobin in neonates. Preterm newborns are particularly at risk because their stratum corneum is thinner, causing increased absorption and higher serum prilocaine levels. However,this appears mainly to be a theoretical concern because the incidence of clinically significant methemoglobinemia is strikingly low, even among the preterm neonates exposed to repeated daily doses of EMLA (up to four times a day). The use of EMLA and sucrose is effective in reducing venipuncture pain.

Couper RT. Methaemoglobinaemia secondary to topical lignocaine/prilocaine in a circumcised neonate. J Paediatr Child Health 2000;36:406–7.

Biran V, Gourrier E, Cimerman P, et al. Analgesic effects of EMLA cream and oral sucrose during venipuncture in preterm infants. Pediatrics 2011;128:e63–70.

16. How do sweet solutions produce analgesia in newborns?

Nonpharmacologic interventions are useful for minor pain and as adjunct therapy for severe pain. Sucrose solutions block the nociceptive transmission in the ascending pathways that transmit noxious stimuli to the brain, while activating the descending inhibitory pathways that modulate pain. Additionally, animal studies show that the gustatory receptors stimulated by sucrose lead to an activation of the endogenous opioid systems in the newborn brainstem, with reduced pain transmission to the thalamocortical circuits. These mechanisms are unlikely to lead to increased beta-endorphin levels in peripheral plasma, as noted in preterm newborns. Additional evidence for this mechanism is demonstrated by the fact that naloxone blocks the analgesic effects of sucrose. Until further evidence becomes available, the consensus opinion remains that sucrose induces effective analgesia for acute pain resulting from skin-breaking procedures in term and preterm newborns. Recently, however, safety of the long-term repeated use of sucrose solutions has been called into question, and protocols should be developed to limit sucrose dosing.

Bhattacharjee M, Mathur R. Antinociceptive effect of sucrose ingestion in the human. Indian J Physiol Pharmacol 2005;49:383–94.

Mitchell A, Waltman PA. Oral sucrose and pain relief for preterm infants. Pain Manag Nurs 2003;4:62–9.

Harrison D, Bueno M, Yamada J, et al. Analgesic effects of sweet-tasting solutions for infants: current state of equipoise. Pediatrics 2010;126:894–902.

Holsti L, Grunau RE. Considerations for using sucrose to reduce procedural pain in preterm infants. Pediatrics 2010;125:1042–7.

Mokhnach L, Anderson M, Glorioso R, et al. NICU procedures are getting sweeter: development of a sucrose protocol for neonatal procedural pain. Neonatal Netw 2010;29:271–9.

17. What are the major goals for postoperative analgesia in neonates?

The goals of perioperative analgesic approaches are the relief of pain, the maintenance of physiologic stability, and the prevention of adverse events such as hypoventilation or shallow respiration owing to diaphragmatic splinting, paralytic ileus, protein catabolism, and pulmonary hypertension. The management of postoperative pain should ideally start before the operative procedure, with consideration given to the size and alignment of the surgical incision; the choice of anesthetic agents; infiltration of the surgical site with lidocaine or bupivacaine; and, if possible, the placement of an epidural catheter before or after surgery. Use of analgesics may improve postoperative outcomes with fewer adverse events, shorter duration of mechanical ventilation, rapid return of gastrointestinal function, and reduced incidence of postoperative apnea and other complications. Opiates are the mainstay of therapy; however, because of their known side effects, including respiratory depression, other drugs such as ketorolac and acetaminophen are being studied.

Truog R, Anand KJS. Management of pain in the postoperative neonate. Clin Perinatol 1989;16:61–78.

Anand KJS, Sippell WG, Aynsley-Green A. Randomised trial of fentanyl anaesthesia in preterm babies undergoing surgery: effects on the stress response. [erratum appears in Lancet 1987 Jan 24;1(8526):234]. Lancet 1987;1(8524):62–6.

Papacci P, De Francisci G, Iacobucci T, et al. Use of intravenous ketorolac in the neonate and premature babies. Paediatr Anaesth 2004;14:487–92.

18. What are the options for safe and effective postoperative analgesia in neonates?

Postoperative analgesia is usually provided with opioids (e.g., morphine, fentanyl, methadone), antipyretic analgesics including acetaminophen or its intravenous analog propacetamol, or the nonspecific cyclooxygenase (COX) inhibitors (e.g., ibuprofen, ketorolac, diclofenac). The newer COX-2 inhibitors (e.g., parecoxib, valdecoxib, celecoxib, meloxicam) have not been studied in or approved for newborns and small children. Other options include epidural or caudal anesthesia with bupivacaine, or bupivacaine mixed with fentanyl infusions continued into the postoperative period. The use of nurse-controlled analgesia using a patient-controlled analgesia pump is also under investigation.

Papacci P, De Francisci G, Iacobucci T, et al. Use of intravenous ketorolac in the neonate and premature babies. Paediatric Anaesth 2004;14:487–92.

19. Are the doses of morphine and fentanyl for postoperative analgesia in neonates similar to the doses used for older children?

Neonates may receive lower morphine infusion rates than older children after surgery, starting as low as 0.005 mg/kg/h for preterm neonates and 0.01 mg/kg/h for term neonates. Neonates with cyanotic congenital heart defects also require lower morphine infusion rates than neonates undergoing noncardiac surgery. Depending on the dose and other patient characteristics, fentanyl and sufentanil provide variable degrees of suppression of autonomic and hormonal/metabolic responses to major surgery in neonates, although fentanyl may increase the risk of postoperative hypothermia. Critically ill neonates, whose vascular tone depends on sympathetic outflow, may become hypotensive after bolus doses of fentanyl or morphine. In preterm neonates undergoing ductal closure, higher fentanyl doses (>10.3 mg/kg) were associated with a decrease in an unstable postoperative respiratory course. Randomized controlled trials show no differences in the postoperative analgesia produced by bolus doses versus continuous infusions of morphine; however, apnea or other complications were greater in the bolus-dosing groups. Intravenous boluses of opioids should be given slowly (over 15 to 30 minutes) to postoperative neonates.

Bouwmeester NJ, Anderson BJ, Tibboel D, et al. Developmental pharmacokinetics of morphine and its metabolites in neonates, infants and young children. Br J Anaesth 2004;92:208–17.

Sammartino M, Garra R, Sbaraglia F, et al. Experience of remifentanil in extremely low-birth-weight babies undergoing laparotomy. Pediatr Neonatol 2011;52:176–9.

Janvier A, Martinez JL, Barrington K, et al. Anesthetic technique and postoperative outcome in preterm infants undergoing PDA closure. J Perinatol 2010;30:677–82.

20. How does the metabolism of morphine differ in the neonate?

The majority of preterm neonates are capable of glucuronidating morphine, but birth weight and gestational and postnatal age influence the hepatic capacity for glucuronidation. Term and preterm neonates and older infants produce relatively greater proportions of morphine-3-glucuronide, which acts as an opioid antagonist and has a prolonged half-life. Older children and adults produce morphine-6-glucuronide, which is a potent analgesic, with 20 times the analgesic potency of morphine itself. Morphine-6-glucuronide was not detected in the plasma of any neonate, which may explain why neonates require relatively high plasma concentrations of unchanged morphine for effective analgesia.

Sammartino M, Garra R, Sbaraglia F, et al. Experience of remifentanil in extremely low-birth-weight babies undergoing laparotomy. Pediatr Neonatol 2011;52:176–9.

Anand KJS, Anderson BJ, Holford NHG, et al. Morphine pharmacokinetics and pharmacodynamics in preterm and term neonates: secondary results from the NEOPAIN trial. Br J Anaesth 2008 Nov;101(5):680-9.

20a. How do the pharmacokinetics of morphine differ in the neonate?

A meta-analysis performed from the reported pharmacokinetics parameters showed an increased volume of distribution for morphine, estimated to be 2.8 ± 2.6 L/kg, which seems to be unaffected by age. In contrast, the half-life and plasma clearance rates for morphine are clearly related to age, secondary to maturational changes in hepatic and renal function. Morphine half-life was estimated to be 9.0 ± 3.4 hours in preterm neonates, 6.5 ± 2.8 hours in term neonates ages 0 to 57 days and 2.0 ± 1.8 hours for older infants and children. Clearance was estimated to be 2.2 ± 0.7 mL/min/kg for preterm neonates, 8.1 ± 3.2 mL/min/kg for term neonates ages 0 to 57 days, and 23.6 ± 8.5 mL/min/kg for older infants and children. The prolonged half-life explains why effective analgesia can be maintained, following a loading dose, with very low infusion rates of morphine (5-15 μg/kg/h). Doses must be further decreased for neonates with impaired hepatic or renal functions, and a pharmacist should be consulted for these patients.

Anand KJS, Anderson BJ, Holford NHG, et al. Morphine pharmacokinetics and pharmacodynamics in preterm and term neonates: secondary results from the NEOPAIN trial. British Journal of Anaesthesia 2008;101:680–9.

21. **How do the pharmacokinetics of fentanyl differ in the newborn infant?**

    Fentanyl is highly lipophilic. It crosses the blood–brain barrier, rapidly accumulates in fatty tissues, and is metabolized in the liver to norfentanyl and other compounds, which are excreted by the kidneys. Fentanyl undergoes first-pass metabolism in the liver and the elimination half-life is predictably prolonged in the presence of increased abdominal pressure, which may limit hepatic blood flow. The plasma clearance of fentanyl increases with gestational and postnatal age, secondary to maturing hepatic and renal function. The volume of distribution also increases with age, whereas the elimination half-life is prolonged in very-low-birth-weight and extremely-low-birth-weight preterm infants and stable thereafter.

22. **What are the long-term outcomes of neonates who received morphine while being ventilated?**

    It is important to remember that preterm neonates are exposed to repeated invasive procedures that induce pain at a time of rapid brain growth and developmental programming of stress responses. In the few experiments that used opioids for surgical or inflammatory pain, no detrimental effects resulting from morphine exposure in infancy could be demonstrated. The long-term outcomes of former preterm children at 5 to 6 years of age who received morphine during their NICU course showed no differences in their cognitive, neuromotor, or behavioral outcomes, but there was a trend toward better performance in those receiving morphine. In children who were 5-years-old, de Graaf found that morphine-exposed neonates (compared with those in the placebo group) rated lower on a visual analysis subset. Other IQ subsets demonstrated no change when adjusted for other covariates using propensity scoring. Pilot data from the NEOPAIN cohort randomized to morphine or placebo groups in the NICU showed no differences in neuropsychologic outcomes at 5 to 7 years of age, but decreased body weight and head circumference, reduced socialization, and adaptive behaviors occurred in the morphine group. These children also had longer choice response latencies and 27% less task completion during a short-term memory task. However, in this same cohort at school age, the authors found a significant benefit of preemptive morphine analgesia compared with placebo controls among ventilated preterm neonates in math skills (8 to 10 years of age). Literacy placement was similar in the morphine and placebo groups. Limited data are available on the long-term developmental outcomes for neonates exposed to fentanyl therapy in the NICU.

MacGregor R, Evans D, Sugden D, et al. Outcome at 5-6 years of prematurely born children who received morphine as neonates. Arch Dis Childhood Fetal Neonatal Ed 1998;79(1):F40–3.

de Graaf J, van Lingen RA, Simons SHP, et al. Long-term effects of routine morphine infusion in mechanically ventilated neonates on children's functioning: five-year follow-up of a randomized controlled trial. Pain 2011;152:1391–7.

✓ KEY POINTS: PAIN MANAGEMENT IN NEONATES

1. All neonates feel pain, and the clinician must effectively deal with the potential for pain during any procedure performed during the neonatal period.

2. Premature infants have a greater sensitivity to pain than do term infants.

3. Although children may not directly recall painful experiences from their NICU stay, they may demonstrate altered behavioral states resulting from painful experiences that were not well managed.

4. Morphine and fentanyl appear to be equally effective for pain relief in neonates and appear to have similar outcomes in short-term follow-up studies.

5. Methadone and some of the newer narcotic agonists (e.g., buprenorphine), as well as a number of other agents, appear to be optimal treatments for narcotic withdrawal in neonates. Paregoric and phenobarbital are no longer drugs of choice.

6. Nonpharmacological approaches, including sucrose, pacifier, swaddling, and breastfeeding, are effective against the acute pain caused by skin or tissue injury.

PULMONOLOGY

Reese H. Clark, MD

CHAPTER 18

DIFFERENTIAL DIAGNOSIS OF NEONATAL PULMONARY DISORDERS

1. **Although apnea in premature infants is often caused by the degree of immaturity (so-called apnea of prematurity), what are other causes of apnea in this population?**
    See Table 18-1.

2. **Is apnea of prematurity correlated with an increased incidence of sudden infant death syndrome (SIDS)?**
    No. Although apnea is often believed to be a provocative factor for SIDS, this relationship has never been causally established. It appears that premature infants with apnea of prematurity are no more likely to die as a result of SIDS than those of comparable gestational age who do not have apnea of prematurity. Premature infants do, however, have a higher SIDS rate than do term infants, suggesting that immaturity of respiratory control may be a component of SIDS. Furthermore, several studies have indicated that unless respiratory patterns of premature infants are recorded, apnea will not be detected because the respiratory abnormalities in these babies are very difficult to see clinically.

    American Academy of Pediatrics. Apnea, sudden infant death syndrome, and home monitoring. Pediatrics 2003;111(4 Pt 1):914–7.

3. **Of all newborn infants who die as a result of culture-proven bacteremia, what proportion has pneumonia?**
    Of infants who die as a result of bacteremia, 90% have evidence of pneumonia on postmortem examination. Many of these infants, however, will not have positive blood cultures during life, making the bacteriologic diagnosis of pneumonia difficult. If pneumonia is suspected on the basis of the clinical examination or chest x-ray, it should be treated aggressively until it has clinically resolved or until the child has been treated for a minimum of 10 days.

4. **What are the most common radiographic features of group B streptococcal (GBS) pneumonia in premature infants? In term infants?**
    In premature infants GBS often mimics respiratory distress syndrome (RDS) with a diffuse reticulogranular pattern and air bronchograms. It is unclear whether this pattern indicates simultaneous disease processes (RDS and GBS) or whether GBS disease causes a secondary surfactant deficiency that produces a radiographic appearance similar to that of RDS when a premature infant is infected.

    In term neonates the most common GBS appearance mimics that of transient tachypnea of the newborn, with increased perihilar interstitial markings, hyperexpanded lung fields, and small pleural effusions.

5. **In a neonate who is breathing normally, is a low partial pressure of oxygen (arterial PO_2) and normal partial pressure of carbon dioxide ($PaCO_2$) more consistent with cyanotic heart disease or severe lung disease?**
    Neonates who have low oxygen saturations or arterial oxygen levels (arterial PO_2), normal carbon dioxide levels ($PaCO_2$), and no signs of respiratory distress usually have cyanotic congenital heart disease. Low arterial PO_2 and a rising $PaCO_2$ in a neonate with labored breathing (e.g., grunting, retractions, tachypnea) suggest intrinsic lung disease and its attendant intrapulmonary shunt. A high

TABLE 18-1. CAUSES OF APNEA IN PREMATURE INFANTS

SYSTEM	PERTURBATION
Central nervous	Intracranial hemorrhage, hypoxic-ischemic encephalopathy, seizures, congenital anomalies, maternal drugs, drugs used to treat the infant
Respiratory	Pneumonia, airway obstruction with lesions, anatomic obstruction (e.g., pharynx or tongue blocking airway), upper airway collapse (e.g., tracheal or laryngomalacia), severe respiratory distress syndrome, atelectasis
Infectious	Septicemia or meningitis caused by bacterial, fungal, or viral agents
Gastrointestinal	Necrotizing enterocolitis, gastroesophageal reflux, positive result to Valsalva maneuver during bowel movements
Metabolic	Hypoglycemia, hypocalcemia, hyponatremia or hypernatremia, inborn errors of metabolism, increased or decreased ambient temperature, hypothermia
Cardiovascular	Hypotension, congestive heart failure, hypovolemia, patent ductus arteriosus
Hematologic	Anemia

level of $PaCO_2$ in association with severe retractions, normal arterial PO_2 in minimal oxygen support, and signs of gas trapping on chest radiograph is most consistent with upper airway obstruction. Therefore if an infant is easy to oxygenate and impossible to ventilate, think airway; if the infant is easy to ventilate and impossible to oxygenate, think heart; and if both oxygenation and ventilation are problems, think lung disease.

NEONATAL RESUSCITATION

6. **What is the most important aspect of neonatal resuscitation?**
   Airway, airway, airway: Managing the airway is always the most critical aspect of resuscitation. Most neonates who require support in the delivery room will respond to stimulation, opening of the airway, and gentle ventilation with a bag and mask.

7. **What is the maximum concentration of oxygen that a self-inflating anesthesia bag not connected to an oxygen reservoir can deliver?**
   Only about 40% oxygen can be delivered without a reservoir. Each time a self-inflating bag is squeezed, room air is drawn into the bag, diluting any oxygen that is connected. When a reservoir is connected, concentrations up to 90% or more of oxygen may be delivered. One of the limitations of the self-inflating bag is that the desired concentration of oxygen cannot be altered easily.

✓ KEY POINTS: DIFFERENTIAL DIAGNOSIS OF NEONATAL PULMONARY DISORDERS

1. If a patient is easy to oxygenate but impossible to ventilate, airway disease should be considered the most likely pulmonary problem.

2. If a patient is easy to ventilate but impossible to oxygenate, cyanotic congenital heart disease is the most likely cause for the gas exchange problem.

3. If both oxygenation and ventilation are problems, intrinsic lung disease is the most likely problem.

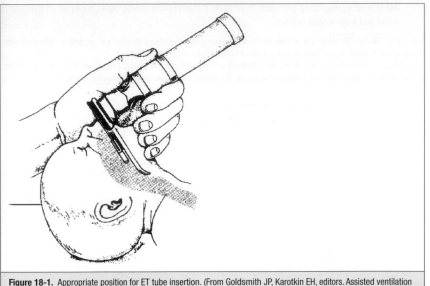

Figure 18-1. Appropriate position for ET tube insertion. (From Goldsmith JP, Karotkin EH, editors. Assisted ventilation of the neonate. 3rd ed. Philadelphia: Saunders; 1996. p. 108.)

8. **What are the approximate endotracheal (ET) tube sizes that would be appropriate for premature infants of varying birth weights?**
   - 2.5-mm internal diameter (ID) for infants weighing <1000 g
   - 3.0-mm ID for infants 1000 to 2000 g
   - 3.5-mm ID for infants 2000 to 3500 g
   - 4.0-mm ID for infants >3500 g

   These sizes are reasonable approximations for most infants, but attention should be paid to the ease of introduction of the ET tube into the airway. A 2.5-mm ET tube may be too small for some babies weighing less than 1000 g, and it may be too large for a few infants with birth weights greater than 1000 gm. The ET tube should slide easily into the airway, and a small leak should be audible around the ET tube when pressures of 25 to 30 cm H_2O are exceeded. An ET tube that is too snug may lead to tracheal inflammation and stenosis, whereas an ET tube that is too small simply may not allow adequate gas delivery to the lungs.

9. **Before radiographic verification, how far should an ET tube be inserted to be in the appropriate position for infants of varying birth weight?**
   The "tip-to-lip" rule for placement is the distance from the ET tube tip to the centimeter marking on the tube itself (Fig. 18-1). Good approximations are as follows:
   - 6 to 7 cm for a child of 1000-g birth weight
   - 7 to 8 cm for a child of 2000-g birth weight
   - 8 to 9 cm for a child of 3000-g birth weight
   - 9 to 10 cm for a child of 4000-g birth weight

10. **Does the vigorous neonate born with thick meconium amniotic fluid need to have the trachea suctioned to remove meconium that may have been aspirated?**
    No. Compared with expectant management, intubation and suctioning of the apparently vigorous meconium-stained infant does not result in a decreased incidence of meconium aspiration syndrome

(MAS) or other respiratory disorders. In addition, it may provoke airway injury, especially if the child is active and moving after delivery.

Wiswell TE, Gannon CM, Jacob J, et al. Delivery room management of the apparently vigorous meconium-stained neonate: results of the multicenter, international collaborative trial. Pediatrics 2000;105(1 Pt 1):1–7.
Kattwinkel J, Bloom RS, American Academy of Pediatrics. American Heart Association. Textbook of neonatal resuscitation. [Elk Grove Village, Ill.]; [Dallas, Tex.]: American Academy of Pediatrics; American Heart Association; 2011.

11. **Which of the following is currently recommended by the neonatal resuscitation program: (A) calcium chloride for asystole, (B) atropine for bradycardia, (C) epinephrine for heart rate below 60 bpm, (D) 5% albumin for hypovolemia?**

    Only (C), epinephrine for heart rate below 60 bpm is currently recommended by the Neonatal Resuscitation Program. The other therapies have their advocates, but most studies have not shown them to be effective adjuncts for neonatal resuscitation.

    Two meta-analyses of several randomized controlled trials comparing neonatal resuscitation initiated with room air versus 100% oxygen showed increased survival when resuscitation was initiated with room air.

Kattwinkel J, Bloom RS, American Academy of Pediatrics. American Heart Association. Textbook of neonatal resuscitation. [Elk Grove Village, Ill.]; [Dallas, Tex.]: American Academy of Pediatrics ; American Heart Association; 2011.
    Davis PG, Tan A, O'Donnell CP, et al. Resuscitation of newborn infants with 100% oxygen or air: a systematic review and meta-analysis. Lancet 2004;364:1329–33.
    Rabi Y, Rabi D, Yee W. Room air resuscitation of the depressed newborn: a systematic review and meta-analysis. Resuscitation. 2007;72:353–63.

12. **Name some important historical figures who needed resuscitation after birth.**

    Voltaire, Samuel Johnson, Johann Wolfgang von Goethe, Thomas Hardy, Pablo Picasso, and Franklin D. Roosevelt—the world would have been a very different place had these individuals not had the benefit of resuscitation, rudimentary as it was. Remember, there were no board-certified neonatologists until the mid-1970s.

13. **Who was the first to use a mechanical device for intubation and resuscitation of neonates?**

    James Blundell (1790-1878), a Scottish obstetrician, used a "silver tracheal pipe" that had a blunt distal end with two side holes. He would slide his fingers over the tongue to feel the epiglottis and guide the tube into the trachea. Blundell would blow air into the tube approximately 30 times per minute to ventilate the baby.

14. **What three characteristics can be used to identify infants who do not require resuscitation?**

    Term gestation, crying or breathing, and good muscle tone are three useful characteristics identifying infants who do not require resuscitation.

15. **Name the initial steps in neonatal resuscitation.**

    1. Thermal management: The infant should be dried and kept warm.
    2. The airway should be assessed and cleared of fluid and birth debris if there are signs of obstruction. *Neonatal Resuscitation Textbook* recommends "suctioning immediately following birth (including suctioning with a bulb syringe) should be reserved for babies who have obvious obstruction to spontaneous breathing or who require positive-pressure ventilation."
    3. The baby should receive tactile stimulation. The baby's bottom should not be spanked; gentle stroking and rubbing of the skin of the legs and buttocks should suffice. The thorax should not be rubbed because it may interrupt a respiratory effort.

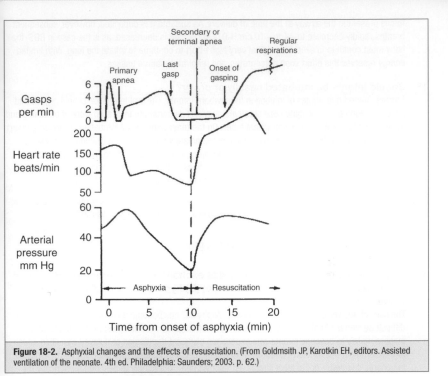

Figure 18-2. Asphyxial changes and the effects of resuscitation. (From Goldmsith JP, Karotkin EH, editors. Assisted ventilation of the neonate. 4th ed. Philadelphia: Saunders; 2003. p. 62.)

16. **What is primary apnea? How is it distinguished from secondary apnea?**

A regular sequence of events occurs when an infant becomes hypoxemic and acidemic. Initially, gasping respiratory efforts increase in depth and frequency for up to 3 minutes, followed by approximately 1 minute of primary apnea (Fig. 18-2). If oxygen (along with stimulation) is provided during the apneic period, respiratory function spontaneously returns. If asphyxia continues, gasping then resumes for a variable period of time, terminating with the "last gasp" and is followed by secondary apnea. During secondary apnea the only way to restore respiratory function is with positive pressure ventilation and high concentrations of oxygen. Thus a linear relationship exists between the duration of asphyxia and the recovery of respiratory function after resuscitation. The longer that artificial ventilation is delayed after the last gasp, the longer it will take to resuscitate the infant. Clinically, however, the two conditions are indistinguishable, although an infant's cyanosis will become progressively worse over time.

✓ KEY POINTS: NEONATAL RESUSCITATION

1. Airway, airway, airway—the most important aspect of neonatal resuscitation is managing the airway.

2. Most neonates who require support in the delivery room will respond to stimulation, opening of the airway, and gentle ventilation with a bag and mask.

17. **How much pressure does it take to inflate the lungs of a healthy infant at the moment of birth?**

The first breath of an infant has been measured in the delivery room and is reported to be between −30 and −140 cm H_2O. These pressures are needed to overcome the substantial fluid and elastic forces present in the airway at the time of delivery. As surfactant is deposited, however, subsequent breaths rapidly decrease to -4 to -10 cm H_2O. If surfactant is decreased, as is the case in RDS, the baby must continue to exert the original very high effort to continue to inflate the lung. With limited energy reserves this effort soon deteriorates, and respiratory failure ensues.

18. **Should infants be intubated nasally or orally?**
Studies support both routes of intubation for newborn infants. The oral intubation school argues that because neonates are obligate nose breathers, they will demonstrate increased work of breathing and atelectasis after removal of nasotracheal tubes. On the other hand, nasal intubation proponents assert that orotracheal intubation results in grooving of the palate with subsequent orthodontic problems. Nasal tubes, however, have been associated with injury to the nasal cartilage. Therefore operator skill and institutional tradition are primary considerations in this clinical decision. After extubation, however, there does appear to be a higher incidence of atelectasis with nasal ET tubes.

Kattwinkel J, Bloom RS, American Academy of Pediatrics. American Heart Association. Textbook of neonatal resuscitation. [Elk Grove Village, Ill.]; [Dallas, Tex.]: American Academy of Pediatrics; American Heart Association; 2011.

TRANSITIONAL PHYSIOLOGY AND THE ASPHYXIATED FETUS

19. **Asphyxia is a condition of impaired gas exchange best characterized by what blood gas abnormalities: (A) hypoxemia, (B) hypercapnia, or (C) metabolic acidosis?**
The correct answer is (C), metabolic acidosis. "Asphyxia" has become a controversial term because difficult deliveries of babies have resulted in so much litigation. The term *asphyxia* often is used inappropriately to describe infants who experience transient depression or delayed transition, much to the dismay of obstetricians, because of the medicolegal problems associated with birth asphyxia. In general, it is better not to label infants as "asphyxiated," but simply to describe numerically the metabolic derangements in the blood gases that are present after birth.

20. **A child is depressed and requires vigorous resuscitation in the delivery room. Subsequently, he demonstrates labile oxygenation and right-to-left shunting. A heart murmur is auscultated. What is the most likely anatomic or physiologic basis for the murmur?**
Tricuspid regurgitation is the most likely source of the murmur. Tricuspid regurgitation is due to increased pulmonary pressure and the backflow of blood into the right atrium. Although two fetal channels often remain open in this situation of transitional circulation (i.e., the foramen ovale and the ductus arteriosus), the source of heart murmurs is most likely from the associated tricuspid regurgitation.

✓ KEY POINTS: TRANSITION AND ASPHYXIA

1. Most infants with CP do not have a history to suggest an intrapartum event as the cause for their CP.

2. The use of the term *asphyxia* is not recommended. Instead, it is much more useful and appropriate to describe the events and symptoms and assign more definitive diagnoses.

21. **In the American Academy of Pediatrics–American College of Obstetricians and Gynecologists' guidelines regarding intrapartum asphyxia as a cause of brain injury, what criteria must be present?**
A neonate who has had hypoxia proximal to delivery that was sufficiently severe to result in hypoxic-ischemic encephalopathy should show evidence of all of the following:
- Profound metabolic or mixed acidemia (pH <7) on an umbilical cord arterial blood sample
- Early onset of neonatal encephalopathy
- Multisystem organ involvement

- Cerebral palsy (CP) of the spastic quadriplegic or dyskinetic type and no evidence of other potential causes for neonatal encephalopathy, such as trauma, coagulation or genetic disorders, and infectious conditions
- Exclusion of other identifiable etiologies, such as trauma, coagulation disorders, infectious conditions, and genetic disorders

Hankins GDV, Speer M. Defining the pathogenesis and pathophysiology of neonatal encephalopathy and cerebral palsy. Obstet Gynecol 2003;102(3):628-36.

22. **What are the established relationships between Apgar scores and subsequently diagnosed CP?**
    - Of children who develop CP, 73% have 5-minute Apgar scores of 7 to 10.
    - A child with a 1-minute Apgar score of 0 to 3 but a 10-minute Apgar score of 4 or higher has a 1% chance of subsequently developing CP.
    - Of children with a 15-minute Apgar score of 0 to 3, 53% die and 38% of survivors will subsequently develop CP.
    - Of children with a 20-minute Apgar score of 0 to 3, 59% die, and 57% of survivors will subsequently develop CP.

Lie KK, Groholt EK, Eskild A. Association of cerebral palsy with Apgar score in low and normal birthweight infants: population based cohort study. BMJ 2010;341:c4990.

23. **True or false? Mental retardation or seizures that are not associated with CP are not likely to be caused by asphyxia or other intrapartum events.**
    True. The etiology of mental retardation and seizures is not known in most cases.

24. **In 1862 William John Little concluded that "spastic rigidity" (i.e., CP) was exclusively caused by perinatal events. This led to the general belief for the next 100 years that CP was a preventable disorder caused by obstetric events. What was Dr. Little's medical specialty?**
    Dr. Little was an orthopedic surgeon. He saw children with the spasticity and mobility problems associated with CP. Only in the past two decades has it been recognized that only 4% to 10% of CP can be attributed to intrapartum events. That understanding has not, however, prevented the initiation of litigation in many cases of CP, even when no obstetric or neonatal malpractice exists.

25. **What prominent neurologist in 1897 came to the conclusion that most cases of CP were not caused by intrapartum events?**
    Sigmund Freud. Although he is most famous for his work in psychiatry, Freud was a prominent neurologist who made many astute observations in the field.

26. **True or false? Electronic fetal monitoring of the fetal heart rate has resulted in decreased deaths and a decrease in the incidence of CP.**
    False. Electronic fetal monitoring has not been shown to be any better than intermittent auscultation of the fetal heart rate. There are no well-controlled trials that show any decline in deaths or CP rates that can be attributed to electronic fetal heart rate monitoring. Although the use of fetal heart rate monitoring has become a standard practice, its prognostic value is currently unclear.

27. **What are the arterial PO_2 levels in a fetus?**
    If arterial blood gases were taken from a fetus, the PaO_2 (arterial PO_2) would be in the range of 25 to 35 mm Hg. Although seemingly low, the strong affinity of fetal hemoglobin for oxygen results in a highly saturated blood that is sufficient to meet the metabolic needs of the fetus. There is, however, little additional room for the PO_2 to decrease, and the fetus whose oxygen level begins to decrease even a small amount may develop problems quickly.

TABLE 18-2. APGAR SCORE

ASSESSMENT	0	1	2
Breathing	No spontaneous respirations	Weak respiratory effort	Vigorous respiratory effort
Heart rate	No HR	HR <100 bpm	HR >100 bpm
Color	Generalized cyanosis	Acrocyanosis	Pink, including extremities
Reflex irritability	None	Weakly responsive	Vigorously responsive
Tone	Flaccid	Weak tone	Good tone

HR, Heart rate

28. **Is fetal distress the same thing as "asphyxia" of the fetus?**
    No. Fetal distress often manifests as nonreassuring fetal heart rate patterns, meconium staining of the amniotic fluid, or a low 1-minute Apgar score. None of these has any predictive value for long-term neurologic outcome. However, the presence of signs of fetal distress is a good predictor of the need for resuscitation after delivery.

29. **Is "asphyxia" reversible?**
    Shorter and less severe periods of asphyxia often reverse spontaneously and may not lead to any long-term damage unless they occur repeatedly. However, complete failure of gas exchange can cause death in as little as 10 minutes.
    The outcome of infants with asphyxia depends on several factors:
    - Speed of onset of asphyxia
    - Duration and extent of asphyxia
    - Presence of ischemia in addition to hypoxia
    - Resuscitative efforts
    The significance of ischemia, in particular, cannot be overstated. Unless circulation is restored, the administration of oxygen will not be effective, and acidemia will increase. The ABCs of resuscitation—airway, breathing, and circulation—remain the key to successful outcome in resuscitation.

30. **Who was Virginia Apgar?**
    Virginia Apgar, an anesthesiologist at Columbia Presbyterian Medical Center in New York City, introduced the Apgar scoring system in 1953 to assess newborn infants' responses to the stress of labor and delivery.

31. **If Apgar scores are not useful in predicting long-term outcome, why do we even bother recording them?**
    Apgar scores are useful for assessing and describing the condition of neonates after birth and their subsequent transition to an extrauterine state (Table 18-2). The Apgar scores are generally obtained and totaled at 1 minute and 5 minutes after birth; however, scores should be recorded for longer periods (at 10, 15, and even 20 minutes) if they are low (until the score is ≥7). Low Apgar scores are useful in identifying neonates who are depressed, and the change in score at 1 minute, 5 minutes, and subsequent time intervals is often helpful in assessing the efficacy of resuscitation. Low Apgar scores (<3) that persist beyond 5 minutes have a better correlation with a poor long-term outcome than Apgar scores at 1 minute.

Kent A. Apgar scores and cerebral palsy. Rev Obstet Gynecol 2011;4(1):33–4.

32. **What is the long-term outcome of infants who are severely asphyxiated?**
    The mortality among severely asphyxiated infants is high and can vary from 50% to 75%. Among survivors, long-term neurodevelopmental sequelae are common and occur in approximately one third

TABLE 18-3. SARNAT CLASSIFICATION OF POSTANOXIC ENCEPHALOPATHY			
From Sarnat HB, Sarnat MS. Neonatal encephalopathy following fetal distress: a clinical and electroencephalographic study. Arch Neurol 1976;33:696–705; and Jain L, Ferre C, Vidyasagar D, et al. Cardiopulmonary resuscitation of apparently stillborn infants. J Pediatr 1991;118:778–82.			
SARNAT STAGE	**SIGNS/SYMPTOMS**	**EEG RESULTS**	**OUTCOME**
I	Lasts <24 hours; hyperalert; uninhibited Moro and stretch reflexes; sympathetic effects	Normal	Normal
II	Obtundation; hypotonia; strong distal flexion	Periodic EEG pattern, occasionally preceded by multifocal seizures	Normal if <5 days; abnormal if continuous delta activity >7 days
III	Stuporous; flaccid; suppressed autonomic and brainstem functions	Isopotential EEG or burst suppression	Probable neurologic impairment or death
EEG, Electroencephalography.			

of infants. Currently, there are no dependable predictors of long-term outcome. The presence and extent of neurologic abnormalities in the early postasphyxial phase and the persistence of abnormal neurologic findings at the time of discharge are the simplest and most effective predictors of long-term outcome. One measure of the severity of early neurologic dysfunction is the clinical staging system developed by Sarnat. Infants with Sarnat stage I encephalopathy are the ones who have mild asphyxia and recover without any significant neurologic sequelae. However, among infants with Sarnat stages II and III encephalopathy, the incidence of long-term neurodevelopmental handicaps can range anywhere from 50% to 100%. In one study of infants who had no detectable heart rate at birth and at 1 minute of age, two thirds died before discharge and 33% of the survivors had severe neurologic handicaps (Table 18-3).

33. **Are newborn brains more resistant to perinatal hypoxic and ischemic injury?**
Younger animals have been shown to have greater resistance to hypoxic-ischemic injury than older animals. Certain areas of the brain, however, appear to be more vulnerable to injury in neonates than in adults and in preterm compared with term infants. The neonatal brain is often described as having some degree of "plasticity," in which some areas may assume the function of other areas of the brain after injury. To what degree this phenomenon actually takes place is not known, but it may explain why prediction of outcome after neurologic injury in neonates is so fraught with error.

34. **What are the differences in the pattern of neurologic injury after hypoxic-ischemic insult in preterm and term infants?**
In preterm infants who survive with hypoxic-ischemic injury, periventricular leukomalacia is the most common (and most devastating) neuropathologic lesion. A large percentage of infants with periventricular leukomalacia develop spastic diplegia later in life. In term infants patterns of neuropathologic injury commonly seen are "watershed infarcts" and diffuse cortical necrosis. These infants are at high risk for developing spastic monoplegia, hemiplegia, or quadriplegia.

35. **Asphyxiated infants who are successfully resuscitated often show signs of injury to multiple organ systems. What other organs are involved? Is the injury permanent?**
In asphyxiated infants who have been successfully resuscitated, the central nervous system (CNS) is the most frequently involved site (72%), followed by the kidneys (62%), heart (29%), intestines (29%), and lungs (26%). Multiple organ involvement occurs even as an asphyxiated fetus or neonate tries to

redistribute blood to vital organs as a part of the "diving reflex." Fortunately, injury to these organs (except the CNS) is not permanent, and complete recovery of function can be expected in most infants who survive. However, the presence of multiorgan failure can seriously jeopardize chances of survival in the immediate postnatal period.

Martin-Ancel A, Garcia-Mix A, Gaya F, et al. Multiple organ involvement in perinatal asphyxia. J Pediatr 1995;127:786–93.

36. **What is the cause of oliguria in infants with hypoxic-ischemic perinatal injury?**
Oliguria is commonly seen in asphyxiated infants and can result from one or more of the following causes:
- Acute renal failure (either acute tubular necrosis or acute cortical necrosis)
- Asphyxiated bladder syndrome (bladder muscle injury)
- Syndrome of inappropriate antidiuretic hormone secretion (SIADH)

Although recovery from acute tubular necrosis is common, acute cortical necrosis is usually fatal. Infants with asphyxiated bladder syndrome, with marked distention, usually recover within a few days, as do most infants with SIADH, unless there has been a pituitary infarct.

37. **Prolonged resuscitation in the delivery room often makes resuscitated infants very cold. Is hypothermia harmful to these infants?**
Until recently, the presence of hypothermia in resuscitated infants was thought to correlate with poor survival and a higher occurrence of complications. However, recent studies have shown that selective cooling of the brain in infants suspected of having severe hypoxic-ischemic brain damage can improve long-term outcome. Multicenter trials from nurseries around the world have been very promising in this regard. It appears, however, that the primary beneficiary is a child with mild to moderate perinatal asphyxia. Infants with more severe forms of injury do not appear to benefit as much. In addition to improving neurodevelopmental outcomes, cooling reduces mortality risk. Analysis of data from all 10 trials that reported mortality rates showed that infants treated with prolonged moderate hypothermia were less likely to die than those who received normal care. A total of 169 (26%) of the 660 infants treated with therapeutic hypothermia died, compared with 217 (33%) of the 660 infants who received standard care (relative risk 0.78, 95% CI 0.66 to 0.93, P=0.005), with a number needed to treat of 14 (95% CI 8 to 47).

Edwards AD, Brocklehurst P, Gunn AJ, et al. Neurological outcomes at 18 months of age after moderate hypothermia for perinatal hypoxic ischaemic encephalopathy: synthesis and meta-analysis of trial data. BMJ 2010;340:c363.

Higgins RD, Raju T, Edwards AD, et al. Hypothermia and other treatment options for neonatal encephalopathy: an executive summary of the Eunice Kennedy Shriver NICHD workshop. J Pediatr 2011;159(5):851–8.

38. **What is the outcome of infants receiving various forms of resuscitation?**
The outcome of depressed infants is usually determined by the degree of resuscitative efforts that are necessary. In one study infants who required chest compressions and epinephrine had the worst outcome, with up to 56% dying in the neonatal period and 21% having an intracranial hemorrhage. Other complications noted in recipients of chest compressions included seizures (18%), respiratory distress (68%), and pneumothorax (24%).

Jain L, Vidyasagar D. Cardiopulmonary resuscitation of newborns: its application to transport medicine. Pediatr Clin North Am 1993;40:287–301.

39. **How is the outcome of resuscitation affected by prematurity and birth weight?**
Very-low-birth-weight (VLBW) infants have the greatest need for resuscitation at birth, with up to two thirds of infants weighing less than 1500 g requiring some form of resuscitation. The morbidity and mortality rates in VLBW infants requiring cardiopulmonary resuscitation are inversely related to their birth weight. Recent data indicate that VLBW infants do better if they are delivered and cared for at tertiary care centers. The speed of an in-house response team to the delivery room for resuscitation unquestionably is a great advantage of the tertiary care center compared with a community hospital.

40. **What are the absolute indications for initiating positive pressure ventilation through a bag-and-mask apparatus in a newborn?**
    - Apnea
    - Bradycardia (heart rate <100 bpm)
    - Ineffective or gasping respirations
    - Intractable cyanosis

41. **What are two contraindications to immediate bag-and-mask ventilation?**
    Immediate bag-and-mask ventilation is contraindicated when there is thick meconium in the hypopharynx and trachea or if a congenital diaphragmatic hernia is known or suspected. In all instances, however, the resuscitator must weigh the advantages of bag-and-mask therapy with the risks. At times, immediate intubation for suctioning or to avoid abdominal distention may be required.

42. **What are some indications for ET intubation during the resuscitation of a newborn?**
    - Need for prolonged bag-and-mask ventilation
    - Prolonged chest compressions (>1 minute)
    - Ineffective bag-and-mask ventilation
    - Congenital diaphragmatic hernia (do not insufflate the bowel with bag-and-mask ventilation, if possible)

43. **What causes persistent bradycardia or cyanosis in an infant who is receiving bag-and-mask ventilation?**
    - Improper mask size or fit (the mask should fit snugly from the bridge of the baby's nose to the base of the chin)
    - Poor seal of mask over the baby's face
    - Improper positioning of the infant (remember to place the baby in the "sniffing" position, with the neck slightly extended and the chin up)
    - Airway obstruction or need for suctioning
    - Ineffective manual ventilation (remember to watch for that chest rise and use just enough positive pressure ventilation—about 15 to 20 cm H_2O pressure for an average term infant—to see good chest rise)

    Make sure the oxygen source is turned on to the bag apparatus ("The heart and lungs can't run if there's no gas").

44. **What are the appropriate steps for the intubation of a neonate?**
    - Always check the equipment to ensure proper functioning (e.g., laryngoscope blade bulb works, suction is on, 100% free-flow oxygen is turned on, tape for ET tube is available).
    - Be sure that the warmer bed is flattened and not at an angle; the latter position of the bed will distort airway landmarks.
    - Choose the appropriately sized ET tube.
    - Position the baby with the neck slightly extended and the chin up (use a roll under the shoulders to achieve proper extension if necessary). Do not hyperextend the neck (Fig. 18-3).
    - Make sure the hypopharynx has been suctioned to clear debris.
    - Using the laryngoscope blade to visualize the vocal cords, insert the ET tube to the appropriate depth. (Limit intubation attempts to approximately 20 seconds to avoid reflex bradycardia.)
    - Institute manual ventilation while holding the tube in a secure position.
    - Listen for equal breath sounds on both sides of the chest.
    - Auscultate over the stomach to make sure there is not an esophageal intubation.
    - Watch for symmetric chest rise. Give just enough positive pressure to initiate chest rise.
    - Use of a CO_2 detector may assist in reassuring that you are in the airway.

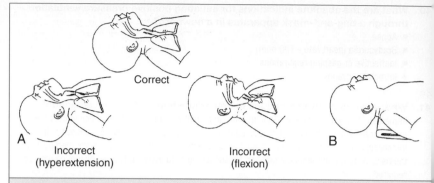

Figure 18-3. A, Correct and incorrect head positions for resuscitation. **B,** Optimal shoulder roll use for maintaining correct head position. (From Goldsmith JP, Karotkin EH, editors. Assisted ventilation of the neonate. 4th ed. Philadelphia: Saunders; 2003. p. 68.)

45. **When should epinephrine be given during a resuscitation in the delivery room?**
In a depressed infant with gasping or absent respirations, 100% oxygen should be given by positive pressure ventilation. Depending on the extent of asphyxia (and depression of heart rate), cardiac compressions are usually initiated within 30 seconds. If there is no response (i.e., increased heart rate) after at least 30 seconds of positive pressure ventilation with 100% oxygen and chest compressions, epinephrine is indicated. As Kattwinkel et al. explain, "The recommended IV dose is 0.01 to 0.03 mg/kg per dose. Higher IV doses are not recommended because animal and pediatric studies show exaggerated hypertension, decreased myocardial function, and worse neurologic function after administration of IV doses in the range of 0.1 mg/kg. If the endotracheal route is used, doses of 0.01 or 0.03 mg/kg will likely be ineffective. Therefore, IV administration of 0.01 to 0.03 mg/kg per dose (0.1-0.3 mL of the 1:10,000 solution), is the preferred route."

Kattwinkel J, Perlman JM, Aziz K, et al. Neonatal resuscitation: 2010 American Heart Association guidelines for cardiopulmonary resuscitation and emergency cardiovascular care. Pediatrics 2010;126(5):e1400–e1413.

46. **Why is sodium bicarbonate not administered to treat respiratory acidosis?**
Unless ventilation is adequate, the carbon dioxide produced by the buffering reaction will not be eliminated and will act as a weak acid, further reducing the pH ("closed flask" phenomenon). It is therefore inappropriate and even dangerous to give bicarbonate until ventilation has been established and is found to be adequate.

47. **Are there complications of sodium bicarbonate therapy in infants?**
The relative risks of sodium bicarbonate therapy in infants are related to dosage (higher > lower), rapidity of administration (faster > slower), and osmolality (higher > lower). Physiologic complications include a transient increase in $PaCO_2$ and fall in arterial PO_2. The sudden expansion of blood volume and increase in cerebral blood flow may increase the risk of periventricular and intraventricular hemorrhage in preterm infants. Other potential complications include the development of hypernatremia and metabolic alkalosis. For these reasons sodium bicarbonate is not recommended as a routine part of the Neonatal Resuscitation Program (NRP).

48. **If a newborn is stabilized and the extent of acidosis is determined by an arterial blood gas, how is the therapeutic correction calculated?**

$$\text{dose of } NaHCO_3 \text{ (mEq)} = \text{base deficit (mEq/L)} \times \text{body weight (kg)} \times 0.3 \text{ (bicarbonate space)} \times 0.5 \text{ (half correction)}$$

Generally, it is safest to correct half the base deficit initially and then reassess acid–base status to determine whether further correction is necessary. Administration of bicarbonate to improve acidosis will often expand the circulation and provide additional acid washout, reducing the need for further therapy. Under optimal circumstances, sodium bicarbonate should be infused in small doses over 10 to 20 minutes as a dilute solution (0.5 mEq/mL). It is sometimes not possible to take that much time to administer bicarbonate.

49. What are the side effects of naloxone?

Naloxone has a history of being remarkably free of adverse effects, except for the possible precipitation of sudden drug withdrawal in infants born to drug-addicted mothers. Other reported side effects relate to the sudden release of catecholamines, which can cause hypertension, sudden cardiac arrest, and cardiac dysrhythmias. It is important to remember that the half-life of naloxone is significantly shorter than that of opioids. As a result, new guidelines from NRP are as follows: "Administration of naloxone is not recommended as part of initial resuscitative efforts in the delivery room for newborns with respiratory depression. Heart rate and oxygenation should be restored by supporting ventilation."

50. What is the primary way by which an infant regulates cardiac output?

Heart rate is the main variable through which an infant can increase cardiac output. A baby cannot significantly change stroke volume. Bradycardia will therefore significantly reduce a newborn's cardiac output.

51. What are the indications for chest compressions in an infant, and how should they be done?

NRP 2010 states that "chest compressions are indicated for a heart rate that is less than 60 per minute despite adequate ventilation with supplementary oxygen for 30 seconds. Because ventilation is the most effective action in neonatal resuscitation and because chest compressions are likely to compete with effective ventilation, rescuers should ensure that assisted ventilation is being delivered optimally before starting chest compressions. Compressions should be delivered on the lower third of the sternum to a depth of approximately one third of the anterior-posterior diameter of the chest. Two techniques have been described: compression with 2 thumbs with fingers encircling the chest and supporting the back (the 2 thumb–encircling hands technique) or compression with 2 fingers with a second hand supporting the back. Because the 2 thumb–encircling hands technique may generate higher peak systolic and coronary perfusion pressure than the 2-finger technique, 76–80, the 2 thumb–encircling hands technique is recommended for performing chest compressions in newly born infants."

Kattwinkel J, Perlman JM, Aziz K, et al. Neonatal resuscitation: 2010 American Heart Association guidelines for cardiopulmonary resuscitation and emergency cardiovascular care. Pediatrics 2010;126(5):e1400–e1413.

52. What is a good source of emergent venous access in the newborn?

An umbilical venous catheter (UVC) can be placed quickly by trimming the umbilicus to approximately 0.5 to 1 cm in length and inserting the catheter just far enough to obtain blood flow (usually about 3 to 5 cm in term infants). All medications (including vasopressor agents) and fluids can be given through this line. This source of access is often available for many days after birth with appropriate preparation of the cord. The catheter, however, should not be left in this position for a prolonged period of time. If the field has remained sterile (a not terribly common situation in the haste of resuscitation), the catheter should soon be advanced into the inferior vena cava, just below the level of the right atrium. A chest radiograph should be obtained to determine the position. If the catheter has been contaminated, it should be replaced after sterile preparation of the field.

53. What are the common medications used for newborn resuscitation? How are they given, and in what doses?

If the heart rate remains below 60 beats per minute despite adequate ventilation with 100% oxygen and chest compressions, administration of epinephrine or volume expansion (or both) may be indicated. Rarely, buffers, narcotic antagonists, or vasopressors may be useful after resuscitation; they are not recommended in the delivery room. The recommended IV dose of epinephrine is 0.01 to 0.03 mg/kg per dose. Higher doses are not recommended.

54. **What fluids are appropriate to use in newborn resuscitation?**
"Volume expansion should be considered when blood loss is known or suspected (pale skin, poor perfusion, weak pulse) and the baby's heart rate has not responded adequately to other resuscitative measures. An isotonic crystalloid solution or blood is recommended for volume expansion in the delivery room. The recommended dose is 10 mL/kg, which may need to be repeated. When resuscitating premature infants, care should be taken to avoid giving volume expanders rapidly, because rapid infusions of large volumes have been associated with intraventricular hemorrhage."

Kattwinkel J, Perlman JM, Aziz K, et al. Neonatal resuscitation: 2010 American Heart Association guidelines for cardiopulmonary resuscitation and emergency cardiovascular care. Pediatrics 2010;126(5):e1400-e1413.

55. **Why is it important to check blood glucose concentration during resuscitation?**
Hypoglycemia can be very damaging to the developing nervous system. It can result when hepatic glycogen stores are depleted as a result of stress. A blood glucose level below 40 mg/dL warrants treatment. The clinician should infuse 10% dextrose in water at a dose of 2 mL/kg over 10 to 15 minutes in an attempt to correct hypoglycemia. The target glucose concentration is greater than 45 to 50 mg/dL before each feeding. It is *not necessary* to use higher concentrations of glucose (e.g., $D_{25}W$) in such circumstances. After the hypoglycemia has been corrected, normoglycemia can usually be maintained by an infusion rate of 5 to 8 mg/kg/min. In some circumstances hypoglycemia may not be corrected until the infusion rate is 8 to 12 mg/kg/min. Infants receiving levels this high who continue to demonstrate hypoglycemia may have an islet cell adenoma of the pancreas that is producing hyperinsulinemia.

Committee on Fetus and Newborn. Postnatal glucose homeostasis in late-preterm and term infants. Pediatrics 2011;127(3):575–9.

56. **Why is measurement of hematocrit after acute blood loss not a good indicator of blood volume?**
The immediate response to acute blood loss is vasoconstriction to maintain blood pressure. The blood that has been lost contains the same percentage of red blood cells as the blood that is retained. The hematocrit will not drop until fluid repletion of the intravascular volume occurs.

57. **What are the important clinical signs used to assess tissue perfusion?**
These clinical signs are pulse rate and quality, capillary refill time, and urine output.

✓ KEY POINTS: RESPIRATORY DISTRESS SYNDROME

1. Prevention is better than rescue treatment in promoting a healthy outcome for a neonate with RDS.

2. The most well-studied and effective way to improve outcomes of neonates with RDS is instilling surfactant into the trachea.

58. **After a traumatic delivery, what are the most commonly injured systems?**
   - Cranial injuries: caput succedaneum, subconjunctival hemorrhage, cephalohematoma, subgaleal hemorrhage, skull fractures, intracranial hemorrhage, cerebral edema
   - Spinal injuries: spinal cord transection
   - Peripheral nerve injuries: brachial palsy (Erb–Duchenne palsy, Klumpke paralysis), phrenic nerve and facial nerve paralysis
   - Visceral injuries: liver rupture or hematoma, splenic rupture, adrenal hemorrhage
   - Skeletal injuries: fractures of the clavicle, femur, and humerus

59. **When should neonatal resuscitation be stopped?**
No precise answer is possible because clinical circumstances and responses are variable. However, in one study of 58 newborns with an Apgar score of 0 at 10 minutes despite appropriate resuscitative

efforts, only 1 of 58 survived, and that infant had profound CP. Studies of therapeutic hypothermia, however, show that initiaton of cooling within 6 hours improves outcomes. According to NRP guidelines (see first reference below), "In a newly born baby with no detectable heart rate, it is appropriate to consider stopping resuscitation if the heart rate remains undetectable for 10 minutes. The decision to continue resuscitation efforts beyond 10 minutes with no heart rate should take into consideration factors such as the presumed etiology of the arrest, the gestation of the baby, the presence or absence of complications, the potential role of therapeutic hypothermia, and the parents' previously expressed feelings about acceptable risk of morbidity."

Prolonged resuscitation has a very high risk of ischemic injury to the brain, resulting in cystic encephalomalacia, CP, severe microcephaly, and developmental delay. Failure of response after more than 10 to 15 minutes should prompt the clinician to consider cessation of therapy, as difficult as that always is to do.

Kattwinkel J, Perlman JM, Aziz K, et al. Neonatal resuscitation: 2010 American Heart Association guidelines for cardio-pulmonary resuscitation and emergency cardiovascular care. Pediatrics 2010;126(5):e1400–e1413.

Kattwinkel J, Bloom RS, American Academy of Pediatrics. American Heart Association. Textbook of neonatal resuscitation. [Elk Grove Village, Ill.]; [Dallas, Tex.]: American Academy of Pediatrics; American Heart Association; 2011.

Jain L. Cardiopulmonary resuscitation of apparently stillborn infants: survival and long-term outcome. J Pediatr 1991;118:778–82.

60. **An infant who requires extensive resuscitation should be observed closely for the development of hypoxic-ischemic encephalopathy. What are the acute neurologic components of this syndrome?**
    - Persistent and prolonged hypotonia
    - Depressed reflexes
    - Altered level of consciousness
    - Convulsions

RADIOLOGY OF PULMONARY DISORDERS OF THE NEONATE

61. **Where should the tip of an umbilical arterial catheter in satisfactory position project on an anteroposterior (AP) radiograph of the chest and abdomen?**
    There are two major schools of thought on this subject. For many years the preferred position was between the third and fourth lumbar vertebrae, as projected on an AP radiograph. The tip lies below the take-off points for the renal and mesenteric arteries, theoretically reducing the risk of injecting fluids or drugs directly into those vessels. With this catheter placement, however, it has been shown that even with relatively low pressure, injectable material can ascend retrograde into the aorta for quite some distance. Other neonatologists prefer a higher placement, in the thoracic aorta at approximately T10 to T12, again avoiding placement of the catheter near the major tributaries off of the descending aorta. Positioning the tip there, however, means that anything injected will flow past major vessels. Several papers have argued for one placement instead of the other, but both are probably safe as long as the clinician takes the following precautions:
    - Careful placement under sterile conditions
    - Daily evaluation of ease of injection and withdrawal of blood
    - Assessment of the pressure waveform on the monitor screen
    - Inspection of the site for erythema and induration
    - Daily evaluation of urine output and blood pressure
    - Prompt removal of the line as soon as it is no longer needed

    Umbilical catheters may be left in place for many days as long as the aforementioned conditions are satisfactorily met. The typical goal is to remove umbilical lines within 7 days of birth. In extreme cases a catheter can be kept in place for 3 weeks without complication. One of the most common errors that is made in neonatal medicine, however, is to leave a catheter in place that is no longer necessary. Because it is not needed, the catheter is often not checked religiously and the risk of complications rises dramatically.

62. **Where should the tip of an umbilical venous catheter (UVC) be placed for satisfactory projection on an AP radiograph of the chest and abdomen?**
The UVC should be kept at the lower margin of the cardiac silhouette, approximately at the level of the right diaphragm, which would correspond to the junction of the inferior vena cava and right atrium of the heart. UVCs should not be allowed to remain below this level or within any of the branches of the portal system of the liver. Infusion of calcium or hyperalimentation into catheters in these incorrect positions may lead to liver toxicity, portal necrosis, cirrhosis, and cavernous transformation of the portal vein. Umbilical venous lines may also inadvertently cross the foramen ovale and enter the left side of the heart if inserted too far. Catheters in this location occasionally cause rhythm disturbances of the heart. This incorrect placement can be detected by the high levels of PO_2 obtained on a venous sample of blood. A single AP film can be misleading because the left atrium is posterior to the right atrium. Line placement may appear to be appropriate because the AP film does not demostrate how far posterior the line is placed. Lateral films of the chest and abdomen and echocardiograms can be used to confirm appropriate placement.

63. **What is the best position, as seen on an AP radiograph of the chest, for the tip of an ET tube in an intubated neonate?**
The optimal position for an ET tube is approximately halfway between the thoracic inlet (look for the medial ends of the baby's clavicles to get a good approximation) and the carina or level of tracheal bifurcation. In small neonates ET tubes often enter the right mainstem bronchus and produce left-sided atelectasis. They may also exert vagal effects and cause bradycardia or irritation if they strike the carina. Tubes that are excessively high also may produce vagal effects and loss of effective ventilation.

64. **What is the most common radiographic appearance of the lungs in a premature neonate with RDS?**
The classic RDS picture in a premature neonate has a diffuse increase in lung density (opacity) with a fine, reticulogranular (grainy) or ground-glass appearance, air bronchograms (a darker appearance to the branching central airway in contrast to the opacity of the lungs), and low lung volumes (Fig. 18-4).

65. **What disease process can produce a radiographic appearance of the lungs identical to that of RDS?**
GBS pneumonia in a premature infant is reported to have an appearance similar to that of RDS. However, premature babies with GBS disease may also have surfactant inactivation or deficiency with true RDS as well as GBS septicemia. Although Sir William Osler might not like the concept of two diagnoses in one little patient, it probably happens more often than not.

✓ KEY POINTS: MECONIUM-STAINED AMNIOTIC FLUID AND MECONIUM ASPIRATION SYNDROME

1. Vigorous meconium-stained infants do not need to be intubated and suctioned in the delivery room.

2. Those who have an initial heart rate above 100 bpm, good respiratory effort, and reasonable tone will not benefit from intubation and suctioning.

3. In fact, some vigorous infants may be injured in the process of suctioning because they are so difficult to restrain.

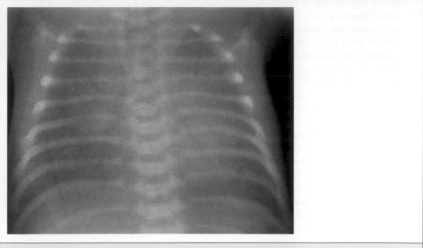

Figure 18-4. Radiograph of a baby with severe respiratory distress syndrome. Note the generalized haziness caused by atelectasis and the air bronchograms throughout the lung.

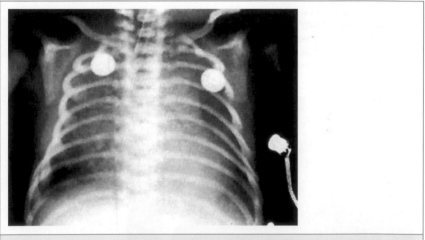

Figure 18-5. Radiograph of an infant with severe meconium aspiration syndrome, marked by hazy densities throughout the lung.

66. **What would be a typical appearance of the lungs in a newborn with significant meconium aspiration?**
   Affected babies often have a coarse, irregular increase in lung markings accompanied by hyperinflation of the lungs. The pneumonic process here is one of patchy atelectasis and overdistention (Fig. 18-5). Pneumomediastinum and pneumothorax are frequent accompanying abnormalities as well.

67. **In a newborn with suspected transient tachypnea of the newborn (e.g., wet lung syndrome, transient respiratory distress of the newborn, delayed reabsorption of fetal lung fluid), approximately how long should it take for the**

chest radiograph to return to a normal appearance to be consistent with this diagnosis?

The textbook description of this clinical condition is a hazy-appearing lung, often with fluid in the right horizontal fissure and increased perihilar markings. The babies have rapid, shallow breathing, in contrast to the retractions of RDS or MAS. It usually is reported to last approximately 24 hours, with 48 to 72 hours considered the maximum. Some infants, however, seem to have this clinical problem for many more days, with subsequent uneventful recovery. What turns off fetal lung fluid production at birth has not been established. One theory is that certain babies may continue to produce a low level of lung fluid for some time after they are born.

68. **What should the clinician look for on the chest radiograph of a newborn in whom congenital diaphragmatic hernia is suspected (usually by antenatal sonography of the fetus)?**

A patient with congenital diaphragmatic hernia rarely presents at birth as the diagnostic dilemma in the delivery room, as once was the case. With fetal ultrasound most of these infants are diagnosed before birth. Radiographically, they have a complex pattern of lucency in one hemithorax (usually the left side, and reflecting air-containing loops of intestine), contralateral shift of the heart and other mediastinal structures, and a lack of expected air-containing intestine in the abdomen.

69. **If a unilateral pneumothorax is suspected in a newborn, what is the best projection of the chest to confirm or exclude this diagnosis?**

Early air leaks are often difficult to diagnose. The most obvious finding is a separation of the edge or margin of the lung from the inner margin of the chest wall, with no lung markings definable in that space. An AP decubitus view of the chest with the side of suspected pneumothorax to the top (non-dependent) is also helpful. For example, if you suspect a left-sided pneumothorax, you should order a "right decubitus AP chest radiograph," which means the right side of the patient will be dependent and the left side nondependent. If a pneumothorax is present, look for a zone of lucency representing pleural air collecting between the lateral chest margin and the adjacent lung (Fig. 18-6).

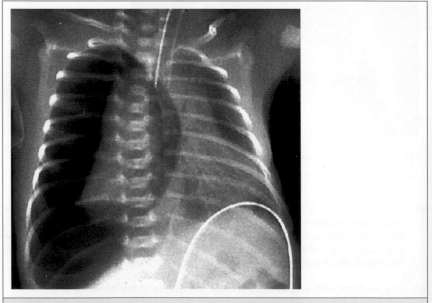

Figure 18-6. Radiograph of a child with a tension pneumothorax on the right.

RESPIRATORY DISTRESS SYNDROME

70. **Which collapses more quickly: a small bubble or a larger one?**
The small one collapses more quickly because of surface tension. The LaPlace relationship states $P = 2T/R$, where P is the pressure across the wall of the sphere, T is surface tension of the substance forming the bubble (i.e., its tendency to collapse), and R is the radius of the sphere. The smaller the radius, the greater the collapsing pressure (Fig. 18-7).

When the bubbles are alveoli without surfactant, pressure on the alveolar surface is quite high because the surface tension is high. As the alveolus collapses without surfactant during exhalation, pressure increases as the radius of the alveolus decreases.

Avery and Mead described the absence of a surface tension–reducing substance in the alveolar fluid of infants who died of hyaline membrane disease. The substance turned out to be the complex substance known as surfactant, which greatly lowers the alveolar surface tension and therefore the tendency of the alveolus to collapse. Surfactant also lowers surface tension as the diameter of the alveolus decreases, allowing for stable alveoli at end-expiratory volumes.

71. **What are the physiologic, physical, and biochemical factors that result in pulmonary vasodilation at the time of birth?**
Within minutes after delivery, pulmonary artery pressure falls, and blood flow increases in response to birth-related stimuli, such as ventilation, increased PO_2, and shear stress. Physical stimuli, including increased shear stress, lung inflation, ventilation, and increased oxygen, cause pulmonary vasodilation in part by increasing production of vasodilators, nitric oxide, and prostacyclin. Pretreatment with the nitric oxide synthase inhibitor, nitro-L-arginine, attenuates pulmonary vasodilation after delivery by 50% in near-term fetal lambs. These findings suggest that a significant part of the rise in pulmonary blood flow at birth may be related directly to the acute release of nitric oxide. Each of the birth-related stimuli can stimulate nitric oxide release independently, followed by vasodilation through cyclic guanosine monophosphate kinase–mediated stimulation of K channels. Although the endothelial isoform of nitric oxide synthase III has been presumed to be the major contributor of nitric oxide at birth, recent studies suggest that other isoforms (neuronal type I and inducible type II) may be important sources of nitric oxide release *in utero* and at birth. Other vasodilators, especially

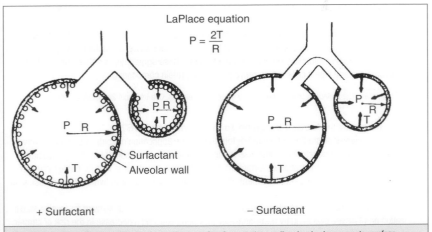

LaPlace equation

$$P = \frac{2T}{R}$$

Surfactant
Alveolar wall

+ Surfactant

− Surfactant

Figure 18-7. The LaPlace relationship. In the absence of surfactant, the smaller alveolus has a greater surface tension and tends to empty into the larger alveolus. In the presence of surfactant, the compacting of surface tension–reducing surfactant acts to "splint" the lung against further collapse. (Courtesy F. Netter, CIBA-Geigy Corp., Ardsley, New York.)

prostacyclin, also modulate changes in pulmonary vascular tone. Rhythmic lung distention and shear stress stimulate both prostacyclin and nitric oxide production in late gestation. Increasing oxygen tension also triggers nitric oxide activity and overcomes the effects of prostacyclin inhibition at birth. Thus, although nitric oxide does not account for the entire fall in pulmonary vascular resistance at birth, nitric oxide synthase activity appears important in achieving postnatal adaptation of lung circulation.

More recently, vasculoendothelial growth factor (VEGF), which is really a family of growth factors, and angiopoietins 1 through 4 have been also shown to have important angiogenic roles during fetal development of the pulmonary vascular bed. These agents also appear to be closely related to the release and influence of nitric oxide in pulmonary development and vasodilation. Additional proteins have been elaborated that may play critical roles in this entire process, demonstrating the increasing complexity of our understanding of neonatal lung development.

Konduri GG. The role of nitric oxide in lung growth and function in the newborn lung. In: Bancalari E, editor. 2nd ed. Philadelphia: Saunders; 2012. p. 111–32.

72. What is the composition of surfactant?

Surfactant, from "surface active material," is 80% phospholipids and 8% neutral lipids. The phospholipid most responsible for surface tension reduction is dipalmitoylphosphatidylcholine. About 12% of surfactant is protein, half of which most likely comprises serum contaminants. Surfactant proteins A, B, C, and D (SP-A, SP-B, SP-C, SP-D) are active in surfactant's surface tension reduction, secretion, absorption, and immune function. SP-A works with other proteins and lipids to improve surface actions and regulate secretion and reuptake. It also works with host defense in the alveolus. Lipophilic SP-B and SP-C facilitate adsorption and spread of lipid across the alveolar surface. SP-D is known to be a ligand for pathogens.

73. Where is surfactant manufactured in the lung?

Surfactant is made in alveolar type II cells. The endoplasmic reticulum and Golgi apparatus package the lipid and protein precursors. Lamellar bodies are formed, including more protein with increasing gestational age. Catecholamines, corticosteroids, and other hormones stimulate the type II cells to secrete lamellar bodies. These unravel to form tubular myelin. Tubular myelin then adsorbs as a lipid-protein monolayer on the alveolar surface, giving maximum surface support to the alveolus. The interaction between intact protein and phospholipid allows optimal surfactant functioning.

Surfactant is inactivated in the alveolar space without large changes in amounts of its components. The monolayer does break down as protein and lipid dissociate. Surfactant changes to a small aggregate form that minimally reduces surface tension. These aggregates are then absorbed by macrophages and type II cells, which recycle lipid and protein components.

Carey B, Trapnell BC. The molecular basis of pulmonary alveolar proteinosis. Clin Immunol 2010;135(2):223–35.

74. When should surfactant be given to an infant with RDS?

The meta-analysis of studies conducted before the routine application of continuous positive airway pressure (CPAP) demonstrated a decrease in the risk of air leak and neonatal mortality associated with prophylactic administration of surfactant. By prophylaxis, most agree that for babies younger than 27 to 29 weeks' gestation, treatment should be given soon after birth (within 20 minutes), after initial stabilization.

Analyses of more recent studies challenge this view. When studies that allowed for routine stabilization on CPAP are evaluated by meta-analysis, they demonstrated a decrease in the risk of chronic lung disease or death in infants stabilized on CPAP. Recent large trials that reflect current practice (including greater utilization of maternal steroids and routine postdelivery stabilization on CPAP) do not support the differences seen in earlier studies and demonstrate less risk of chronic lung disease or death when using early stabilization on CPAP with selective surfactant administration to infants requiring intubation.

Engle WA, Committee on Fetus and Newborn. Surfactant-replacement therapy for respiratory distress in the preterm and term neonate. Pediatrics 2008;121(2):419–32.

Rojas-Reyes MX, Morley CJ, Soll R. Prophylactic versus selective use of surfactant in preventing morbidity and mortality in preterm infants. Cochrane Database Syst Rev 2012 Mar 14;3:CD000510:CD000510.

75. What other therapies are effective in infants with RDS?

The goal of therapy is to maintain minute volume by maintaining functional, open alveoli for gas exchange. When atelectasis occurs in infants with RDS, CO_2 cannot get out and O_2 cannot get in. To maintain alveolar volume and therefore gas exchange, positive end-expiratory pressure (PEEP) is essential. CPAP can be used to maintain alveolar volume during exhalation despite inadequate surfactant. It works if the pressure delivered to the alveoli prevents closing pressure (remember, $P = 2T/R$) from completely collapsing alveoli, but it should not be so great that it hinders adequate exhalation. Early institution of CPAP appears to prevent the need for intubation in a significant percentage of VLBW infants.

When alveolar collapse is too rapid or widespread, positive pressure ventilation is the best tool. Positive pressure opens the alveoli for inhalation. End-expiratory pressure maintains alveolar volume during exhalation. Positive pressure ventilation will be necessary until adequate surfactant reduces surface tension and a sufficient number of alveoli are recruited for adequate minute ventilation.

Should infants with RDS receive high-frequency ventilation? The primary pathology of RDS comes from an inability to maintain lung inflation and fluid leak into the alveolar space. Secondary pathology originates from positive pressure reexpansion of collapsed alveoli. A ventilation strategy that maintains lung volume and avoids large distending pressure seems ideal. That is the idea behind high-frequency ventilation for RDS. The lung is inflated, and lung volumes are maintained while gas exchange occurs, using tidal volumes less than dead space. High-frequency ventilator technology is improving, and its applicability as the first-line treatment for RDS continues to be evaluated. Consensus has not yet been reached, however.

Cools F, Askie LM, Offringa M, et al. Elective high-frequency oscillatory versus conventional ventilation in preterm infants: a systematic review and meta-analysis of individual patients' data. Lancet 2010;375(9731):2082–91.

Courtney SE, Durand DJ, Asselin JM, et al. High-frequency oscillatory ventilation versus conventional mechanical ventilation for very-low-birth-weight infants. N Engl J Med 2002;347:643–52.

Johnson AH, Peacock JL, Greenough A, et al. High-frequency oscillatory ventilation for the prevention of chronic lung disease of prematurity. N Engl J Med 2002;347:633–42.

76. Are there complications and problems with surfactant therapy?

U.S. mortality rates associated with RDS and prematurity declined significantly with the introduction of exogenous surfactant. By 1994 the combination of congenital and chromosomal defects had become the leading cause of infant mortality, and RDS with prematurity fell, for the first time, to number two on the list. Although bronchopulmonary dysplasia (BPD) has not significantly decreased in frequency, the severity of this chronic lung disease has declined for most surviving premature infants with RDS.

The only pulmonary complication that appears to have increased with therapy is a small but detectable rise in pulmonary hemorrhage. Other nonpulmonary complications have not been significantly affected.

77. What is CPAP?

CPAP is continous positive airway pressure. CPAP is applied to an infant's airway using a variety of devices to maintain positive pressure in the airway during spontaneous breathing. These devices include a head hood, face chamber, face mask, several types of nasal cannulae, nasopharyngeal tube, and ET tube. Nasal cannulae inserted into the nares are used most often. Not all CPAP devices are equal, and they have varying degrees of success. They have been associated with a number of problems, such as difficulty with gaining access to the baby and maintaining connection to the airway, increase in dead space, and increase in airway resistance.

78. **What is the effect of CPAP?**
As with many things in life, the right amount is beneficial and too much is detrimental. When the proper amount of positive pressure is used, CPAP will accomplish the following:
- Increase transpulmonary pressure and functional residual capacity
- Prevent alveolar collapse and decrease intrapulmonary shunting
- Increase compliance
- Conserve surfactant
- Increase airway diameter and splint the airway
- Splint the diaphragm

If too much CPAP is applied, however, it can cause overdistention of the alveoli; worsen ventilation–perfusion match; increase pulmonary vascular resistance; decrease compliance; and impede venous return to the right side of the heart, thereby decreasing cardiac output.

79. **What are the indications for using CPAP in neonates?**
These include but are not limited to the following:
- Diseases with a low functional residual capacity (e.g., RDS)
- Apnea and bradycardia of prematurity
- MAS
- Airway closure disease (e.g., bronchiolitis, BPD)
- Tracheomalacia
- Partial paralysis of the diaphragm
- Respiratory support after extubation

80. **What are the complications of nasal CPAP?**
- Pneumothorax (<2%): usually occurs in the acute phase and is usually more benign than when it occurs during mechanical ventilation. Pneumothorax is not a contraindication for CPAP therapy.
- Nasal obstruction: obstruction caused by secretions or improper positioning of CPAP prongs. Secretions in nasal cavities should be suctioned every 4 hours or as needed.
- Abdominal distention from swallowed air: This is usually benign and occurs more commonly in the chronic than acute phase. Abdominal distention can be treated by intermittent aspiration of the stomach. For severe distention an indwelling orogastric tube may be required.
- Nasal or septal erosion or necrosis: This finding is a concern in a VLBW premature infant with sensitive skin who may need CPAP therapy for weeks. However, this can be prevented by choosing a properly sized CPAP cannula and avoiding compression of the septum. A snug cap is used to hold the tubings securely in place, and self-adhesive Velcro is used to keep the cannulae away from the septum.

81. **What is the oxygenation index?**
The oxygenation index (OI) is used to express the severity of the respiratory disease.

$$OI = (MAP \times FiO_2)/PaO_2 \text{ and MAP can be calculated}$$
$$= (PIP - PEEP) \times T_I/(T_IT_E) \text{ PEEP,}$$

where MAP = mean airway pressure, FiO_2 = fractional concentration of oxygen in inspired gas, PaO_2 = partial pressure of oxygen in arterial blood, PIP = peak inspiratory pressure, $PEEP$ = positive end-expiratory pressure, T_I = inspiration time, and T_E = expiration time.

Note that the MAP is influenced by all respirator controls except the FiO_2. However, without a uniform ventilation strategy, the oxygenation index cannot be universally applied as an expression of severity of respiratory disease. This statement is especially true in the NICU, where patients may be hyperventilated; in these patients the MAP, and thus the oxygenation index, is elevated regardless of the severity of disease.

MECONIUM-STAINED AMNIOTIC FLUID AND MECONIUM ASPIRATION SYNDROME

82. **Do vigorous meconium-stained infants need to be intubated and suctioned in the delivery room?**
    No. Those who have an initial heart rate greater than 100 bpm, good respiratory effort, and reasonable tone will not benefit from intubation and suctioning. In fact, some vigorous infants may be injured in the process of suctioning because they are so difficult to restrain.

Vain NE, Szyld EG, Prudent LM, et al. Oropharyngeal and nasopharyngeal suctioning of meconium-stained neonates before delivery of their shoulders: multicentre, randomised controlled trial. Lancet 2004;364:597–602.

Wiswell TE, Gannon CM, Jacob J, et al. Delivery room management of the apparently vigorous meconium-stained neonate: results of the multicenter, international collaborative trial. Pediatrics 2000;105(1 Pt 1):1–7.

83. **How long has meconium been present in the amniotic fluid if an infant has evidence of meconium staining?**
    Gross staining of the infant is a surface phenomenon proportional to the length of exposure and meconium concentration. With heavy meconium, staining of the umbilical cord begins in as little as 15 minutes, and with light meconium, it begins after 1 hour. Yellow staining of the newborn's nails requires 4 to 6 hours. Yellow staining of the vernix caseosa takes between 12 and 14 hours.

84. **Is meconium staining a good marker for neonatal asphyxia?**
    Because between 10% and 20% of all deliveries have *in utero* passage of meconium, meconium staining alone is not a good marker for neonatal asphyxia. For an infant to pass meconium, there does need to be a period of hypoxemia that initiates increased bowel contractility before birth. Simply having hypoxemia, however, is not the same thing as having perinatal asphyxia.

85. **What pulmonary disorder is most frequently associated with persistent pulmonary hypertension of the newborn (PPHN)?**
    MAS is associated with the majority of cases of PPHN. Other associated disorders include RDS, sepsis or pneumonia, idiopathic PPHN, and lung hypoplasia (including congenital diaphragmatic hernia). In all instances the pulmonary artery pressure remains near systemic levels and results in right-to-left shunting of blood.

86. **What factors are involved in the pathophysiology of MAS?**
    Causes of aspirated meconium are as follows:
    - Airway obstruction
    - Alveolar and parenchymal inflammation
    - Alveolar and parenchymal edema
    - Altered pulmonary vasoreactivity leading to pulmonary vasoconstriction, increased pulmonary resistance, and right-to-left shunting
    - Direct toxicity of meconium constituents on pulmonary parenchyma leading to ischemia and necrosis
    - Surfactant dysfunction (inactivation and decreased production of SP-A and SP-B)
    - Pulmonary vascular remodeling
    - Altered lung elastic forces (increased resistance, decreased compliance) (Fig. 18-8)

✓ KEY POINTS: PPHN AND CONGENITAL DIAPHRAGMATIC HERNIA

1. The most studied and effective therapy for neonates with pulmonary hypertension is inhaled nitric oxide.

2. Ventilator-induced alkalosis, bicarbonate infusions, and prostaglandin products have not been adequately studied and are not recommended.

3. Inhaled nitric oxide does not reduce the need for extracorporeal membrane oxygenation in neonates with congenital diaphragmatic hernia.

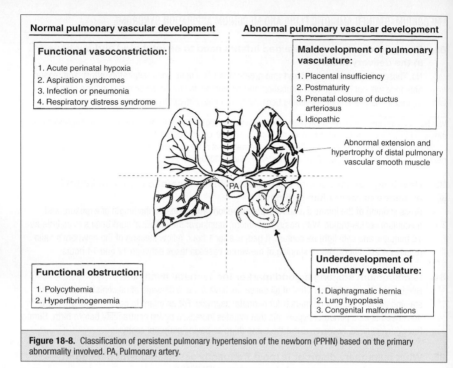

Figure 18-8. Classification of persistent pulmonary hypertension of the newborn (PPHN) based on the primary abnormality involved. PA, Pulmonary artery.

87. **What disorder makes up the largest proportion of neonates who are treated with extracorporeal membrane oxygenation (ECMO)?**

Infants with MAS make up between 30% and 40% of infants who are treated with ECMO. Unfortunately, the circumstances that lead to MAS in many cases are precipitous and unavoidable. As a result, by the time therapy can be started, the pathophysiology is sufficiently far advanced and can be halted only by the use of ECMO. Other disorders that are managed with ECMO include sepsis, pneumonia, pulmonary hypoplasia (most often caused by congenital diaphragmatic hernia), and RDS. Patients with MAS tend to have the shortest ECMO courses and the highest survival rates, approaching 97% in the most experienced ECMO centers. However, the use of ECMO in recent years has declined significantly with the introduction of inhaled nitric oxide and improved ventilatory management.

88. **Meconium-stained amniotic fluid (MSAF) is found across all races and socioeconomic strata in humans. Additionally, MSAF and MAS are noted frequently in domestic animals. How do farmers and veterinarians manage MSAF in an effort to prevent MAS?**

Farmers and veterinarians grab newborn animals by their hindquarters and swing them in a circular motion. Centrifugal forces move MSAF outward into the upper airway and oropharynx. Caretakers then manually remove the material. Of course, it is not recommended that infants be swung by the legs to remove meconium from the airway.

89. **Is thin-consistency MSAF more likely to enter the airways and cause MAS or other forms of respiratory distress compared with thick-consistency MSAF?**

No. The thicker the consistency of MSAF, the greater the likelihood of MAS or other respiratory distress. There is at least a sevenfold increase in the incidence of respiratory disorders among infants born through "pea-soup" MSAF compared with those born through watery-consistency MSAF.

90. **What mechanisms of meconium aspiration into the lungs contribute to ventilatory failure, and what is the role of surfactant therapy in the treatment of this condition?**

Meconium-induced lung injury is associated with many pulmonary changes that contribute to respiratory failure. These include airway obstruction, inflammation with release of vasoactive substances, and surfactant dysfunction. Meconium has the ability to inactivate surfactant both *in vivo* and *in vitro* and has direct effects on type II pneumocyte function. In both animal models and human infants who have aspirated meconium and who are undergoing pulmonary fluid analysis, inflammatory cell numbers and total protein are significantly elevated compared with infants in the control group. Various inflammatory mediators, including myeloperoxidase and interleukin-8, are increased. Maximal influx of inflammatory cells occurs by 16 hours of age with some recovery by 72 hours. These findings support the role of surfactant replacement in infants with MAS that requires ventilatory support.

Wiswell TE. Advances in the treatment of the meconium aspiration syndrome. Acta Paediatr Suppl 2001;90(436):28–30.
  Soll RF, Dargaville P. Surfactant for meconium aspiration syndrome in full term infants. Cochrane Database Syst Rev 2000;(2):CD002054.

PERSISTENT PULMONARY HYPERTENSION OF THE NEWBORN

91. **What is PPHN?**

Successful transition from intrauterine to extrauterine life requires that the pulmonary vascular resistance decreases precipitously at birth. In infants with PPHN, this decrease does not occur. Pulmonary arterial pressure remains elevated, and blood continues to shunt right to left across the ductus arteriosus and foramen ovale, resulting in significant hypoxemia.

92. **When was PPHN first described? Why is persistent fetal circulation not an accurate term to describe PPHN?**

In 1969 Gersony and coworkers described a group of term infants without structural heart disease who became cyanotic shortly after birth and who had only mild respiratory distress. These infants all had suprasystemic pulmonary arterial pressures with right-to-left shunting across persistent fetal pathways (ductus arteriosus and foramen ovale). Hence this condition was called persistent fetal circulation.

The shunting across the foramen ovale and ductus arteriosus as a result of suprasystemic pulmonary arterial pressure seen in PPHN is very similar to fetal circulation. However, the exclusion of placental circulation and the fact that ductus venosus may or may not be patent preclude the use of the term *persistent fetal circulation* to describe this condition. The term *persistent pulmonary hypertension of the newborn* describes the pathophysiology of the disease more accurately, indicating that the critical problem in this situation is the failure of the pulmonary circulation to decrease to normal pressures.

Gersony WM, Due GV, Sinclair JC. "PFC" syndrome (persistence of fetal circulation). Circulation 1969;40:3–9.
  Askie LM, Ballard RA, Cutter GR, et al. Inhaled nitric oxide in preterm infants: an individual-patient data meta-analysis of randomized trials. Pediatrics 2011 Oct;128(4):729–39.
  Tissot C, Beghetti M. Review of inhaled iloprost for the control of pulmonary artery hypertension in children. Vasc Health Risk Manag 2009;5(1):325–31.
  Abman SH, Chatfield BA, Hall SL, et al. Role of endothelium-derived relaxing factor during transition of pulmonary circulation at birth. Am J Physiol 1990;259(6 Pt 2):H1921–H1927.

93. **What are the clinical features of PPHN?**

Infants with PPHN are usually delivered at term or post term. Often they are born through MSAF. The typical clinical manifestations of a neonate with PPHN are as follows:

- Labile hypoxemia or cyanosis disproportionate to the level of respiratory distress may be present. These infants are extremely sensitive to environmental stimuli.
- Infants with significant ductal shunting have higher oxygen saturation in the right hand (preductal) than in the legs (postductal). Similarly, arterial PO_2 in the right radial artery is significantly greater

than that obtained from the umbilical artery. Infants with predominant shunting at the level of foramen ovale have similar preductal and postductal oxygen levels.

- Cardiac murmur compatible with tricuspid insufficiency is present.
- Chest radiograph may reveal cardiomegaly. The underlying disease (e.g., congenital diaphragmatic hernia, RDS) alters the radiologic picture. Infants with idiopathic PPHN have clear and undervascularized lung fields ("black-lung" PPHN).
- Echocardiography is important to rule out cyanotic congenital heart disease and establish the diagnosis. In infants with PPHN, shunting at the atrial and ductal level can be demonstrated. Tricuspid insufficiency, right ventricular hypertrophy, septal deviation to the left, and prolonged right ventricular systolic intervals support the diagnosis of PPHN.

94. **What are the common causes of PPHN?**
The common causes of PPHN are summarized in the mnemonic DIAPHRAGMATIC:
- Diaphragmatic hernia (hypoplastic lungs)
- Infection (including pneumonia), especially GBS
- Aspiration syndromes (e.g., meconium, amniotic fluid)
- Postmaturity
- Hyperviscosity (polycythemia, hyperfibrinogenemia)
- RDS (i.e., hyaline membrane disease)
- Asphyxia
- Growth retardation (placental insufficiency)
- Maternal nonsteroidal antiinflammatory drug ingestion
- Air leak
- Transient tachypnea of newborn
- Idiopathic ("black lung" PPHN)
- Congenital anomalies of the lung, alveolar-capillary dysplasia

The causes of PPHN can also be classified according to the predominant abnormality involved (see Fig. 18-2).

95. **Why is the right hand a preferred site to obtain preductal pulse oximetry readings?**
In some infants the left subclavian artery arises from the arch of the aorta just distal to the level of the insertion of the ductus arteriosus. In these infants a pulse oximetry probe applied to the left hand indicates postductal saturations. Therefore it is always better to obtain preductal oxygen saturation from the right upper limb, a site that indicates preductal saturation.

96. **What is the pathophysiology of PPHN?**
Persistent elevation of pulmonary arterial pressure in PPHN results from active constriction of pulmonary vessels (as in pneumonia), underdevelopment of the pulmonary vessels (as in congenital diaphragmatic hernia), or maldevelopment of the pulmonary vasculature (as in prenatal ductal closure caused by maternal ingestion of nonsteroidal antiinflammatory drugs and idiopathic PPHN).

Vascular remodeling: In infants dying as a result of PPHN caused by maldevelopment of the pulmonary vessels, pulmonary arterial smooth muscle hypertrophies and extends from pre-acinar arteries into normally nonmuscular intra-acinar arteries, even to the level of the alveolus. This thickened muscle encroaches on the vessel lumen and results in mechanical obstruction to blood flow.

Functional abnormalities in the pulmonary vessels (e.g., reduced nitric oxide synthase, reduced soluble guanylyl cyclase, and increased levels of vasoconstrictors such as endothelin) have been described.

Persistently elevated pulmonary vascular resistance increases right ventricular afterload and oxygen demand and impairs oxygen delivery to cardiac muscle. Ischemic damage to the myocardium, papillary muscle necrosis, and tricuspid regurgitation can occur. Increased right ventricular pressure displaces the septum into the left ventricle, impairs left ventricular filling, and decreases cardiac output. Myocardial dysfunction is an important cause for mortality in PPHN (Fig. 18-9).

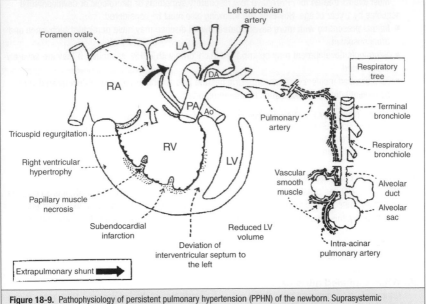

Figure 18-9. Pathophysiology of persistent pulmonary hypertension (PPHN) of the newborn. Suprasystemic pulmonary arterial pressure results in right ventricular (RV) hypertrophy and deviation of the intraventricular septum to the left. This reduces the left ventricular (LV) volume and decreases systemic output. Extrapulmonary right-to-left shunting occurs at the foramen ovale from the right atrium (RA) to the left atrium (LA) and at the level of the ductus arteriosus (DA) from the pulmonary artery (PA) to the aorta (Ao). Normally, PAs distal to the level of terminal bronchioles are not muscular. Abnormal extension and hypertrophy of distal pulmonary vascular smooth muscle (shown as interrupted lines), sometimes to the level of intra-acinar arteries, is seen in severe PPHN.

97. **How are infants with a cyanotic congenital heart disease differentiated from those with PPHN?**

It is often very difficult clinically to differentiate between these two conditions. Patients with PPHN are more labile and exhibit wide swings in oxygen saturations. A significant difference between the pre-ductal and postductal oxygen saturations is also a clinical finding in favor of PPHN. An additional test that is sometimes used in this clinical situation is the hyperoxia test. The child to be tested is placed on an inspired oxygen level of 100%. On an arterial blood gas determination, if the arterial PO_2 level rises above 100 mm Hg, it is unlikely that the infant has significant cyanotic heart disease and more likely has pulmonary hypertension or pulmonary parenchymal disease. This test, however, is not infallible, and some children with PPHN may not be able to increase their arterial PO_2 above 100 mm Hg. In addition, it may be necessary to give positive pressure ventilation to a baby to be sure that one is ventilating the lungs of a child with pulmonary disease adequately to maximize the arterial oxygen levels. The best way to differentiate between these two entities is by echocardiography.

98. **What is the long-term outcome of infants treated for PPHN?**

In the past the mortality for infants with PPHN ranged from 20% to 40%, and the incidence of neurologic handicap ranged from 12% to 25%. With recent advances in conservative management, survival and neurodevelopmental outcome have improved considerably. In most centers inhaled nitric oxide and ECMO have further reduced mortality associated with severe PPHN. Survival rates between 76% and 93% have been reported for infants with pneumonia, meconium aspiration, and idiopathic PPHN who require ECMO. The outlook for infants with diaphragmatic hernia requiring ECMO has not been as dramatic, and survival is still only about 60% to 80%.

Most infants treated for PPHN have few respiratory symptoms or neurologic or developmental sequelae by 1 year of age. However, the following also must be considered:

- Infants presenting with more severe parenchymal disease may have persistent tachypnea and bronchospasm.
- Neurologic development may be impaired in children with PPHN, especially if they are severely asphyxiated.
- An increased incidence of sensorineural hearing loss among infants with PPHN treated with hyperventilation and alkalization has been reported.

Levison J, Halliday R, Holland AJ, et al. A population-based study of congenital diaphragmatic hernia outcome in New South Wales and the Australian Capital Territory, Australia, 1992-2001. J Pediatr Surg 2006;41(6):1049–53.

Davis PJ, Firmin RK, Manktelow B, et al. Long-term outcome following extracorporeal membrane oxygenation for congenital diaphragmatic hernia: the UK experience. J Pediatr 2004;144(3):309–15.

99. **What are the future prospects for treating infants with PPHN?**
Although ECMO has considerably reduced the mortality rates associated with PPHN, it is an invasive procedure limited to a few tertiary care centers. Inhaled nitric oxide has reduced the use of ECMO. Unfortunately, this reduction has not been associated with an improvement in long-term outcome.

INHALED NITRIC OXIDE

100. **What is inhaled nitric oxide?**
Nitric oxide is an important regulator of vascular muscle tone at the cellular level. Nitric oxide is generated enzymatically by nitric oxide synthases from L-arginine. Nitric oxide activates guanylyl cyclase by binding to its heme component, leading to the production of cyclic guanosine monophosphate (GMP). The mechanism by which cyclic GMP relaxes vascular smooth muscle is not clear. It appears to involve inhibition of activation-induced elevation in cytosolic calcium concentration.

Several randomized control trials indicate that inhaled nitric oxide reduces the incidence of the combined end point of death or need for ECMO compared with patients not offered treatment with inhaled nitric oxide. This reduction seems to be entirely due to a reduction in the use of ECMO insofar as mortality is not reduced.

Finer NN, Barrington KJ. Nitric oxide for respiratory failure in infants born at or near term. Cochrane Database Syst Rev 2001;2:CD000399.

✓ KEY POINTS: MAJOR ANOMALIES THAT ALTER PULMONARY FUNCTION

1. Both intrinsic defects in the larynx or trachea and extrinsic compression of the trachea can cause airway obstruction syndrome.

2. Lung function is normal in most of these disorders so that airway management, which relieves the obstruction, usually normalizes gas exchange.

101. **Inhaled nitric oxide acts like an endothelium-relaxing factor and is a major regulator of vascular smooth muscle tone. Why doesn't it also dilate the systemic vascular system?**
Nitric oxide has a high affinity for the iron of all heme proteins, including reduced hemoglobin, with which it forms nitrosyl hemoglobin (NOHb). The NOHb is then oxidized to methemoglobin with the production of nitrate. As a result, when given by inhalation, nitric oxide is inactivated before acting on any systemic vascular bed, while relaxing the pulmonary vascular smooth muscle through the cyclic GMP production. In normal development endogenous nitric oxide produced in endothelial cells from

oxygen and L-arginine diffuses into smooth cells in the vascular wall and causes vasodilation. Nitric oxide that diffuses into the blood vessel lumen is avidly bound by hemoglobin and does not cause systemic vasodilatation.

102. Does inhaled nitric oxide reduce the use of ECMO in neonates with congenital diaphragmatic hernia?

Meta-analysis showed that infants with diaphragmatic hernia do not appear to share the benefits of inhaled nitric oxide that infants with other causes of hypoxemic respiratory failure experience. Indeed, there are suggestions that outcomes may be worse in infants with congenital diaphragmatic hernia who received inhaled nitric oxide compared with control subjects. This analysis showed that the incidence of death or requiring ECMO was 40 of 46 among control patients and 36 of 38 among patients treated with nitric oxide (relative risk, 1.09; 95% confidence interval [CI], 0.95 to 1.26). Mortality rates were similar in control and treatment patients (18 of 46 in the control group compared with 18 of 38 in the treatment group; relative risk of death, 1.20; 95% CI, 0.74 to 1.96), but there was a significant increase in the requirement for ECMO in infants treated with inhaled nitric oxide (31 of 46 in the control group compared with 32 of 38 in the treatment group; relative risk, 1.27; 95% CI, 1.00 to 1.62).

Finer NN, Barrington KJ. Nitric oxide for respiratory failure in infants born at or near term. Cochrane Database Syst Rev 2001;2:CD000399.

103. What are the major concerns regarding the weaning of nitric oxide and oxygen in infants with PPHN?

When nitric oxide and O_2 come into contact, peroxynitrite ($ONOO^-$), a potent oxidant, is formed. The relative amount of nitric oxide, O_2^-, $ONOO^-$, and antioxidants in the airway will determine whether nitric oxide will be beneficial or potentially toxic. These oxidants can contribute to lung injury by enhancing lung inflammation, producing pulmonary edema, and reducing surfactant function. Furthermore, recent findings have shown that abrupt withdrawal of inhaled nitric oxide, even in infants with minimal or no response, can induce worsening pulmonary hypertension. The potential for pulmonary inflammatory injury can be decreased as the concentrations of inhaled nitric oxide and O_2 are lowered. Most late preterm and term infants can be weaned off inhaled nitric oxide within 4 days.

Clark RH, Kueser TJ, Walker MW, et al. Low-dose nitric oxide therapy for persistent pulmonary hypertension of the newborn. Clinical Inhaled Nitric Oxide Research Group. N Engl J Med 2000;342(7):469–74.

104. What are the indications and the risks associated with the use of inhaled nitric oxide for the treatment of ventilatory failure in preterm infants?

An individual patient meta-analysis indicated that routine use of inhaled nitric oxide for treatment of respiratory failure in preterm infants cannot be recommended. Further research is necessary to determine the optimal starting dose and duration of therapy.

One population that may be an exception is preterm infants born after prolonged rupture of membranes. Multiple small studies suggest that preterm infants with severe respiratory failure born after premature and prolonged rupture of membranes may benefit from inhaled nitric oxide

Askie LM, Ballard RA, Cutter GR, et al. Inhaled nitric oxide in preterm infants: an individual-patient data meta-analysis of randomized trials. Pediatrics 2011;128(4):729–39.
Ball MK, Steinhorn RH. Inhaled nitric oxide for preterm infants: a marksman's approach. J Pediatr 2012;161(3):379–80.

MAJOR ANOMALIES THAT ALTER PULMONARY FUNCTION

105. Infants with fetal akinesia syndrome (Pena–Shokeir phenotype) frequently have pulmonary anomalies. Describe the pulmonary anomalies in this disorder.

Infants with Pena–Shokeir phenotype (also termed arthrogryposis multiplex congenita with pulmonary hypoplasia) have gracile ribs and reduced thoracic volume. Also present are a lack of fetal breathing activity; polyhydramnios resulting from a lack of fetal swallowing; and intrauterine

constraint, resulting in muscular hypoplasia involving both intercostal and diaphragmatic musculature. Thoracic wall weakness, hypotonia of the muscles of respiration, and anterior horn cell atrophy
or deficiency lead to reduced ventilatory drive, which may improve over time for some infants.

106. **Fetal airway obstruction can be the direct result of intrinsic defects in the
larynx or trachea, resulting in congenital high airway obstruction syndrome.
What is the differential diagnosis of extrinsic fetal obstruction?**
- Cervical teratoma
- Lymphangioma
- Vascular rings
- Occipital encephalocele
- Cervical myelomeningocele
- Thyroglossal duct cyst
- Thyroid cyst or tumor
- Congenital goiter
- Branchial cleft cysts

The major causes of extrinsic fetal airway obstruction are cervical lymphangioma, teratoma, and
vascular rings (e.g., double aortic arch, pulmonary vascular sling).

107. **What precautions should be taken for a child with suspected fetal airway
obstructive syndromes during pregnancy and at the time of delivery?**
As fetuses with fetal airway obstruction reach viability, they should be monitored closely for development or progression of hydrops (for intrinsic obstruction cases) or polyhydramnios (when extrinsic
obstruction is present). The fetus should be delivered by using the *ex utero* intrapartum treatment
procedure, with maintenance of uteroplacental circulation and gas exchange. This approach provides
time to perform procedures such as direct laryngoscopy, bronchoscopy, or tracheostomy to secure
the fetal airway, thereby converting an emergent airway crisis into a controlled situation.

MECHANICAL VENTILATION OF THE NEONATE

108. **What are the two basic ways of cycling conventional mechanical ventilators?**
- Time-cycled, pressure-limited ventilators have become the standard in neonatal mechanical
ventilation because of the problems associated with volume-cycled ventilators. Time-cycled,
pressure-limited ventilators have the advantage of providing continuous flow through the circuit,
which allows the infant to take spontaneous breaths of fresh gas between mechanical breaths
(the mechanical breaths are referred to as intermittent mandatory ventilation [IMV]). The system
gives the operator direct control over the delivered peak inspiratory pressure (PIP) and allows
for easier compensation for leakage around ET tubes, and the decelerating flow pattern allows
better gas distribution within the lungs.
- Volume-cycled ventilators deliver a preset tidal volume, usually in a constant-flow fashion,
generating whatever pressure is necessary to deliver the gas into the lungs. This results in a
triangular pressure and volume waveforms with maximum volume and pressure being reached
just before the onset of exhalation.

109. **What are the disadvantages of time-cycled, pressure-limited ventilators?**
The chief disadvantage is the fact that tidal volume is not directly controlled. The delivered tidal
volume is determined by the interaction between PIP and lung compliance. Consequently, as compliance changes, so will the delivered tidal volume. Improving lung compliance can lead to excessive
tidal volume and can cause lung injury. Conversely, worsening compliance can lead to hypoventilation and loss of lung volume. In addition, if an infant is breathing asynchronously with the ventilator,
peak pressures are reached quickly, and volume is reduced. This situation may result in a serious
deterioration of blood gases.

110. **What unique problems make volume-cycled ventilation difficult in newborn infants?**

Uncuffed ET tubes that are used in newborn infants result in a variable degree of air leakage around the tube, causing variable loss of tidal volume. Additional tidal volume is lost through gas compression within the relatively large volume of gas in the ventilator circuit and humidifier and to stretching of the relatively compliant circuit during inspiration. As a result, the tiny premature infant with poorly compliant lungs receives only a small and variable fraction of the tidal volume generated by the ventilator. In essence, the circuit is ventilated rather than the baby.

111. **What are the ways to increase ventilation (improve CO_2 removal) in an infant on time-cycled, pressure-limited ventilation?**

- Increase IMV
- Decrease PEEP
- Increase PIP
- Decrease dead space (e.g., by shortening the ET tube).

There is an upper limit to the effective respiratory rate. An excessively rapid IMV rate may lead to inadequate expiratory time with incomplete exhalation and air trapping. Thus, paradoxically, when the IMV is greater than 90 to 120 breaths per minute, further increases in rate may lead to CO_2 retention. This situation is most likely to occur in infants with increased airway resistance and prolonged time constants. In such infants the best way to improve ventilation is to decrease the IMV rate.

Tidal volume is proportional to the difference between PIP and PEEP. This is referred to as ΔP. Thus lowering PEEP will increase ΔP and improve ventilation (although it can lead to loss of lung volume with deterioration of oxygenation). Occasionally, excessively high PEEP in a patient with relatively compliant lungs can lead to incomplete exhalation and CO_2 retention. This is not a common problem but should be considered in a patient with improving oxygenation and a worsening respiratory acidosis.

112. **Name the two major factors that affect oxygenation in neonatal mechanical ventilation.**

- Mean airway pressure (Paw)
- FiO_2

Paw has been shown to be a major determinant of oxygenation. Adequate distending pressure is needed to maintain lung volume and prevent the diffuse microatelectasis that leads to ventilation–perfusion imbalance with consequent hypoxemia.

Clark RH, Gerstmann DR, Jobe AH, et al. Lung injury in neonates: causes, strategies for prevention, and long-term consequences. J Pediatr 2001;139(4):478–86.

113. **List the key ventilator variables that affect Paw in conventional time-cycled, pressure-limited ventilation.**

- PIP
- Inspiratory to expiratory ratio
- PEEP
- Inspiratory flow

Paw is the area under the pressure curve (Fig. 18-10). Increasing the PEEP is usually the most effective means of increasing the Paw. The least recognized factor affecting the area under the curve is the slope of the upstroke of pressure, which determines the shape of the pressure waveform. Higher flow leads to more rapid upstroke and a more square-shaped curve, which has a larger area than one with a gradual upstroke and a more triangular shape.

114. **When placing an infant on conventional time-cycled, pressure-limited ventilation, how do you choose the initial PIP?**

For any given PIP the delivered tidal volume will be determined by the compliance of the baby's lungs. Select a pressure based on the best estimate of what the infant will need, and observe the result. If adequate chest rise, good breath sounds, and oxygenation are apparent, the pressure is

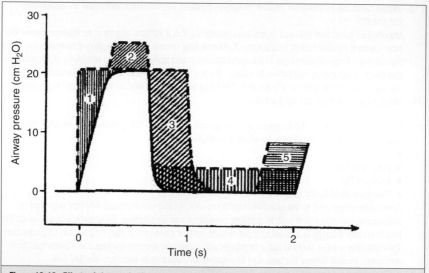

Figure 18-10. Effects of changes in airway pressures and timing on the respiratory waveform and mean airway pressure (Paw). Different waveforms will have different associated blood gases in many instances. (From Reynolds EOM. Pressure waveform and ventilator settings for mechanical ventilation in severe hyaline membrane disease. Int Anesthesiol Clin 1974;12:259.)

appropriate. If the chest rise is excessive, reduce the PIP, and if the chest movement is inadequate, higher PIP is needed (assuming the ET tube is correctly positioned).

Most modern infant ventilators now have the means to directly measure tidal volume (V_T), eliminating the dependence on subjective assessment of adequacy of chest wall movement and allowing more accurate determination of optimal PIP. The target V_T measured at the airway opening should be 4 to 6 mL/kg in the acute phase of the disease.

Note: Some devices measure V_T at the point where the circuit attaches to the ventilator. This position is undesirable because it will give an artificially large V_T measurement, ignoring the loss of V_T to compression of gas in the circuit and circuit stretching. Furthermore, gadgets do malfunction, so continue to use your eyes and ears to verify that the "numbers" are believable.

Klingenberg C, Wheeler KI, Davis PG, et al. A practical guide to neonatal volume guarantee ventilation. J Perinatol 2011;31(9):575–85.

Keszler M. Volume-targeted ventilation. Early Hum Dev 2006;82(12):811–8.

115. List as many possible causes of acute CO_2 retention in an infant on mechanical ventilation as you can. (There are many more than you may think.)
    - The ET tube is dislodged.
    - The ET tube is occluded with secretions.
    - The ET tube is up against the carina.
    - There is an accumulation of secretions in the airways (patient needs suctioning).
    - The patient has a pneumothorax and some other condition that acutely decreased lung compliance.
    - Acute bronchospasm is present.
    - Oversedation with suppression of spontaneous respiratory effort is occurring.
    - The ventilator is malfunctioning (e.g., leak in circuit, partial disconnection).
    - There has been an acute onset of sepsis with loss of spontaneous respiratory effort.
    - Acute abdominal distention or the presence of a large abdominal mass is leading to decreased diaphragmatic excursion.

Most of these should be readily recognizable clinically. If the chest is not moving, the first priority is to make sure that the airway is patent, the ET tube is in place, and the ventilator is cycling. Many modern infant ventilators have the ability to display flow and pressure waveforms, which should help diagnose or confirm the problem. When in doubt, the clinician should reintubate. Manual ventilation may be appropriate if a circuit or ventilator problem is suspected, but be careful not to use excessive pressure, which may cause lung injury.

116. What are some adverse effects associated with mechanical ventilation?
- Acute lung injury (barotrauma or volutrauma, such as pneumothorax, pneumomediastinum, pneumopericardium, pulmonary interstitial emphysema)
- Chronic lung injury (chronic lung disease, BPD)
- Hemodynamic impairment caused by increased intrathoracic pressure
- Intraventricular hemorrhage and periventricular leukomalacia
- Tracheitis or pneumonia
- Tracheal damage with subglottic stenosis
- Palatal groove and damage to tooth buds of the upper incisors

Some degree of impairment of venous return to the heart is inevitable because, unlike spontaneous breathing, intrathoracic pressure rises above ambient pressure during positive pressure ventilation. The problem becomes more severe when high or excessive pressures are used. Intraventricular hemorrhage can be triggered by hemodynamic instability, elevated venous pressure, and sudden increases in cerebral blood flow (as might occur with retention of CO_2). Periventricular leukomalacia is associated with hypotension and with marked respiratory alkalosis.

117. Which of the following infants, each ventilated and with PIP of 25 cm H_2O, PEEP of 5 cm H_2O, IMV of 90 breaths per minute, and an inspiratory time of 0.3 seconds, is least likely to experience hypercarbia, hemodynamic impairment, and air leakage resulting from incomplete exhalation (air trapping): (A) A 12-hour-old, 760-g premature infant of 26 weeks' gestation who has RDS; (B) a 2-hour-old, 3.8-kg infant of 41 weeks' gestation who has MAS; or (C) a 6-week-old, 1420-g, former 25 weeks' gestation premature infant with severe chronic lung disease?
(A) is correct. Hypercarbia, hemodynamic impairment, and air leak caused by incomplete exhalation occur when the expiratory time is too short to allow complete exhalation before the next mechanical breath occurs. This situation is most likely to occur in infants who have increased airway resistance, such as is seen in meconium aspiration with acute airway obstruction or in chronic lung disease in which airway edema, copious secretions, and bronchospasm are present.

118. What is a time constant, and why is it important to consider when ventilating a newborn infant?
A time constant is the product of lung compliance and airway resistance (Tc = R × C). Conceptually, time constants reflect the time it takes for gas flow to cease and pressure to be fully equilibrated between the large airways and the alveoli when a sudden pressure change is applied to the airway opening (three time constants are needed for 95% equilibration) (Fig. 18-11).

In acute RDS, compliance is low and airway resistance is also low (normal). Therefore short inspiratory times can be used. In addition, time constants are also a function of size (total compliance, not compliance per kilogram, is used). Consequently, large subjects such as adults or horses have long time constants, and small premature infants and hummingbirds have short time constants. Time constants are a major determinant of resting respiratory rate, which turns out to fall exactly where work of breathing is lowest. This is why adults at rest breathe at a rate of 14 breaths per minute, term infants breathe at 40 breaths per minute, and small premature infants breathe at about 60 breaths per minute. Mice and hummingbirds breathe significantly more quickly. In infants with acute respiratory distress, tachypnea is a reflection of shorter time constants as lung compliance decreases because of various causes. Asthmatics, on the other hand, prefer to breathe rather slowly because of their prolonged expiratory phase. The bottom line is this: Consider the underlying disease process and its pathophysiology before making decisions about ventilator settings.

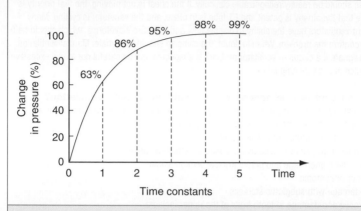

Figure 18-11. Time constants in the lung. A percentage change in pressure in relation to the time (in time constants) allowed for equilibration. As a longer time is allowed for equilibration, a higher percentage change in pressure occurs. (From Carlo WA, Martin RJ. Principles of assisted ventilation. Pediatr Clin North Am 1986;33:321.)

119. What are some of the advantages of synchronized mechanical ventilation?
- Avoidance of asynchrony (baby "bucking" or "fighting" the ventilator)
- Less need for sedation, neuromuscular blockade, or both
- Lower airway pressures because the baby and the ventilator work in tandem
- Decreased risk of barotrauma, volutrauma, and intraventricular hemorrhage
- Preservation of respiratory muscle training (compared with muscle paralysis)
- Greater ease of weaning from mechanical ventilation

✓ KEY POINTS: MOST EFFECTIVE WAYS TO AVOID INJURY IN NEONATES WHO REQUIRE MECHANICAL VENTILATION

1. Optimize oxygen delivery and prevent hyperoxia and hypoxia (by carefully adjusting FiO_2 levels).

2. Normalize functional residual capacity to prevent lung collapse (by giving surfactant to patients with RDS and using end-expiratory pressure to maintain lung volume).

3. Avoid volutrauma (by limiting the tidal volume used to support ventilation).

120. What is assist-controlled (A/C) ventilation? How does it differ from synchronized intermittent mandatory ventilation (SIMV)? When should it be used?
A/C ventilation is a form of mechanical ventilation in which the infant triggers the ventilator to cycle with each breath (Fig. 18-12). With a small triggering effort, therefore, the baby can achieve a much higher level of ventilatory support than with spontaneous breathing. In general, A/C ventilation can be used very successfully to treat VLBW babies with RDS or pulmonary insufficiency of prematurity. It has become the most common way to initiate mechanical ventilation therapy in these clinical situations. It often enables patients to be ventilated at lower PIP levels than with conventional mechanical ventilation or SIMV. It differs from SIMV in that, with A/C, the baby will trigger a ventilator breath with each respiratory effort. In SIMV the ventilator is synchronized to the baby's respiratory cycle so as to avoid stacking of the ventilator and infant breaths, but the baby is given only a preset amount of synchronized breaths. With modern ventilators, if the baby becomes apneic during either A/C ventilation or SIMV, the machine will deliver a preset number of breaths per minute.

Goldsmith JP, Karotkin EH, editors. Assisted ventilation of the neonate. Philadelphia: Saunders; 2004.

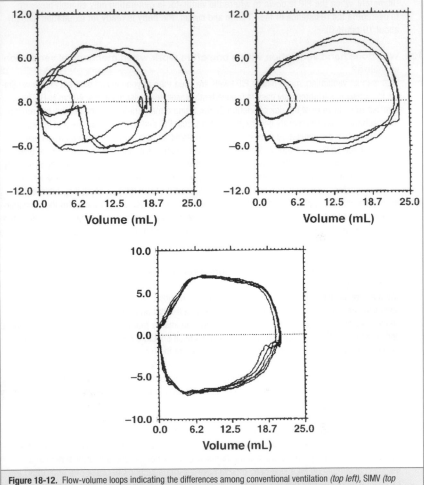

Figure 18-12. Flow-volume loops indicating the differences among conventional ventilation *(top left)*, SIMV *(top right)*, and assist-controlled ventilation *(bottom)*. The loops are erratic with conventional ventilation. With synchronized intermittent mandatory ventilation, the loops are either triggered by the patient or the ventilator. In assist-controlled mode, all loops are ventilator generated, either triggered by the patient (if breathing above the set rate) or by the ventilator (if the infant's respiratory rate falls below the set level). (From Goldmsith JP, Karotkin EH, editors. Assisted ventilation of the neonate. 4th ed. Philadelphia: Saunders; 2003. p. 208.)

121. **An infant is now on PIP of 18 cm H₂O, IMV rate of 30 breaths per minute, and FIO₂ of 0.3. Which is the correct way of weaning the infant from mechanical ventilation in A/C mode: (A) progressively decrease the PIP and IMV; (B) progressively lower the IMV, leaving the PIP unchanged; or (C) progressively lower the PIP, leaving the IMV unchanged?**

C is correct. In A/C mode, every breath that the infant takes triggers a ventilator breath—that is, every breath is supported. As a result, the baby is in control of the ventilatory rate. The IMV rate is only a back-up rate in case the infant is apneic or the triggering mechanism is not functioning. Decreasing the IMV rate does not actually decrease the level of support the infant is receiving. Weaning occurs by lowering the degree of support for each breath (i.e., the PIP).

Ultimately, when the PIP is down to where the ventilator is generating only enough pressure to overcome the resistance of the ET tube and circuit, the baby is ready for extubation (usually about 10 cm H_2O).

122. Why does hand ventilation with a bag often work when mechanical ventilation is failing?

With manual ventilation, much higher PIP levels are used than anyone would dare set on the ventilator. In a crisis it is frighteningly easy to inadvertently generate pressures above 40 cm H_2O. The clinician must beware of the risk of pneumothorax. Using a manometer may be helpful, but most of the mechanical gauges grossly underestimate the actual PIP and the actual duration of inspiration, especially when the ventilatory rate is rapid. This explains, in part, why it is that when you place the baby back on the ventilator, ostensibly on the same settings as the pressures that were used with hand ventilation, the saturation usually drifts down again (because the ventilator PIP is actually lower than that with which you were bagging). It is sometimes preferable to maintain the infant on the ventilator and simply increase the level of support (PIP and IMV) as needed to achieve the desired result. This approach allows you to continue to use the monitoring function of the ventilator to provide feedback regarding the tidal volume and other parameters, and it provides controlled and accurate pressure delivery. However, if the baby is still doing poorly, hand ventilation is an acceptable alternative.

123. What do you do when an infant's condition seems to deteriorate on a ventilator?

When a baby is doing poorly on a ventilator, the clinician should remove the baby from the machine and hand ventilate with an anesthesia (preferably) or self-inflating bag. The chest excursion should be carefully examined and breath sounds auscultated to ensure that the ET tube is still well positioned and not plugged. If there is any question about the tube, it should be replaced promptly. A chest radiograph is often helpful to ensure proper positioning of the tube and to confirm that no air leak is present. Transillumination of the chest can also be helpful in detecting pneumothoraces. If the tube seems fine and there are no radiologic changes, the ventilator itself must be carefully checked for malfunction. Respiratory therapists should be available around the clock in any intensive care nursery in which infants are ventilated.

124. How should a baby be prepared for extubation?

Although there is a great deal of literature on neonatal intubation, few articles describe the risks of extubation. Nothing is more frustrating than successfully completing a course of neonatal mechanical ventilation on a sick baby only to have a serious setback because of a poor effort at extubation. When a child has reached the predetermined levels for extubation, the following should be done:

- A chest radiograph should be obtained as a baseline so that postextubation changes can be compared.
- The child should be given nothing by mouth for at least 4 hours before extubation and should be given intravenous fluids during that time.
- A CPAP setup or oxygen should be available to help the child's transition to spontaneous breathing.
- A laryngoscope and a new ET tube should be at hand in case the child does poorly.
- It is not necessary to initiate steroids or methylxanthines before extubation in all children. However, these adjuncts may be useful if one or two prior attempts at extubation have failed. Bear in mind that the evidence for the value of steroids is mostly anecdotal.

125. How does the clinician proceed to extubate the infant after these preparations?

When the child is ready to be extubated, the tube should be carefully untaped from the face to prevent any abrasions. An anesthesia bag should be attached to the ET tube, and a long, slow,

low-level (15 cm H_2O), positive pressure breath should be administered as the ET tube is withdrawn from the airway. This breath overcomes the natural negative pressure created as the tube is withdrawn from the airway. The child should be given CPAP or oxygen and observed closely. Stridor or hoarseness is common and typically indicates upper airway edema. Marked retractions also may be seen and are worrisome, indicating either volume loss in the lung or upper airway obstruction. Adequate humidification of inspired gas is essential after extubation. Because of the initial inability to oppose the vocal cords, feeding should not be resumed for at least 6 to 12 hours after extubation. Clinical deterioration that occurs 24 to 48 hours after extubation may be caused by a number of factors, including increased atelectasis, upper airway edema and obstruction, and muscular fatigue. If reintubation is deemed necessary, it should be carried out promptly.

NEONATAL HIGH-FREQUENCY VENTILATION

126. What is neonatal high-frequency ventilation?
Neonatal high-frequency ventilation uses devices that provide respiratory support for critically ill neonates with the use of small tidal volume, rapid rate assisted ventilation. Generally, this means rates above 150 breaths per minute and tidal volumes below 2 to 3 mL/kg.

127. What are the three types of high-frequency ventilation, and how are they distinct from one another?
- High-frequency oscillation (Sensormedics)
- High-frequency jet ventilation (Bunnell, Inc.)
- High-frequency flow interruption (Infant Star)

Oscillation exchanges gas by producing positive and negative flow in the ventilator circuit through the use of a vibrating diaphragm. Jet ventilation delivers high-frequency breaths through the interruption of a continuous gas flow directly into the airway through a unique ET tube located in the airway. The interruption takes place in a patient box located close to the baby, by a pinch valve that opens and closes on a piece of plastic tubing. With jet ventilation, inspiration is active; exhalation is passive. High-frequency flow interruption generates the signal by interrupting the flow of gas. It is similar to the jet ventilator except that the interruption of the gas flow occurs at a site much farther from the infant.

128. Have the three types of high-frequency ventilation been compared in clinical trials?
No. Because there have been no comparison trials, each type has its advocates and critics.

129. What happens to tidal volume delivery to the alveolus when frequency is increased during high-frequency oscillation?
It decreases. Impedance of the airway and ET tube are frequency dependent. As rate is increased, impedance to transmission of pressure swings increases. Thus tidal volume decreases as frequency is increased.

130. How is minute ventilation estimated on high-frequency ventilation?
With standard mechanical ventilation or spontaneous breathing, minute ventilation = frequency × tidal volume. In high-frequency ventilation, minute ventilation = (frequency) × (tidal volume)^2

This question emphasizes the importance of understanding the differences between high-frequency oscillation and conventional ventilation. In conventional ventilation increasing the rate will increase carbon dioxide elimination in most cases. With high-frequency ventilation turning up the rate generally causes a decrease in minute ventilation owing to the loss of tidal volume delivery. When ventilation is inadequate during high-frequency ventilation, turning the rate down can increase carbon dioxide elimination.

131. How does high-frequency ventilation work?

No one really knows. Modeling of the wave flow in high-frequency ventilation is exceedingly complex. Several theories have been proposed, however, to explain high-frequency ventilation:

- Spike theory: This theory postulates that the resistance along the periphery of the airway is higher than in the center so that a spike is produced that extends far down the center of the airway, bypassing much of the lung's dead space.
- Pendelluft: The rapid to-and-fro movement of air between lungs or between lung segments may be enhanced at higher frequencies.
- Brownian diffusion: This may increase at higher frequencies.
- Coaxial flow: This theory speculates that gas flow in the airway is not simply a to-and-fro movement. Rather, inhaled gas spikes down the center of the airway, whereas the exhaled carbon dioxide moves along the periphery in a circuitous fashion. As frequencies increase, a whirlpool may actually arise within the airway that literally pulls the small-volume puffs of gas to a very deep region of the lung (Fig. 18-13).

132. What factors affect ventilation during high-frequency ventilation?

Just as in conventional ventilation, changes in respiratory system impedance affect carbon dioxide elimination during high-frequency ventilation. The important distinction is that high-frequency

✓ KEY POINTS: HIGH-FREQUENCY VENTILATION IN NEONATES

1. There are several types of high-frequency ventilation, but the device used may be less important than the ventilatory strategy with which the device is used.

2. If the lung is poorly inflated, a strategy of lung recruitment (increased mean airway pressure compared with that being used on a conventional ventilator) is appropriate.

3. If air leakage is present or the lung is overinflated, a strategy that minimizes intrathoracic pressure is important, and a lower mean airway pressure may be the most appropriate approach.

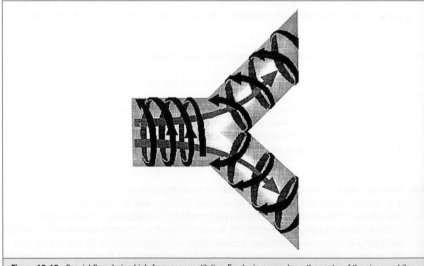

Figure 18-13. Coaxial flow during high-frequency ventilation. Fresh air moves down the center of the airway, while exhaled CO_2 is removed along the periphery. (From Spitzer AR, editor. Intensive Care of the Fetus and Neonate. 2nd ed. Philadelphia: Saunders; 2005.)

ventilation is more sensitive to changes in impedance than conventional modes of ventilation. Changes in ET tube size, respiratory system compliance, airway patency, and mucus plugging all can have a profound effect on tidal volume delivery and therefore ventilation. Because of the frequencies used and the small tidal volumes, these changes seem to be significantly magnified with high-frequency ventilation compared with conventional ventilation.

133. In neonates with poor lung inflation, should high-frequency oscillation be used at lower, the same, or higher Paw than that being used on conventional ventilation?

The strategy with which high-frequency oscillation is used is important. Patients with diffuse loss of lung volume (i.e., atelectasis) should be treated with a lung recruitment strategy. High-frequency oscillation allows the use of higher Paws than conventional ventilation because the small tidal volumes promote ventilation without causing lung overinflation. This approach has been studied in animal models of hyaline membrane disease and has been shown to improve lung inflation, decrease acute lung injury, decrease pulmonary air leaks, and promote survival. Often referred to as a "high mean airway pressure strategy," the real goal is not a high Paw but rather optimal lung inflation. Unfortunately, measures of optimal lung inflation are not available. Clinically, the goal is to promote lung recruitment while avoiding lung overinflation, cardiac compromise, and lung atelectasis.

Cools F, Askie LM, Offringa M, et al. Elective high-frequency oscillatory versus conventional ventilation in preterm infants: a systematic review and meta-analysis of individual patients' data. Lancet 2010;375(9731):2082–91.

Krebs J, Pelosi P, Tsagogiorgas C, et al. Open lung approach associated with high-frequency oscillatory or low tidal volume mechanical ventilation improves respiratory function and minimizes lung injury in healthy and injured rats. Crit Care 2010;14(5):R183.

134. When high-frequency ventilation is used, what measurements help guide choice of ventilation settings?

The chest radiograph and the arterial PO_2/FiO_2 ratio can be used to help guide therapy. If the chest radiograph shows more than nine posterior ribs of inflation, flattened diaphragms, a small heart, or very clear lung fields, the lung may be overinflated. Similarly, if the Paw is high and the FiO_2 is low, then Paw should be decreased before FiO_2. If the chest radiograph shows fewer than seven posterior ribs of inflation, domed diaphragms, a normal heart size, or diffuse radiopacification, the lung may be underinflated. Therefore the Paw should be increased if the Paw is low and the FiO_2 is high. The assessment of cardiac function is also important for the safe use of high-frequency ventilation. Monitoring heart rate, blood pressure, urine output, and capillary refill can help alert the care provider to changes in cardiac output.

135. What adverse events have been reported with the use of high-frequency ventilation?

Several studies have shown evidence of increased brain injury (i.e., periventricular leukomalacia and intraventricular hemorrhage) associated with high-frequency ventilation, particularly when initiated as an initial treatment modality in a VLBW baby. Although meta-analysis does not confirm this finding, the concern remains, and further studies are needed in this regard. The complication of necrotizing tracheobronchitis was reported with early models of high-frequency ventilation. This complication has disappeared with the development of improved humidification systems.

136. What are the variables used to alter oxygenation during high-frequency ventilation?

Altering Paw to optimal levels will change lung volume, improve ventilation–perfusion matching, and decrease intrapulmonary shunt. FiO_2 is used to change the alveolar oxygen concentration.

In oscillatory ventilation Paw can be altered directly by changing that setting on the ventilator. With jet ventilation Paw is a measured value that is a combination of several factors: PIP, PEEP, duration of inspiratory phase (jet valve on time), and background sigh rate.

137. **Has high-frequency ventilation been conclusively shown to reduce the use of ECMO in neonates with MAS?**

No. Only anecdotal evidence exists to support the efficacy of high-frequency ventilation in neonates with MAS. In fact, in neonates with MAS and signs of air trapping, high-frequency ventilation may be dangerous. Reported success in MAS with high-frequency ventilation is between 30% and 40%.

Henderson-Smart DJ, De Paoli AG, Clark RH, et al. High frequency oscillatory ventilation versus conventional ventilation for infants with severe pulmonary dysfunction born at or near term. Cochrane Database Syst Rev 2009;3:CD002974.

138. **Theoretically, how does high-frequency ventilation prevent acute lung injury in hyaline membrane disease?**

Volutrauma occurs most rapidly when the lung is repeatedly cycled from a low volume to a high volume. Use of zero end-expiratory pressure and excessive tidal volumes can create acute lung injury within minutes. Application of end-expiratory pressure reduces "atelectotrauma" by preserving functional residual capacity at the end of each assisted breath. Lung overinflation is avoided by using small tidal volumes. Thus the extremes of low and high lung volumes are avoided with high-frequency ventilation.

139. **What other tools are used in neonatology to promote better lung inflation and reduce the injury associated with ventilating a collapsed lung?**

The use of end-expiratory pressure, surfactant, prone positioning, and liquid ventilation all promote lung recruitment over time. They work by stabilizing recruited alveoli at the end of exhalation.

140. **To use high-frequency ventilation safely, what factors must be carefully monitored?**

Hyperventilation must be avoided. Data on brain injury in neonates suggest that hyperventilation may cause brain injury through ischemia as CO_2 is lowered. This finding has been observed in a number of published studies, both with conventional and high-frequency ventilation.

Lung overinflation or underinflation also may have adverse affects on the baby. Currently, no good methods are available for defining optimal lung volume during high-frequency ventilation. Evaluating cardiac performance, chest radiographs, and arterial PO_2/FiO_2 ratio can help the clinician avoid extremes, but the Holy Grail of high-frequency ventilation is defining when the lung is optimally inflated.

141. **In what pulmonary disease states has high-frequency ventilation been shown to promote improved oxygenation compared with conventional modes of ventilation?**

The most dramatic improvements in oxygenation have been reported in patients with poor lung inflation. In general, this means neonates with RDS or pneumonia. Lung disease in which there is a significant amount of airway debris or resistance does not seem to respond as well to high-frequency ventilation.

NEONATAL EXTRACORPOREAL MEMBRANE OXYGENATION

142. **What is ECMO?**

ECMO is a modification of standard cardiopulmonary bypass techniques used in the operating room during open heart surgery. It was adapted in a simplified circuit to provide artificial life support to pulmonary patients in an intensive care unit setting. Neonatal ECMO was the first clinically successful application of this technology to treat severe and progressive cardiorespiratory failure caused by MAS and complicated by persistent pulmonary artery hypertension occurring in the first week of life. At the core of ECMO technology are the heart–lung pump (a semiocclusive roller device) and the innovative Kolobow polycarbonate-spooled, silicone membrane oxygenator (Fig. 18-14). Both devices are sufficiently powerful to completely support cardiac output and lung function in neonates.

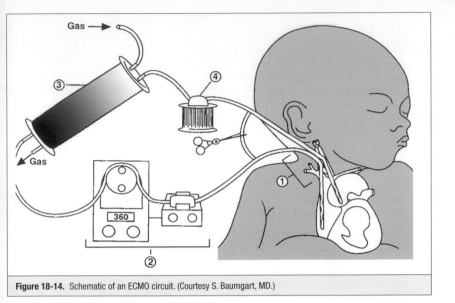

Figure 18-14. Schematic of an ECMO circuit. (Courtesy S. Baumgart, MD.)

143. What is extracorporeal life support (ECLS)?

ECLS includes ECMO, hemofiltration, hemodialysis, and indwelling oxygenator filaments (i.e., intravenous oxygenator). Many of these other techniques can be incorporated with an ECMO circuit or can be applied separately.

Kim K, Mazor RL, Rycus PT, et al. Use of venovenous extracorporeal life support in pediatric patients for cardiac indications: a review of the Extracorporeal Life Support Organization registry. Pediatr Crit Care Med 2012;13(3):285–9.

Lazar DA, Cass DL, Olutoye OO, et al. The use of ECMO for persistent pulmonary hypertension of the newborn: a decade of experience. J Surg Res 2012;177(2):263–7.

Haines NM, Rycus PT, Zwischenberger JB, et al. Extracorporeal Life Support Registry Report 2008: neonatal and pediatric cardiac cases. ASAIO J 2009;55(1):111–6.

144. What evidence suggests that ECMO actually works?

The definitive randomized trial establishing the effectiveness of neonatal ECMO was conducted by the National Health Service in the United Kingdom. Of 93 infants referred to ECMO centers, 30 (or 32%) died compared with 54 of 92 (59%) receiving conventional care. The relative risk for reduced mortality with ECMO was 0.55 (95% CI, 0.39 to 0.77; P <0.0005). Of the survivors, one child in each group was severely disabled at 1 year, and ten ECMO patients (compared with six conventionally treated infants) were disabled to a lesser degree. The UK Collaborative ECMO Trial Group concluded that ECMO support should be actively considered for mature neonates with severe but potentially reversible respiratory failure.

UK Collaborative ECMO Trial Group: UK collaborative randomised trial of neonatal extracorporeal membrane oxygenation. Lancet 1996;348:75–82.

Petrou S, Bischof M, Bennett C, et al. Cost-effectiveness of neonatal extracorporeal membrane oxygenation based on 7-year results from the United Kingdom Collaborative ECMO trial. Pediatrics 2006;117(5):1640–9.

145. Who is a neonatal ECMO candidate?

The success of ECMO relies on the physician's ability to recognize, within the first week of illness, those near-term or term newborn infants with reversible pulmonary disease and to exclude infants with irreversible pulmonary disease. According to the ECLS Organization's Registry data estimates,

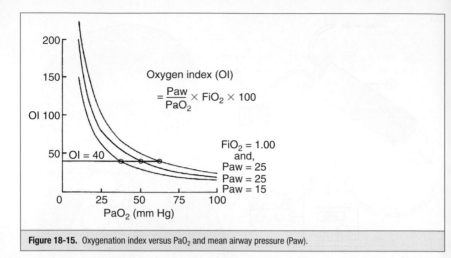

Figure 18-15. Oxygenation index versus PaO$_2$ and mean airway pressure (Paw).

only one in approximately 1700 infants can benefit from ECMO. Criteria for ECMO patient selection have been widely debated during the past decade, and two controversial questions have arisen: (1) Is less invasive therapy likely to succeed? (2) With constantly improving neonatal ventilatory and pharmacologic techniques, must physicians continually reassess ECMO criteria? In general, the earlier the ECMO physician can identify the infant with a high probability of dying as a result of disease (before iatrogenic consequences of conventional therapy), the better the patient selection and outcome will be. The following inclusion and exclusion criteria provide general neonatal ECMO guidelines that are currently widely accepted:

- >34 weeks' gestational age
- >2 kg birth weight
- <2 weeks' postnatal age (or ≤10 days' high-pressure mechanical ventilation, relative age)
- Reversible cardiopulmonary condition
- No major cardiac malformation
- No syndromes with an unsurvivable prognosis
- No uncontrollable bleeding diathesis (e.g., disseminated intravascular coagulation with bleeding uncontrolled despite multiple component transfusions or progressive parenchymal brain hemorrhage)
- No irrevocable brain injury

146. What pulmonary indices are used to identify ECMO candidates?

Once the aforementioned inclusion and exclusion criteria have been considered, one of several pulmonary indices is used to assess the severity of respiratory illness and the likelihood of death if the infant is treated conventionally. The simplest and most popular index is the oxygenation index (Fig. 18-15). Briefly, the oxygenation index is equivalent to the Paw generated during mechanical ventilation multiplied by the FiO$_2$ (both of these values indicate the level of conventional ventilatory support) divided by the postductal arterial oxygen tension in the blood (a sensitive indicator of both ventilation and perfusion of the baby's lung). The resulting value is multiplied by 100. The relative importance of the ratio between Paw and arterial oxygen tension in the calculation of oxygenation index performed at 1.00 (FiO$_2$) is further demonstrated graphically in Figure 18-15. Once the arterial PO$_2$ is below 40 mm Hg in the denominator of the oxygenation index equation, a geometric rise in the oxygenation index occurs. This rise parallels increased pulmonary vascular resistance with increased right-to-left shunting in the patient with severe pulmonary arterial hypertension.

147. **How may vascular access for ECMO be achieved, and what are the benefits and liabilities of venoarterial (VA) versus venovenous (VV) bypass?**

VA Bypass: The gold standard for ECMO therapy is VA bypass. An internal jugular drainage cannula and a second common carotid arterial infusion cannula are placed surgically through a right neck incision performed at the bedside. VA ECMO provides complete cardiopulmonary support to an infant's native heart and lungs when either or both are failing.

Advantages:
- Complete cardiopulmonary support
- Used for heart and lung failure
- Cardiac function not essential

Disadvantages:
- Carotid artery ligation
- Embolism (clot, air) infused into arterial circulation
- Potential hyperoxic reperfusion injury

VV Bypass: A less invasive technique for augmenting systemic oxygenation using ECMO is VV bypass. In neonates a novel double-lumen cannula (12 or 14 French) is surgically inserted into the internal jugular vein and positioned within the right atrium. Blood is withdrawn from the lateral lumen, reoxygenated, and infused back into the medial lumen. The right atrial admixture of oxygenated and deoxygenated blood then crosses through fetal channels (the foramen ovale and the ductus arteriosus) in the infant with severe pulmonary arterial hypertension to supply systemic oxygenation via shunt flow. Because systemic blood supply is delivered entirely by the infant's native left ventricle, sufficient ventricular force must be available to circulate this oxygenated admixture against systemic vascular resistance, which is usually increased in critically ill patients. Frequently, both cardiotonic pressors and generous volume infusions of saline, albumin, or plasma along with blood transfusions are required to maintain an infant's circulation on VV ECMO. VV access does not require invasion of the carotid artery; therefore systemic embolism is less risky, and the right common carotid artery is left intact after decannulation from bypass.

Advantages:
- Spares carotid artery
- Embolism less risky
- One double-lumen cannula sufficient

Disadvantages:
- Less effective cardiac support
- Lower arterial PO_2 with mixing in right atrium
- Recirculation into double-lumen cannula
- Mixed venous saturation (SvO_2) and SaO_2 monitors unreliable; must follow arterial PO_2, pH to judge oxygen sufficiency

148. **What is the single most important parameter for monitoring the effectiveness of ECMO?**

SvO_2 from the jugular venous cannula drain is monitored continuously during bypass using a fiber-optic device inserted directly into the blood path coming out of the patient. SvO_2 does not so much reflect pulmonary function (as does the systemic arterial saturation) as it represents the adequacy of tissue oxygen delivery from the native heart and the ECMO circuit combined. If the oxygen delivered by ECMO is sufficient to meet tissue oxygen demand, then the SvO_2 is generally greater than 70%. Failure to meet tissue oxygen demand results in the progressive desaturation of venous blood returning from the capillary beds into the right atrium. An SvO_2 below 65% to 70% indicates marginal oxygen delivery, and an SvO_2 below 60% may be associated with lactic acid production through anaerobic metabolism. Therefore the single most important parameter monitored during ECMO and used to assess the adequacy of bypass is the SvO_2. Notably, during VV ECMO the SvO_2 may be artificially elevated because of recirculation of arterialized blood back into the drainage side of the double-lumen cannula; however, trends in SvO_2 may still be useful, and the patient may be taken off bypass briefly to assess a true SvO_2.

149. How long do babies stay on bypass? How do you know when to wean ECMO flow?

The typical ECMO course transpires over 3 to 7 days, while awaiting spontaneous lung recovery.

 KEY POINTS: NEONATAL EXTRACORPOREAL MEMBRANE OXYGENATION

1. A definitive randomized trial established the effectiveness of neonatal ECMO. It showed that survival in neonates offered ECMO was better than in neonates receiving conventional care.

2. The relative risk reduction in mortality with ECMO was 0.55 (95% CI, 0.39 to 0.77; P <0.0005). ECMO is one of the few therapies that has been shown to save the lives of critically ill neonates.

3. Clinicians should be careful not to place children at unnecessary risk by using therapies that have not been established to improve outcome.

Cardiac recovery and mobilization of capillary leak edema usually precede lung recovery and weaning the ECMO pump flow rate. As the tissue edema is mobilized, fluid is transferred back into the intravascular space, increasing the baby's native cardiac output. Therefore the infant's systemic arterial saturation and arterial PO_2 may actually decrease during recovery (as ECMO support is weaned and the infant's native cardiac output drives right-to-left shunting of deoxygenated blood through fetal channels in an accelerated fashion). During this early improvement phase on ECMO, diuretic therapy (e.g., furosemide, mannitol) or hemofiltration may assist in reducing this native circulation of desaturated blood. Thereafter, as the mixed venous saturation improves in the jugular venous cannula (above 80%), the ECMO pump flow is reduced in 10 mL/min decrements until a pump idle rate is reached of approximately 100-mL/min minimum flow (to prevent stasis and clotting within the circuit). Frequent arterial and venous blood gas assessments are important during the weaning process. Recent reports have suggested that pulmonary function testing demonstrating increased functional residual capacity (>15 mL/kg) and improved dynamic lung compliance may be useful in determining more exactly when lung recovery is sufficient to warrant coming off bypass.

AIR LEAK SYNDROMES

150. Which respiratory conditions in newborn infants have the highest incidence of air leak?

Infants with RDS and MAS are at highest risk for air-leak syndrome, and it is estimated that between 1% and 2% of all newborns may have a spontaneous pneumothorax. The incidence of air leak increases with decreasing birth weight and gestational age, and it increases with more severe lung disease. The reason for the increase with MAS is the viscosity of meconium, which results in a ball-valve mechanism that leads to air trapping. Newborns in general have a higher incidence of air leaks than the general population because of the high transpulmonary pressure (−30 to −150 cm H_2O) associated with the onset of breathing.

151. What is the least common form of neonatal air-leak syndrome?

Pneumothorax is the most common form of air leak, and, fortunately, pneumopericardium is the least common. Pneumopericardium must be recognized promptly because of its high morbidity and mortality risk. In the era before surfactant, pulmonary interstitial emphysema was more common and in many cases preceded other forms of air leak. Pneumomediastinum is uncommon but the most difficult to treat because there is no easy way to evacuate mediastinal air.

152. Why has the incidence of neonatal air leak syndromes declined?

One of the major factors has to be the "kinder, gentler" approach to neonatal ventilation. Permissive hypercapnia was a popular approach during the 1990s, and this led to more conservative ventilatory management strategies.

A second important change was the introduction of surfactant replacement therapy toward the end of the 1980s. Most of the early surfactant trials documented a 30% to 50% reduction in the rate of neonatal air leaks.

153. You are called to the bedside of a baby who has suddenly become cyanotic while on a ventilator. You listen to the chest, and you hear better breath sounds on the right side. You call for a chest radiograph, but the x-ray technician is on a break. Neither the senior resident nor the neonatologist is available, and you are on your own. What do you suspect, and how can you tell whether you are correct?

Your suspicion should be high for a tension pneumothorax in this clinical situation. Before you place a needle into the chest, however, consider the following:

- You could transilluminate the chest with a high-intensity fiberoptic light. If a pneumothorax is present, the left side should light up, whereas the right will transilluminate less.
- Also, check the position of the ET tube. Make sure it is in a good position and has not changed (look at the numeric value of the ET tube and compare with where it is supposed to be). If there is evidence that the position of the ET tube has changed and it is out or has been pushed in too far, secure the airway and make sure it is in appropriate position. If the acute deterioration is caused by ET tube malposition, repositioning of the tube should lead to rapid improvement in gas exchange. Repositioning that does not lead to improvement supports the diagnosis of air leak as a possible cause for the deterioration.

154. A baby is breathing asynchronously on a conventional ventilator, and you are concerned that she is at risk for a pneumothorax. What can you can do to decrease the risk of air leak in this patient?

- Increasing the gas temperature may slightly decrease the incidence of air leak.
- Decreasing the inspiratory time will decrease Paw and could decrease the risk of pneumothorax, but it may reduce oxygenation.
- Increasing the ventilatory rate may allow you to take over ventilation and decrease the baby's effort, but you need to watch for air trapping.
- Use of a synchronized mode of ventilation (SIMV or A/C) will help the baby breathe with the ventilator breaths.
- Sedation and pain relief may help significantly.

155. What are some possible ways to treat unilateral pulmonary interstitial emphysema?

The primary treatment goal unilateral pulmonary interstitial emphysema is to allow the affected lung to deflate. Selective bronchial intubation will allow the contralateral lung to deflate (of course, selective left mainstem intubation may be technically difficult), but it may pose problems because the perfusion to the ventilated lung may not be sufficient for gas exchange in all cases. A randomized trial of high-frequency jet ventilation did show effectiveness in treating pulmonary interstitial emphysema by lowering the Paw, which may allow the emphysema to resolve. In infants the lung in the superior position will receive more of the ventilation. Placing the affected lung in the downward position may be helpful in deflating that lung.

Keszler M, Donn SM, Bucciarelli RL, et al. Multicenter controlled trial comparing high-frequency jet ventilation and conventional mechanical ventilation in newborn infants with pulmonary interstitial emphysema. J Pediatr 1991;119(1 Pt 1):85–93.

Keszler M, Durand DJ. Neonatal high-frequency ventilation. Past, present, and future. Clin Perinatol 2001;28(3):579–607.

156. What important sign distinguishes a tension pneumothorax from one without tension?

There is no specific sign. In a tension pneumothorax an ongoing air leak contributes to a progressive Increase In Intrathoraclc pressure. Shift of the trachea or the point of maximal impulse, decreased breath sounds, pallor, or cyanosis and retractions may occur in either tension or nontension pneumothorax. In a tension pneumothorax the critical factor is the ongoing increase in cardiopulmonary embarrassment to the patient. When a pneumothorax is first detected, it is usually very difficult to tell whether a pneumothorax is under tension. If the child appears clinically stable for the moment, the clinician can wait for a time (30 to 60 minutes) and repeat a chest radiograph before inserting a chest tube. In some cases, however, waiting is impossible, and a thoracentesis must be done immediately.

157. Why do neonates have an increased susceptibility to alveolar rupture?

Neonates are subject to air leaks because of uneven alveolar ventilation in RDS or MAS. Air trapping also frequently occurs because of small airway plugs. The areas that are more distensible receive more ventilation, which leads to high transpulmonary pressure that in turn increases the likelihood of alveolar rupture. An additional factor is that the neonate has fewer alveolar connecting channels (pores of Kohn), which allow air to redistribute between ventilated and nonventilated alveolar spaces. Lastly, resuscitation by an overzealous, inexperienced practitioner also increases the newborn's susceptibility to air leaks.

158. Where is a chest tube best placed for the best drainage of an air leak?

Ideally, a chest tube should be placed in that part of the thoracic cavity where it will do the most good with the least risk to the infant. Positioning of the infant is the key to the entire procedure. All too commonly, the baby is allowed to remain supine. When the clinician enters the chest in that position, the catheter hits the lung and moves posteriorly (Fig. 18-16). However, if the child is placed nearly vertical to start the procedure, it is easy to angle the catheter anteriorly for optimal placement. The thoracostomy tube is inserted through an incision made in the fifth interspace in the midaxillary line. After the incision is made, the clinician tunnels up an interspace with a hemostat, which is used to pop through the strong muscular wall of the chest (a remarkably tough structure even in a tiny premature infant). If a pneumothorax is present, a gush of air should be seen when the chest is opened. The catheter should be advanced so that no end holes lie outside the chest wall. If the catheter is

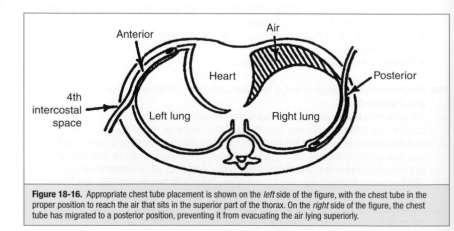

Figure 18-16. Appropriate chest tube placement is shown on the *left* side of the figure, with the chest tube in the proper position to reach the air that sits in the superior part of the thorax. On the *right* side of the figure, the chest tube has migrated to a posterior position, preventing it from evacuating the air lying superiorly.

inserted too far, it must be pulled back. The chest tube is then connected to a suction apparatus. The suction rarely needs to be greater than −10 to −15 cm H_2O.

159. Why should the second intercostal space be avoided for chest tube placement?

The use of anterior catheter insertions in the second interspace is not recommended, except in rare circumstances. It is too easy to hit the breast bud, which may damage future breast development or leave unsightly scars in any patient.

160. How can renal malformations increase the likelihood of pneumothorax in newborns?

Obstructive uropathies lead to oligohydramnios. Insufficient amniotic fluid volume leads to pulmonary hypoplasia. The mechanism is not completely understood but in part is due to external compression of the neonate's thorax, which impedes fetal lung growth. It is also believed that fetal breathing movements against an intrauterine fluid volume may be critical for normal lung development.

161. A term infant with a nontension air leak may be treated by placing the infant in 30% oxygen. How does this work?

The air in a spontaneous or nontension pneumothorax will have the same nitrogen concentration as room air. By allowing the baby to breathe pure oxygen, a gradient for nitrogen is created from the extrapulmonary to the intrapulmonary spaces. Nitrogen will naturally diffuse across this gradient, allowing the pneumothorax to reabsorb more rapidly. Caution should be used when considering this approach in preterm infants, who are more subject to oxidant injury. Recent work suggests that supplemental oxygen use may not be associated with faster resolution of spontaneous pneumothorax in term infants. Term infants with tachypnea associated with a spontaneous pneumothorax who were placed in room air did not require supplemental oxygen and did not have longer recovery times compared with infants placed in more than 60% oxygen.

BRONCHOPULMONARY DYSPLASIA

162. What is BPD?

BPD is the chronic lung disease that often follows RDS in VLBW babies. First described by Northway in 1967, it has become the greatest foe of all neonatologists and the focal point of perhaps more studies than any other clinical syndrome in neonatology. BPD was not a disease until the neonate became a patient. Once people attempted to save critically ill neonates with lung disease, a certain percentage developed BPD. In most nurseries the BPD rate is between 20% and 30% in infants who weigh less than 1500 g. BPD is defined as a need for oxygen at either 28 days of life or, more recently, at 36 weeks' postconception, with radiographic changes consistent with chronic lung disease. The incidence of BPD increases with decreasing gestational age at birth, decreasing birth weight, and increasing severity of lung disease at birth. In addition, testing (physiologic test) to determine if an infant is able to tolerate being in room air at 36 weeks' postconceptional age influences the use of the term BPD.

Northway WH Jr, Rosan RC, Porter DY. Pulmonary disease following respiratory therapy of hyaline membrane disease. N Engl J Med 1967;276:357–68.

Walsh MC, Wilson-Costello D, Zadell N, et al. Safety, reliability, and validity of a physiologic definition of bronchopulmonary dysplasia. J Perinatol 2003;23:451–6.

163. What are the histopathologic features of BPD in the lungs of newborn infants?

In a series of open lung biopsies from VLBW infants ages 14 days to 7 weeks who were receiving ventilatory support with radiographic changes consistent with chronic lung disease, Coalson and colleagues described a consistent lack of alveolarization with variably widened alveolar septae and minimal changes in the airways. Mild to moderate septal fibrosis was also apparent. These widened alveolar septae were hypercellular with disordered capillary growth. Typically, the alveolar spaces were laden with numerous alveolar macrophages and neutrophils.

Transmission electron microscopy demonstrated poor differentiation of type I and type II lung epithelial cells. These epithelial cells had relatively abundant cytoplasm and extensive glycogen stores; however, lamellar bodies were extremely rare to totally absent. There was no progression of alveolarization with enlarged simplified terminal air spaces or minimal and focal saccular fibroplasia. The interstitium of the lung contained myofibroblasts, and there was focal deposition of elastin and collagen fibers. Most saccular walls showed blunted "outpouchings" or secondary crest formation.

Coalson JJ, Winter VT, Siler KT, et al. Neonatal chronic lung disease in extremely immature baboons. Am J Respir Crit Care Med 1999;160:1333–46.

Coalson JJ. Pathology of new bronchopulmonary dysplasia. Semin Neonatol 2003 Feb;8(1):73–81.

Coalson JJ. Pathology of bronchopulmonary dysplasia. Semin Perinatol 2006 Aug;30(4):179–84.

Ambalavanan N, Carlo WA. Ventilatory strategies in the prevention and management of bronchopulmonary dysplasia. Semin Perinatol 2006;30(4):192–9.

164. How does BPD develop?

The etiology of BPD is not clear, but several factors likely contribute to its development (the six Ps of BPD):

- Prematurity
- Positive pressure ventilation
- Prolonged oxygen exposure
- Protracted use of ET tubes
- Pulmonary edema (resulting from a patent ductus arteriosus, overhydration, or delayed diuresis)
- Pulmonary air leak (e.g., interstitial emphysema, pneumothorax)

Other factors, such as free oxygen radical exposure and sepsis, also seem to be contributory in many instances. Sepsis, in particular, has recently become an increasingly important piece of the BPD puzzle. The key to this disease, however, appears to be the chronic exposure that babies have to the six Ps.

In extremely-low-birth-weight infants, BPD appears to be caused by a combination of nutritional failure and failure of alveolarization, resulting in both diminished somatic and lung growth. These factors lead to oxygen and ventilator dependency in a manner different from the original etiology of BPD.

165. Do steroids administered postnatally have an adverse effect on the nervous system?

Both animal and human studies indicate that chronic steroid use may result in reduced amounts of neural tissue mass. Neurologic handicap rates are higher in infants treated with dexamethasone. Somatic growth may also be adversely affected.

Yeh TF, Lin YJ, Lin HC, et al. Outcomes at school age after postnatal dexamethasone therapy for lung disease of prematurity. N Engl J Med 2004;350:1304–13.

Watterberg KL. Policy statement—postnatal corticosteroids to prevent or treat bronchopulmonary dysplasia. Pediatrics 2010;126(4):800–8.

166. Why is it that a child can recover from BPD, but an adult cannot repair the lung injury seen in emphysema?

Children continue to add new alveoli until approximately 8 years of age. After that time surface area and volume within the lung continue to increase with growth, but new alveoli are no longer added. Although scarring does occur in the lungs of patients with BPD, there appears to be sufficient healthy tissue to regenerate an adequate new alveolar volume.

167. What other treatments besides steroids help in the treatment of BPD?

The key to recovery from BPD is growth of alveoli and overall growth. As a result, optimal nutritional support is critical in BPD, perhaps more so than anything else. The following are other therapeutic adjuncts that help:

- Optimal ventilator management
- Provision of optimal PEEP for tracheobronchomalacia

- Bronchodilators
- Fluid restriction (it is difficult in neonates to give many calories and restrict fluids at the same time)
- Diuretic therapy (short-term therapy may be helpful, but long-term use has not been shown to improve outcomes)
- Chloride supplementation to prevent metabolic alkalosis from diuretics if they are used
- Methylxanthines (both caffeine and theophylline decrease work of breathing and apnea)
- Sedation and pain relief

168. What are BPD spells? How should they be treated?

BPD spells are acute episodes of deterioration encountered during the course of treatment of a child with BPD. The baby typically becomes increasingly cyanotic, agitated, and inconsolable, with a marked deterioration in overall pulmonary status. Oxygen and ventilatory assistance often need to be increased during these episodes. At times they may be quite acute and severe, occasionally resulting in sudden death.

BPD spells frustrate even the best neonatologists with respect to management issues. Bronchospasm is often cited as the cause of this deterioration, but personal experience suggests that many such episodes, especially the more acute, severe forms, are more commonly the result of airway collapse caused by tracheobronchomalacia. Increasing the PEEP to stabilize an airway (assuming the child is intubated) can be beneficial in such cases. If the clinician does suspect bronchospasm, prebronchodilator and postbronchodilator therapy can be evaluated with pulmonary function testing. Flexible fiberoptic bronchoscopy is also valuable to detect granulomas or tracheobronchial malacia that might be causing airway obstruction.

169. Why are chlorothiazide and spironolactone preferred as diuretics in BPD as opposed to furosemide? Isn't furosemide a more powerful diuretic?

Furosemide is a more potent diuretic than either chlorothiazide or spironolactone. In chronic situations such as BPD in a neonate, however, calcium sparing is important to prevent rickets, and thiazide diuretics are thought to be more effective in this regard. Spironolactone helps prevent potassium loss and reduces the severity of metabolic alkalosis resulting from diuretics. It is always a good idea, however, to initiate potassium chloride supplementation whenever diuretics are initiated for BPD because so many of these children develop a significant metabolic alkalosis. Furosemide also has a greater tendency to produce nephrocalcinosis when used on a chronic basis, which is less likely to occur with thiazide diuretics. There are no randomized control trials that demonstrate the efficacy and safety of diuretics in the management of BPD.

APNEA OF PREMATURITY

170. What is apnea of prematurity?

Apnea is the cessation of breathing. Although this problem affects people of all ages in many different forms, it is most prevalent in premature infants younger than 36 weeks' gestation. *Pathologic apnea* refers to cessation of breathing for more than 20 seconds; cessation of breathing for less than 20 seconds and accompanied by bradycardia 20% below the baseline heart rate; or cessation of breathing for less than 20 seconds with oxygen desaturation below 80%. Apnea in a newborn is classified as central, obstructive, or mixed. Most apnea of prematurity is classified as central apnea (Fig. 18-17), in which there is complete absence of respiratory effort. Obstructive apnea occurs when an infant makes a respiratory effort but no airflow is present because of the presence of obstruction (see Figure 18-17, *bottom*). Obstructive apnea can be associated with gastroesophageal reflux. Mixed apnea is a combination of central and obstructive apnea.

171. What is periodic breathing?

Periodic breathing is a type of central apnea characterized by brief pauses in breathing of less than 10 seconds, followed by periods of regular respiration of less than 20 seconds' duration. This pattern

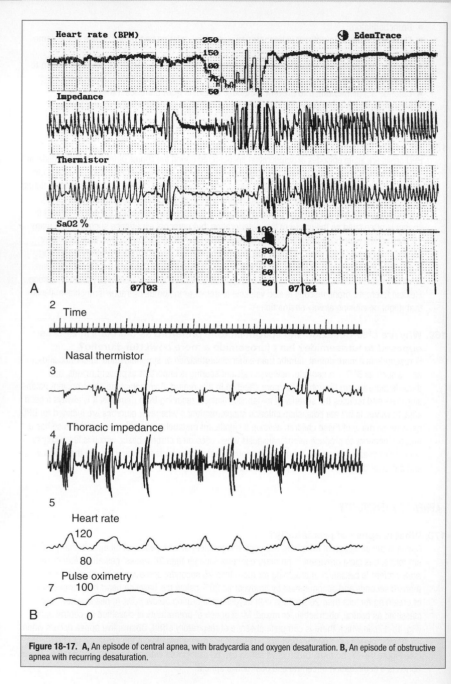

Figure 18-17. A, An episode of central apnea, with bradycardia and oxygen desaturation. **B,** An episode of obstructive apnea with recurring desaturation.

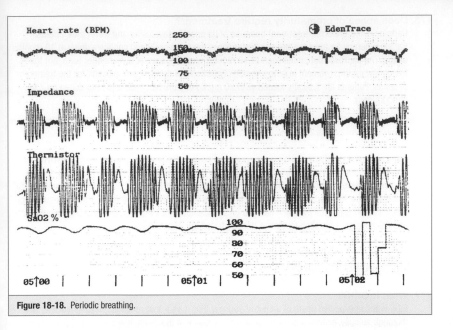

Figure 18-18. Periodic breathing.

repeats itself for at least three cycles and often many more times (Fig. 18-18). The significance of this form of breathing is unknown at present. Many prematurely born infants demonstrate periodic breathing for as much as 20% to 30% of total sleep time. Because of the frequency of this finding, some neonatologists consider periodic breathing to be a normal maturational process. On the other hand, it also may be a reflection of significant immaturity of respiratory control and a variant of apnea.

172. What is the incidence of apnea of prematurity?

Virtually all premature infants have some degree of apnea. At 34 to 35 weeks' postconceptional age, about 65% of infants have demonstrable apnea. About two thirds of these children have central apnea or periodic breathing, and one third have obstructive or mixed apnea.

173. What is the significance of apnea of prematurity?

In the short term, particularly in the NICU, extremely premature infants can have prolonged apneic episodes that may be fatal. As they mature, most infants will have more self-limited episodes. Less clear are the long-term effects on infants who have had a history of severe apnea of prematurity. Clinical studies suggest apnea of prematurity, particularly with oxygen desaturation, may affect learning and other aspects of childhood development.

Hunt CE, Corwin MJ, Baird T, et al. Cardiorespiratory events detected by home memory monitoring and one-year neurodevelopmental outcome. J Pediatr 2004;145:465–71.

Mattia FR, deRegnier RA. Chronic physiologic instability is associated with neurodevelopmental morbidity at one and two years in extremely premature infants. Pediatrics 1998;102:E35.

174. When does apnea of prematurity resolve?

Although in most cases apnea of prematurity is gone by 37 weeks' postconceptional age, in many cases it can persist even beyond 45 weeks' postconceptional age (and occasionally longer). Recent evidence indicates that apnea persists longest in the most immature infants.

Lorch SA, Srinivasan L, Escobar GJ. Epidemiology of apnea and bradycardia resolution in premature infants. Pediatrics 2011;128(2):e366–e373.

175. Does apnea of prematurity require treatment?
Caffeine is the preferred treatment because of its once-a-day dosing and fewer side effects. Caffeine therapy for apnea of prematurity reduces the rates of CP and cognitive delay at 18 months of age. The improved outcomes seen at 18 months were not seen at 5 years after birth, but the trends toward improvement in outcome still favored use of caffeine over placebo for the treatment of apnea. Patients are typically loaded with 20 mg/kg of caffeine citrate and maintained on 7 to 8 mg/kg daily.

Schmidt B, Anderson PJ, Doyle LW, et al. Survival without disability to age 5 years after neonatal caffeine therapy for apnea of prematurity. JAMA 2012;307(3):275–82.

176. Do premature infants with apnea need to be discharged with home monitors?
Home cardiorespiratory monitoring is a technology that was developed in the 1970s after several studies suggested a possible relationship between apnea and sudden infant death syndrome (SIDS). Since that time hundreds of thousands of premature infants have been discharged with these monitors. Although anecdotal evidence has shown that these devices are effective in decreasing the rate of SIDS, no large, controlled study has demonstrated this conclusively.

SUDDEN INFANT DEATH SYNDROME

177. What is SIDS?
SIDS is the unexpected death of an infant younger than 1 year that remains unexplained after a thorough autopsy, history, and investigation of the scene of the death. It was named SIDS in 1969. Although people of all ages die suddenly, the rate of sudden death is highest for those younger than 1 year of age. The 1-year cutoff has been arbitrarily assigned; actually, the overwhelming majority of SIDS deaths occur before 6 months of life.

178. How many infants die of SIDS each year?
In the United States approximately 3000 deaths resulted from SIDS in 1998. This represents a rate of approximately 0.75 deaths caused by SIDS per 1000 live births. The peak age of SIDS is 2 to 5 months. The rate is substantially higher in urban areas, particularly among African-American infants. Interestingly, the SIDS rates in the Hispanic and Asian populations are equal to or lower than that of the Caucasian population in the United States. In the developed nations of Europe and Asia, SIDS rates are slightly lower than in the United States. SIDS rates are also lower in Australia and New Zealand.

179. Has the rate of SIDS changed since 30 years ago, when it was first recognized as an entity?
The SIDS rate slowly declined from 1985 to 1994, then it began to drop precipitously from about 2 deaths per 1000 births in 1992 to the present 0.55 per 1000 births. This rapid decline paralleled the institution of the "Back to Sleep" campaign sponsored by the National Institutes of Health, the SIDS Alliance, and the American Academy of Pediatrics. This initiative followed the discovery that the simple act of changing infants' sleeping positions from the stomach to the back was responsible for a dramatic reduction in the SIDS rate in England and Australia. In the United States the rate of infants sleeping on their backs has risen from 15% to over 70% in the past 5 years. It is likely that the SIDS rate will decrease even more as increasing numbers of infants sleep on their backs.

Moon RY. SIDS and other sleep-related infant deaths: expansion of recommendations for a safe infant sleeping environment. Pediatrics 2011;128(5):e1341–e1367.

180. How did such a simple change have such a great effect?
In medicine, as in all aspects of life, uncomplicated and elegant observations can make great differences. Although the exact physiology is unclear, it is likely that sleeping on the back reduces

the rebreathing of carbon dioxide; adjusts the position of the airway, thus reducing obstruction; and reduces the possibility of poor oxygenation and ventilation through the mattress. The effects on the baby's thermal environment and the ability to eliminate heat may also be important.

181. Is SIDS a form of child abuse?

There has been a great deal of publicity about infants originally diagnosed with SIDS who were ultimately found to be the victims of a homicidal parent. These children included the case that established the supposed link between SIDS and apnea. Again, like many news stories, this represents an extremely small number of cases and is the exception rather than the rule. Although it is impossible to quantify, it is thought that fewer than 2% of SIDS cases are probable homicides.

✓ KEY POINTS: SUDDEN INFANT DEATH SYNDROME

1. The SIDS rate in the United States has dropped precipitously from about 2 deaths per 1000 births in 1992 to the present 0.55 per 1000 births.

2. This rapid decline paralleled the institution of the "Back to Sleep" campaign, sponsored by the National Institutes of Health, the SIDS Alliance, and the American Academy of Pediatrics.

3. This initiative followed the discovery (in England and Australia) that the simple act of changing infants' sleeping positions from the stomach to the back was responsible for a dramatic reduction in the SIDS rate.

182. What are the risk factors for SIDS?

The greatest known risks for SIDS appear to be prone sleeping and maternal smoking, both prenatally and postnatally. The American Academy of Pediatrics' "Back to Sleep" program, which encourages parents to put their infants to sleep lying on their backs, has led to a decrease in the number of SIDS cases reported in the United States. Other apparent risk factors include African-American race, low socioeconomic status, young maternal age, winter season, and prematurity. More recently, some evidence has suggested that there are genetic markers for SIDS in some families. The SIDS rate for premature infants is about 2.25 times that for term infants. Infants with apnea of prematurity are at no greater risk for SIDS than premature infants without apnea of prematurity.

LUNG ABNORMALITIES

183. What are the different types of congenital cystic lesions of the lung?

Congenital cystic lesions of the lung generally include those diseases that result from a problem in the formation of mesodermal and ectodermal tissue during lung development. These lesions include pulmonary sequestrations, congenital cystic adenomatoid malformations, congenital lobar emphysema, and bronchogenic pulmonary cysts.

184. What is the most common congenital lung malformation?

Pulmonary sequestration is thought to be the most common congenital lung malformation. A pulmonary sequestration is an area of nonfunctioning lung tissue with no connection to the tracheobronchial tree but with a systemic arterial supply. Pulmonary sequestrations can be diagnosed antenatally. They can be asymptomatic in the newborn or can cause respiratory distress caused by lung compression or congestive heart failure. Resection is generally recommended, even if asymptomatic, to reduce the secondary risk of recurrent infection.

185. How are pulmonary sequestrations classified?

Pulmonary sequestrations are either extralobar or intrapulmonary. Extralobar pulmonary sequestrations include lesions with lung tissue surrounded by its own pleura. Intrapulmonary sequestrations, also known as intralobar sequestrations, have no discernible pleural tissue.

186. **What is a congenital cystic adenomatoid malformation of the lung? How does it generally present?**

Congenital cystic adenomatoid malformation originates as an adenomatous growth in the terminal bronchioles early in gestation. In most cases there is a connection with the tracheobronchial tree that causes these lesions to increase in size. Only one lobe of the lung is usually involved. Congenital cystic adenomatoid malformations are now frequently diagnosed in the antenatal period by sonography. The most common presentation in the postnatal period is respiratory distress. Surgical removal of the affected lobe is the treatment of choice.

187. **What is the most common cause of mortality resulting from congenital lung malformations?**

PPHN is the most common cause. Lung malformations such as congenital diaphragmatic hernia and congenital cystic adenomatoid malformation can lead to lung hypoplasia and concomitant PPHN. Recent efforts have been made to identify infants at greatest risk of mortality who might be candidates for fetal surgical intervention.

188. **When are congenital lung malformations diagnosed in the antenatal period? What are some poor prognostic signs?**

The presence of nonimmune hydrops fetalis, shift of the mediastinum, bilateral lesions, and the presence of other associated congenital abnormalities all portend a poor prognosis for infants with congenital lung lesions.

189. **Are there any congenital lung malformations that have been successfully treated antenatally?**

Congenital cystic adenomatoid malformation has been treated with some success in the antenatal period. Antenatal surgical repair of congenital cystic adenomatoid malformations is generally limited to infants with fetal hydrops. One series of 13 infants had 8 survivors; 5 infants died in the intraoperative or perioperative period. In all survivors resection of the malformation led to resolution of fetal hydrops and increased lung growth. The principal operative concern is the initiation of maternal labor. Antenatal treatment of congenital diaphragmatic hernia has been ineffective.

190. **What is the cause of congenital lobar emphysema?**

Congenital lobar emphysema is caused by antenatal bronchial obstruction. This obstruction can be either intrinsic or extrinsic to the bronchiole and causes an overinflation of the pulmonary lobe. Intraluminal obstruction can result from a cartilaginous deficiency or inflammatory changes. Extrinsic causes include compression from an adjacent vascular structure or mass. Infants can present with respiratory distress or be asymptomatic in the newborn period. This lesion is more common in males, is usually seen in the left upper lobe, and is frequently associated with other congenital abnormalities of the heart and kidney. The treatment of congenital lobar emphysema is usually lobectomy.

191. **What is a bronchogenic cyst?**

A bronchogenic cyst results from abnormal budding of bronchial tissue during development. Bronchogenic cysts are single unilocular lesions of 2 to 10 cm in diameter. The cysts may or may not communicate with the remainder of the tracheobronchial tree. Bronchogenic cysts can be found in the mediastinum or in the peripheral lung tissue. Mediastinal cysts are thought to arise earlier in the development than those found in the periphery. Bronchogenic cysts can be asymptomatic at birth and may not present until adulthood. Other lesions are symptomatic because of compression or infection. Surgical resection is generally recommended.

CHAPTER 19

SURGERY

Alejandro Garcia, MD, and William Middlesworth, MD

PRENATAL CONSULTATION AND FETAL INTERVENTIONS

1. **Which congenital malformations can be detected prenatally?**
   Numerous structural congential malformations can be detected prenatally, including the following: anencephaly, encephalocele, spina bifida, hydrocephalus, transposition of the great arteries, hypoplastic left heart syndrome, limb reduction defect, bilateral renal agenesis, diaphragmatic hernia, omphalocele, and gastroschisis. Prenatal diagnosis of gastrointestinal atresia and obstruction is suggested by the presence of polyhydramnios and dilated bowel loops, which develop proximal to the obstructed site. The overall prenatal detection rate for gastrointestinal obstruction is 34%; it is 52% for duodenal, 40% for small intestine, 29% for large intestine, 25% for esophageal, and 7% for anal atresia.

2. **What fetal surgical interventions are currently available?**
   Congenital diaphragmatic hernia (CDH): A few centers are reporting early trials using techniques that permit expansion of the affected lung prenatally. Most trials involve internal or external obstruction of the trachea, which allows expansion of the lungs *in utero*. Trials have been limited by concerns regarding maternal safety, premature labor, and miscarriage. The results of recent randomized control trials using tracheal occlusion show survival benefits for fetuses with severe CDH compared with those receiving standard postnatal management, but with higher rates of premature rupture of membranes and preterm delivery. Multicenter trials of temporary tracheal occlusion are planned.

   Myelomeningocele: Prenatal repair for myelomeningocele reduced the need for shunting and improved motor outcomes at 30 months but was associated with maternal and fetal risks.

   Twin-twin transfusion syndrome: In monochorionic twins with evidence of unequal distribution of blood flow between fetuses, fetoscopic laser surgery can be performed to disconnect some of the communicating blood vessels *in utero*. This procedure stops the flow of blood from the donor to the recipient and halts the progression of twin-twin transfusion. Occasionally, one twin is lacking a functioning cardiac system, and reversed arterial perfusion occurs, with blood flow traveling from the normal twin to the abnormal twin leading to cardiac failure in the normal twin; this is known as the twin reversed arterial perfusion (TRAP) sequence. Fetal laser surgery can be used to interrupt blood supply to the nonviable twin.

   Congenital cystic adenomatoid malformation (CCAM): Infants with prenatally diagnosed CCAM with hydrops are at very high risk for fetal or neonatal demise. This has led to the performance of either fetal surgical resection of the massively enlarged pulmonary lobe (fetal lobectomy) for cystic or solid lesions or thoracoamniotic shunting for lesions with a dominant cyst. It was discovered that administration of betamethasone, performed preoperatively to induce fetal lung maturity, also caused regression of these lesions. The role for fetal intervention in fetuses with CCAM and hydrops refractory to medical treatment is currently unknown.

   Sacrococcygeal teratoma: Fetuses with evidence of hydrops have been treated with trials of radiofrequency ablation of feeding vessels or fetal resection of the teratoma. The benefit of these treatment modalities is unknown.

Ruano R, Yoshisaki CT, daSilva MM, et al. A randomized controlled trial of fetal endoscopic tracheal occlusion versus postnatal management of severe isolated congenital diaphragmatic hernia. Ultrasound Obstet Gynecol 2012;39:20–7.

Deprest JA, Gratacos E, Nicolaides K, et al. Changing perspectives on the perinatal management of isolated congenital diaphragmatic hernia in Europe. Clin Perinatol 2009;36:329–47.

Adzick NS, Thorn EA, Spong CY, et al. A randomized trial of prenatal versus postnatal repair of myelomeningocele. N Engl J Med 2011;364:993–1004.

Adzick NS. Fetal surgery for myelomeningocele: trials and tribulations. J Pediatr Surg 2012;47:273–81.

Danzer E, Hubbard AM, Hedrick HL, et al. Diagnosis and characterization of fetal sacrococcygeal teratoma with prenatal MRI. AJR Am J Roentgenol 2006;187:350–6.

CONGENITAL DIAPHRAGMATIC HERNIA (CDH)

3. **What are the embryologic events that lead to the development of a CDH?**
   The posterolateral portion of the diaphragm is the last to form, when the pleuroperitoneal canal closes. If it has remained open by the time the extruded midgut returns to the peritoneal cavity between the ninth and tenth weeks of gestation, the viscera will pass into the chest, and a CDH will result.

4. **What are three causes of respiratory distress in a baby born with a CDH?**
   - Associated pulmonary hypoplasia
   - Pulmonary hypertension resulting from abnormally high pulmonary vascular resistance caused by the paucity of pulmonary arterioles and their abnormal vascular reactivity
   - Mechanical compression of the lungs caused by the herniated viscera

5. **What is the common clinical presentation of a baby with a CDH?**
   Although affected infants will occasionally be asymptomatic, they usually present with moderate to severe respiratory distress. There are diminished breath sounds on the side of the hernia and usually a shift of the heart and trachea to the opposite side. The abdomen is characteristically scaphoid. Increasingly, CDH is being diagnosed *in utero* by antenatal ultrasound.

✓ KEY POINTS: MOST COMMON CHARACTERISTICS OF A NEWBORN INFANT WITH CDH

1. Dyspnea

2. Cyanosis

3. Scaphoid abdomen

4. Diminished breath sounds on the side of the hernia (usually the left)

6. **What prenatal tests are available to help predict mortality in infants with CDH?**
   Many studies have looked at lung-to-head ratio (LHR, the ratio of contralateral lung diameter to head circumference measured during 24-28 weeks' gestation), liver position, and mediastinal shift as tools to predict mortality. Although reports have been conflicting, LHR is increasingly used to predict mortality in infants with left-sided CDH. Recent studies of infants with left-sided CDH have shown that an LHR value of less than 0.85 carries a very poor prognosis and is predictive of mortality 95% of the time. An LHR greater than 1.4, however, is virtually always associated with survival.

Aspelund G, Fisher JC, Simpson LL. Prenatal lung-head ratio: threshold to predict outcome for congenital diaphragmatic hernia. J Matern Fetal Neonatal Med 2012;25:1011–6.

Hedrick HL, Danzer E, Merchant A, et al. Liver position and lung-to-head ratio for prediction of extracorporeal membrane oxygenation and survival in isolated left congenital diaphragmatic hernia. Am J Obstet Gynecol 2007;197:422.e1–422.e4.

7. **If a baby is suspected of having a CDH, which study is most useful?**
   The most useful tool is a chest x-ray, which will usually demonstrate air-filled intestinal loops in the chest (once the baby has had time to swallow air); the diaphragmatic contour on the affected side is

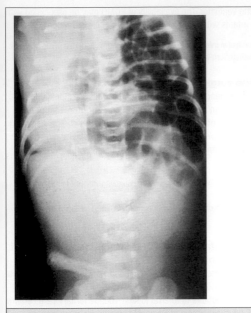

Figure 19-1. Left-sided diaphragmatic hernia with air-filled loops of intestine on the left side of the chest and deviation of the mediastinum to the right.

obliterated, and the mediastinum is often shifted to the opposite side (Fig. 19-1). In babies with the less common right-sided CDH, the findings may be more confusing, with opacification of the right lower chest from the herniated liver; in these cases, ultrasonography will provide clarification.

8. **What is the initial management strategy for an infant with a CDH?**
Endotracheal intubation with mechanical ventilation, supplemental oxygen, and orogastric decompression are used immediately in the presence of respiratory distress. Positive pressure ventilation through a face mask is not recommended because gas will enter the gastrointestinal tract and further compress the lungs. Exogenous surfactant, high-frequency ventilation, and inhaled nitric oxide are occasionally used but have no proven benefit. Barotrauma to the lungs caused by aggressive ventilation should be avoided. The level of PCO_2 may be allowed to rise to 50 to 60 mmHg (permissive hypercapnia) as long as the arterial pH remains greater than 7.25. The arterial PaO_2 should be kept between 50 and 80 mmHg but not above 100 mm Hg.

Antonoff MB, Hustead VA, Groth SS, et al. Protocolized management of infants with congenital diaphragmatic hernia: effect on survival. J Pediatr Surg 2011;46:39–46.

Garcia AV, Stolar CJH. Congenital diaphragmatic hernia and protective ventilation strategies in pediatric surgery. Surg Clin North Am 2012;92:659–68.

Guidry CA, Hranjec T, Rodgers BM, et al. Permissive hypercapnia in the management of congenital diaphragmatic hernia: our institutional experience. J Am Coll Surg 2012;214:640–7.

9. **What is the role of extracorporeal membrane oxygenation (ECMO) in babies with CDH?**
ECMO, the use of a modified heart–lung machine to provide cardiorespiratory support independent of the lungs, may be used before or after corrective surgery if the baby does not respond to the ventilatory therapy described previously. Supporting an infant on ECMO and delaying surgery allow time for pulmonary hypertension to improve while avoiding lung damage caused by barotrauma and

excessive oxygen concentrations from the ventilator. The availability of ECMO may be associated with an increased chance of survival among infants with CDH.

Kattan J, Godoy L, Zavala A, et al. Improvement of survival in infants with congenital diaphragmatic hernia in recent years: effect of ECMO availability and associated factors. Pediatr Surg Int 2010;26:671–6.

10. **What is the optimal timing for the surgical repair of a CDH?**
    CDH was once thought to be a surgical emergency, but now repair is deferred intentionally to allow for normal physiologic changes to occur in the postnatal circulation. Current recommendations are for resuscitation followed by a period of stabilization until the neonate's clinical condition improves. If the baby requires ECMO preoperatively, surgical repair is usually delayed until the ECMO settings have been lowered and the patient is considered ready to come off ECMO, but before decannulation.

Chiu P, Hedrick HL. Postnatal management and long-term outcome for survivors with congenital diaphragmatic hernia. Prenat Diagn 2008;28:592–603.

Tsao K, Lally KP. Surgical management of the newborn with congenital diaphragmatic hernia. Fetal Diagn Ther 2011;29:46–54.

11. **What is the current survival rate for infants with CDH? Which factors are most responsible for the recent improvements?**
    Several institutions are now reporting survival rates of 80% to 90% (compared with historical survival rates of 50% to 60%) for infants with left-sided CDH and approximately 55% for right-sided CDH. Most of the improvement is believed to be attributable to referral to high-volume tertiary care centers for management of these babies, as well as minimization of iatrogenic pulmonary injury through the avoidance of high ventilatory settings. However, many single institution–based reports are confounded by case selection bias, which fails to consider those CDH patients who do not reach referral centers. This is referred to as the "hidden mortality" of CDH.

Valfre L, Braguglia A, Conforti A, et al. Long-term follow-up in high risk congential diaphragmatic hernia survivors: patching the diaphram affects outcome. J Pediatr Surg 2011;46:52–6.

Mah VK, Chiu P, Kim PCW. Are we making a real difference? Update on 'hidden mortality' in the management of congenital diaphragmatic hernia. Fetal Diagn Ther 2011;29:40–5.

Logan JW, Cotton CM, Goldberg RN, et al. Mechanical ventilation strategies in the management of congenital diaphragmatic hernia. Semin Pediatr Surg 2007;16:115–25.

Fisher JC, Jefferson RA, Arkovitz MS, et al. Redefining outcomes in right congenital diaphragmatic hernia. J Pediatr Surg 2008;43:373–9.

ECMO

12. **What are the options available for extracorporeal support in a neonate?**
    ECMO support can provide heart–lung bypass (venoarterial support) or simply lung bypass (venovenous support). For infants with signs of hemodynamic instability such as in sepsis, heart failure, or CDH, venoarterial support is most commonly used. A cannula is placed into the right atrium via the right internal jugular vein for venous return, and a second cannula is placed into the aortic arch by way of the right common carotid artery for arterial delivery. In cases of isolated respiratory failure such as in meconium aspiration, venovenous support can be used. A double-lumen cannula is placed into the right internal jugular vein, and the tip of the cannula lies in the right atrium. Blood is removed from the right atrium, gas exchange occurs in the ECMO circuit (Fig. 19-2), and the blood is returned to the right atrium.

13. **What are the contraindications for ECMO support in a neonate?**
    The selection of neonates as potential ECMO candidates remains controversial and varies according to the institution. Relative contraindications that must be considered are the presence of an irreversible cardiopulmonary disorder, coexisting anomalies incompatible with life (e.g., trisomy 13 or 18), uncorrectable bleeding diathesis, and existing intracranial hemorrhage (above grade II). Infants who

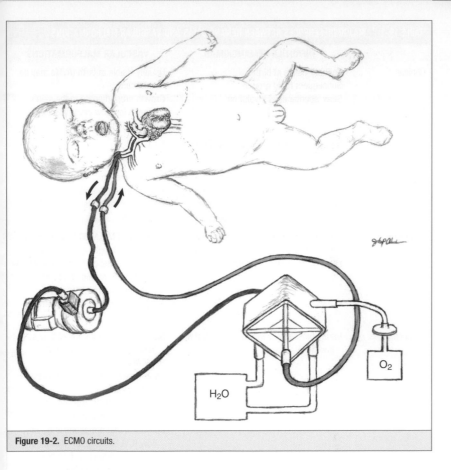

Figure 19-2. ECMO circuits.

are younger than 35 weeks' gestation are at a high risk of developing intracranial hemorrhage with systemic heparinization.

VASCULAR ANOMALIES

14. **What is the classification system for vascular anomalies?**

Vascular anomalies represent a spectrum of conditions that result from focal aberrations of blood vessel development. According to the International Society for the Study of Vascular Anomalies (ISSVA), vascular anomalies are classified as hemangiomas (proliferating endothelial tumors) and congenital vascular malformations (Table 19-1). Hemangiomas are proliferative lesions that typically undergo periods of rapid growth and involution after birth. Hemangiomas can be distinguished from congenital vascular malformations by immunoreactivity for the glucose-1 transporter (GLUT-1). Congenital vascular malformations have been defined as lesions that are present at birth that do not further proliferate postnatally, although more recent data suggest that remodeling and growth can occur in some settings. Congenital vascular malformations can be subclassified further according to hemodynamic characteristics. Fast-flow lesions include arteriovenous fistulas and malformations, and slow-flow lesions include venous, lymphatic, and mixed malformations.

Lang SS, Beslow LA, Bailey RL, et al. Follow-up imaging to detect recurrence of surgically treated pediatric arteriovenous malformations. J Neurosurg Pediatr 2012;9:497–504.

TABLE 19-1. MAJOR DIFFERENCES BETWEEN HEMANGIOMAS AND VASCULAR MALFORMATIONS

	INFANTILE HEMANGIOMAS	VASCULAR MALFORMATIONS
Clinical	Variably visible at birth Subsequent rapid growth Slow, spontaneous involution	Usually visible at birth (AVMs may be quiescent) Growth proportionate to the skin's growth (or slow progression); present lifelong
Sex ratio (female : male)	3 : 1 to 5 : 1 and 9 : 1 in severe cases	1 : 1
Pathology	Proliferating stage: hyperplasia of endothelial cells and SMC-actin cells Multilaminated basement membrane Higher mast cell content in involution	Flat endothelium Thin basement membrane Often irregularly attenuated walls (VM, LM)
Radiology	Fast-flow lesion on Doppler sonography Tumoral mass with flow voids on MRI Lobular tumor on arteriogram	Slow flow (CM, LM, VM) or fast flow (AVM) on Doppler sonography MR: Hypersignal on T2 when slow flow (LM, VM); flow voids on T1 and T2 when fast flow (AVM) Arteriography of AVM demonstrates AV shunting
Bone changes	Rarely mass effect with distortion but no invasion	*Slow-flow VM*: distortion of bones, thinning, underdevelopment *Slow-flow CM*: hypertrophy *Slow-flow LM*: distortion, hypertrophy, and invasion *High-flow AVM*: destruction, rarely extensive lytic lesions Combined malformations (e.g., slow-flow [CVLM = Klippel–Trénaunay–Weber syndrome] or fast-flow [CAVM = Parkes Weber syndrome]): overgrowth of limb bones, gigantism
Immunohisto-chemistry on tissue samples	*Proliferating hemangioma*: high expression of PCNA, type IV collagenase, VEGF, urokinase, and bFGF *Involuting hemangioma*: high TIMP-1, high bFGF (at all growth stages) Express GLUT-1, merosin, FcγRII and Lewis Y antigen	Lack expression of PCNA, type IV collagenase, urokinase, VEGF, and bFGF Lack expression of GLUT-1, merosin, FcγRII, and Lewis Y antigen One familial (rare) form of VM linked to a mutated gene on 9p (VMCM1)
Hematology	No coagulopathy (Kasabach–Merritt syndrome is a complication of other vascular tumors of infancy, e.g., kaposiform hemangioendothelioma and tufted angioma, with an LM component)	Slow-flow VM or LM or LVM may have an associated LIC with risk of bleeding (DIC)

AV, arteriovenous; AVM, arteriovenous malformation; bFGF, basic fibroblast growth factor; CAVM, capillary arteriovenous malformation; CM, capillary malformation/port-wine stain; CLVM, capillary lymphatic venous malformation; DIC, disseminated intravascular coagulation; GLUT-1, glucose transporter protein-1; LIC, localized intravascular coagulopathy; LM, lymphatic malformation; MRI, magnetic resonance imaging; PCNA, proliferating cell nuclear antigen; SMC, smooth muscle cell; TIMP, tissue inhibitor of metalloproteinase; VEGF, vascular endothelial growth factor; VM, venous malformation.

Litzendorf M, Hoang K, Vaccaro P. Recurrent and extensive vascular malformations in a patient with Bannayan–Riley–Ruvalcaba syndrome. Ann Vasc Surg 2011;25;1138.e15–9.

Ernemann U, Kramer U, Miller S, et al. Current concepts in the classification, diagnosis and treatment of vascular anomalies. Eur J Radiol 2010;75:2–11.

15. **What is the etiology of lymphatic malformations?**

Formerly known as cystic hygromas, lymphatic malformations are congenital vascular anomalies that can develop in areas of lymphatic drainage and are occasionally diagnosed *in utero*. Lymphatic malformations are hypothesized to develop from primitive lymphatic sacs that arise from mesenchyme or embryologic endothelial networks. Contraction of thickened muscular linings may increase intramural pressure and cause cystic dilation. Children can present with macrocystic or microcystic disease or a mixture of the two. Lymphatic malformations most commonly occur in the cervicofacial and cervicothoracic regions, although they can arise in virtually any location. They can cause complications such as obstruction of airway or vital organs, recurrent infection, bleeding, destruction of involved bones, and disfigurement.

16. **How are vascular anomalies treated?**

Treatment of hemangiomas is selective, with intervention reserved for lesions that threaten vital functions, such as vision or respiration, or cause deformity or pain (Box 19-1). Current first-line medical therapy for common hemangiomas of infancy has shifted in recent years from corticosteroids to beta blockers. The molecular mechanisms of response are still not fully defined, but both agents appear to induce or accelerate involution.

Treatment of congenital vascular malformations is highly dependent on the type of lesion and its location. Some lymphatic malformations, such as unilocular macrocystic malformations of the neck, may be amenable to surgical excision; other macrocystic lesions can often be treated successfully by sclerotherapy with doxycycline or other agents. Arteriovenous and venous malformations are generally treated using interventional radiologic techniques, such as transarterial embolization or sclerotherapy. Others, such as Klippel–Trénaunay–Weber syndrome, are in general treated conservatively and supportively. Current trials examining the role of oral therapy for diffuse, extensive, refractory, and recurrent lymphatic or mixed lesions with agents such as sirolimus [http://clinicaltrials.gov/ct2/show/NCT00975819] and sildenafil are currently under way.

Blei F. Congential lymphatic malformations. Ann N Y Acad Sci 2008;1131:185–94.

Swetman GL, Berk DR, Vasanawala SS, et al. Sildenafil for severe lymphatic malformations. N Engl J Med 2012;366:384–6.

BOX 19-1 INDICATIONS FOR CONSIDERING EARLY HEMANGIOMA TREATMENT

- Life-threatening or function-threatening hemangiomas, including those causing impairment of vision, respiratory compromise, or congestive heart failure
- Hemangiomas in certain anatomic locations (nose, lip, glabellar area, and ear) that may cause permanent deformity or scars
- Large facial hemangiomas, particularly those with a large dermal component
- Ulcerated hemangiomas
- Pedunculated hemangiomas that are virtually certain to leave fibrofatty residua

---

17. **How are severe cases of cervical vascular anomalies with tracheal compression treated at the time of delivery?**

The *ex utero* intrapartum treatment (EXIT) procedure is available at selected centers for fetuses with evidence of airway compression *in utero*. A standard cesarean section is performed, and the baby is partially delivered but remains attached by its umbilical cord to the placenta. While the infant is maintained on placental circulation, an airway can be established, the mass resected, or extracorporeal life support can be initiated. Studies have shown that the EXIT procedure can be performed with minimal maternal morbidity and effective rescue of threatened infants.

Olutoye OO, Olutoye OA. EXIT procedure for fetal neck masses. Curr Opin Pediatr 2012;24:386–93.

CONGENITAL LUNG ABNORMALITIES

18. **What are the various types of congenital lung malformations in newborn infants?**
    - Pulmonary sequestration: This malformation of the lung usually receives its blood supply from anomalous systemic vessels; they may be intralobar (i.e., incorporated within the normal lung) or extralobar (i.e., separate from the normal lung) and do not communicate with the bronchial tree.
    - Congenital pulmonary airway malformations (CPAMs): These are benign lesions that result from an overgrowth of the bronchial structures and may consist of large cysts, small cysts, or a solid lesion within the lung.
    - Congenital lobar emphysema: This represents overinflation of a lobe or segment of the lung usually caused by cartilaginous deficiency of the bronchial tree, leading to distal air trapping. It may also result from trauma caused by mechanical ventilation (Fig. 19-3).

Correia-Pinto J, Gonzaga S, Huang Y, et al. Congenital lung lesions—underlying molecular mechanisms. Semin Pediatr Surg 2010;19:171–9.

19. **What are the ways in which lung malformations present?**
    Increasingly, lung malformations are being discovered *in utero* by ultrasonography. These anomalies may be asymptomatic and discovered incidentally on an imaging study for another condition. They may produce symptoms related to respiratory compromise in neonates. Later in life, symptoms may be attributed to compression (e.g., chest pain, wheezing, dyspnea) or infection (e.g., chest pain, fever, cough, dyspnea). Occasionally, cross-sectional imaging is necessary because these lung malformations might be missed with traditional radiographs.

20. **What is the treatment of lung malformations?**
    The treatment is almost always surgical excision, although the timing of surgery remains controversial. Increasingly, thoracoscopic resection is safe and feasible in infancy. CPAMs may resolve after a course of prenatal steroids with bethamethasone given during the second trimester. Some evidence suggests that CPAMs may develop into pleuropulmonary blastoma if left untreated. Asymptomatic congenital lobar emphysema may be observed, and many cases will regress over time.

Morris LM, Lim F, Livingston JC, et al. High-risk fetal congenital pulmonary airway malformations have a variable response to steroids. J Pediatr Surg 2009;44:60–5.

ESOPHAGEAL ATRESIA AND TRACHEOESOPHAGEAL FISTULA

21. **What is the embryologic etiology of esophageal atresia and tracheoesophageal fistulas?**
    The precise etiology is unknown, but it is believed that the septation process that normally separates the foregut into the trachea and esophagus by the seventh week of gestation is incomplete. The more rapidly dividing trachea separates the upper and lower portions of the esophagus into discontinuous segments.

22. **Describe the five possible configurations of esophageal atresia and tracheoesophageal fistulas. Which is the most common?**
    Esophageal atresia and tracheoesophageal fistula usually occur in combination but may occur in isolation.
    - Type A: isolated esophageal atresia (rare)
    - Type B: esophageal atresia with a proximal fistula (rare)
    - Type C: The upper esophagus ends blindly with a fistulous connection between the distal esophagus and the trachea (by far the most common type, accounting for approximately 85% of cases)

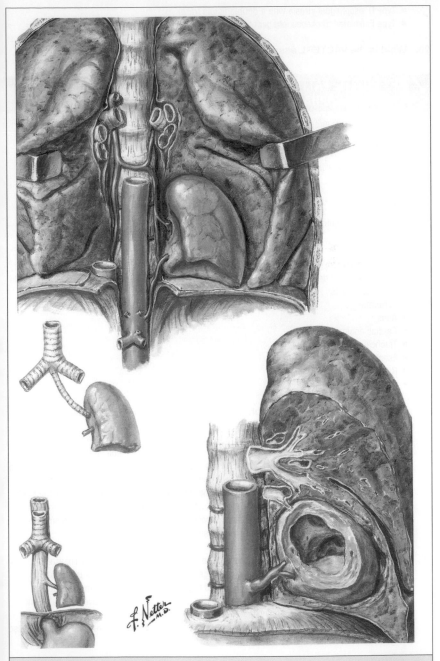

Figure 19-3. Bronchopulmonary sequestration. (Netter illustration from www.netterimages.com. © **Elsevier Inc**. All rights reserved.)

- Type D: esophageal atresia with a double fistula (rare)
- Type E: isolated tracheoesophageal fistula (rare)

23. **What is the VACTERL association?**

✓ KEY POINTS: PATTERNS OF ESOPHAGEAL ATRESIA AND TRACHEOESOPHAGEAL FISTULA

1. Isolated esophageal atresia (5% to 10% of cases)

2. Esophageal atresia with a tracheal fistula to the upper esophageal segment (rare)

3. Esophageal atresia with a tracheal fistula to the lower esophageal segment (most common, in 85% of cases)

4. Esophageal atresia with tracheal fistulas to both esophageal segments (rare)

5. Isolated tracheoesophageal ("H" type) fistula (5% to 10% of cases)

VACTERL is an acronym for a combination of congenital abnormalities that frequently occur together; the presence of one or more should prompt a search for the others. These anomalies may involve the following structures:
- Vertebrae
- Anus
- Cardiac anomalies
- Trachea
- Esophagus
- Renal anomalies
- Limb

24. **How do babies born with esophageal atresia usually present? How can the diagnosis be established?**
Infants with esophageal atresia drool excessively because they cannot swallow their oral secretions. If feeding is attempted, the baby may develop respiratory distress as a result of aspiration from the blind-ending upper esophageal pouch. The clinician should attempt to pass a nasogastric tube, which will encounter resistance. A chest radiograph will demonstrate the tip of the tube coiled in the upper chest, confirming the diagnosis of esophageal atresia. Air visualized in the gastrointestinal tract indicates the presence of a fistula distal to the trachea, whereas a gasless abdomen implies an isolated esophageal atresia. Infants with an isolated tracheoesophageal fistula may exhibit symptoms later in life related to soiling of the lungs and respiratory distress.

25. **What is the initial management plan for a baby with esophageal atresia?**
The prevention of aspiration is most crucial. A nasogastric or orogastric sump tube is placed into the blind upper esophageal segment and connected to suction while the baby is maintained in a head-up position to minimize gastroesophageal reflux into the distal fistula. Intravenous fluids and broad-spectrum antibiotics are administered, and the baby is investigated for additional VACTERL abnormalities (see answer to Question 23). Positive pressure ventilation is not recommended because it can cause abdominal distention through the fistula.

26. **When is a primary repair performed? When is the surgical repair done in stages?**
If the baby is stable and the gap between esophageal segments is short, operative division of the fistula and a primary esophageal anastomosis is performed. When the infant is extremely premature or sick or has a long esophageal gap (as frequently occurs in isolated esophageal atresia without a

fistula), the repair is done in stages. Division of any fistula and placement of a feeding gastrostomy are the initial procedures. Numerous classification systems have been developed to predict the outcome of infants with tracheoesophageal fistulas, such as the Waterson and Spitz criteria. Generally, infants weighing less than 1.5 kg and those with cardiac abnormalities carry a poor prognosis. Infants with one risk factor generally have good outcomes; those with both factors have a poor prognosis.

Sinha CK, Haider N, Marri RR, et al. Modified prognostic criteria for oesophageal atresia and tracheo-oesophageal fistula. Eur J Pediatr Surg 2007;17:153–7.

27. **List the common complications that may develop after repair of esophageal atresia.**
   Complications include anastomotic leak, stricture formation, recurrence of the tracheoesophageal fistula, and gastroesophageal reflux. Infants with evidence of reflux require acid suppression because of the long-term risk of esophageal cancer. These babies may also have underlying tracheomalacia.

CONGENITAL OBSTRUCTION OF THE INTESTINAL TRACT

28. **What are some clinical findings indicating that a newborn infant may have an obstruction of the intestinal tract?**
   - Polyhydramnios: The fetus swallows large quantities of amniotic fluid, which is absorbed in the upper intestinal tract in the latter stages of pregnancy; an obstruction in the proximal intestine will cause this fluid to back up and accumulate in excessive quantities.
   - Bilious vomiting: Regurgitation of feedings is common in newborn infants, but vomiting significant quantities of bile may be evidence of mechanical obstruction.
   - Abdominal distention: Progressive abdominal distention in the first 24 to 48 hours after birth as the infant swallows air may indicate a relatively distal intestinal blockage.
   - Failure to pass meconium: If there is no passage of meconium within 24 to 48 hours after birth, the clinician must consider the possibility of a congenital obstruction.
   - Not all of these clinical manifestations may occur, and the presence of any of them may signify the presence of an obstruction.

29. **If congenital obstruction is suspected on the basis of the scenarios just mentioned, what should be done next?**
   A careful history and physical examination is the next important step. A prenatal ultrasound may have demonstrated a dilated intestine proximal to an obstruction. Was prenatal genetic testing performed? (Down syndrome and other chromosomal abnormalities are associated with duodenal atresia and Hirschsprung disease.) Is there a family history of cystic fibrosis (which may point to meconium ileus) or siblings with intestinal atresia (which may be familial)? On examination the baby's overall condition should be noted (sepsis is in the differential diagnosis and has several features in common with obstruction). Are there features of Down syndrome? Is there abdominal distention? Is the abdominal wall red? (This may signify an antenatal perforation.) Are there any palpable hernias? Is the anal opening in the normal location and patent?

✓ **KEY POINTS: SIGNS OF CONGENITAL OBSTRUCTION OF THE INTESTINAL TRACT IN NEONATES**

1. Polyhydramnios

2. Bilious vomiting

3. Abdominal distention

4. Failure to pass meconium within 24 to 48 hours after birth

30. **Which imaging study should be performed first if congenital intestinal obstruction is suspected?**

Plain abdominal radiographs (supine and decubitus) are most useful and should be performed first. A normal gas pattern with no dilation of intestinal loops and air in the rectum lowers the likelihood of obstruction. A "double bubble" sign is pathognomonic for complete duodenal obstruction. Several dilated loops of intestine with air fluid levels and a lack of distal gas are indicative of a high intestinal obstruction. Many dilated loops of intestine suggest a distal small bowel or colonic obstruction.

31. **What is the role of contrast radiographs if congenital obstruction is suspected?**

In some instances contrast radiographs may be unnecessary—air is an excellent contrast medium, and if there is evidence of complete duodenal or jejunal obstruction on the plain films, further imaging studies are not necessary. If there is a dilated proximal intestine and some distal gas, suggesting a partial obstruction or a volvulus, an upper gastrointestinal tract contrast series is indicated. If there appears to be a distal obstruction, a contrast enema should be performed to differentiate meconium plug, meconium ileus, intestinal atresia, and Hirschsprung disease.

32. **What are the causes of duodenal obstruction in infants?**

Duodenal obstruction is most commonly caused by atresia or congenital duodenal obstruction of malrotation. Atresia may take the form of stenosis, a web, or complete separation of the duodenal segments. One cause of atresia is the failure of complete recanalization of the lumen of the duodenum after the solid phase of embryologic development, when the epithelial lining occludes the lumen; another is an annular pancreas, wherein the ventral and dorsal pancreatic buds fuse around the duodenum and compress it during development. Most commonly, duodenal atresia occurs distal to the ampulla of Vater, accounting for the bilious nature of the vomiting.

33. **What is the etiology of malrotation?**

Normal rotation consists of a 270-degree turning of the midgut on the axis of the superior mesenteric artery, resulting in the duodenojejunal junction being fixed in the left upper quadrant and the cecum attached in the right lower quadrant. In malrotation this process does not occur or is incomplete, resulting in a narrow base mesentery that puts the child at risk for development of a volvulus and obstruction (Fig. 19-4).

34. **How do patients with malrotation and midgut volvulus present?**

The most common scenario is bilious vomiting for no apparent reason in an infant who has been otherwise well and has a flat abdomen. Clinical deterioration, acidosis, abdominal tenderness, and rectal bleeding are late and ominous signs.

35. **If an infant has bilious vomiting, what should be done?**

Unexplained bilious vomiting in an infant is a surgical emergency until proved otherwise. If no other explanation is apparent (e.g., bilious vomiting with profuse diarrhea and fever may signify a systemic infection, such as gastroenteritis), an immediate evaluation for malrotation should be performed. Because plain abdominal radiographs are often nonspecific, an urgent upper gastrointestinal tract contrast study is mandatory to determine the position of the ligament of Treitz and look for a possible twist.

36. **If the diagnosis of midgut volvulus is delayed, what are the potential consequences?**

The twisting of the mesentery leads to vascular compromise and intestinal ischemia. Gangrene of the entire small intestine may occur within as short a period as several hours from the onset of symptoms.

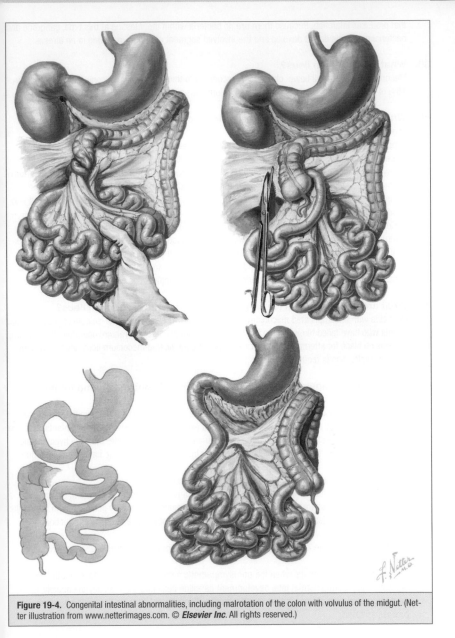

Figure 19-4. Congenital intestinal abnormalities, including malrotation of the colon with volvulus of the midgut. (Netter illustration from www.netterimages.com. © *Elsevier Inc*. All rights reserved.)

37. **How can the etiology of jejunal and ileal atresia be differentiated from that of duodenal atresia?**

The leading theory is that duodenal atresia results from a failure of recanalization in the eighth through tenth week of fetal development; there is no similar solid phase of development of the jejunum or ileum. Jejunal and ileal atresia are believed to result from an intrauterine vascular accident that produces infarction. Because there are no bacteria within the intestine at this time, gangrene and bacterial peritonitis do not develop and the involved segment atrophies, resulting in an atresia.

39. What is meconium ileus?
Meconium ileus is small bowel obstruction secondary to thick, tenacious meconium. Approximately 15% of infants with cystic fibrosis have meconium ileus at the time of birth.

40. What is the difference between simple meconium ileus and complicated meconium ileus?
Simple meconium ileus is the mechanical blockage of the distal ileum by the sticky, inspissated meconium characteristically found in babies with cystic fibrosis. Radiographs often demonstrate a foamy appearance of the dilated meconium-filled bowel loops and a lack of air-fluid levels. A barium enema will demonstrate multiple filling defects in the distal ileum and should be followed by the administration of Gastrografin. Its high osmolarity causes fluid to pass into the bowel lumen and will often relieve the obstruction nonoperatively.

Complicated meconium ileus refers to an *in utero* perforation resulting from the initial intestinal obstruction, leading to meconium peritonitis, ascites, a meconium cyst, segmental volvulus, or intestinal atresia. Infants are usually distended at the time of birth (unlike with simple meconium ileus, in which distention is initially minimal and progresses over 24 to 48 hours). Infants with meconium peritonitis may have erythema of the abdominal wall and calcifications on abdominal radiographs.

41. What are the indications for surgery in patients with meconium ileus?
Neonates with uncomplicated meconium ileus are initially treated with water-soluble contrast enema. Infants who have failed to respond to two or three therapeutic enemas require operative intervention. There is no place for attempted contrast treatment of complicated meconium ileus because urgent surgical exploration is required.

42. What are the dangers associated with attempted contrast enema treatment of simple meconium ileus?
The hydrostatic pressure of the enema can perforate the intestine, so it is imperative that the procedure be performed by a radiologist who is skilled and experienced in treating newborn infants. Also, the fluid shift into the intestinal lumen from the hyperosmolar contrast can render the baby hypovolemic, and it is essential that the baby be well hydrated with intravenous fluids at the time of the procedure.

43. How do intestinal duplications produce obstruction?
Duplications are endothelial-lined cystic or tubular structures found on the mesenteric side of the intestine that usually share a common wall. Mucous secretions or stool may accumulate in the duplication, causing it to distend, which may compress the adjacent bowel and cause obstruction.

44. Why does the zone of aganglionosis in Hirschsprung disease always involve the rectum?
Hirschsprung disease results when the parasympathetic nervous system fails to invest the entire digestive tract. During normal fetal development ganglion cells migrate cranially to caudally, so premature cessation of this process results in aganglionic bowel distal to the point where the process arrested.

45. How does Hirschsprung disease cause obstruction?
The abnormally innervated distal bowel is unable to relax and propagate a peristaltic wave, producing a functional obstruction.

46. Where is the transition zone found in infants with Hirschsprung disease?
Two thirds of the time the transition zone is in the rectosigmoid region, but the zone of aganglionosis may involve the entire colon or even extend into the small intestine (i.e., total colonic Hirschsprung

disease). Although Hirschsprung disease affects boys four times as often as girls, long-segment disease affects boys and girls equally.

47. **How do patients with Hirschsprung disease typically present?**
Failure to pass meconium in the first 24 hours after birth is highly suggestive of Hirschsprung disease. There is a wide spectrum of presentations, ranging from complete functional distal obstruction with bilious vomiting and a distended abdomen to chronic constipation (in which case the diagnosis is usually not made until after the neonatal period). Sepsis resulting from enterocolitis can occur at any time.

48. **How is the diagnosis established?**
The gold standard is a rectal biopsy that typically demonstrates an absence of ganglion cells and hypertrophy of parasympathetic nerve fibers, which stain intensively for acetylcholinesterase. This biopsy can be done at the bedside in the neonate. A contrast enema is suggestive of Hirschsprung disease if it shows a change in the caliber of the colon at the transition zone (Fig. 19-5). It is important that the study be delayed if the baby has had an enema or a digital rectal examination or even if a rectal thermometer was inserted because any rectal manipulation may temporarily obliterate the radiographic appearance of the transition zone. The contrast enema may identify a transitional zone, which may be useful for operative planning.

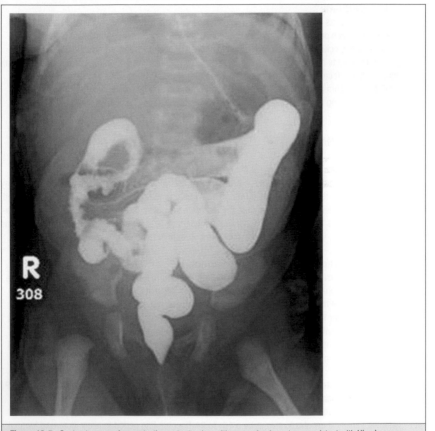

Figure 19-5. Contrast enema demonstrating patent colon with narrowing in rectum consistent with Hirschsprung disease.

49. What is the treatment for Hirschsprung disease?

Even in instances in which there is significant abdominal distention, the proximal intestine can almost always be decompressed by rectal irrigation and rectal exams, allowing time for a diagnostic work-up. Surgical repair involves resection of the aganglionic segment of bowel. Various surgical procedures have been developed to address this. The traditional surgical repair is a staged operation with a temporary diverting colostomy constructed above the transition zone, followed several months later by a "pull-through" operation in which the ganglionic bowel is brought down and anastomosed to the anal canal. In full-size babies without enterocolitis, the pull-through procedure is performed as a single operation, often with laparoscopic assistance.

50. What is Hirschsprung enterocolitis?

Patients with Hirschsprung disease may develop enterocolitis, the precise cause of which is not well understood but which involves stasis, bacterial overgrowth, and translocation through the wall of the colon. Enterocolitis may be the first recognized manifestation of Hirschsprung disease but may also occur after surgery. It can be mild or severe with explosive diarrhea, dehydration, peritonitis, and sepsis. Enterocolitis is the most common cause of mortality from Hirschsprung disease. Treatment must be immediate and consists of bowel rest, broad-spectrum antibiotics, and thorough colonic irrigations.

51. How does one differentiate meconium ileus from meconium plug and small left colon syndrome?

Meconium ileus, as previously described, is obstruction of the distal ileum by thick and viscid meconium, which occurs in 10% to 20% of neonates with cystic fibrosis. Meconium plug is caused by meconium blocking the left colon in otherwise healthy babies. Small left colon syndrome is most common in infants of diabetic mothers and produces an obstruction from a temporarily dysfunctional, small-caliber left colon. A contrast enema with barium is usually diagnostic as well as therapeutic for both meconium plug and small left colon syndrome (through its mechanical effect), although subsequent testing for Hirschsprung disease or cystic fibrosis may be indicated.

ANORECTAL MALFORMATIONS

52. What is an anorectal malformation?

Anorectal malformations comprise a spectrum of disorders in which the rectum is deflected anteriorly and fails to reach its normal perineal termination. When the rectum and urinary system end in a blind pouch, this is classified as a cloaca. When the rectum ends above the levator muscles, the malformation is classified as high; when it passes through these muscles, the malformation is low. High lesions are more common in males; low lesions are more common in females.

53. How are anorectal malformations diagnosed?

The diagnosis is usually obvious on inspection of the perineum, which should be standard procedure for a newborn examination. Either no perineal opening is present or an external fistula is visible. In male newborns this fistula is usually a small opening anterior to the normal anal location in the perineum or as far forward as the scrotal raphe. Female newborns may also have an external fistula draining into the anterior perineum, or else in the posterior vulva behind the hymen (the vaginal "fourchette"). A single perineal opening signifies a cloaca, where the rectum, vagina, and urethra all open into one common chamber.

54. What are the steps for the evaluation of a baby with an anorectal malformation?

Inspection and urinalysis allow the clinician to determine the anatomy in most cases. A perineal fistula always means the lesion is low and a colostomy is not necessary. If such a fistula cannot be detected initially, there should always be a 16- to 24-hour waiting period to allow increased luminal pressure to force meconium through a possible fistula so that it becomes visible on examination. If there is meconium in the urine, an internal fistula to the urinary tract is confirmed. If there is no visible fistula, a cross-table lateral film with the baby in the prone position can be used to measure the most distal aspect of the rectum relative to the perineal skin. The work-up should also include a search for other possible components of the VACTERL association (see answer to Question 23).

55. When is a colostomy not necessary as the initial operative procedure? Is surgery always necessary?

If there is an external fistula to the perineum, or bucket-handle deformity in a male (i.e., a vertical raphe in the perineum with indentations on both sides), the lesion is low, and a primary anoplasty can be performed in the neonatal period. Otherwise, the lesion is probably high or intermediate, and an initial colostomy is recommended, followed by a pull-through procedure within the next several months. If there is a large fistulous opening only slightly anterior to the normal anal location ("anterior anus"), function may be normal and surgery may be unnecessary.

56. How are anorectal malformations surgically corrected?

Alberto Peña devised the posterior sagittal anorectoplasty (PSARP) in which the anal and rectal sphincter muscles are divided posteriorly in the midline; this operative approach has become the standard procedure for the pull-through procedure because it allows for excellent visualization. Recently, a laparoscopic pull-through operation has become feasible.

57. What is the main determination of continence in persons who have had an imperforate anus? What should parents be told?

Continence depends on the coordinated actions of the external sphincter, internal sphincter, and levator muscles. Because the levators are most important, infants with low lesions in whom the bowel has descended normally within the levator sling have an excellent functional outlook. Children with high anomalies frequently have underdeveloped sphincter muscles, and their results are mixed, with many having at least occasional soiling. Finally, children with a flat bottom (which implies very poorly developed muscles) without a developed gluteal fold and those having sacral anomalies on radiograph have the worst prospects for normal continence. These patients require a structured bowel management program, including daily enemas, to achieve "functional" continence. All children with anorectal malformations suffer from constipation, and parents must be informed of bowel regimens.

NECROTIZING ENTEROCOLITIS (NEC)

58. What is NEC?

NEC is a condition that most commonly affects premature infants after the institution of oral feedings; however, it also occurs in term babies who have other comorbidities (e.g., congenital heart disease). It is a hemorrhagic necrosis that initially affects the mucosa but may progress to involve full-thickness injury. Manifestations vary considerably, from mild abdominal distention with hematochezia to fulminant sepsis with necrosis of the entire intestinal tract.

59. What are the factors that are believed to predispose a patient to the development of NEC?

Although the precise etiology is unknown, three factors seem to act in concert in promoting the development of NEC:

- Damage to the intestinal mucosa, which may result from ischemia caused by perinatal hypoxia, low-flow states (e.g., premature infants with patent ductus arteriosus), or reperfusion injury
- The combination of intestinal immaturity and the presence of feedings in the intestinal tract, which acts as a substrate for bacterial proliferation (NEC is highly uncommon among infants who have not received enteral feeds.)
- Impaired host defense mechanisms, as is the case in premature infants, allowing intestinal bacteria to invade the wall of the intestine (It is believed that the excessive immature inflammatory response associated with abnormal intestinal microbiota is the most likely basis for the pathogenesis of NEC.) (Fig. 19-6)

Neu J, Walker WA. Necrotizing enterocolitis. N Engl J Med 2011;364:255–64.

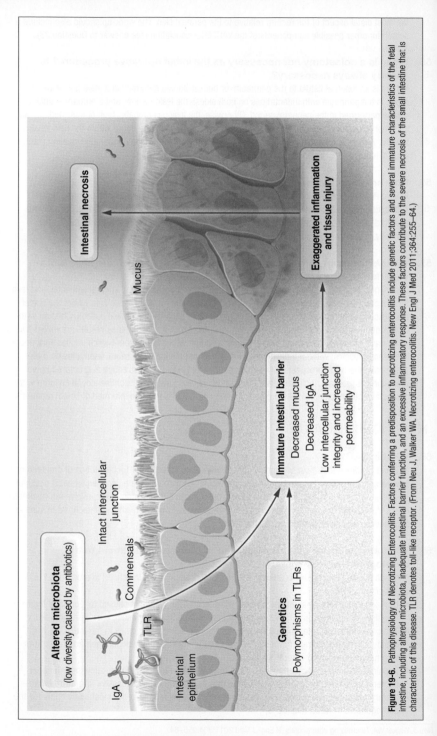

Figure 19-6. Pathophysiology of Necrotizing Enterocolitis. Factors conferring a predisposition to necrotizing enterocolitis include genetic factors and several immature characteristics of the fetal intestine, including altered microbiota, inadequate intestinal barrier function, and an excessive inflammatory response. These factors contribute to the severe necrosis of the small intestine that is characteristic of this disease. TLR denotes toll-like receptor. (From Neu J, Walker WA. Necrotizing enterocolitis. New Engl J Med 2011;364:255–64.)

Within the figure:

Altered microbiota (low diversity caused by antibiotics)

IgA

TLR

Commensals

Intact intercellular junction

Intestinal epithelium

Mucus

Intestinal necrosis

Immature intestinal barrier
Decreased mucus
Decreased IgA
Low intercellular junction integrity and increased permeability

Genetics
Polymorphisms in TLRs

Exaggerated inflammation and tissue injury

60. **Which portion of the gastrointestinal tract is affected by NEC?**
NEC may involve any portion of the gastrointestinal tract, but the ileocecal region is the most commonly affected.

61. **Is there a specific type of bacteria associated with NEC?**
No. Although affected patients may be clustered in place and time, no consistent agent has been isolated from all reported epidemics, and it is considered that a variety of the enteric flora may contribute to NEC's pathogenesis.

62. **How do babies with NEC typically present?**
Clinical signs are initially nonspecific and may consist of lethargy, apnea, temperature instability, and feeding intolerance. Gastrointestinal manifestations follow and include vomiting, bloody stools, abdominal distention, and abdominal tenderness. Generalized sepsis may supervene.

63. **How is the diagnosis of NEC established?**
Although the diagnosis may be strongly suspected by the clinical findings outlined in the previous passages, the presence of bubbly lucencies in the intestinal wall on x-ray, called pneumatosis intestinalis, is pathognomonic. Pneumatosis represents gas in the bowel wall produced by enteric organisms and is seen in 80% of NEC cases (Fig. 19-7). Other radiographic features may include irregularly dilated air-filled loops of bowel and the visualization of branching lucencies in the liver, which may signify gas in the portal venous system.

64. **Do all infants who develop NEC require surgery?**
No. Most infants with NEC will respond to medical treatment consisting of withholding all enteral feeds, nasogastric decompression, broad-spectrum systemic antibiotics, and general supportive measures to optimize tissue oxygenation and perfusion. Frequent clinical examinations are mandatory, and serial abdominal radiographs are obtained to assess for static loops or perforation.

65. **When is surgery indicated in an infant with NEC?**
Absolute indications for surgical intervention include pneumoperitoneum and intestinal gangrene (as demonstrated by abdominal wall erythema, unchanging bowel gas pattern, or failure to respond to medical therapy). Relative indications include progressive clinical deterioration, abdominal wall erythema, tender abdomen, metabolic acidosis, ventilatory failure, oliguria, thrombocytopenia, and portal vein gas.

✓ KEY POINTS: INDICATIONS FOR SURGERY IN INFANTS WITH NEC

1. Absolute indication: free air in the abdomen on radiograph

2. Relative indications: clinical deterioration with erythema of the abdominal wall, a distended and tense abdomen, portal venous gas, static loops on abdominal x-ray, refractory metabolic acidosis, and thrombocytopenia

66. **What are the surgical options for patients with NEC that require surgical intervention?**
Traditionally, a laparotomy is performed with inspection of the entire intestinal tract. Necrotic or perforated segments are resected, and an ostomy is performed. Bedside placement of an abdominal drain has been shown to have similar outcomes with regard to mortality, dependence on total parenteral nutrition, and length of hospital stay compared with laparotomy. Peritoneal drainage can be used as a temporizing procedure followed by subsequent operation. Close observation is required after any operative intervention.

Moss RL, Dimmitt RA, Barnhart DC, et al. Laparotomy versus peritoneal drainage for necrotizing enterocolitis and perforation. N Engl J Med 2006;354:2224–34.

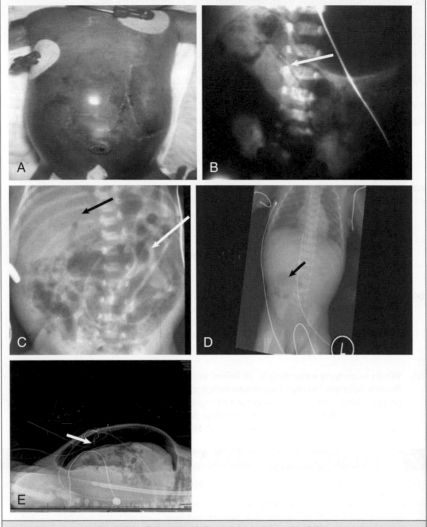

Figure 19-7. Features of Necrotizing Enterocolitis. **A,** Tense abdominal distension. **B,** Pneumaosis intestinalis. **C,** Portal venous gas and thickened bowel wall. **D,** Featureless, fixed loop of bowel. **E,** Pneumoperitoneum, or free air.

67. When should the stoma be closed?

Ideally, stomas are reversed months later, when the patient is thriving and the elective procedure is very low risk. In reality, malabsorption or skin breakdown often necessitates earlier closure. A distal contrast study should always be obtained before reversing an ostomy to ensure that there is no silent stricture in the defunctionalized bowel. Approximately 10% to 15% of patients with NEC who do not develop full-thickness necrosis and perforation will develop an obstructive intestinal stricture.

68. How does spontaneous intestinal perforation (SIP) differ from NEC?

Babies with SIP are generally younger (<1 week old) and more premature than NEC babies and often have not been fed. The exact etiology is unknown, but a very localized area of ischemia may be causative. Unlike with NEC, the surrounding bowel is not affected. Treatment consists of a localized resection with either an ostomy or possibly a primary anastomosis.

Gorson PV, Attridge JT. Understanding clinical literature relevant to spontaneous intestinal perforations. Am J Perinatol 2009;26:309–16.

ABDOMINAL WALL DEFECTS: OMPHALOCELE AND GASTROSCHISIS

69. **What are the different embryologic events that result in the development of an omphalocele and a gastroschisis?**
Between the fifth and tenth weeks of embryologic development, the intestine protrudes out of the umbilical ring and into the yolk sac. An omphalocele results when the lateral abdominal folds do not close and the exteriorized viscera remain in the sac (Fig. 19-8). The etiology of gastroschisis is unknown. (Table 19-2)

69a. **What are the differences between gastroschisis and omphalocele?**
See Table 19-3.

70. **How does the previously described embryology account for the anatomic appearances of omphalocele and gastroschisis?**
   - Omphalocele: This is a centrally located defect of the umbilical ring that has not closed, and the viscera are covered with a sac composed of peritoneum and amnion (Fig. 19-9).
   - Gastroschisis: This defect is always lateral to the cord, usually on the right, and has no covering sac (Fig. 19-10).
   The defects in the abdominal wall are generally larger in omphalocele than in gastroschisis. Extracelomic liver is almost always present with omphalocele.

71. **Which entity, omphalocele or gastroschisis, is more often associated with other syndromes?**
Babies with an omphalocele have a higher incidence of associated anomalies, such as trisomy 13 and 18 syndromes, Beckwith–Wiedemann syndrome, pentalogy of Cantrell, bladder and cloacal exstrophy, and congenital cardiac abnormalities.
   Gastroschisis is associated with younger maternal age but not associated with genetic syndromes. However, approximately 10% of these infants do have intestinal atresias, perhaps related to compression of the developing intestine against the edge of the abdominal opening.

72. **What is the importance of prenatal diagnosis?**
Detection of abdominal wall defects *in utero* is important for several reasons. It can help prepare the family and assist in triaging the patient to a prenatal center. In the case of an omphalocele, associated defects can be searched for; their presence may affect prenatal care; timing and mode of delivery; and, in the case of multiple severe anomalies, potential termination of pregnancy.

73. **What is the best method for delivering a child with an abdominal wall defect?**
Most studies show that cesarean section provides no significant advantage over vaginal delivery. One exception is the fetus with a very large omphalocele, for which several case reports have documented dystocia and liver damage during vaginal delivery.

74. **What should the immediate postnatal management of infants with abdominal wall defects involve?**
Infants born with abdominal wall defects are prone to three serious problems: hypovolemia, hypothermia, and sepsis. Exposed bowel leads to increased loss of insensible fluid as well as heat loss. Immediate management includes placing the lower half of the infant, including exposed viscera, in a plastic wrapping or moist, sterile gauze; maintaining the infant in a warmer; initiating intravenous

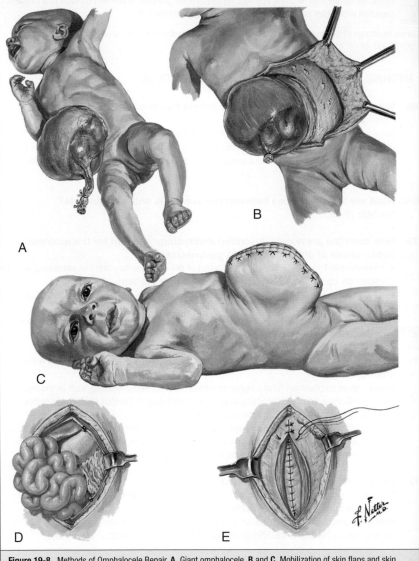

Figure 19-8. Methods of Omphalocele Repair. **A,** Giant omphalocele. **B** and **C,** Mobilization of skin flaps and skin closure, leaving large hernia. **D** and **E,** Layered fascial closure. (Netter illustration from www.netterimages.com. © *Elsevier Inc.* All rights reserved.)

access and fluids; and providing nasogastric decompression to minimize bowel distention. Parenteral antibiotics are administered to decrease the risk of sepsis.

75. **How urgent is surgical closure? What are the surgical options?**
   Babies with gastroschisis require urgent intervention because the viscera are exposed and vascular compromise may be present. In an infant with omphalocele, surgery is not urgent, and there is time for stabilization and evaluation of potential associated anomalies.

TABLE 19-2. DIFFERENCES BETWEEN GASTROSCHISIS AND OMPHALOCELE

From Chabra S, Gleason CA. Gastroschisis: embryology, pathogenesis, epidemiology. NeoReviews 2005;6:e493–e499.

	GASTROSCHISIS	OMPHALOCELE
Incidence	1 in 10,000 (now increasing)	1 in 5000
Defect location	Right paraumbilical	Central
Covering sac	Absent	Present (unless sac ruptured)
Description	Free intestinal loops	Firm mass including bowel, liver, etc.
Associated with prematurity	50% to 60%	10% to 20%
Necrotizing enterocolitis	Common (18%)	Uncommon
Common associated anomalies	Gastrointestinal (10% to 25%)	Intestinal atresia
Malrotation	Cryptorchidism (31%)	Trisomy syndromes (30%)
Cardiac defects (20%)	Beckwith–Wiedemann syndrome	Bladder exstrophy
Prognosis	Excellent for small defect	Varies with associated anomalies
Mortality	5% to 10%	Varies with associated anomalies (80% with cardiac defect)

TABLE 19-3. CHARACTERISTICS OF GASTROSCHISIS AND OMPHALOCELE

	OMPHALOCELE	GASTROSCHISIS
Sac	Present	Absent
Associated anomalies	Common	Uncommon
Location of defect	Umbilicus	Right of umbilicus
Maternal age	Average	Younger
Mode of delivery	Vaginal/cesarean	Vaginal
Surgical management	Not urgent	Urgent
Prognostic factors	Condition of bowel	Associated anomalies

Volume 16, Issue 3 <http://www.sciencedirect.com/science/journal/09575839/16/3> June 2006. p. 192–8 [accessed 27.06.2013].

The two surgical options are primary closure or, if there is tension that might compromise respiratory function or the viscera itself, staged closure with a silo. A silo prevents dessication of the exposed viscera and resultant fluid losses.

76. **How does staged closure work?**
Staged closure involves placing prosthetic material, usually a reinforced Silastic silo, over the viscera and attaching it to the fascia at the edges of the defect (Fig. 19-11). The silo is manually compressed daily to gradually reduce the viscera and expand the peritoneal cavity. Most infants can be closed within 7 to 10 days with this method. Staged closure decreases the risk of long-term bowel dysfunction and need for reoperation.

Riboh J, Abrajano CT, Garber K, et al. Outcomes of sutureless gastroschisis closure. J Pediatr Surg 2009;44:1947–51.

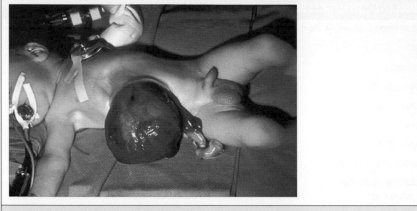

Figure 19-9. Omphalocele.

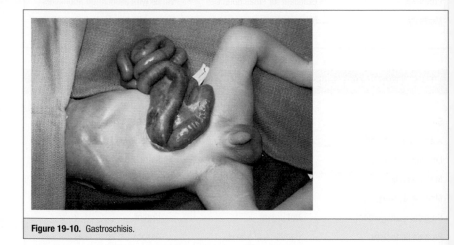

Figure 19-10. Gastroschisis.

77. **Is nonoperative treatment ever appropriate in a baby with an omphalocele?**
Yes. The omphalocele sac can be painted with an antiseptic, such as silver sulfadiazine or povidone-iodine. The sac will eventually epithelialize and contract, leaving a ventral hernia (which may be quite large) that can be repaired electively if the baby survives. This also allows for shorter duration of mechanical ventilator support and earlier feeds.

Ein SH, Langer JC. Delayed management of giant omphalocele using silver sulfadiazine cream: an 18-year experience. J Pediatr Surg 2012;47:494–500.

ABDOMINAL MASSES

78. **What is the origin of most neonatal abdominal masses?**
More than half of all abdominal masses in neonates arise from the urinary tract.

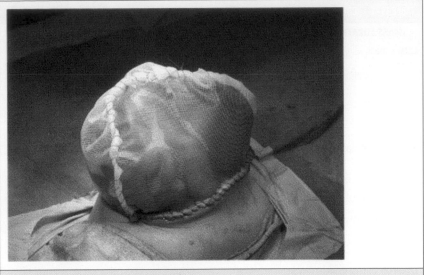

Figure 19-11. Prosthetic silo applied for staged omphalocele closure.

79. **List the two most common causes of abdominal masses of urologic origin in the neonate.**
    - Hydronephrosis secondary to ureteropelvic junction (UPJ) obstruction
    - Multicystic kidney disease

80. **How do the location and other physical characteristics of the common abdominal masses in newborn infants provide clues for their identification?**
    Physical examination may significantly narrow the diagnostic possibilities, even if it does not provide any absolute answer (Table 19-4). The following are of particular note:
    - Large masses may fill the entire abdomen, making it impossible to determine the site of origin on examination.
    - Hard, nodular masses are usually malignant tumors.
    - A highly mobile mass is usually a mesenteric cyst, a duplication, or an ovarian cyst.

81. **What is the recommended treatment for a newborn girl with an ovarian cyst that has been detected on antenatal ultrasound?**
    The management of ovarian cysts in a neonate is somewhat controversial. Most arise in response to antenatal hormonal stimulation and may subsequently resolve after birth. Potential complications such as torsion, hemorrhage into the cyst, and rupture are somewhat related to the size of the cyst; the risk of malignancy depends on whether the cyst is simple (homogeneous) or complex.

    Most authors advise observation of simple cysts that are less than 5 cm in diameter with serial ultrasound exams. Excision is recommended for cysts that are larger than 5 cm, have solid components, or cause compressive symptoms. Cysts larger than 5 cm carry a higher risk of torsion. Many ovarian cysts are amenable to laparoscopic excision.

82. **What imaging studies are most useful in investigating a newborn with an abdominal mass?**
    A plain abdominal radiograph might reveal a mass effect or bowel obstruction; can help localize the mass; and can sometimes provide useful information about the mass itself, such as the presence of calcifications or stool. An abdominal ultrasound is useful in the majority of cases because it can

TABLE 19-4. COMMON ABDOMINAL MASSES IN NEONATES

MASS LOCATION	TYPE	CHARACTERISTICS
Lateral mass	Multicystic kidney or hydronephrosis	Smooth, moderate mobility, transilluminates
	Renal tumor (Wilms or mesoblastic nephroma)	Smooth, minimal mobility, does not transilluminate
	Neuroblastoma	Irregular contour, minimally mobile, frequently crosses the midline, does not transilluminate
Midabdominal mass	Mesenteric cyst	Smooth, mobile, transilluminates
	Gastrointestinal duplication cyst	Smooth, mobile, does not transilluminate; may be associated with obstruction
	Ovarian cyst	Smooth, mobile, transilluminates
Upper abdominal mass	Hepatic tumors	Hard, immobile, does not transilluminate
	Choledochal cyst	Smooth, immobile, does not transilluminate; may be associated with jaundice
Lower abdominal mass	Hydrometrocolpos	Smooth, immobile, does not transilluminate; may be associated with imperforate hymen
	Bladder	Smooth, fixed; associated with lower urinary obstruction
	Urachal cyst	Smooth, fixed to abdominal wall, extends to umbilicus
	Sacrococcygeal teratoma	Hard, fixed, does not transilluminate; often associated with external sacral component

show whether the mass is cystic or solid, can reveal the effect on adjacent anatomic structures, and often can identify the exact anatomic location of the mass. Further information can be provided with abdominal computed tomography, magnetic resonance imaging, or urologic imaging.

83. **What is the differential diagnosis of a mass arising from the liver in a neonate?**
    - Hemangioma (benign)
    - Hemangioendothelioma (benign)
    - Hepatoblastoma (malignant)

    Ultrasound appearance is characteristic and often diagnostic. Serum alpha-fetoprotein is usually elevated in hepatoblastoma. Small to moderate hemangiomas can be observed or treated medically with corticosteroids. Most large or symptomatic hemangiomas (causing pain, heart failure, thrombocytopenia) and all hemangioendotheliomas and hepatoblastoma require hepatic resection.

84. **What is the most common cause of bilateral abdominal masses in the neonate?**
    Hydronephrosis secondary to ureteropelvic junction obstruction or posterior urethral valves.

85. **A newborn infant has a large mass below the spine arising from the presacral region, compressing the rectum and anus anteriorly. What is the most likely diagnosis?**
    Sacrococcygeal teratomas are the most common congenital tumor (Fig. 19-12). They can appear alarming because of their large size and compressive effects, but 90% are benign and can be

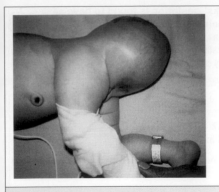

Figure 19-12. Sacrococcygeal teratoma.

completely resected. The Altman classification system is used to describe the morphology of the tumors relative to their location.

- Altman type I: entirely external, sometimes attached to the body only by a narrow stalk
- Altman type II: mostly outside the body with some intrapelvic extension
- Altman type III: mostly inside the body with some intraabdominal extension
- Altman type IV: entirely internal, also known as a presacral teratoma

HERNIAS AND CRYPTORCHIDISM

86. **What are the embryologic causes of an indirect inguinal hernia? Why are they more common in premature infants?**
When the testes descend from the abdomen during embryologic development, there is a resulting communication between the scrotum and the peritoneal cavity, the processus vaginalis, which usually becomes obliterated between the seventh and ninth months of gestation. Failure of this processus to close allows viscera to protrude into the groin or scrotum as an indirect inguinal hernia. Premature infants are less likely to have had time for the processus vaginalis to close.

87. **Do all inguinal hernias need to be repaired?**
Yes. Inguinal hernias will not resolve spontaneously, and there is a serious risk of incarceration (inability to be reduced), which can lead to strangulation.

88. **When should an asymptomatic inguinal hernia that is discovered in a newborn infant be repaired?**
This issue is somewhat controversial. If an inguinal hernia is asymptomatic, some surgeons will wait several months until the baby is older, but most recommend repairing it before the baby's discharge from the nursery to prevent complications. If the infant is premature and has diminished respiratory reserve (e.g., bronchopulmonary dysplasia), the operative procedure can be performed under spinal or epidural anesthesia, in most cases without having to intubate the baby.

89. **Which structure is most likely to be contained in an inguinal hernia in a girl?**
The ovary is the most likely structure.

90. **If a newborn infant has an umbilical hernia, should operative repair be performed at this time?**
No. The vast majority of umbilical hernias will close spontaneously by 4 to 5 years of age. The risk of incarceration in the interim is extremely small, and recurrences for early repair are likely.

91. A newborn infant delivered at 34 weeks' gestation is found to have an undescended right testicle. What should be done?

Undescended testes are very common in newborn males, especially when they are born prematurely. Observation only is indicated at this time. If the testicle cannot be brought down easily into the scrotum upon subsequent follow-up examinations, surgery can be performed between 9 and 15 months of age.

UROLOGIC CONDITIONS

92. What is the incidence of hypospadias?

The incidence of hypospadias is approximately 1 in 300 live male births.

Ardavan A, Stock JA. Long-term follow-up and late complications following treatment of pediatric urologic disorders. Med Clin North Am 2011;95:15–25.

93. Which additional abnormalities are usually associated with classical bladder exstrophy?

Epispadias, abnormal gait, anteriorly displaced anus, and vesicoureteral reflux are often associated with bladder exstrophy.

Stec AA, Baradaran N, Tran C, et al. Colorectal anomalies in patients with classic bladder exstrophy. J Pediatr Surg 2011;46:1790–3.

Stec AA, Baradaran N, Gearhart JP. Congenital renal anomalies in patients with classic bladder exstrophy. Urology 2012;79:207–9.

94. What are the embryologic events that lead to classical bladder exstrophy?

Bladder exstrophy is caused by a persistence of the cloacal membrane after the fourth gestational week and a lack of medial migration of the lateral mesoderm.

Cheng L, Lopez-Beltran A, Bostwick DG. Congenital disorders and pediatric neoplasms, in bladder pathology. Hoboken, NJ: John Wiley & Sons; 2012.

95. What are the major components of prune-belly syndrome (also known as Eagle–Barrett syndrome)?

Prune-belly syndrome consists of deficient abdominal wall musculature, hydronephrosis, and undescended testes.

96. What is the most common genitourinary malformation associated with imperforate anus?

Renal agenesis is the most common malformation.

97. What is the approximate percentage of children with spina bifida who have abnormal bladder innervation?

Approximately 90% of children with spina bifida have abnormal bladder innervation.

CIRCUMCISION

98. Why is retraction of the foreskin in uncircumcised boys not recommended in neonates?

The undersurface of the foreskin is fused with the glans at birth, and it is not until later in childhood that the foreskin is truly retractable.

99. Is the American Academy of Pediatrics in favor of or against routine circumcision in newborn males?

The Academy has recently revised its guidelines on circumcision, now favoring the procedure, though stopping short of recommending it for all male infants. The recent change has been prompted by growing evidence that favors several health benefits including prevention of urinary tract infections, human immunodeficiency virus (HIV), and penile cancer. Circumcision also prevents transmission of certain sexually transmitted infections, including HPV and herpes.

100. What are the potential advantages and disadvantages of neonatal circumcision?

Advantages:
- Prevents phimosis
- Prevents paraphimosis (i.e., inability to pull the foreskin back over the glans after it is retracted)
- Lowers the incidence of urinary infections
- Prevents balanoposthitis (i.e., infection of the glans and foreskin)
- Prevents cancer of the penis
- Decreases the risk of contracting HIV, human papilloma virus (HPV), and herpesvirus

Disadvantages:
- Medically unnecessary for most boys
- Painful
- Risks of complications (e.g., bleeding, infection, ulcers, damage to glans)

Xu X, Patel DA, Dalton VK, et al. Can routine neonatal circumcision help prevent human immunodeficiency virus transmission in the United States? Am J Mens Health 2009;3:79–84.

101. What are the contraindications to circumcision in neonates?

Neonatal circumcision should not be performed if the baby is otherwise ill or there are congenital anomalies of the penis (e.g., hypospadias, in which case the foreskin may be needed for eventual reconstruction).

INDEX

Page numbers followed by f indicate figures; t, tables; b, boxes.